A Comprehensive Guide to Hidradenitis Suppurativa

Vivian Y. Shi, MD

Associate Professor
Department of Dermatology
University of Arkansas for Medical Sciences
Little Rock, AR, United States

Jennifer L. Hsiao, MD

Assistant Professor
Division of Dermatology
University of California, Los Angeles
Santa Monica, CA, United States

Michelle A. Lowes, MBBS, PhD

Visiting Associate Attending Physician
The Rockefeller University
New York, NY, United States

Iltefat H. Hamzavi, MD

Senior Staff Physician
HS Multidisciplinary Clinic
Multicultural Dermatology Center
Department of Dermatology Henry Ford Hospital
Hamzavi/Dermatology Specialists
Clinical Associate Professor
Wayne State University School of Medicine
President, Hidradenitis Suppurativa Foundation
Detroit, MI, United States

ELSEVIER

Elsevier
1600 John F. Kennedy Blvd.
Ste 1800
Philadelphia, PA 19103-2899

A COMPREHENSIVE GUIDE TO HIDRADENITIS SUPPURATIVA   ISBN: 978-0-323-77724-7
Copyright © 2022, by Elsevier Inc. All Rights Reserved.

Notices

Library of Congress Control Number: 2021946979

Senior Content Strategist: Charlotta Kryhl
Content Development Specialist: Erika Nisin
Director, Content Development: Ellen Wurm-Cutter
Publishing Services Manager: Shereen Jameel
Senior Project Manager: Umarani Natarajan
Design Direction: Bridget Hoette

Printed in the United States of America

Last digit is the print number: 9   8   7   6   5   4   3   2   1

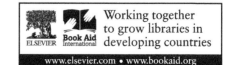

Foreword

Hidradenitis suppurativa (HS) is a chronic skin disease causing multiple inflammatory lesions typically in the flexural sites, with profound impact on quality of life because of pain, pus production, scarring, and the unpredictability of flares. It causes cumulative life course impairment due to effects on relationships, education, and employment prospects. Prevalence estimates vary from 0.1% to 4% depending on the methodology used and population studied. Despite being a relatively straightforward clinical diagnosis, recognition of HS is highly variable, leading to an average diagnostic delay of 7 years, compared to less than 2 years for psoriasis.

Lack of recognition has limited HS care up until recently. Fortunately, advances in HS research and translation into clinical practice are gathering pace. A PubMed search for 2020 reveals 644 HS articles, compared to 83 articles in 2010 and 16 in 2000. The challenge is then to integrate the new knowledge into a single, easily accessible source. I commend the authors of "A Comprehensive Guide to Hidradenitis Suppurativa" for ensuring that their textbook lives up to its name and is truly "comprehensive"!

There are chapters covering etiology, pathophysiology, epidemiology, and medical and non-medical treatment. Comorbidities and consequences of HS (particularly the effects on mental health and links with cardiovascular disease) are also discussed. The textbook goes further and includes special populations such as children and people with skin of color. Importantly, it considers HS multidisciplinary management and patient support to encourage holistic care. Management of pain and itch are considered, as well as lifestyle modification and alternative therapies. It also provides a window into the future in terms of the HS therapeutic pipeline, advances in outcome measure instruments, and the key challenges ahead to improve the lives of people with HS.

By spreading authorship of chapters across a large group of HS experts—including a patient advocate—the textbook incorporates multiple perspectives from those who are actively publishing in each aspect of HS research. Geographical comprehensiveness is ensured by giving an overview and comparison of management guidelines from across the globe, including North America, South America, and Europe. The book's structure encourages the reader to take an understanding of the pathophysiology of HS and translate this into practical therapeutic approaches, covering medical and laser treatment and a range of surgical options.

Unlike some chronic inflammatory skin conditions such as psoriasis, HS is a scarring condition; thus, preventing disease progression is a key aim of treatment. Identifying those people with HS at risk of rapid progression and providing personalized treatment that will slow progression is one of the challenges identified by the final chapter. "A Comprehensive Guide to Hidradenitis Suppurativa" provides an excellent summary of the state of play of current evidence and, by identifying evidence gaps, gives us a springboard in to the future innovations in HS care. Substantial progress has been made; still, there is a lot more to do to ensure that HS disease control is on a par with other chronic inflammatory conditions, while minimizing quality-of-life impact and lifecourse impairment.

Dr. John Ingram, MA, MSc, DM(Oxon), FRCP(Derm), FAcadMEd
Clinical Reader & Consultant Dermatologist
Division of Infection & Immunity
Cardiff University, Cardiff, United Kingdom

Contributors

Afsaneh Alavi, MD, FRCPC
Department of Dermatology
Mayo Clinic
Rochester, Minnesota
United States

Maria Aleshin, MD
Department of Dermatology
Stanford University School of Medicine
Redwood City, California
United States

Falk G. Bechara, Professor, MD
Department of Dermatologic Surgery
Ruhr-University
Bochum
Germany

Richard G. Bennett, MD
Department of Dermatology
University of Southern California
Division of Dermatology
University of California
Los Angeles, California
United States

Ron Birnbaum, MD
Division of Dermatology
Harbor-UCLA Medical Center
West Carson, California
United States

Nicholas Brownstone, MD
Department of Dermatology
University of California, San Francisco
San Francisco, California
United States

Connor R. Buechler, MD
Departments of Internal Medicine and Dermatology
University of Minnesota
Minneapolis, Minnesota
United States

Angel Shree' Byrd, MD, PhD
Department of Dermatology
Howard University College of Medicine
Washington, District of Columbia
Department of Dermatology
Johns Hopkins University School of Medicine
Baltimore, Maryland
United States

Alexandra P. Charrow, MD, MBE
Department of Dermatology
Brigham and Women's Hospital
Harvard Medical School
Boston, Massachusetts
United States

Emily F. Cole, MD, MPH
Department of Dermatology
Emory University School of Medicine
Atlanta, Georgia
United States

Erin K. Collier, MD, MPH
Kaiser Permanente Los Angeles Medical Center
Los Angeles, California
United States

Steven D. Daveluy, MD
Department of Dermatology
Wayne State University
Detroit, Michigan
United States

Jennifer M. Fernandez, MD, RD
Department of Medicine
University of Arizona
Phoenix, Arizona
United States

John W. Frew, MBBS (Hons), MMed (Clin Epi), Mac, FACD
Department of Dermatology
Liverpool Hospital
Laboratory of Translational Cutaneous Medicine
Ingham Institute of Applied Medical Research
University of New South Wales
Sydney, Australia

Amit Garg, MD
Department of Dermatology
Zucker School of Medicine at Hofstra/Northwell
Center for Health Innovations & Outcomes Research
Feinstein Institutes for Medical Research
Dermatology Service Line
Northwell Health
New Hyde Park, New York
United States

Ralph George, MD
Department of Surgery
University of Toronto
Toronto, Canada

Stephanie R. Goldberg, MD
Mary Washington Hospital Center
Fredericksburg, Virginia
United States

Noah Goldfarb, MD
Departments of Medicine and Dermatology
University of Minnesota
Departments of Medicine and Dermatology
Minneapolis Veteran Affairs Health Care System
Minneapolis, Minnesota
United States

Sandra Guilbault
Hope for HS
Troy, Michigan
HS Foundation
Santa Monica, California
United States

Iltefat H. Hamzavi, MD, FAAD
Hamzavi/Dematology Specialists
Department of Dermatology
Henry Ford Health System
Detroit, Michigan
United States

Paul G. Hazen, MD, MD, FAAD, Fellow-ASMS
Department of Dermatology
Case-Western Reserve University School of Medicine
Cleveland, Ohio
United States

Marsha Henderson, MD
Hamzavi/Dematology Specialists
Department of Dermatology
Henry Ford Hospital
Detroit, Michigan
United States

Aleksi J. Hendricks, MD
Department of Medicine
University of Arizona College of Medicine
Tucson, Arizona
United States

Jennifer L. Hsiao, MD
Division of Dermatology
University of California
Los Angeles, California
United States

Tarannum Jaleel, MD, MHSc
Department of Dermatology
Duke University
Durham, North Carolina
United States

Lydia J. Johnson, MD
Department of Dermatology
Virginia Commonwealth University Health System
Richmond, Virginia
United States

Olivier Join-Lambert, Sr., MD, PhD
Research Group on Microbial Adaptation
Caen Normandie University
Department of Microbiology
Caen Normandie Hospital
Caen, France

Michelle L. Kerns, MD
Department of Dermatology
Johns Hopkins University School of Medicine
Baltimore, Maryland
United States

Alexa B. Kimball, MD, MPH
Department of Dermatology
Clinical Laboratory for Epidemiology and Applied Research in Skin (CLEARS)
Beth Israel Deaconess Medical Center and Harvard Medical School
Boston, Massachusetts
United States

Joslyn S. Kirby, MD, MS, MEd
Department of Dermatology
Penn State Hershey Medical Center
Hershey, Pennsylvania
United States

Indermeet Kohli, PhD
Department of Dermatology
Henry Ford Health System, Detroit
Department of Physics and Astronomy
Wayne State University
Detroit, Michigan
United States

Joi Lenczowski, MD
Department of Dermatology
Virginia Commonwealth University Health System
Richmond, Virginia
United States

Hadar Lev-Tov, MD, MAS
Dr. Phillip Frost Department of Dermatology &
    Cutaneous Surgery
University of Miami—Miller School of Medicine
Miami, Florida
United States

Wilson Liao, MD
Department of Dermatology
University of California, San Francisco
San Francisco, California
United States

Michelle A. Lowes, MBBS, PhD
The Rockefeller University
New York, New York
United States

Alexis B. Lyons, MD
Department of Dermatology
Henry Ford Health System
Detroit, Michigan
United States

Neeta Malviya, MD
Department of Dermatology
Zucker School of Medicine at Hofstra/Northwell
New Hyde Park, New York
United States

Robert G. Micheletti, MD
Departments of Dermatology and Medicine
University of Pennsylvania
Philadelphia, Pennsylvania
United States

Peyton C. Morss-Walton, BA
Clinical Laboratory for Epidemiology and Applied
    Research in Skin (CLEARS)
Department of Dermatology
Beth Israel Deaconess Medical Center
Boston, Massachusetts
United States

Bridget Myers, BS
Department of Dermatology
University of California, San Francisco
San Francisco, California
United States

Haley B. Naik, MD, MHSc
Department of Dermatology
University of California, San Francisco
San Francisco, California
United States

Shanthi Narla, MD
Department of Dermatology
Henry Ford Health System
Detroit, Michigan
United States

Aude Nassif, MD
Centre Médical
Institut Pasteur, Paris
Ile de France
France

Tien Viet Nguyen, MD
Pacific Medical Centers
Seattle, Washington
United States

Georgios Nikolakis, Dr. Med.
Departments of Dermatology, Venereology, Allergology, and
    Immunology
Dessau Medical Center, Brandenburg Medical School Theodor
    Fontane and Faculty of Health Sciences
Brandenburg, Dessau
Germany

Elizabeth O'Brien, MD, FRCPC
Departments of Internal Medicine and Dermatology
McGill University
Montreal, Québec
Canada

Lauren A.V. Orenstein, MD
Department of Dermatology
Emory University School of Medicine
Atlanta, Georgia
United States

Angie Parks-Miller, CCRP, CWCA
Hope for HS
Troy, Michigan
Department of Dermatology
Henry Ford Hospital
Detroit, Michigan
United States

Zarine S. Patel, PhD
The Motherhood Center of New York
New York, New York
United States

Martina L. Porter, MD
Clinical Laboratory for Epidemiology and Applied Research in
    Skin (CLEARS)
Department of Dermatology
Beth Israel Deaconess Medical Center and Harvard Medical
    School
Boston, Massachusetts
United States

Kyla N. Price, MD
College of Medicine
University of Illinois—Chicago
Chicago, Illinois
United States

Mayur Ramesh, MD
Division of Infectious Diseases
Henry Ford Health System
Detroit, Michigan
United States

Barry I. Resnik, MD, MD, FAAD
Dr. Phillip Frost Department of Dermatology &
    Cutaneous Surgery
University of Miami Miller School of Medicine
Resnik Skin Institute, Miami
Jackson Memorial Hospital/University of Miami Hospital
Miami, Florida
United States

Monica Rosales Santillan, MD
Department of Dermatology
Boston University School of Medicine
Clinical Laboratory for Epidemiology and Applied Research
    in Skin (CLEARS)
Beth Israel Deaconess Medical Center
Boston, Massachusetts
United States

Muskaan Sachdeva, BHSc
Faculty of Medicine
University of Toronto
Toronto, Canada

Daniela P. Sanchez, MD
Dr. Phillip Frost Department of Dermatology &
    Cutaneous Surgery
University of Miami—Miller School of Medicine
Miami, Florida
United States

Kevin T. Savage, MD
Beth Israel Deaconess Medical Center
Boston, Massachusetts
United States

Chris Sayed, MD
Department of Dermatology
University of North Carolina
Chapel Hill, North Carolina
United States

Monica Shah, BSc
Faculty of Medicine
University of Toronto
Toronto, Canada

Rob Leland Shaver, BS
School of Medicine
University of Minnesota-Twin Cities
Minneapolis, Minnesota
United States

Vivian Y. Shi, MD
Department of Dermatology
University of Arkansas for Medical Sciences
Little Rock, Arkansas
United States

Jan M. Smogorzewski, MD
Division of Dermatology
Harbor-UCLA Medical Center
Torrance, California
United States

Farah Succaria, MD
Department of Dermatology
Johns Hopkins University School of Medicine
Baltimore, Maryland
United States

Ryan M. Svoboda, MD, MS
Department of Dermatology
Penn State Hershey Medical Center
Hershey, Pennsylvania
United States

Alyssa M. Thompson, BS
College of Medicine, University of Arizona
Tuscon, Arizona
United States

Aristeidis G. Vaiopoulos, Dr. Med.
Departments of Dermatology, Venereology, Allergology, and
    Immunology
Dessau Medical Center, Brandenburg Medical School Theodor
    Fontane and Faculty of Health Sciences
Brandenburg, Dessau
Germany

Surya A. Veerabagu, BA
Tulane University School of Medicine
New Orleans, Louisiana
United States

Joseph R. Walsh, BS
Medical College of Wisconsin School of Medicine
Milwaukee, Wisconsin
United States

Maximillian A. Weigelt, MD
Dr. Phillip Frost Department of Dermatology and Cutaneous
    Surgery
University of Miami—Miller School of Medicine
Miami, Florida
United States

Ximena Wortsman, MD
Department of Imaging
IDIEP—Institute for Diagnostic Imaging and Research of the Skin
    and Soft Tissues
Department of Dermatology
Faculty of Medicine, University of Chile
Department of Dermatology
Faculty of Medicine, Pontifical Catholic University of Chile
Santiago, Chile

Christos C. Zouboulis, Prof., Dr. Med., Prof., HC, Dr. HC
Departments of Dermatology, Venereology, Allergology, and
    Immunology
Dessau Medical Center, Brandenburg Medical School Theodor
    Fontane and Faculty of Health Sciences
Brandenburg, Dessau
Germany

Contents

Section 6: On the Horizon

Video Contents

Introduction to Hidradenitis Suppurativa

1

Historical Perspective on Hidradenitis Suppurativa

ERIN K. COLLIER, JENNIFER L. HSIAO, AND VIVIAN Y. SHI

CHAPTER OUTLINE

Introduction

Hidradenitis suppurativa (HS) has a convoluted history with conflicting bodies of knowledge and a complicated pathogenesis. Since HS was first described in the 19th century, it has taken on various names and treatment strategies, leading to further confusion among researchers, physicians, and affected individuals. Alfred Velpeau and Aristide Verneuil are prominent historical figures who are credited with the discovery and characterization of HS centuries ago. Since then, many prominent physicians and researchers have contributed to our knowledge of this disease. Despite the longstanding history of investigation on HS, 150 years passed before development of the first staging system and there still remains no consensus on HS pathophysiology. As our understanding of HS grows, targeted therapies continue to evolve and help to clarify aspects of the pathogenesis as well as allow for optimal treatment of HS patients. Improved knowledge of the pathomechanisms in HS has slowly helped to reduce the controversy and mysticism surrounding this disease.

Historic Figures in Hidradenitis Suppurativa

The chronicle of HS began in 19th century France, where it was first described by Velpeau and Verneuil. Karl Marx, a famous 19th century German philosopher, is now also thought to have had HS,[1] with earliest records of his disease dating just a few years after Verneuil's first publications.

Alfred-Armand-Louis-Marie Velpeau (1795–1867)

Alfred-Armand-Louis-Marie Velpeau (Fig. 1.1) was born in the Touraine village of Bréches, France on May 18, 1795.

Born of humble beginnings, he was expected to follow in his father's footsteps, who was a farrier and "veterinary-artist." However, Velpeau developed a strong interest in medicine, purchasing his first medical textbooks from money raised selling chestnuts while tending to his father's cattle.[2–4] After reading some "do-it-yourself"-type medical texts, he began providing opinions on his neighbors' afflictions.[5] Attempting to extinguish the sadness from a depressed young girl, he succeeded only in poisoning her with hellebore, which marked the turning point of his life.[2–4]

When the local physician, Dr. Bodin, arrived to treat the girl, he became so impressed by Velpeau's knowledge and determination that he introduced him to another member of the aristocracy, M. Duncan. Duncan shared in the fascination of Velpeau and invited him to join the tutoring lessons given to his children. After a year of demonstrating remarkable progress, Duncan introduced Velpeau to Vincent Gourand, surgeon at a hospital in Tours, and later to Piérre-Fidele Bretonneau, the head doctor of the hospital. Velpeau was only 21 years old (year 1816) at this point and was now an assistant to a renowned French physician of the time. Bretonneau treated Velpeau as a son over the next four years, training him in clinical medicine and pathology.[2–4]

By 1820, at the age of 25, Velpeau accepted a position in the Saint Louis Hospital where he achieved awards in anatomy and physiology. In 1823, he was appointed "agrégé en médecine" (associate of medicine) with honors and in 1824 took appointments as junior surgical staff in various hospitals. After passing a higher degree in surgery, the "Chirurgical," Velpeau was hired as surgeon of La Pitié in 1828. Five years later, at 38 years old, he was appointed as university chair of clinical surgery and went on to hold this position for the next 33 years.[2–4]

During Velpeau's tenure, he was said to have published works of over 340 titles and 10,000 pages. He authored texts on several topics, including surgical anatomy (1825), obstetrics (1830), operative medicine (1832), embryology (1833), as well as uterine and breast diseases (1854). Velpeau also gave his eponym to various anatomical structures, conditions, and innovations, notably

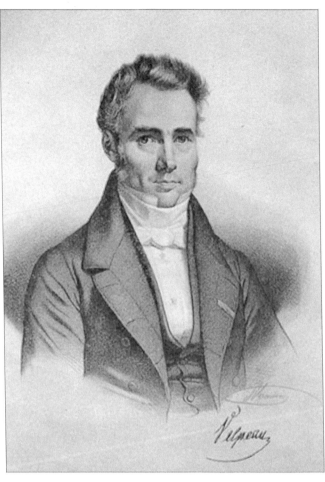

• **Fig. 1.1** Image of Velpeau.

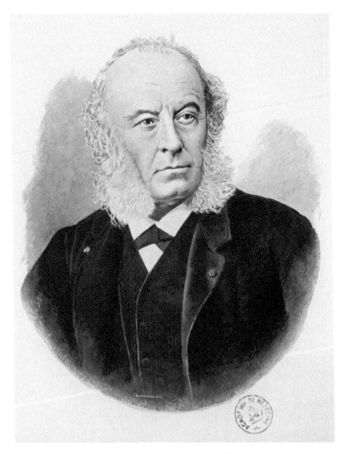

• **Fig. 1.2** Image of Verneuil. (From Jermac GE, Revuz J, Leyden J. *Hidradenitis Suppurativa*. Berlin: Springer; 2006.)

Velpeau's "canal," "deformity," "hernia," and "pressure bandage."[2-4]

Furthermore, Velpeau is credited with being the first person to recognize and attempt to describe HS as a distinct disease process. In 1833, Velpeau described a "phlegmon tubériforme" (tuberiform phlegmnon) of the axilla, which he observed as inflammation of sebaceous follicles (frequently arising from rubbing irritation), which is occasionally painful and ends in suppuration. Velpeau also described an alternative but similar clinical aspect of HS, called "phlegmon érysipélateux" (erysipelas phlegmon), which included induration and tumors, and was always painful. Velpeau lamented the ignorance of authors in underestimating the dire consequences of this axillary inflammation.[6]

Velpeau died on August 24, 1867, at the age of 72. He was a man of humble origins who ascended the ranks of the medical profession to become one of the prominent surgeons of his time.[2-4] His contribution to dermatology is etched in history, as we credit him for his discovery of HS.

Aristide Auguste Stanislas Verneuil (1823–1895)

Aristide Auguste Stanislas Verneuil (Fig. 1.2) was born in Paris, France on November 29, 1823.

In 1843 Verneuil was appointed Interne des Hôpitaux de Paris (Intern of Paris hospitals) and went on to graduate as a Doctor in Medicine in 1852. He became Professeur Agrégé (Associate Professor) at the Paris Faculty of Medicine in 1853 and appointed Surgeon of the Paris Hospitals in 1856, where he was the first official teacher of syphilis and other venereal diseases.[6]

Verneuil held several successive appointments throughout his medical career, notably head of Lourcine Hospital, Le Midi Hospital (1865), Hôpital Lariboisière (1865), La Pitié (1872), and Hôtel-Dieu (1889), serving as Professor of Clinical Surgery (1872–1889) in La Pitié hospital, and Chair of Surgery at Hôtel-Dieu Hospital (1889–1892). Verneuil is also known for his positions as President of the Société de Chirurgie (1869), Charter member and later President of the Congress of Surgery, Member of the Académie de Médecine (1869), Member of the Académie des Sciences (1887), and Commander of the Legion of Honour.[6-8]

Between 1854 and 1865, Verneuil published a number of articles on skin tumors and took particular interest in sudoral (sweat gland) tumors. This interest led him to Velpeau's discovery. Although Velpeau had postulated that the origin of the abscesses found in HS patients was the sebaceous follicles, Verneuil hypothesized that they instead originated from the sweat glands. It is said that Verneuil had only personally observed a single case of acute inflammation of the sudoral glands, which was on a cadaver of a young girl. In his recorded notes, he observed inflammation of the sacral and gluteal region, multiple circumscribed and subcutaneous abscesses probably located in the sweat glands, and noted several pinhead-sized pustules filled with liquid but without any sign of inflammation. He reported unroofing the pustule to reveal a tiny red cavity in which a thin boar bristle or stylet could be introduced. The underlying channel was approximately one fifth to one third of a millimeter in depth, crossing the dermis and leading to a larger subdermal cavity filled with the same fluid, likely the early description of what is now known as a sinus tract.[6]

Verneuil suspected that the suppuration was a result of necrosis of the sudoral glands with purulent excretion from the sudoral ducts, leading to accumulation of pus beneath the epidermis. Through clinical and histologic observation, Verneuil localized these abscesses to the sweat glands, with the caveat that he could not infer the etiology of the disease with so few observations.[6] Verneuil died on June 11, 1895, leaving behind a rich legacy within the fields of surgery and dermatology. He was also the first to attempt describing the pathogenesis of HS.[6]

Terminology

The 19th century's identification of HS as a unique entity marked the start of debate regarding the proper naming convention for this disease. Sifting through the medical literature, one can find several different names to reference this one condition, including hidradenitis suppurativa, apocrine acne, apocrinitis, Velpeau's disease, Verneuil's disease, Fox-den disease, pyodermia sinifica fistulans, and acne inversa.[9] (Box 1.1) However, many of these names have since been abandoned or described as misnomers.

In 1864, Verneuil named the disease "hidrosadénite phlegmoneuse,"[10] the French term for "hidradenitis suppurativa." This name was given based on Verneuil's observation that the anatomical distribution of the disorder mirrored the characteristic distribution of sweat glands.[6] The name was derived using Greek "hidros" meaning "sweat" and "aden" meaning "glands."[11] However, the proceeding indecision and controversy surrounding whether this condition was in fact its own separate disease led to the creation of various other names and eponyms.

In 1891, French physician Barthélémy regarded HS as part of a folliculitis and he introduced the new terms "acnitis" and "folliclis" to describe follicular and perifollicular inflammation of unknown origin.[6,12] However, in 1893, French dermatologist Dr. Dubreuilh rejected the new terms in favor of "hidrosadenitis."[6,13]

At the beginning of the 20th century, nosological discussions arose regarding the connection between HS and acne conglobata, at which point French physician Dr. Spitzer proposed the name "dermatitis folliculitis et perifolliculitis conglobata" (dermatitis folliculitis and perifolliculitis conglobate).[6,14] In 1949, another French physician, Dr. Degos, insisted that a distinction between acne conglobata and HS was nearly impossible

to establish.[6,15,16] Recognizing the difference between English and French views and noting that English literature commonly used the designation of "Verneuil's disease," French author Mouly encouraged others to acknowledge the work of Verneuil and named the condition "maladie de Verneuil" (Verneuil disease) in 1959.[6,17]

In 1956, American dermatologists Pillsbury, Shelley, and Kligman named the coexistence of acne conglobata, hidradenitis suppurativa, and dissecting cellulitis of the scalp, the "follicular occlusion triad." This decision was based on the common features of follicular hyperkeratinization, retention of keratin products, and secondary bacterial infection within all three conditions.[6,18] Almost 20 years later, they proposed adding pilonidal sinus disease and updating the term to "acne tetrad" (also known as "follicular occlusion tetrad").[6,19]

More recently, the moniker "acne inversa" has gained favor based on histologic evaluations of the disease. In 1989, Plewig and Steger, two German dermatologists, suggested the name upon observing that the four components of the acne tetrad affected anatomical areas that were the *inverse* of the localizations of acne vulgaris.[20,21] In 2005, American dermatologists Sellheyer and Krahl demonstrated histopathological evidence of the occlusion of hair follicles as well as observations of clinical and therapeutic similarities to acne. As a result, the authors insisted that "hidradenitis suppurativa" should be abandoned as a misnomer and replaced with "acne inversa."[21] However, opponents to the name "acne inversa" argue that histology alone does not define dermatology and that more research into the pathogenesis should be conducted.[22] Thus, despite centuries of investigation, a general consensus regarding terminology for this disease had yet to be reached. "Hidradenitis suppurativa (HS)" is currently the most commonly used and recognized name for this disease.

Uncovering Hidradenitis Suppurativa Pathogenesis Studies Throughout History

Apocrine Gland Theory of Pathogenesis

A 1889 publication by Italian physician Dr. Giovannini was likely the first histopathological study to support Verneuil's hypothesis of the origin of HS by demonstrating the existence of an inflammatory process around the sweat glands associated with complete glandular destruction.[6,23] In 1893, Dubreuilh agreed that HS lesions originated from the sweat coil.[6,13] Apocrine glands were further implicated in HS pathogenesis in 1939 as Brunsting, an American dermatologist, studied the histology of several of his patients. Brunsting's histologic observations led him to the theory that the apocrine structures and surrounding connective tissue were the initial locations of inflammation in HS. Furthermore, in his clinical description of the disease, he emphasized that lesions were located around the same anatomic regions that apocrine glands are situated.[6,24,25]

HS was first attempted to be replicated in humans by American dermatologists Drs. Shelley and Cahn in 1955. Occlusion of the axillary skin of their subjects with belladonna tape for 2 weeks caused a quarter of them to develop subcutaneous nodules as seen in HS. Shelley and Cahn viewed histologic specimens of the subjects with clinical lesions, showing inflammation, keratinous plugging, and dilatation of the apocrine sweat duct without

---

• BOX 1.1   **Common English Names Given to Hidradenitis Suppurativa**

Velpeau's disease	Apocrine acne
Verneuil's diseas	Acne inversa
Apocrinitis	Hidradenitis suppurativa

involvement of proximal hair follicles or sebaceous and eccrine glands. Shelley and Cahn concluded that hormonal dysregulation of the apocrine glands caused the hair follicle to become blocked that promoted inflammation with occasional secondary infection.[26]

The work by Shelley and Cahn further supported the involvement of apocrine glands, and now, hormonal dysregulation in HS pathogenesis. This conclusion was due to histologic observations of known inflammatory changes within and around apocrine glands in HS patients. In addition, the increase in sex hormones during puberty, and young adulthood was thought to stimulate sex hormone receptors within apocrine glands to cause inflammatory changes in predisposed patients. Finally, HS and apocrine gland distribution in humans were similar: axillary, inguinal, perianal, perineal, mammary, inframammary, buttock, pubic, chest, scalp, retroauricular, and eyelid areas.[26]

However, more recent studies suggest apocrine glands are not always involved in primary HS pathogenesis. American dermatologists Anderson and Dockerty were the first to provide evidence against apocrine glands being involved with primary pathogenesis of HS in 1958. They examined tissue samples from 64 individuals with HS and found that not all specimens had inflammation of the apocrine glands. Apocrine gland inflammation only occurred when there was also widespread inflammation involving eccrine and sebaceous glands, hair follicles, and blood vessels. Finally, there were no tissue samples with apocrine gland inflammation that spared the surrounding tissues. For these reasons, Anderson and Dockerty determined that apocrine glands were not essential for the primary pathogenesis of HS.[27] In addition, two Welsh surgeons, Drs. Morgan and Hughes, found no difference in size or density of apocrine glands in HS subjects compared with control subjects.[28]

English pathologists Drs. Yu and Cook conducted a study in 1990 that focused on examining the axillae of their HS patients. Most of the histologic specimens had atypical hair follicles, cysts, and dermal sinuses. The cysts had stratified squamous epithelium, laminated keratin, and most had hair follicles. A third of the subjects had apocrine gland inflammation when extensive inflammation was present throughout the subcutaneous tissue. This supported the findings of Anderson and Dockerty in that adnexal involvement did not always include apocrine glands.[29] Findings by Attanoos et al. and Larralde et al. support Yu and Cook's conclusion.[30,31]

Pilosebaceous Follicle Theory of Pathogenesis

Danish dermatologist Dr. Jemec and pathologists Drs. Thomsen and Hansen studied sebaceous glands in the pathogenesis of HS in 1997. Some of their patient's histologic specimens showed no involvement of sebaceous glands and minimal axillary, genital, inguinal, and facial seborrhea. They concluded that the pathogenesis of HS was not the same as acne, in which dysfunctional sebum production is typical.[32]

One of the most accepted theories of HS pathogenesis today is that primary follicular plugging causes inflammation and dilatation of the pilosebaceous unit. This causes inflammatory nodules and abscesses to form containing corneocytes, bacteria, sebum, and hair. Eventual rupture of these nodules and abscesses into the dermis propagates the spread of inflammation by invasion of

neutrophils, lymphocytes, and histiocytes. Recurrent inflammation and secondary infection of the subcutaneous tissue creates sinus tracts and fistulas. Despite the evidence of follicular plugging being an important factor of HS pathogenesis, it is not a universally accepted theory and the cause of follicular plugging remains undetermined. The two most commonly proposed mechanisms are hyperparakeratosis or parakeratosis and anatomic abnormalities of the pilosebaceous unit.[26,29,31,33,34]

To test these theories, Jemec and Gniadecka used ultrasonography to study hair follicles in subjects with HS. They found marked differences between control (from patients without HS) and HS follicles. In addition, structure and distribution of follicles were different for the axillary and genitofemoral regions. Interestingly, areas of skin that appeared to not be affected by HS still showed structural abnormalities of the follicle including distorted shapes and increased width variability. Genitofemoral areas had more variability to follicle width than axillary. Conversely, axillary areas had an overall increase in skin thickness and follicle distribution compared with genitofemoral areas. Despite their findings, Jemec and Gniadecka could not determine whether increased skin thickness and structural abnormalities of the hair follicles are primary factors of HS pathogenesis or secondary changes due to chronic inflammation.[35]

Additional Theories of Past and Present

Today, additional theories of HS pathogenesis include genetic alterations and immune dysregulation. In the 1980s, English geneticists Drs. Fitzsimmons and Guilbert performed a series of studies that demonstrated the familial inheritance pattern of HS.[36,37] Genome sequencing in Chinese families has since uncovered mutations in genes (NCSTN, PSENEN, PSEN1) that code for gamma-secretase, which cleaves the transmembrane receptor (Notch) involved in epidermal and follicular development.[38–40] Other studies hypothesize that autoinflammation plays a role in disease pathogenesis, with notable elevations in several inflammatory cytokines (IL-1β, IL-10, IL-11, IL-17A, and CXCL9) observed in HS patients.[41] A study by van der Zee et al. discovered that the cytokines IL-1β, and TNF-α, were elevated in HS lesions as well as in perilesional skin. The levels of these cytokines also showed trends toward a positive correlation with HS disease severity, making these markers suitable targets for medical therapy.[42]

Hormonal influences have also been suspected to be a factor in HS pathogenesis by both clinicians and patients since the early 20th century. However, most of these reports are anecdotal with a limited number of studies supporting this theory. Beginning in 1986, two English studies found that antiandrogen therapy was an effective treatment for HS. Mortimer et al. found most subjects with HS had long-term improvement or complete remission of symptoms by reducing androgen levels.[43] The same year, Sawers et al. found mixed results of antiandrogen therapy, in which some subjects had complete, long-term remission, while others experienced no benefit and excessive estrogenic side effects.[44] In 2007, Canadian dermatologists Drs. Kraft and Searless reported results from a retrospective chart review, finding that the response to antihormonal therapy was superior to that of antibiotics.[45] These findings support the theory that androgens could be a factor in HS pathogenesis. Despite all these discoveries, much remains unknown regarding the pathogenesis of HS and other mediators of this disease. The updated understanding of HS pathogenesis is discussed in Chapters 10 to 12.

The Birth of Hidradenitis Suppurativa Staging Systems

The first staging system for HS was developed by Dr. Harry James Hurley Jr., an American dermatologist, in 1989. Hurley developed a staging system for HS by separating patients into three groups based on the extent of scar tissue and sinuses. Since its inception, the Hurley staging has been the most used system to assess HS severity.[46] Hurley's staging system was first introduced in a textbook chapter, not as a journal article.

The simplicity of the Hurley system has made its use convenient for clinicians. In 2003, Sartorius et al. suggested that the Hurley system is too basic to accurately evaluate treatment effects in clinical studies. Furthermore, the Hurley staging is not dynamic; a patient's stage cannot be lowered if clinical signs improve. They proposed additions to the current Hurley staging system by including anatomic regions, number and types of lesions, distance between lesions, and the presence of normal skin in between lesions. Points are accumulated in each of these categories and added to give both a regional and total score. In addition, Sartorius suggested adding a visual scale for pain or using the dermatology life quality index (DLQI) when evaluating patients with HS.[47] Hidradenitis Suppurativa Physician's Global Assessment (HS-PGA) and Hidradenitis Suppurativa Clinical Response (HiSCR) are newer tools used to assess HS clinical severity and response to treatment. HS evaluation tools are discussed in greater detail in Chapter 13.

A Historical Note on Hidradenitis Suppurativa Treatment

Currently, there are no single global standardized management guidelines for HS (see Chapter 14). There have been very few Level I evidence-based studies (randomized controlled trials or meta-analyses) for medical or surgical HS treatments, which adds to the difficulty in determining the most efficacious strategies. However, therapeutic approaches have been developed in response to evolving understanding of HS pathogenesis. Throughout history, various treatment modalities have been attempted to stop the progression of this disease, including medical therapies, surgical and in-office procedures, and lifestyle modifications. One can find a variety of therapies suggested for the treatment of HS in the literature, such as topical applications (e.g., hydrocortisone[48] or clindamycin[49]), dry or wet warm compresses, ultraviolet light treatments, x-ray therapy, incision and drainage, antibiotics, exteriorization and curettage, electrocoagulation, and excision.[50]

Lessons From the Past

The history of HS, though complicated and convoluted, can offer a wealth of information. Hidradenitis suppurativa, first named over 150 years ago, still remains a clinical conundrum today. The etiology of the disease has evolved from early understandings of primary apocrine gland inflammation to theories of primary follicular plugging, autoinflammation, and immune dysregulation (Fig. 1.3). However, our lack of consensus on the underlying pathogenesis, as well as a standard naming convention, serves as a reminder of the many unknowns still surrounding this disease. As we move into an era of more targeted therapies for HS, it is important to review past and present studies to guide strategies for drug development. Research looking into the genetic profile of HS has provided additional insight into HS pathogenesis and inheritance patterns. Identifying causative mutations could allow for future studies on gene therapy and development of drugs targeted toward gamma-secretase. Similarly, further research into the autoinflammatory state and cytokine profile of HS has provided important implications for the management of HS with immunosuppressants, biologics, and small molecule inhibitors. Antiandrogen therapy has also shown efficacy in reducing HS symptoms and can be further explored. Diagnostic advances, along with surgical and procedural advances, will also allow for expeditious diagnosis and early treatment of HS to avoid devastating long-term sequelae.

Conclusion

One must know the history of a disease in order to better understand the disease itself. As we move into a new era of technological and scientific advances, having a more thorough understanding of the theories of HS pathogenesis, attempted and failed therapies, and the tenacity for knowledge of prior physicians and researchers help build our understanding of HS. These historic perspectives will guide future management and research strategies.

Acknowledgments

The authors would like to thank Joshua Buchtel for his assistance with literature review.

Historic Timeline on Hidradenitis Suppurativa

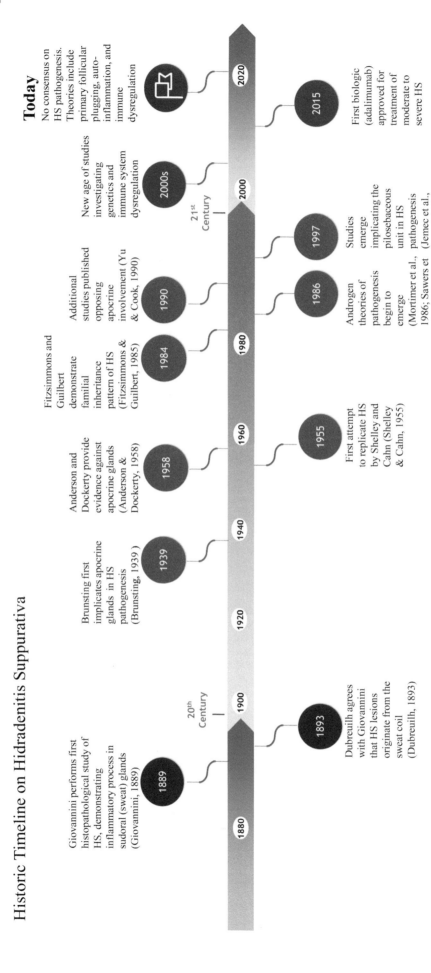

Today
No consensus on HS pathogenesis. Theories include primary follicular plugging, auto-inflammation, and immune dysregulation

2020

2015
First biologic (adalimumab) approved for treatment of moderate to severe HS

2000s
New age of studies investigating genetics and immune system dysregulation

2000

21st Century

1997
Studies emerge implicating the pilosebaceous unit in HS pathogenesis (Jemec et al., 1997)

1990
Additional studies published opposing apocrine involvement (Yu & Cook, 1990)

1986
Androgen theories of pathogenesis begin to emerge (Mortimer et al., 1986; Sawers et al., 1986)

1984
Fitzsimmons and Guilbert demonstrate familial inheritance pattern of HS (Fitzsimmons & Guilbert, 1985)

1980

1960

1958
Anderson and Dockerty provide evidence against apocrine glands (Anderson & Dockerty, 1958)

1955
First attempt to replicate HS by Shelley and Cahn (Shelley & Cahn, 1955)

1940

1939
Brunsting first implicates apocrine glands in HS pathogenesis (Brunsting, 1939)

1920

1900

20th Century

1893
Dubreuilh agrees with Giovannini that HS lesions originate from the sweat coil (Dubreuilh, 1893)

1889
Giovannini performs first histopathological study of HS, demonstrating inflammatory process in sudoral (sweat) glands (Giovannini, 1889)

1880

• **Fig. 1.3** Timeline of Hidradenitis Suppurativa Pathogenesis Studies.

References

1. Shuster S. The nature and consequence of Karl Marx's skin disease. *Br J Dermatol.* 2008;158(1):1–3. https://doi.org/10.1111/j.1365-2133.2007.08282.x.

2. Dunn PM. Dr Alfred Velpeau (1795–1867) of Tours: The umbilical cord and birth asphyxia. *Arch Dis Child Fetal Neonatal Ed.* 2005;90(2):184–186. https://doi.org/10.1136/adc.2004.060244.

3. Aron E. Alfed Velpeau (1795–1867). Une carrie`re exceptionnelle. *Hist Sci Med.* 1994;28:1–7.

4. Dickson Wright A. Two great French Surgeons. *Hist Med.* 1970;2:11–13.

5. Hall MH. The Velpeau Bandage. *Canad Med Ass J.* 1963;88(7):223.

6. Tilles G. Verneuil and Verneuil's disease: an historical overview. 2006. https://doi.org/10.1007/978-3-540-33101-8_2.

7. Huguet F. *Les Professeurs de La Faculté de Médecine de Paris, Dictionnaire Biographique 1794–1939*; 1991. https://doi.org/10.11588/fr.1993.2.58396.

8. Décès de M. Verneuil. *Bull Acad Med.* 1895;627–629. Published online.

9. About this Disease: Hidradenitis Suppurativa—explained. *HS-usa.org.* Published 2020. http://www.hs-usa.org/hidradenitis_suppurativa.htm.

10. Verneuil A. De l'hidrosadénite phlegmoneuse et des abcès sudoripares. *Arch Gen Med.* 1864;115:327–337.

11. Shah N. Hidradenitis suppurativa: a treatment challenge. *Am Fam Physician.* 2005;72(8):1547–1552.

12. Barthélémy T. De l'acnitis ou d'une variété spéciale de folliculites et périfolliculites disséminées et généralisés. *Ann Dermatol Syphil.* 1891;2:1.

13. Dubreuilh W. Hidrosadénites suppuratives disséminées. *Arch Med Exp Ana Path.* 1893;5:63–101.

14. Spitzer L. Dermatitis folliculitis et perifollicultis conglobata. *Dermatolog Z.* 1901;10:8.

15. Degos R, Garnier G, Caron J. Acné conglobata très améliorée par l'auréomycine. *Bull Soc Fran Dermatol Syphil.* 1949;489–490. Published online.

16. Degos R, Garnier G, Niel J. Acné conglobata à localisation hétérotypique et avec infiltration profondes, péri anales, pseudo tuberculeuses. *Bull Soc Fran Dermatol Syphil Dermatol Syphil.* 1949;489–490. Published online. 346–347.

17. Mouly R. Hidrosadénites inguino périnéo fessières. *Bull Soc Fran Dermatol.* 1959;184–190. Published online.

18. Pillsbury D, Shelley W, Kligman A. Bacterial infections of the skin. In: Pillsbury D, Shelley W, Kligman A, eds. *Dermatology.* 1st ed. Saunders; 1956:459–498.

19. Plewig G, Kligman A. Acne: morphogenesis and Treatment. *Acne.* 1975;192. Published online.

20. Plewig G, Steger M. Acne inversa (alias acne triad, acne tetrad or hidradenitis suppurativa). In: Marks R, Plewig G, eds. *Acne and Related Disorders.* Martin Dunitz; 1989:345–357.

21. Sellheyer K, Krahl D. "Hidradenitis suppurativa" is acne inversa! An appeal to (finally) abandon a misnomer. *Int J Dermatol.* 2005;44(7):535–540. https://doi.org/10.1111/j.1365-4632.2004.02536.x.

22. Scheinfeld N. Hidradenitis should not be renamed acne inversa. *Dermatol Online J.* 2006;12(7):6.

23. Giovannini S. Un caso d'hidrosadenite. *Giorn Ital Mal Vene e dellle Pelle.* 1889;302–305. Published online.

24. Brunsting H. Hidradenitis and other variants of acné. *Arch Dermatol Syphil.* 1952;65:303–315.

25. Brunsting H. Hidradenitis suppurativa; abscess of apocrine sweat glands—a study of clinical and pathological features with a report of 22 cases of and a review of the literature. *Arch Dermatol Syphilol.* 1939;108–120. Published online.

26. Shelley W, Cahn M. The pathogenesis of suppurativa in man. *Arch Dermatol Syphil.* 1955;72:562–565.

27. Anderson MJ, Dockerty MB. Perianal hidradenitis suppurativa—A clinical and pathologic study. *Dis Colon Rectum.* 1958;1(1):23–31. https://doi.org/10.1007/BF02616510.

28. Morgan WP, Hughes LE. The distribution, size and density of the apocrine glands in hidradenitis suppuritiva. *Br J Surg.* 1979;66(12):853–856. https://doi.org/10.1002/bjs.1800661206.

29. Yu CC, Cook M. Hidradenitis suppurativa: a disease of follicular epithelium, rather than apocrine glands. *Br J Dermatol.* 1990;122:763–769.

30. Attanoos R, Appleton M, Douglas-Jones A. The pathogenesis of hidradenitis suppurativa: a closer look at apocrine and apoeccrine glands. *Br J Dermatol.* 1995;133:254–258.

31. Larralde M, Abad M, Munoz A, Luna P. Childhood flexural comedones: a new entity. *Arch Dermatol.* 2007;143(7):909–911.

32. Jemec GBE, Thomsen B, Hansen U. The homogeneity of hidradenitis suppurativa lesions: a histological study of intra-individual variation. *Apmis.* 1997;105(1–6):378–383.

33. Alikhan A, Lynch P, Eisen D. Hidradenitis suppurativa: a comprehensive review. *J Am Acad Dermatol.* 2009;60(4):539–561. https://doi.org/10.1016/j.jaad.2008.11.911.

34. Jemec GBE. Histology of hidradenitis suppurativa. *J Am Acad Dermatol.* 1996;34(6):994–999.

35. Jemec GBE, Gniadecka M. Ultrasound examination of hair follicles in hidradenitis suppurativa. *Arch Dermatol.* 1997;133(8):967–970.

36. Fitzsimmons J, Guilbert P. A family study of hidradenitis suppurativa. *J Med Genet.* 1985;22:367–373.

37. Fitzsimmons J, Fitzsimmons E, Guilbert P. Familial hidradenitis suppurativa: evidence in favour of single gene transmission. *J Med Genet.* 1984;21:281–285.

38. Yamamoto N, Tanigaki K, Han H, et al. Notch/RBP-J signaling regulates epidermis/hair fate determination of hair follicular stem cells. *Curr Biol.* 2003;13:333–338.

39. Wang B, Yang W, Wen W, et al. γ-secretase gene mutations in familial acne inversa. *Science.* 2010;330(6007):1065.

40. Ingram J. The Genetics of Hidradenitis Suppurativa. *Dermatol Clin.* 2016;34:23–28.

41. Smith M, Nicholson C, Parks-Miller A, Hamzavi I. Hidradenitis suppurativa: an update on connecting the tracts. *F1000Research.* 2017;6:1272.

42. van der Zee H, de Ruiter L, van den Broecke D, et al. Elevated levels of tumour necrosis factor (TNF)-α, interleukin (IL)-1β and IL-10 in hidradenitis suppurativa skin: a rationale for targeting TNF-α and IL-1β. *Br J Dermatol.* 2011;164(6):1292–1298.

43. Mortimer P, Dawber R, Gales M, Moore R. A double-blind controlled cross-over trial of cyproterone acetate in females with hidradenitis suppurativa. *Br J Dermatol.* 1986;115(3):263–268.

44. Sawers R, Randall VA, Ebling F. Control of hidradenitis suppurativa in women using combined antiandrogen (cyproterone acetate) and oestrogen therapy. *Br J Dermatol.* 1986;115(3):269–274.

45. Kraft J, Searless G. Hidradenitis suppurativa in 64 female patients: retrospective study comparing oral antibiotics and antiandrogen therapy. *J Cutan Med Surg.* 2007;11(4):125–131.

46. Hurley H. Axillary hyperhidrosis, apocrine bromhidrosis, hidradenitis suppurativa, and familial benign pemphigus: surgical approach. In: Roenigk R, Roenigk Jr H, eds. *Roenigk and Roenigk's Dermatologic Surgery: Principles and Practice.* 2nd ed. Marcel Dekker; 1996:623–645.

47. Sartorius K, Lapins J, Emtestam L, Jemec GBE. Suggestions for uniform outcome variables when reporting treatment effects in hidradenitis suppurativa. *Br J Dermatol.* 2003;149(1):211–213.

48. Kipping HF. How I treat hidradenitis suppurativa. *Postgrad Med.* 1970;48(3):291–292. https://doi.org/10.1080/00325481.1970.11693572.

49. Clemmensen OJ. Topical treatment of hidradenitis suppurativa with clindamycin. *Int J Dermatol.* 1983;22(5):325–328. https://doi.org/10.1111/j.1365-4362.1983.tb02150.x.

50. Mustafa EB, Ali SD, Kurtz LH. Hidradenitis suppurativa: review of the literature and management of the axillary lesion. *J Natl Med Assoc.* 1980;72(3):237–243.

2

Hidradenitis Suppurativa Epidemiology

PEYTON C. MORSS-WALTON, ALEXA B. KIMBALL, AND MARTINA L. PORTER

Introduction

This chapter will focus on the epidemiology of hidradenitis suppurativa (HS), examining the body of evidence available for estimating the incidence and prevalence of HS, and the distribution of HS by gender, age, and race.

Epidemiology is a broad subject that also encompasses the risk factors for disease development and the impact of a disease on societal metrics, such as the likelihood of people with a disease to be unemployed. The intersection of risk factors and disease comorbidities can be difficult to separate, and in this chapter we will discuss correlation and causation studies and how they can provide an idea of which patients are most at risk for the development of HS.

Hidradenitis Suppurativa Epidemiology

Prevalence and Incidence

Prevalence and incidence are the most common metrics used to assess the burden of disease in a population. Prevalence assesses the proportion of a population with a disease over a point in time.

In contrast, incidence is the rate of new, or newly diagnosed, cases of a disease over a period of time (typically 1 year). Taken together, incidence and prevalence can show the rate at which a disease is being diagnosed and the duration of time that patients carry the diagnosis. The ability to determine these statistics is affected by data source, coding, and other biases.

Estimates of the overall prevalence of HS range from 0.03% to 4% with a likely prevalence of around 1% (Table 2.1). Several types of datasets such as those from patient-facing surveys, cohort, and population-based studies have noted differences in prevalence that may be attributed to study design or regional study population differences. Typically, the threshold of 47 cases per 100,000 people or below is defined "rare."[1] While HS has been classified as a rare disease in the past, increasing data suggest that it should no longer be considered rare.

Large cohort studies using claims databases or billing codes may underestimate prevalence, as they only capture patients who seek medical care, while survey studies may report higher rates of prevalence, as patients with the disease may be more incentivized to respond. Several methods of analysis exist. Claims database studies use large databases derived from either the provider side or the insurer side. A population-based observational and case-control study using the U.K. Clinical Practice Research Datalink found an overall point prevalence of HS diagnosis to be 0.77%; however, when probable cases (individuals confirmed by primary care physician to have a history of between one and four skin boils in flexural regions) were also included, the prevalence rose to 1.19%.[2] Some studies control for incorrect coding by performing a full or partial chart review to estimate the positive predictive value of each coded diagnosis. For example, a 2017 US population analysis used a chart-verified billing code model to estimate HS prevalence at 0.10% in the US population (98 per 100,000 persons).[3]

Several smaller cohort studies have used dermatologist-rendered diagnosis instead of billing code diagnosis resulting in prevalence estimates ranging from 0.03 to 0.2% (see Table 2.1).[4–7] Survey studies report a higher estimate of prevalence on average, with the notable caveat that survey validation may influence the resultant reporting. Studies performed in Denmark and Australia used previously validated HS surveys to report a general prevalence of 0.67–2.1%.[8–10] Other survey studies, using unvalidated questionnaires, have reported prevalence ranging from 0.41% to 4%.[11–13]

Breakdown of prevalence by disease severity is rarely reported, as it is difficult to ascertain through billing codes and patient surveys. However, one US analysis of predominantly white patients in Olmsted County, Minnesota, reported a distribution of Hurley stage as Hurley I 59.7%, Hurley II 38.1%, and Hurley III

TABLE 2.1 Prevalence and Incidence of Hidradenitis Suppurativa by Country/Study

Country	Study	Population Queried	Overall Prevalence Estimates	1-Year Incidence Estimates	Method
North America					
US	Lookingbill et al. (1988)[5]	1,157	0.09%		Dermatologist-diagnosed
US	Cosmatos et al. (2013)[83]	7,927	0.053%		Insurance claims database (ICD) codes
US	Kimball and Sung (2013)[84]	429,329 563,931	0.11% in 2007 0.2% in 2011		Billing codes
US	Shlyankevich et al. (2014)[85]	2 million	0.078%		Chart-verified billing codes
US	Shahi et al. (2014)[86]	144,000	0.13%		Billing codes
US	Garg et al.[3] (2017)	48 million	0.10%	0.01%[17]	Chart-verified International Classification of Diseases (ICD) codes
South America					
Brazil	Ianhez et al.[13] (2018)	17,004	0.41%		Survey
Argentina	Zimman et al. (2019)[87]	143,245	0.02%		Chart-verified billing codes
Europe					
Denmark	Jemec (1988)[11]	100	4%		Survey
Denmark	Jemec et al.[4] (1996)	507	1% 1-year prevalence		Dermatologist-diagnosed
France	Revuz et al.[12] (2008)	6,887	0.97%		Survey
Spain	Albares et al. (2012)[7]	1,071	0.2%		Dermatologist diagnosed
Denmark	Vinding et al. (2014)[8]	16,404	2.10%		Validated survey
Denmark	Riis et al. (2019)[9]	27,765	1.8%		Validated survey
Germany	Kirsten et al. (2020)[18]	2.3 million	0.04%	0.03%	ICD codes
Sweden	Killasli et al. (2020)[88]	9 million	0.14%		Registry
Africa					
Mali	Mahé et al. (2002)[6]	10,575	0.03%		Dermatologist-diagnosed
Middle East					
Israel	Shalom et al. (2015)[89]	3,207	0.7%		(ICD) codes
Asia					
Korea	Lee et al. (2018)[23]	50 million	0.06%		(ICD) codes
Oceania					
Australia	Calao et al. (2018)[10]	11,433	0.67%		Validated survey

2.2%.[14] Smaller studies of HS patient cohorts have observed a higher burden of moderate to severe HS with over half of patients in Hurley stages II and III,[15,16] and high-severity patients may be overrepresented in samples drawn from patients seeking care.

As awareness of the diagnosis rises, there may also be an increase in incidence. Only two studies have reported HS incidence (see Table 2.1). Through a US dataset, the 1-year incidence of HS in the United States was reported as 11.4 per 100,000 (0.01%), with the 10-year incidence as 8.6 per 100,000.[17] In Germany, the incidence was estimated at 0.03%.[18]

Demographic Factors

When evaluating the epidemiology of a disease, it is important to consider the factors that influence disease prevalence, as they may give insight into the types of populations more susceptible to the disease and help determine populations that should receive increased screening or for whom clinicians should have a higher baseline suspicion of disease. Prevalence of HS has been evaluated against different demographic factors and found to vary based on gender, age group, and race (Table 2.2). Several studies examining this demography in more detail have provided insight as to the types of populations likely to contain the highest disease burden.

TABLE 2.2	Demographic Factors Associated With Hidradenitis Suppurativa
Demographic Factor	Hidradenitis Suppurativa Associations
Gender	• Western studies report female predominance of up to 2:1 • Gender predominance may differ by ethnicity, as some Asian studies suggest a reverse gender predominance
Age	• Highest prevalence at age 30–39 • Early-onset group of age <17 has a decreased prevalence
Race	• Prevalence in patients with skin of color is up to threefold higher than in white patients; 296 per 100,000 compared with 95 per 100,000, respectively.[3] • Less prevalent in Asian populations; for example, 0.06% in Korea vs. 0.10% in US[3,23]

Gender

Most Western studies note an increased prevalence in female versus male HS patients, but, gender predominance may differ based on racial or geographic differences, as researchers studying Asian populations report male predominance.

For example, in the United States, female patients had a prevalence of more than double that of males: 137 per 100,000 compared with male patients at 58 per 100,000.[3] This is echoed in other studies, including a Swedish study, that showed a prevalence of 0.21% in women versus 0.07% in men. Brazilian population surveys also showed a higher prevalence among females, 0.49%, versus a prevalence of 0.30% among males. The proportion of female/male was found to increase with age group from 0.46% female/0.38% male for age below 40 years to 0.56%/0.23% for age above 40 years.[13] In the HS UNITE registry, which draws on populations from North America, Europe, and Australia, 69.7% of registrants were female.[19]

Notably, while most population-based analyses are age-adjusted, in an American analysis limited to the pediatric HS population, there remains an increased prevalence of female versus male patients at 0.045 to 0.012, respectively.[20] This proportion has also been observed in a smaller-scale single-center study of the US pediatric HS population, which reported 85.7% versus 14.3% female to male patients.[21]

One Korean retrospective study of 438 participants noted a higher ratio of male patients, 2.5:1, and noted that male patients had more severe disease.[22] Similarly, a larger Korean population-based analysis found that males predominated with a ratio of 1.6:1.[23] A questionnaire-based study in Japan also noted a higher disease burden in male patients with a ratio of 2:1[24] and a small study of 58 patients in Singapore also reported a higher percentage of males (58.6%).[25] Further population-based studies are needed to clarify this difference, but it may be that the gender differences in HS prevalence are specific to certain populations or genetic variance.

Race

It is increasingly well-documented that HS disproportionately affects non-Asian minorities.[3,26–28] Several studies in the United States support this conclusion.[3,29] Garg et al. found that the prevalence of HS in African Americans was threefold higher than white

patients, 296 per 100,000 compared with 95 per 100,000.[3] While few true prevalence studies exist that examine race, the racial makeup of HS patients has been proxied by comparing the race of patients seeking care for HS versus other conditions. In one US single-center analysis of 476 HS patient charts, 66% were African American, despite making up only 36% of patients seen at the study institution.[28] In another US single-center analysis of 366 HS patients, 6.4% of black patients seeking care were for HS complaints, while only 3.9% of white patients seeking care were for HS.[27] A retrospective review in the United States of 284 HS patients found an even more stark ratio of 7.22:1 African American to white HS patients.[30] Data from the National Ambulatory Medical Care Survey were also examined to show the odds ratio (OR) for African Americans compared with white patients seeking care for HS as 2.00.[31] A 2014 review of data from the National Center for Health Statistics found that 23% of visits for HS are from African American patients, compared with 13% of visits from African American patients overall.[32] In addition, in one retrospective study of 375 patients, African American patients were significantly more likely to present with more advanced Hurley stage II or III disease compared with all other racial groups (OR 2.46, $P = .003$).[33]

Overall, studies in the United States support the higher burden of HS disease in African American patients. It remains to be seen whether this is an example of variations in HS by race that is replicated in other countries. While reported prevalence of HS varies somewhat by region, further population-based analyses are needed before we can concretely determine more affected populations.

Age

Disease prevalence also varies by age, with the highest prevalence in the United States seen between age 30 and 39.[20] This is generally the age range cited as when disease onset most commonly occurs, though one French study reported the typical median age of onset for HS symptoms as between 20 and 24 years.[34]

The age of onset distribution of HS is usually reported as unimodal within the age range of 30 to 39 years,[35] but one study reported a bimodal age distribution observed with a second peak of self-reported disease symptom onset in post-menopausal women.[16] This finding corresponds with an observation from a Brazilian study that the ratio of women to men increases with age, implying that if there is a late-onset group of HS disease, it is predominantly experienced by women.

Several studies have reported that up to 25% of HS cases may present before age 18, which some authors have qualified as "early onset" or "adolescent" disease.[14,36] One Spanish study of 134 HS patients reported 51.5% experiencing adolescent-onset disease,[37] and in Brazil, a higher prevalence of HS was found in adolescents (0.57%) as compared with adults (0.47%).[13] One study also reported that racial differences in age of onset may be observed,[15] suggesting that, similar to the differences seen in gender-based analyses based on country where the study was conducted, age-based prevalence analyses may also be affected by the demographics of the population studied. In a US pediatric analysis, prevalence was highest in female adolescents aged 15 to 17 years.[20] Recently it has also been suggested that early-onset HS patients are more likely to be overweight or obese.[38–40]

There is a documented delay in diagnosis of between 7.2[41] and 10.2 years[42] for HS patients. An association of diagnostic delay of HS with increased disease severity has been suggested.[41] These delays in care may also impact our assessment of HS severity prevalence, as patients have cited that the first 6 years of disease are typically the most severe,[35] and these are the years that are delayed to care.

Considering the overall prevalence of HS in childhood in contrast to adult-diagnosed HS, so-called "early-onset HS" continues to meet the threshold of classification for a rare disease, with fewer than 47 cases per 100,000 people.[1]

Risk Factors

Risk factors are another cornerstone of epidemiology research, as some risk factors may be modifiable. In addition, risk factors also continue to help determine populations who may benefit from increased screenings and other disease-modifying interventions. Several risk factors, both behavioral and genetic, have been associated with HS. In most cases, causation has not yet been established, as the pathogenesis of HS remains under investigation. Most risk factors correlate only to the presence of HS; however, some are associated with an increase in disease severity.

Family History

No dominant genetic pattern has yet been established for HS, although several small genome-wise association studies (GWAS) have now been published.[43] Only one gene, a gamma-secretase, comprising four units—presenilin (PSEN), presenilin enhancer-2 (PSENEN), nicastrin protein (NCSTN), and anterior pharynx defective-2—has been associated with 5% of HS families who exhibit a dominant inheritance pattern. The majority of studies examining this gamma-secretase unit have associated HS disease with mutations in either PSEN, PSENEN, or NCSTN,[44] but these mutations do not account for disease in the vast majority of HS patients.[45] In addition, one other study notes that a higher copy number of defensin genes, which encode for proinflammatory defensins, may be related to HS inheritance.[46] Currently, the consensus regarding HS inheritance is that it is a genetically heterogenous disease.[44]

Up to 35% of HS patients have been reported to have a positive family history of the disease,[34,47] and a positive family history of HS has been associated with an earlier age of disease onset[48] compared with the commonly cited range of 20 to 24 years.[34] There may be overlap between the prevalence of "adolescent onset" disease and a positive family history of HS. Interestingly, there have also been reports that an absence of family history correlates with increased disease severity.[34]

Family history of HS may also vary based on ethnicity, similarly to the observed differences in disease prevalence. A case series of 58 Japanese patients found that only 1.7% of Japanese patients had a family history of HS, which was significantly lower than the 29.1% observed in data the authors amalgamated from Western studies.[49]

Lifestyle

Many different facets of lifestyle, including smoking, obesity, and socioeconomic status, have been linked with HS (Table 2.3). While study design varies, most studies report an "increased risk" of HS in groups with the associated risk factor. This may be reported as an increased likelihood, or in an OR, a measure of association that compares the odds of disease in those with the risk factor to the odds of disease in those without the risk factor.

Smoking

A 2020 meta-analysis of smoking and HS identified 25 studies, with 101,977 patients and 17 million controls.[50] The meta-analysis reported an OR of 4.26 between current smoking status and a

TABLE 2.3 Lifestyle Factors Associated With Hidradenitis Suppurativa

Risk Factor	Hidradenitis Suppurativa Associations
Smoking	• Elevated odds ratio (4.26) links current smoking status and hidradenitis suppurativa (HS) diagnosis.[50] Nonsmokers exhibit better response to HS treatment (odds ratio 2.643).[51]
Obesity	• Elevated body mass index associated with more severe HS • May influence earlier age of onset
Friction and mechanical stress	• May act as a trigger for lesion formation by disrupting the local skin environment
Diet	• More evidence required on specific dietary associations • Increased lesions linked to low vitamin D and Zinc
Socioeconomic status (SES)	• HS associated with low SES

diagnosis of HS, but they did not report a causal relationship between the two factors. While no link between smoking and HS disease severity has been proven, a 2017 study examining first-line HS therapies across a single-center outpatient population ran a multivariate logistic regression that controlled for other factors, such as type of treatment initiated, and found that after treatment, nonsmokers with HS were significantly more likely to have improvement in their disease at follow-up as compared with smokers with HS (OR 2.643).[51]

Body Mass Index

Body mass index (BMI) may also impact HS. A multicenter study of 246 patients concluded that BMI and HS are related, though the relationship between HS severity and BMI increases was not linear. Patients with a high BMI (BMI >35) were shown to have more severe disease, and an increase in BMI, even for patients with a non-obese BMI, statistically increased patient-reported HS severity.[52] In a separate multivariate analysis of 152 cases, BMI was found to independently predict HS disease severity.[53] A systematic review and meta-analysis of dietary and metabolic factors and HS found nine studies on body weight and HS. This meta-analysis concluded that HS patients are four times more likely to be obese than the general population.[54] It is also likely that obesity influences an earlier age of disease onset, as seen in a study of 722 adolescent onset HS patients, which found that pediatric HS patients are 2.5 times as likely as their peers to be obese.[40] HS patients also have been found to have dysregulated adipose hormones such as adiponectin, hinting at a pathologic connection.[55]

Epicardial fat thickness, a marker of cardiovascular disease associated with several systemic inflammatory dermatologic diseases, has also been proportionally associated with increased disease severity in HS, independent of BMI.[56]

Friction and Mechanical Stress

Friction and mechanical stress have also been identified as possible triggers for HS flares.[57] Body sites with high friction or mechanical stress from clothing, belts, and/or skin folds are often implicated in the development of friction-associated lesions.[58] Friction is also a common trigger reported by patients in surveys.[59] Frequent irritation to skin may promote follicular occlusion and HS lesion formation. Similarly, sweating is also implicated in patient surveys as an HS trigger and may support theories on HS pathogenesis regarding microbial dysbiosis.[60] Sweating may change the pH and flora of the local cutaneous microenvironment and contribute to the formation of HS lesions.

Interestingly, bariatric surgery research supports the connection between HS and friction, as some research reports a notable percentage (32%) of patients experience a worsening of disease after surgery despite weight loss, due largely to the remaining presence of skin folds, generating significant friction and triggering nodule formation.[61]

Various forms of hair removal, most commonly shaving with a straight razor, have also been implicated in the formation of HS nodules,[35] and patients report improvement with cessation of the behavior[59] or use of laser hair removal.[62] This improvement is consistent with the follicular occlusion model of HS nodule formation, as the regrowth of hairs may increase rates of follicular occlusion, subsequent follicular inflammation, and stimulation of an atypical HS immune response resulting in lesion formation.

Diet

A systematic review and meta-analysis of the role of dietary interventions in HS showed that diet may play a role in HS activity and severity, highlighting that dairy, brewer's yeast, and processed foods may have an impact on HS severity. However, more studies are needed to concretely determine this relationship.[63] While many patients anecdotally link their disease improvement with variations in diet, the only significant association between diet and HS to date is an increased HS lesion count observed in patients with vitamin D and zinc deficiencies.[63]

Socioeconomic Status

It is well-documented that patients with a lower socioeconomic status (SES) and lower education level living in non-metropolitan areas receive lower access to care than their higher economic status counterparts.[64,65] HS, compared with other dermatologic diseases, has been significantly associated with a lower SES,[66] and HS patients are more likely to be on the US Medicaid healthcare program than commercial insurance or Medicare.[67] Among HS patients, lower SES has been significantly associated with higher Hurley stage disease.[33] HS is also linked to obesity, which is known to have a direct relationship with SES.[68]

Quality of Life and Mental Health

Depression and decreased quality of life have also been associated with HS. Epidemiologically, it is difficult to determine whether depression and other mental health challenges should be considered a comorbidity of HS or if these factors increase risk for the development of HS. Further confounding the link is the knowledge that some mental illnesses are also associated with behaviors that are known risk factors for HS, such as obesity and smoking. Interestingly, one study that found HS to be significantly associated with bipolar disorder observed that the association became insignificant when controlling for body weight,[69] suggesting that if there is a causative link between mental health and HS, it may be not be direct. Mental health comorbidities of HS are discussed in detail in **Chapter 8**.

HS patients have also been shown to struggle with other emotional stressors more than the general population. In addition to

poor quality of life as measured by the Dermatology Life Quality Index (DLQI), HS has been associated with other markers of unhappiness, including poor body image.[70,71] This association was stronger in HS patients than other skin disease patients,[70] and may represent an increased burden of stress in this patient population. Indeed, one study examining HS and psoriasis patients found that after controlling for disease severity and weight, HS patients were willing to trade significantly more years of their life to live at a normal weight.[72] In addition, HS patients experience emotional difficulty in their sexual lives. Quality of life and HS are discussed in detail in **Chapter 21**.

Societal Impact of Disease

It is difficult to disentangle correlation and causation for many of the observed correlations between HS and risk factors. As discussed, HS is associated with a lower SES. One explanation for the lower SES observed in those with severe HS is the impact of HS on their ability to work. Many HS patients, even those with Hurley stage I disease, experience a reduction in work productivity and a reduction in daily activities.[73] In one survey of 100 adults with HS, only 57 patients were employed, and 21% reported missing work due to HS. The remaining 43% were unemployed.[73] In a survey in Denmark, 25% of HS patients were unemployed compared with 6.2% in the general population.[74] The authors speculate that the higher rates of unemployment observed in HS patients is likely twofold, due to the impact of pain and stigma that cause absenteeism, and a longstanding disease burden affecting education prospects. Similarly, as discussed earlier, HS patients in the United States disproportionately are on Medicaid insurance, which provides coverage for populations with lower income level, as well as disabilities,[67] and can act as a proxy for the SES of a population.

Compared with psoriasis, HS patients experience significantly higher scores, indicating higher productivity impairment, on the Total Work Productivity Impairment (TWPI) questionnaire,[75] which measures the impairment of both paid and unpaid household labor due to a health problem.

The prolonged burden of the painful and disfiguring disease may result in cumulative life course impairment (CLCI) for HS patients. CLCI is used to assess the cumulative impact caused by a disease during a lifetime, representing the consequences of choices made that were informed or dictated by the disease and how it can change the course of a patient's life. It represents the sociologic and economic scars of a chronic disease.[76] CLCI is a phenomenon that has been well-documented as negative in psoriasis patients.[77] In comparison, little data on HS's long-term impact are available, but the evidence from patient surveys, interviews, and work productivity of HS patients supports the inference that HS patients may also have a significant negative CLCI.[77]

HS patients facing stigma and a lower income level may be less likely and less able to seek care and propagate a vicious cycle of increasing disease severity. In one US analysis, only 21% of HS patients had one ambulatory encounter with a dermatologist in 5 years,[78] versus 55% of patients having an emergency department (ED) or inpatient care encounter.[79] Patients with HS were significantly more likely than patients with psoriasis to use the ED or inpatient care.[79] In a US analysis, inpatient costs were found to represent a higher proportion of the economic burden of HS costs on the healthcare system.[67]

For an individual HS outpatient, a European study examined the cost per patient of flares, looking at both outpatient costs and inpatient costs. They estimated the cost per flare to an outpatient as €229.80, with a European hospitalization having a similar cost of €220.50.[80] These costs were substantially reduced by the decrease in flares seen with the introduction of adalimumab treatment for HS. The overall implication is that HS patients may not have access to flare-mitigating therapy. The authors concluded that HS flares increase cost of care, requiring urgent outpatient visits and hospitalizations, and increase the impact on the patient's life, such as on work productivity. Costs were reduced by anti-tumor necrosis factor alpha therapy due to the reduction in HS exacerbations achieved by this more efficacious therapy.

Growing the Field

The delay to care seen in HS patients may be a combination of two factors: patient reluctance and/or inability to access care, and a knowledge gap of providers. Many HS patients are misdiagnosed before finally receiving a diagnosis of HS.[81]

It is possible that as research and awareness in the field of HS grow,[82] they will correspond to a rise in diagnosis, and may eventually increase the current prevalence estimates. The field has been growing at a rapid pace; since 2008, annual HS-related publications have grown exponentially, and two phase 3 randomized clinical trials (RCTs) of adalimumab as an effective therapy for HS led to the landmark event of the US Food and Drug Administration approval of adalimumab for HS.[29]

Conclusion

Prevalence estimates for HS continue to vary based on the populations assessed and the study type, and more large-scale population studies, specifically incorporating minority populations, are needed to provide an idea of the true global prevalence.

Greater awareness of HS may accompany an increase in incidence rates and prevalence in the future, and may alter the age distribution if early HS is recognized in younger patients. Increasing use of disease-modifying treatments may also change the severity distribution of the disease if patients are treated and do not progress to the more advanced scarring of Hurley stage III disease.

More information regarding HS prevalence and incidence is required to continue assessing its effect on the population. Future studies focusing on vulnerable populations such as children, minorities, and populations with low SES will continue to add to the body of knowledge regarding the disease. Epidemiologic data will also assist providers in community-based interventions for HS patients, enabling appropriate risk factor identification, public health prevention efforts, and informed screenings for comorbidities.

References

1. Richter T, Nestler-Parr S, Babela R, et al. Rare Disease Terminology and Definitions—A Systematic Global Review: Report of the ISPOR Rare Disease Special Interest Group. *Value Health*. 2015;18(6):906–914. https://doi.org/10.1016/j.jval.2015.05.008.
2. Ingram J, Jenkins-Jones S, Knipe D, et al. Population-based Clinical Practice Research Datalink study using algorithm modelling to identify the true burden of hidradenitis suppurativa. *Br J Dermatol*. 2018;178:e306. https://doi.org/10.1111/bjd.16515.
3. Garg A, Kirby JS, Lavian J, et al. Sex- and age-adjusted population analysis of prevalence estimates for hidradenitis suppurativa in the United States. *JAMA Dermatol*. 2017;153(8):760–764. https://doi.org/10.1001/jamadermatol.2017.0201.
4. Jemec GBE, Heidenheim M, Nielsen NH. The prevalence of hidradenitis suppurativa and its potential precursor lesions. *J Am Acad Dermatol*. 1996;35(2, Part 1):191–194. https://doi.org/10.1016/S0190-9622(96)90321-7.
5. Lookingbill DP. Yield from a complete skin examination: Findings in 1157 new dermatology patients. *J Am Acad Dermatol*. 1988;18(1, Part 1):31–37. https://doi.org/10.1016/S0190-9622(88)70004-3.
6. Mahé A, Cissé IA, Faye O, et al. Skin diseases in Bamako (Mali). *Int J Dermatol*. 1998;37(9):673–676. https://doi.org/10.1046/j.1365-4362.1998.00454.x.
7. Albares. Epidemiologic study of skin diseases among immigrants in Alicante, Spain. *Actas Dermo-Sifiliográficas (English Edition)*. 2012;103(3):214–222. https://doi.org/10.1016/j.adengl.2011.07.007.
8. Vinding GR, Miller IM, Zarchi K, et al. The prevalence of inverse recurrent suppuration: a population-based study of possible hidradenitis suppurativa. *Br J Dermatol*. 2014;170(4):884–889. https://doi.org/10.1111/bjd.12787.
9. Riis PT, Pedersen OB, Sigsgaard V, et al. Prevalence of patients with self-reported hidradenitis suppurativa in a cohort of Danish blood donors: a cross-sectional study. *Br J Dermatol*. 2019;180(4):774–781. https://doi.org/10.1111/bjd.16998.
10. Calao M, Wilson JL, Spelman L, et al. Hidradenitis Suppurativa (HS) prevalence, demographics and management pathways in Australia: a population-based cross-sectional study. De Vita V, ed. *PLoS ONE*. 2018;13(7). https://doi.org/10.1371/journal.pone.0200683, e0200683.
11. Jemec GBE. The symptomatology of hidradenitis suppurativa in women. *Br J Dermatol*. 1988;119(3):345–350. https://doi.org/10.1111/j.1365-2133.1988.tb03227.x.
12. Revuz JE, Canoui-Poitrine F, Wolkenstein P, et al. Prevalence and factors associated with hidradenitis suppurativa: results from two case-control studies. *J Am Acad Dermatol*. 2008;59(4):596–601. https://doi.org/10.1016/j.jaad.2008.06.020.
13. Ianhez M, Schmitt JV, Miot HA. Prevalence of hidradenitis suppurativa in Brazil: a population survey. *Int J Dermatol*. 2018;57(5):618–620. https://doi.org/10.1111/ijd.13937.
14. Vazquez BG, Alikhan A, Weaver AL, et al. Incidence of hidradenitis suppurativa and associated factors: a population-based study of Olmsted County. *Minnesota J Invest Dermatol*. 2013;133(1):97–103.
15. Morss P, Porter M, Savage K, et al. Investigating race and gender in age at onset of hidradenitis suppurativa. *J Eur Acad Dermatol Venereol*. 2019. https://doi.org/10.1111/jdv.16095. Published online November 17. jdv.16095.
16. Naik HB, Paul M, Cohen SR, et al. Distribution of self-reported hidradenitis suppurativa age at onset. *JAMA Dermatol*. 2019. Published online.
17. Garg A, Lavian J, Lin G, et al. Incidence of hidradenitis suppurativa in the United States: a sex- and age-adjusted population analysis. *J Am Acad Dermatol*. 2017;77(1):118–122. https://doi.org/10.1016/j.jaad.2017.02.005.
18. Kirsten N, Petersen J, Hagenström K, Augustin M. Epidemiology of hidradenitis suppurativa in Germany—an observational cohort study based on a multisource approach. *J Eur Acad Dermatol Venereol*. 2020;34(1):174–179. https://doi.org/10.1111/jdv.15940.
19. Prens EP, Lugo-Somolinos AM, Paller AS, et al. Baseline Characteristics from UNITE: An Observational, International, Multicentre Registry to Evaluate Hidradenitis Suppurativa (Acne Inversa) in Clinical Practice. *Am J Clin Dermatol Published online February*. 2020;19. https://doi.org/10.1007/s40257-020-00504-4.
20. Garg A, Wertenteil S, Baltz R, et al. Prevalence estimates for hidradenitis suppurativa among children and adolescents in the United States: a gender- and age-adjusted population analysis. *J Invest Dermatol*. 2018;138(10):2152–2156. https://doi.org/10.1016/j.jid.2018.04.001.

21. Braunberger TL, Nicholson CL, Gold L, et al. Hidradenitis suppurativa in children: The Henry Ford experience. *Pediatr Dermatol.* 2018;35(3):370–373. https://doi.org/10.1111/pde.13466.

22. Yang JH, Moon J, Kye YC, et al. Demographic and clinical features of hidradenitis suppurativa in Korea. *J Dermatol.* 2018;45(12):1389–1395. https://doi.org/10.1111/1346-8138.14656.

23. Lee JH, Kwon HS, Jung HM, et al. Prevalence and comorbidities associated with hidradenitis suppurativa in Korea: a nationwide population-based study. *J Eur Acad Dermatol Venereol.* 2018;32(10):1784–1790. https://doi.org/10.1111/jdv.15071.

24. Kurokawa I, Hayashi N. Questionnaire surveillance of hidradenitis suppurativa in Japan. *J Dermatol.* 2015;42(7):747–749. https://doi.org/10.1111/1346-8138.12881.

25. Choi E, Cook AR, Chandran NS. Hidradenitis Suppurativa: An Asian Perspective from a Singaporean Institute. *Skin Appendage Disord.* 2018;4(4):281–285. https://doi.org/10.1159/000481836.

26. Lee DE, Clark AK, Shi VY. Hidradenitis suppurativa: disease burden and etiology in skin of color. *Dermatology.* 2017;233(6):456–461. https://doi.org/10.1159/000486741.

27. Reeder VJ, Mahan MG, Hamzavi IH. Ethnicity and hidradenitis suppurativa. *J Invest Dermatol.* 2014;134(11):2842–2843. https://doi.org/10.1038/jid.2014.220.

28. Vlassova N, Kuhn D, Okoye GA. Hidradenitis suppurativa disproportionately affects African Americans: a single-center retrospective analysis. *Acta Derm Venereol.* 2015;95(8):990–991. https://doi.org/10.2340/00015555-2176.

29. Kimball AB, Okun MM, Williams DA, et al. Two Phase 3 Trials of Adalimumab for Hidradenitis Suppurativa. *N Eng J Med.* 2016;375(5):422–434. https://doi.org/10.1056/NEJMoa1504370.

30. Vaidya T, Vangipuram R, Alikhan A. Examining the race-specific prevalence of hidradenitis suppurativa at a large academic center; results from a retrospective chart review. *Dermatol Online J.* 2017;23(6).

31. Udechukwu NS, Fleischer AB. Higher risk of care for hidradenitis suppurativa in African American and non-hispanic patients in the United States. *J Natl Med Assoc.* 2017;109(1):44–48. https://doi.org/10.1016/j.jnma.2016.09.002.

32. McMillan K. Hidradenitis suppurativa: number of diagnosed patients, demographic characteristics, and treatment patterns in the United States. *Am J Epidemiol.* 2014;179(12):1477–1483. https://doi.org/10.1093/aje/kwu078.

33. Soliman YS, Hoffman LK, Guzman AK, et al. African American patients with hidradenitis suppurativa have significant health care disparities: a retrospective study. *J Cutan Med Surg.* 2019;23(3):334–336. https://doi.org/10.1177/1203475418803077.

34. Canoui-Poitrine F, Revuz JE, Wolkenstein P, et al. Clinical characteristics of a series of 302 French patients with hidradenitis suppurativa, with an analysis of factors associated with disease severity. *J Am Acad Dermatol.* 2009;61(1):51–57. https://doi.org/10.1016/j.jaad.2009.02.013.

35. von der Werth J, Williams H. The natural history of hidradenitis suppurativa. *J Eur Acad Dermatol Venerol.* 2000;14(5):389–392. https://doi.org/10.1046/j.1468-3083.2000.00087.x.

36. Palmer RA, Keefe M. Early-onset hidradenitis suppurativa. *Clin Exp Dermatol.* 2001;26(6):501–503. https://doi.org/10.1046/j.1365-2230.2001.00876.x.

37. Molina-Leyva A, Cuenca-Barrales C. Adolescent-onset hidradenitis suppurativa: prevalence, risk factors and disease features. *Dermatology (Basel).* 2019;235(1):45–50. https://doi.org/10.1159/000493465.

38. Reichert B, Fernandez Faith E, Harfmann K. Weight counseling in pediatric hidradenitis suppurativa patients. *Pediatr Dermatol.* 2020. https://doi.org/10.1111/pde.14131. Published online March 2.

39. Andersen PL, Kromann C, Fonvig CE, et al. Hidradenitis suppurativa in a cohort of overweight and obese children and adolescents. *Int J Dermatol.* 2019. https://doi.org/10.1111/ijd.14639.

40. Balgobind A, Finelt N, Strunk A, Garg A. Association between obesity and hidradenitis suppurativa among children and adolescents: a population-based analysis in the United States. *J Am Acad Dermatol.* 2020;82(2):502–504. https://doi.org/10.1016/j.jaad.2019.08.034.

41. Saunte DM, Boer J, Stratigos A, et al. Diagnostic delay in hidradenitis suppurativa is a global problem. *Br J Dermatol.* 2015;173(6):1546–1549. https://doi.org/10.1111/bjd.14038.

42. Garg A, Neuren E, Cha D, et al. Evaluating patients' unmet needs in hidradenitis suppurativa: results from the Global VOICE project. *J Am Acad Dermatol.* 2019. https://doi.org/10.1016/j.jaad.2019.06.1301. Published online July 3.

43. Liu M, Degner J, Georgantas RW, et al. A genetic variant in the BCL2 gene associates with adalimumab response in hidradenitis suppurativa clinical trials and regulates expression of BCL2. *J Invest Dermatol.* 2020;140(3). https://doi.org/10.1016/j.jid.2019.06.152. 574–582.e2.

44. Li X, Jiang L, Huang Y, et al. A gene dysfunction module reveals the underlying pathogenesis of hidradenitis suppurativa: an update. *Aust J Dermatol.* 2020;61(1):e10–e14. https://doi.org/10.1111/ajd.13107.

45. Ravn Jørgensen A-H, Brøgger-Mikkelsen M, Ring HC, Thomsen SF. Patients with a familial predisposition to hidradenitis suppurativa have a distinct clinical phenotype. *J Am Acad Dermatol.* 2020. https://doi.org/10.1016/j.jaad.2020.04.022. Published online April 11.

46. Giamarellos-Bourboulis EJ, Platzer M, Karagiannidis I, et al. High copy numbers of β-defensin cluster on 8p23.1, confer genetic susceptibility, and modulate the physical course of hidradenitis suppurativa/acne inversa. *J Invest Dermatol.* 2016;136(8):1592–1598. https://doi.org/10.1016/j.jid.2016.04.021.

47. Canoui-Poitrine F, Le Thuaut A, Revuz JE, et al. Identification of three hidradenitis suppurativa phenotypes: latent class analysis of a cross-sectional study. *J Invest Dermatol.* 2013;133(6):1506–1511. https://doi.org/10.1038/jid.2012.472.

48. Schrader AMR, Deckers IE, van der Zee HH, et al. Hidradenitis suppurativa: a retrospective study of 846 Dutch patients to identify factors associated with disease severity. *J Am Acad Dermatol.* 2014;71(3):460–467. https://doi.org/10.1016/j.jaad.2014.04.001.

49. Omine T, Miyagi T, Hayashi K, et al. Clinical characteristics of hidradenitis suppurativa patients in Okinawa, Japan: differences between East Asia and Western countries. *J Dermatol.* 2020. https://doi.org/10.1111/1346-8138.15411. Published online May 26.

50. Acharya P, Mathur M. Hidradenitis suppurativa and smoking: a systematic review and meta-analysis. *J Am Acad Dermatol.* 2020;82(4):1006–1011. https://doi.org/10.1016/j.jaad.2019.10.044.

51. Denny G, Anadkat MJ. The effect of smoking and age on the response to first-line therapy of hidradenitis suppurativa: an institutional retrospective cohort study. *J Am Acad Dermatol.* 2017;76(1):54–59. https://doi.org/10.1016/j.jaad.2016.07.041.

52. Riis PT, Saunte DM, Benhadou F, et al. Low and high body mass index in hidradenitis suppurativa patients—different subtypes? *J Eur Acad Dermatol Venereol.* 2018;32(2):307–312. https://doi.org/10.1111/jdv.14599.

53. Katoulis AC, Liakou AI, Rotsiamis N, et al. Descriptive epidemiology of hidradenitis suppurativa in Greece: a study of 152 cases. *Skin Appendage Disord.* 2017;3(4):197–201. https://doi.org/10.1159/000475822.

54. Choi F, Lehmer L, Ekelem C, Mesinkovska NA. Dietary and metabolic factors in the pathogenesis of hidradenitis suppurativa: a systematic review. *Int J Dermatol.* 2020;59(2):143–153. https://doi.org/10.1111/ijd.14691.

55. Malara A, Hughes R, Jennings L, et al. Adipokines are dysregulated in patients with hidradenitis suppurativa. *Br J Dermatol.* 2018;178(3):792–793. https://doi.org/10.1111/bjd.15904.

56. Alatas ET, Biteker M, Alatas OD. Epicardial fat thickness is increased and associated with disease severity in hidradenitis suppurativa. *Arch Dermatol Res.* 2020. https://doi.org/10.1007/s00403-019-02032-6. Published online January 1.

57. Boer J, Mihajlovic D. Boils at frictional locations in a patient with hidradenitis suppurativa. *Acta Dermatovenerol Croat.* 2016;24(4):303–304.

58. Boer J, Nazary M, Riis PT. The role of mechanical stress in hidradenitis suppurativa. *Dermatol Clin.* 2016;34(1):37–43. https://doi.org/10.1016/j.det.2015.08.011.

59. Kurzen H, Kurzen M. Secondary prevention of hidradenitis suppurativa. *Dermatol Reports.* 2019;11(2). https://doi.org/10.4081/dr.2019.8243.

60. Loh TY, Hendricks AJ, Hsiao JL, Shi VY. Undergarment and fabric selection in the management of hidradenitis suppurativa. *Dermatology.* 2019;1–6. https://doi.org/10.1159/000501611. Published online August 29.

61. Golbari NM, Lee Porter M, Kimball AB. Response to: remission of hidradenitis suppurativa after bariatric surgery. *JAAD Case Rep.* 2018;4(3):278–279. https://doi.org/10.1016/j.jdcr.2017.11.024.

62. Vossen ARJV, van der Zee HH, Terian M, et al. Laser hair removal alters the disease course in mild hidradenitis suppurativa. *J Dtsch Dermatol Ges.* 2018;16(7):901–903. https://doi.org/10.1111/ddg.13563.

63. Eiken HC, Holm JG, Thomsen SF. Studies on the role of diet in the management of hidradenitis suppurativa are needed. *J Am Acad Dermatol.* 2020;82(4):e137–e138. https://doi.org/10.1016/j.jaad.2019.10.137.

64. Dumont S, Cullati S, Manor O, et al. Skin cancer screening in Switzerland: cross-sectional trends (1997–2012) in socioeconomic inequalities. *Prev Med.* 2019;129:105829. https://doi.org/10.1016/j.ypmed.2019.105829.

65. Tripathi R, Knusel KD, Ezaldein HH, et al. Association of demographic and socioeconomic characteristics with differences in use of outpatient dermatology services in the United States. *JAMA Dermatol.* 2018;154(11):1286–1291. https://doi.org/10.1001/jamadermatol.2018.3114.

66. Deckers IE, Janse IC, van der Zee HH, et al. Hidradenitis suppurativa (HS) is associated with low socioeconomic status (SES): a cross-sectional reference study. *J Am Acad Dermatol.* 2016;75(4). https://doi.org/10.1016/j.jaad.2016.04.067. 755–759.e1.

67. Marvel J, Vlahiotis A, Sainski-Nguyen A, et al. Disease burden and cost of hidradenitis suppurativa: a retrospective examination of US administrative claims data. *BMJ Open.* 2019;9(9). https://doi.org/10.1136/bmjopen-2019-030579, e030579.

68. Sobal J, Stunkard AJ. Socioeconomic status and obesity: a review of the literature. *Psychol Bull.* 1989;105(2):260–275. https://doi.org/10.1037/0033-2909.105.2.260.

69. Tzur Bitan D, Berzin D, Cohen A. Hidradenitis suppurativa and bipolar disorders: a population-based study. *Dermatology (Basel).* 2020;1–7. https://doi.org/10.1159/000504535. Published online January 7.

70. Lindsø Andersen P, Nielsen RM, Sigsgaard V, et al. Body image quality of life in patients with hidradenitis suppurativa compared with other dermatological disorders. *Acta Derm Venereol.* 2020. https://doi.org/10.2340/00015555–3464. Published online April 6.

71. Schneider-Burrus S, Jost A, Peters EMJ, et al. Association of hidradenitis suppurativa with body image. *JAMA Dermatol.* 2018;154(4):447–451. https://doi.org/10.1001/jamadermatol.2017.6058.

72. Storer MA, Danesh MJ, Sandhu ME, et al. An assessment of the relative impact of hidradenitis suppurativa, psoriasis, and obesity on quality of life. *Int J Womens Dermatol.* 2018;4(4):198–202. https://doi.org/10.1016/j.ijwd.2018.08.009.

73. Yao Y, Jørgensen A-HR, Thomsen SF. Work productivity and activity impairment in patients with hidradenitis suppurativa: a cross-sectional study. *Int J Dermatol.* 2020;59(3):333–340. https://doi.org/10.1111/ijd.14706.

74. Riis PT, Thorlacius L, List EK, Jemec GBE. A pilot study of unemployment in patients with hidradenitis suppurativa in Denmark. *Br J Dermatol.* 2017;176(4):1083–1085. https://doi.org/10.1111/bjd.14922.

75. Hamzavi IH, Sundaram M, Nicholson C, et al. Uncovering burden disparity: a comparative analysis of the impact of moderate-to-severe psoriasis and hidradenitis suppurativa. *J Am Acad Dermatol.* 2017;77(6):1038–1046. https://doi.org/10.1016/j.jaad.2017.07.027.

76. Ibler KS, Jemec GBE. Cumulative life course impairment in other chronic or recurrent dermatologic diseases. In: Linder MD, Kimball AB, eds. *Current Problems in Dermatology.* 44. Basel: Karger; 2013:130–136. https://doi.org/10.1159/000350056.

77. Mattei PL, Corey KC, Kimball AB. Cumulative life course impairment: evidence for psoriasis. *Curr Probl Dermatol.* 2013;44:82–90. https://doi.org/10.1159/000350008.

78. Garg A, Lavian J, Strunk A. Low Utilization of the Dermatology Ambulatory Encounter among Patients with Hidradenitis Suppurativa: A Population-Based Retrospective Cohort Analysis in the USA. *Dermatology (Basel).* 2017;233(5):396–398. https://doi.org/10.1159/000480379.

79. Khalsa A, Liu G, Kirby JS. Increased utilization of emergency department and inpatient care by patients with hidradenitis suppurativa. *J Am Acad Dermatol.* 2015;73(4):609–614. https://doi.org/10.1016/j.jaad.2015.06.053.

80. Argyropoulou M, Kanni T, Kyprianou M, et al. Cost-savings of adalimumab in hidradenitis suppurativa: a retrospective analysis of a real-world cohort. *Br J Dermatol.* 2019;180(5):1161–1168. https://doi.org/10.1111/bjd.17151.

81. Loget J, Saint-Martin C, Guillem P, et al. Misdiagnosis of hidradenitis suppurativa continues to be a major issue. The R-ENS Verneuil study. *Ann Dermatol Venereol.* 2018;145(5):331–338. https://doi.org/10.1016/j.annder.2018.01.043.

82. Savage KT, Gonzalez Brant E, Flood KS, et al. Publication trends in hidradenitis suppurativa from 2008 to 2018. *J Eur Acad Dermatol Venereol.* 2020. https://doi.org/10.1111/jdv.16213. Published online January 22.

83. Cosmatos I, Matcho A, Weinstein R, et al. Analysis of patient claims data to determine the prevalence of hidradenitis suppurativa in the United States. *J Am Acad Dermatol.* 2013;68(3):412–419. https://doi.org/10.1016/j.jaad.2012.07.027.

84. Sung S, Kimball AB. Counterpoint: analysis of patient claims data to determine the prevalence of hidradenitis suppurativa in the United States. *J Am Acad Dermatol.* 2013;69(5):818–819. https://doi.org/10.1016/j.jaad.2013.06.043.

85. Shlyankevich J, Chen AJ, Kim GE, Kimball AB. Hidradenitis suppurativa is a systemic disease with substantial comorbidity burden: a chart-verified case-control analysis. *J Am Acad Dermatol.* 2014;71(6):1144–1150. https://doi.org/10.1016/j.jaad.2014.09.012.

86. Shahi V, Alikhan A, Vazquez BG, et al. Prevalence of hidradenitis suppurativa: a population-based study in Olmsted County. *Minnesota Dermatology.* 2014;229(2):154–158. https://doi.org/10.1159/000363381.

87. Zimman S, Comparatore MV, Vulcano AF, et al. Hidradenitis suppurativa: estimated prevalence, clinical features, concomitant conditions, and diagnostic delay in a University Teaching Hospital in Buenos Aires, Argentina. *Actas Dermosifiliogr.* 2019;110(4):297–302. https://doi.org/10.1016/j.ad.2019.01.004.

88. Killasli H, Sartorius K, Emtestam L, Svensson Å. Hidradenitis suppurativa in Sweden: a registry-based cross-sectional study of 13,538 patients. *Dermatology (Basel).* 2020;1–8. https://doi.org/10.1159/000505545. Published online February 3.

89. Shalom G, Freud T, Harman-Boehm I, et al. Hidradenitis suppurativa and metabolic syndrome: a comparative cross-sectional study of 3207 patients. *Br J Dermatol.* 2015;173(2):464–470. https://doi.org/10.1111/bjd.13777.

3

Clinical Manifestation and Phenotypes of Hidradenitis Suppurativa

MUSKAAN SACHDEVA, MONICA SHAH, AND AFSANEH ALAVI

Clinical Manifestation

Morphology of Hidradenitis Suppurativa Lesions

A key component of the diagnosis of an individual with hidradenitis suppurativa (HS) involves examining for the presence of typical HS morphology.[1] The quantity and location of lesions indicate the severity of HS.[2] It is important to consider the possibility of multiple lesion types coexisting simultaneously, together contributing to the severity of HS. Certain lesions (e.g., open comedones, small atrophic scars) suggest quiescent disease, while others (e.g., inflammatory papules, nodules) indicate active inflammation. Additionally, recent research has shown that tunnels (described below) are immunologically active. This chapter will provide an in-depth look at common HS lesions including inflammatory nodules, cysts, abscesses, comedones, draining tunnels or sinus tracts, scars, and several others (Fig. 3.1).

Comedones (Fig. 3.2): Comedones are the skin-colored, small bumps representing dilated hair infundibulum with oxidized black or white keratinous debris (open comedones).[3] There are two main types of comedones: blackheads, due to the oxidation of the pigment melanin; and whiteheads, in which the hair follicle is completely clogged and covered by a thin upper layer of stratum corneum, inhibiting exposure to air (hence the alternate name of

"closed").[4] Double-ended comedones are characteristic for HS, most likely resulting from the keratinization of the residual stump of two adjacent follicles undergoing cicatricial rearrangements (Fig. 3.3).

Pores: Pores are normally 1-mm wide dots that appear on the surface of the skin to indicate the opening of hair follicles.[5] Each hair follicle contains a sebaceous and apocrine gland, which produces the skin's oils and sweat, respectively. When these pores become clogged and full of debris, they become comedones. The dilation of pores may facilitate the accumulation of debris, giving rise to comedones.

Papules (Fig. 3.4): Papules are small, raised cutaneous lesions. They often present as numerous, firm, typically non-scaly lesions, smaller than 1 cm in size. Papules can be the same color as the surrounding skin, yellow-brown, red-brown, or purple-brown, depending on the patient's skin color phenotype. They arise when clogging in a pore causes inflammation of a hair follicle.[6]

Nodules (Fig. 3.5): Inflammatory nodules are one of the first defining characteristics of HS and probably the most characteristic lesion of HS.[7] These tender, deep-seated, rounded lesions more than 1 cm last a mean duration of 7 to 15 days. Patients with inflammatory nodules usually report a burning or stinging sensation, pain, pruritus, a warm feeling, and/or tenderness. Over time, the nodules may rupture, erode, and ulcerate, resulting in painful draining or non-draining tunnels.

Plaques (Fig. 3.6): Plaques in HS are elevated, solid, indurated lesions. Plaques may be flat topped or rounded and may have a cribriform-like surface. They are typically more than 1 cm in diameter and may or may not have defined borders.[8] Plaques can take on many different shapes including circular (round), linear, and polygonal (not geometric).

Pustules (Fig. 3.7): Pustules are superficial pus-filled lesions ≤ 1 cm. They are collections of neutrophils located superficially, usually just below the stratum corneum or in a hair follicle. The pus contents can indicate the presence of an infection or can be sterile inflammation, with the latter commonly seen in HS patients.[9]

Abscesses (Fig. 3.8): An abscess, or a boil, is a fluctuant, commonly painful lesion that appears within or below the skin's surface. The abscess is usually full of pus, or dead white blood cells. The surrounding erythema is a result of increased blood flow to the area of the abscess as part of the body's immune response to fight infection or inflammation. If left untreated, they can open and lead to a draining lesion. Without proper

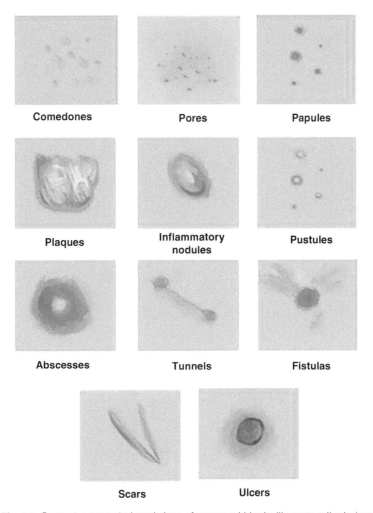

• **Fig. 3.1** Computer-generated renderings of common hidradenitis suppurativa lesions.

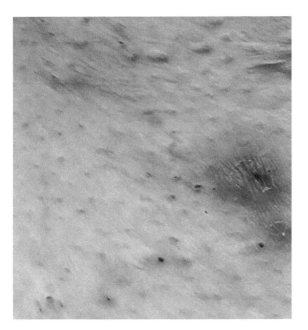

• **Fig. 3.2** Hidradenitis suppurativa-associated comedones.

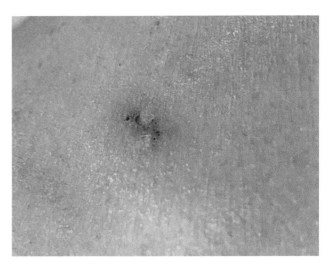

• **Fig. 3.3** Hidradenitis suppurativa-associated double-ended comedones.

application of coverings, this presents as an infection-prone site where environmental pathogens may enter freely and inflict more infection.[10]

Tunnels or tracts (Figs. 3.9 and 3.10): A tunnel or sinus tract is a linear connection that forms beneath the epidermis connecting two sites and may open to the skin surface: skin to skin (both sides open), blunted tunnel (one side open to skin), and closed tunnel (not open to skin).[11] They often contain pus and other bodily fluids rich in bacteria that can aggravate the pain, itchiness, and

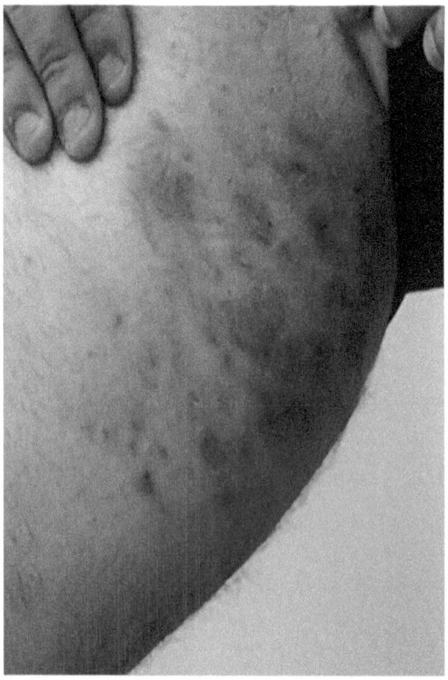

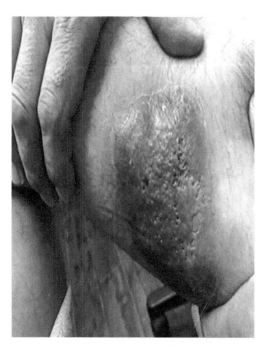

• **Fig. 3.4** Hidradenitis suppurativa-associated papule.

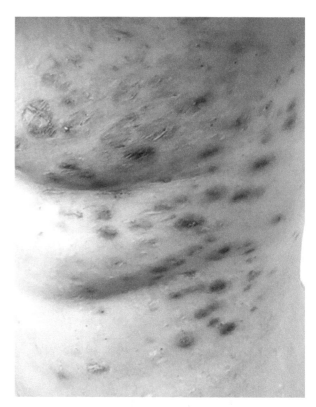

• **Fig. 3.5** Hidradenitis suppurativa-associated inflammatory nodules.

• **Fig. 3.6** Hidradenitis suppurativa-plaque.

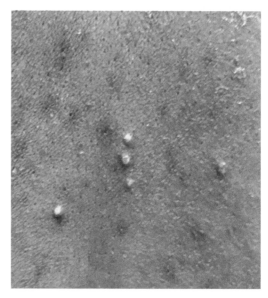

• **Fig. 3.7** Hidradenitis suppurativa-associated pustules.

inflammation associated with HS. They often occur in the later stages of HS and commonly contain biofilms.[12] These tunnels are usually treated by deroofing the tunnel and debriding the base to remove the gelatinous tissue, or by complete surgical excision.[13] Tunnels/tracts are also immunologically active, with a study by Jorgensen et al. demonstrating their immunological profile consisting of increased levels of matrix metalloproteases and tumor necrosis factor (TNF)-positive cells.[14]

Scars (Figs. 3.11 to 3.14): Irreversible tissue damage commonly associated with retraction. The progression of HS is often indicated

by significant scarring that could be cordlike, hypertrophic, keloidal, atrophic, or cerebriform. In many cases, scarring and active lesions are mixed and connected.

Ulcers (Fig. 3.15): Skin ulcers are open wounds that develop on the skin following an injury, poor circulation, and pressure. The poor blood flow delays healing of the injured epidermis and dermis. They differ from erosions in that erosions only involve the superficial epidermis, whereas ulcers have full thickness, impacting the dermis as well.[15] Knife-like ulcers, also known as fissures, are

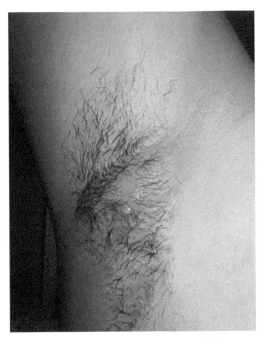

• **Fig. 3.8** Hidradenitis suppurativa-associated abscesses.

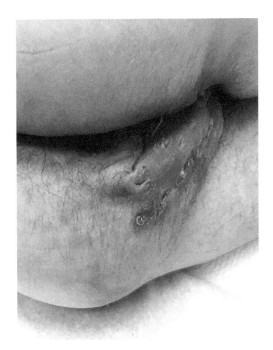

• **Fig. 3.9** Hidradenitis suppurativa-associated tracts/tunnels.

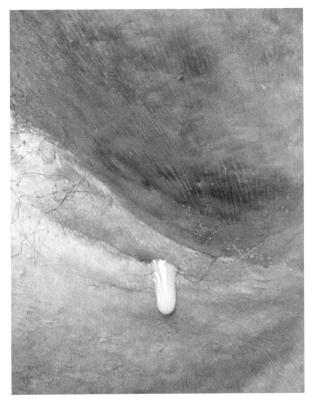

• **Fig. 3.10** Draining tunnel.

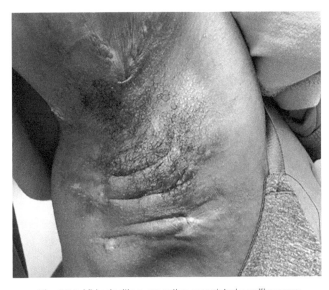

• **Fig. 3.11** Hidradenitis suppurativa associated cordlike scars.

Another key feature of HS lesions is their heterogeneity, which can lead to a range of clinical presentations. Recently, clinicians have begun stratifying patients into subtypes to better classify and study HS.[17] The most currently used subtype classification goes by the body structure affected: axillary-mammary, follicular, and gluteal. This classification system was implemented to study any correlation between genotype and phenotype, if one exists.

Primary lesions versus secondary lesions: Primary lesions occur simultaneously with the onset of disease, while secondary lesions occur as a disease progresses and is often are the result of certain treatments.[18] There are ongoing debates regarding the classification of HS lesions in that some are primary lesions (such as comedones and nodules), while secondary lesions include scars and ulceration.

characteristic of Crohn's disease that can sometimes be present in HS patients without underlying irritable bowel disease (IBD).

Fistulae: Fistulae are tunnels extending from skin to a hollow organ such as rectum, bladder, or vagina.[16].

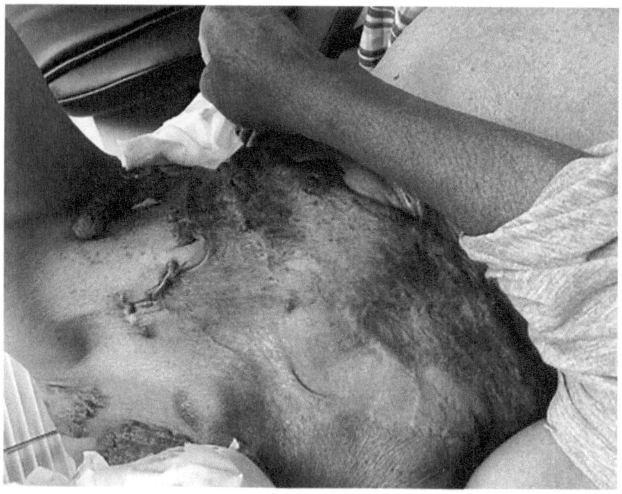

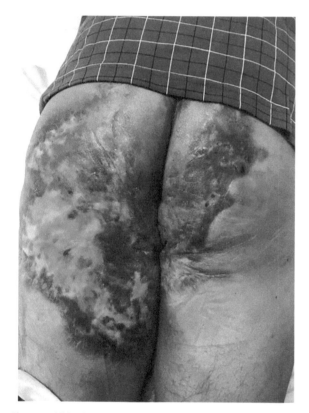

• **Fig. 3.12** Hidradenitis suppurativa associated hypertrophic and keloidal scar.

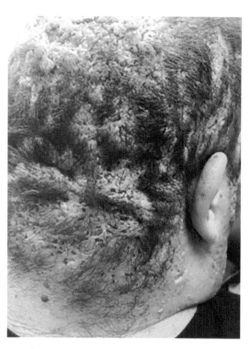

• **Fig. 3.14** Scalp involvement in hidradenitis suppurativa with cribriform scar.

• **Fig. 3.13** Hidradenitis suppurativa-associated atrophic scar (severe).

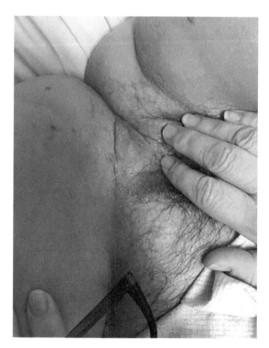

• **Fig. 3.15** Hidradenitis suppurativa "knife-like" ulcers.

Common Locations

HS typically affects the areas of the body where skin touches skin and areas of skin rich in apocrine glands. These include the axilla, groin, buttocks, and others, which are described below (Fig. 3.16). Furthermore, in females, the most commonly impacted areas are the groin (56.9%), axilla (44.8%), and under the breasts (25.9%). In males, the most commonly impacted areas are the groin (43.3%), anal region (36.7%), and axilla (30%).[19,20]

The axillary region (Fig. 3.17) is a common site for HS-related lesions and abscesses due to the high mechanical stress that the skin is under due to friction. This area is also rich in hair follicles and apocrine glands, providing an environment for certain bacteria to grow and induce pain, inflammation, malodor, and pruritus. This warm and moist environment also helps promote the growth of these bacteria, particularly those from the *Staphylococcus lugdunesis*

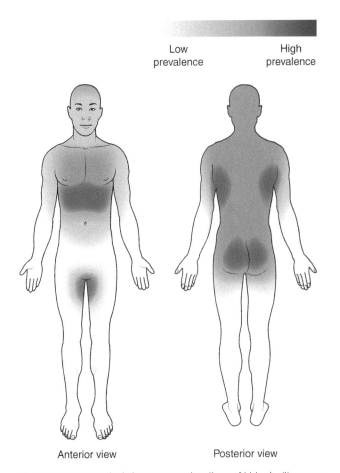

Low prevalence   High prevalence

Anterior view   Posterior view

• **Fig. 3.16** Heat map depicting common locations of hidradenitis suppurativa lesions.

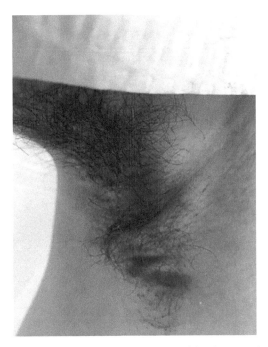

• **Fig. 3.17** Typical hidradenitis suppurativa with involvement of axilla.

family, which constitute 60% of the bacteria usually found in cultures of the axillary area.[21] The microbiome and antimicrobial therapies in HS are discussed in detail in Chapters 11 and 16, respectively.

Similar to the axillary regions, the groin provides an optimal environment for bacteria to promote lesions and abscesses. The skin in the groin experiences increased amounts of friction and sweat brought on by daily activities such as walking and sitting and provides a greater surface area for bacteria to colonize. Undergarments can also be another source of mechanical stress and friction when they rub against the skin as a result of body movements.

HS lesions can also present at the site of the buttocks, specifically the intergluteal cleft, which is an area under high mechanical stress brought on by daily activities. It is also a warm environment to promote the growth of bacteria. Individuals with HS nodules and abscesses in this area find it difficult to perform basic daily tasks such as walking and sitting due to the irritation placed on the nodules in this area. Additionally, pilonidal cysts can occur in the apex of the gluteal cleft. Studies have suggested an association between the presence of perianal fistula and an increased risk for IBD due to the abnormal connection between the anal canal and the perianal skin.[22] Other less commonly involved areas include under breasts and intermammary area, the chest, scalp, neck, abdomen, legs, face, and retro-auricular area.

Studies have shown that the largest factor that determines the location of HS lesions is gender. Women are more likely to present lesions on the anterior body parts, such as chest, breast inframammary, and axillary regions. Men tend to have more posterior and atypical afflicted areas and are also prone to perineal and perianal disease.[20] The presence of HS on areas such as the groin and axillae can negatively impact movement, functionality, sexual health, and overall quality of life.

Symptoms

Pain is the cardinal symptom associated with HS. The majority of disease symptoms begin to show between puberty and age 40. Almost half of patients report feeling burning, stinging, warmth, or pruritus 12 to 48 hours before the appearance of a lesion.[23] Pain is the symptom with the most impact on quality-of-life impairment.[24] The painful boils are most often found near the apocrine glands, such as around the groin or armpits. The average duration of a nodule is 7 to 15 days. Over time, the nodule may lead to dermal abscesses and eventually rupture, releasing a foul odor and pus secretion. As the disease progresses, scarring, fibrosis, and draining tunnels may occur. Overall, pain and pruritus are two hallmark symptoms of HS.

Pain: The first symptom of HS commonly encountered is painful lesions that become inflamed. The pain can last days to months, and the patient may also experience repeated outbreaks of these lesions in the same location or in other parts of the body (refer to section "II. Common Locations").

Pruritus: The lesions that are responsible for pain are also responsible for pruritus. Generally, these lesions fill with pus and burst open. The release of the pus and cytokines stimulates itch receptors. Repeated scratching can also lead to raised, thickened skin and bleeding. In addition, continuous drainage in skin folds also causes irritant contact dermatitis that is commonly associated with itching.

Odor: It has been shown that malodor produces psychological discomfort in both patients and healthcare professionals and contributes to stigmatization and social isolation, although it is established that HS is not contagious. Malodor is a marker of bacterial colonization that is associated with biofilm formation in up to 60% in chronic wounds, and anaerobic bacteria are considered a major producer of this malodor.[25]

Others: Inflammation is common among HS patients due to the most commonly affected areas being those with excess skin folds that provide for a warm and moist environment. This can lead to bacterial colonization, which triggers an inflammatory response. Other symptoms include bleeding that can cause anemia.

Recurrence and Flares

HS is a chronic, recurrent disease. However, the recurrence rates can be lowered with combined medical and surgical therapies. Some studies have shown post-surgical recurrence rates drop to as low as 37% to 50% after a mean follow-up time of 72 months (Ritz et al., 1998)[26]. Another issue with HS that amplifies the burden on the individual is that of flares. There is no consensus on the definition of flare, but the most accepted definition is a 25% increase in the number of lesions from the baseline.[27] A more recent study of flares from the patient perspective suggests that flares should be defined as prominent changes in symptoms, emotions, and functions that cannot be assessed solely by physical exam.[28] While little is known about what causes flare-ups, steps can be taken to prevent them, such as knowing how to identify them and seeking appropriate treatment. The lesions and other clinical manifestations of HS generally follow an evolution of progression. For example, comedones result from quiescent lesions, tunneling forms from adjacent active areas, and scars result from previously inflamed sites.[27]

Current Phenotypic Classifications

Latent Classifications

Using latent classical analysis, HS has been proposed to fall into one of the following three subtypes: axillary-mammary, follicular, and gluteal in descending order of prevalence (48%, 26%, and 26%, respectively). The subtypes were proposed by Gasparic et al. based on a retrospective chart review of 625 patients with HS.[29] Each subgroup has defining characteristics that are discussed below, along with other phenotype classifications. The three main subgroups provide a mean for stratifying HS patients in clinical studies and trials, as well as allowing physicians to choose the most appropriate treatment course tailored to the characteristics of the patient and their clinical manifestations (Table 3.1).

Phenotypes

To overcome the nonspecific nature of conventional classification systems (i.e., Hurley staging), van der Zee proposed dividing HS phenotypes into six classes, one of which falls under "typical" and the other five under "atypical."[30]

Regular (typical): This is the broadest of the phenotypes. It is a long-term state characterized by inflamed, swollen nodules and abscesses under the skin, which are painful and break open to release fluid or pus. The areas affected are diverse, including the axillary, mammary regions, and groin where there are numerous folds in the skin. The axillary-mammary subdivision is characterized by patients with a high probability of breast and armpit lesions and hypertrophic scars. It typically involves the anterior portions of the

TABLE 3.1	Clinical Manifestations of Latent Hidradenitis Suppurativa Subtypes
Latent HS Subtype	Clinical Manifestations
Axillary-Mammary	• Mainly axillary and mammary areas • More common in females • High BMI • More severe hidradenitis suppurativa (HS)
Follicular	• Atypical and follicular lesions • Pilonidal sinus, comedones, and severe acne • More common in males and smokers • Positive family history of HS • Early disease onset • Increased disease severity
Gluteal	• Gluteal and intergluteal cleft areas • More commonly in males • Lower BMIs • Milder disease severity

body and has a higher prevalence in females. The age of onset can be anywhere from 10 to 50 years, with an average age of 23 years old.

Frictional furuncle (atypical): This subtype involves more inflammation of the hair follicle and skin adnexal units, and it occurs at sites under high friction, such as the inner aspects of the thighs and the buttocks. The hair follicles swell and turn into furuncles and carbuncles, which are often red and tender. Pus is also released due to the increased recruitment of leukocytes to the site of lesion.

Scarring folliculitis (atypical): This subtype, also known as folliculitis decalvans, is a rare form of alopecia that involves scarring and inflammation.[31] It is characterized by redness, swelling, and pustules around the hair follicle that leads to the destruction of the follicle and permanent hair loss. It affects both genders, but is more common in males, and specifically affects the scalp.[32] Several hairs are often seen coming out of one follicular ostia, so the scalp looks "tufted." Eventually the hairs fall out as the follicle is destroyed, usually by the accumulation of the *Staphylococcus aureus* bacteria, and leaves behind a scar.[33]

Conglobata (atypical): The (acne) conglobata subtype is a highly inflammatory phenotype presenting with comedones, nodules, abscesses, and draining sinus tracts. The onset of this phenotype is usually after adolescence (between 18 and 30 years of age). It persists for a long time, and gradually starts to dissipate around the age of 40. This phenotype is greatly exacerbated by the excess release of androgens, explaining why it is more common in males.

Ectopic (atypical): This subtype refers to the presence of HS lesions, such as nodules and abscesses, in areas not usually associated with HS, such as the feet, hands, and forearms. The incidence of this phenotype is very uncommon and only presents in very severe cases. As a result, the cause for the appearance of nodules and abscesses in these areas is not well understood, especially since these areas usually lack hair follicles and/or apocrine glands.

Gluteal (atypical): The gluteal subtype presents with lesions in the gluteal region, as well as follicular papules and folliculitis. It typically involves patients with lower body mass indices who are current smokers with a less severe disease course, despite a longer disease duration than the more common axillary-mammary phenotype.

Follicular (atypical): The follicular subtype is characterized by atypical and follicular lesions (i.e., comedones, severe acne, pilonidal sinus) found primarily in the breast, axillary, ears, chest, back, and leg areas. These defining features fit with HS being one of the four diseases making up the "follicular occlusion tetrad" (the other three being acne conglobata, dissecting cellulitis, and pilonidal sinus), given their common pathophysiology. The follicular subtype is also associated with male gender, current smokers, a positive family history of HS, earlier disease onset, and increased disease severity and duration compared with axillary-mammary.[34]

Syndromic Hidradenitis Suppurativa

HS may also occur as part of a syndrome, which is why it is then termed syndromic HS, and helps our understanding of disease pathogenesis. Associated syndromes include Bazex-Dupre-Christol, Down's, keratitis-ichthyosis-deafness (KID), synovitis acne pustulosis hyperostosis osteitis (SAPHO), pyogenic arthritis-acne-pyoderma gangrenosum-suppurativa hidradenitis (PAPASH), pyoderma gangrenosum-acne-spondyloarthritis (PAS), pyoderma gangrenosum-acne-suppurativa hidradenitis (PASH), and Dowling-Degos disease. While these syndromes are rare, it is important to recognize them when they do occur, as treatment approach may need to be altered from regular HS treatment. Genetic syndromes associated with HS further discussed in Chapter 8.

Three subtypes of syndromic HS have been proposed: syndromes with known genetic abnormalities, syndromes characterized by follicular plugging or structural defects, and syndromes with possible autoinflammatory pathogenesis. The first two can be more broadly categorized under keratinocyte abnormalities (Table 3.2). Due to the rareness and complexity of syndromic HS, there is no universally effective treatment and treatment is typically individualized.[35]

Link between Genetics/Biomarkers and Phenotypes

While the exact cause of HS still remains unknown, recent studies have suggested several predisposing factors, including genetic and endocrine factors.[36] In particular, research has proposed that HS is an autosomal dominant genotype, which agrees with the common trend of individuals with HS having at least one parent with the disease. While much research is still ongoing to determine the exact gene responsible for HS, candidate genes that have been proposed include the *NCSTN*, *PSEN1*, and *PSENEN* genes. These genes produce proteins that are components of a complex called gamma secretase, which cleaves many other proteins that are important for several chemical signaling pathways, such as Notch signaling, which is important for the maturation of follicular and skin cells. Genetics and epigenetics of HS are discussed in Chapter 12. Furthermore, an excess of androgens has been proposed to be involved in the development and exacerbation of HS. In women, outbreaks usually occur before their menstrual period. HS specifically pertaining to women is discussed in detail in Chapter 31, "Hidradenitis Suppurativa in Women."

Summary

While the cause of HS is still being debated, much research has been successful in identifying the clinical presentations that are unique to HS and in creating systems for diagnosing and assessing disease severity. However, despite these initiatives, there still remain flaws where HS may be mistaken for other skin diseases, or vice versa. As time passes, there is potential for more definitive tests that can conclusively diagnose HS. In the meantime, it is paramount that medical education programs ensure adequate teaching of the types of lesions found in HS and update the curriculum as new insights are found. Programs have also been put in place to educate the public on what to expect in HS, so that if a patient suspects that they or someone else has HS, this information can be quickly and correctly brought to the attention of their physician. HS-specific organizations can also aid this effort by providing educational resources to both physicians and patients in order for them to be able to distinguish the types of lesions and appropriate treatment. Much progress has also been made in developing treatments with high efficacy for HS, but this still relies on the correct diagnosis of HS. As has been discussed in this chapter, the cause and clinical manifestation of HS vary from other similar skin diseases. As a result, treatments are often tailored to these causes and symptoms, stressing the need for physicians to be aware of the clinical presentation of HS to optimize management and timely prevention of disease progression.

TABLE 3.2	Classification and Description of Syndromic Hidradenitis Suppurativa
Syndromic Hidradenitis Suppurativa (HS) Classification	**Description**
Keratinocyte-associated abnormality	These groups of syndromes are caused mainly by genetic mutations that affect the expression of proteins found in keratinocytes. This reduces their viability and triggers apoptosis more often. The keratinocytes release abnormal amounts of IL-1b, IL-10, and chemokine ligand 5. The combined effects of these hypersecretions and genetic mutations result in follicular plugging, and structural and functional defects of the epithelial barrier.
Autoinflammatory	Characterized by recurrent episodes of fever, painful arthritis, and skin lesions consistent with HS, acne, pyoderma gangrenosum (PG), accompanied by elevated systemic inflammatory markers in blood. The different autoinflammatory syndromes associated with HS share a common pathogenesis involving a dysregulated innate immune system and abnormal IL-1 secretion.

References

1. Scheinfeld N. An atlas of the morphological manifestations of hidradenitis suppurativa. *Dermatol Online J.* 2014;20(4):22373.
2. Vossen AR, van der Zee HH, Prens EP. Hidradenitis suppurativa: A systematic review integrating inflammatory pathways into a cohesive pathogenic model. *Frontiers in Immunology.* 2018;9:2965.
3. Wipperman J, Bragg DA, Litzner B. Hidradenitis suppurativa: Rapid evidence review. *Am Fam Physician.* 2019;100(9):562–569.
4. Pink A, Anzengruber F, Navarini AA. Acne and hidradenitis suppurativa. *Br J Dermatol.* 2018;178(3):619–631.

5. Menderes A, Sunay O, Vayvada H, et al. Surgical management of hidradenitis suppurativa. *Int J Med Sci.* 2010;7(4):240–247.

6. Jain A, Majumdar B, Sen D, et al. Asymptomatic papules over central and pericentral areas of the face. *Indian Dermatol Online J.* 2015; 6(3):198–200. https://doi.org/10.4103/2229-5178.156404.

7. Revuz J. Hidradenitis suppurativa. *J Eur Acad Dermatol Venereol.* 2009;23(9):985–998. https://doi.org/10.1111/j.1468-3083.2009. 03356.x.

8. van Rappard DC, Starink MV, van der Wal AC, et al. Four cases of plaque form hidradenitis suppurativa. *J Eur Acad Dermatol Venereol.* 2016;30(10):e104–e106. https://doi.org/10.1111/jdv.13346.

9. Mengesha YM, Bennett ML. Pustular skin disorders: diagnosis and treatment. *Am J Clin Dermatol.* 2002;3(6):389–400. https://doi. org/10.2165/00128071-200203060-00003.

10. Ball SL, Tidman MJ. Managing patients with hidradenitis suppurativa. *Practitioner.* 2016;260(1793):25–29, 3.

11. Ring HC, Sigsgaard V, Thorsen J, et al. The microbiome of tunnels in hidradenitis suppurativa patients. *J Eur Acad Dermatol Venereol.* 2019;33(9):1775–1780. https://doi.org/10.1111/jdv.15597.

12. Ring HC, Bay L, Nilsson M, et al. Bacterial biofilm in chronic lesions of hidradenitis suppurativa. *Br J Dermatol.* 2017;176(4):993–1000. https://doi.org/10.1111/bjd.15007.

13. Campos E, Bessa H. Managing Hidradenitis suppurativa. *Arch Surg Dermatol.* 2019;2(1):23–33. https://doi.org/10.36959/446/381.

14. Jørgensen AR, Thomsen SF, Karmisholt KE, et al. Clinical, microbiological, immunological and imaging characteristics of tunnels and fistulas in Hidradenitis suppurativa and Crohn's disease. *Exp Dermatol.* 2020;29(2):118–123. https://doi.org/10.1111/exd.14036.

15. Panuncialman J, Falanga V. Unusual causes of cutaneous ulceration. *Surg Clin North Am.* 2010;90(6):1161–1180. 2010 https://doi.org/ 10.1016/j.suc.2010.08.006.

16. Ardon CB, Molenaar C, van Straalen KR, et al. High prevalence of hidradenitis suppurativa in patients with perianal fistula. *Int J Colorectal Dis.* 2019;34(7):1337–1339. https://doi.org/10.1007/ s00384-019-03313-2.

17. Tricarico PM, Boniotto M, Genovese G, et al. An integrated approach to unravel Hidradenitis suppurativa etiopathogenesis. *Front Immunol.* 2019;10:892. https://doi.org/10.3389/fimmu.2019. 00892.

18. Hess CT, Skin IQ. Primary and secondary lesions. *Adv Skin Wound Care.* 2005;18(1):19. https://journals.lww.com/aswcjournal/fulltext/ 2005/01000/skin_iq__primary_and_secondary_lesions.8.aspx.

19. Dufour DN, Emtestam L, Jemec GB. Hidradenitis suppurativa: a common and burdensome, yet under-recognised, inflammatory skin disease. *Postgrad Med J.* 2014;90(1062):216–220. https://doi.org/10. 1136/postgradmedj-2013-131994.

20. Calao M, Wilson JL, Spelman L. Hidradenitis suppurativa (HS) prevalence, demographics and management pathways in Australia: a population-based cross-sectional study. *PloS one.* 2018;13(7), e0200683. https://doi.org/10.1371/journal.pone.0200683.

21. García Colmenero L, Martin-Ezquerra G, Sánchez-Schmidt JM, et al. The role of *Staphylococcus lugdunensis* in skin and soft tissue infections. *Eur J Dermatol.* 2018;28(4):551–553. https://doi.org/10. 1684/ejd.2018.3334.

22. Gee MS, Harisinghani MG. MRI in patients with inflammatory bowel disease. *J Magn Reson Imaging.* 2011;33(3):527–534. https://doi.org/10.1002/jmri.22504.

23. Ballard K, Shuman VL. *Hidradenitis suppurativa.* StatsPearl; 2019. https://www.ncbi.nlm.nih.gov/books/NBK534867/.

24. Napolitano M, Megna M, Timoshchuk EA, et al. Hidradenitis suppurativa: from pathogenesis to diagnosis and treatment. *Clinical, cosmetic and investigational dermatology.* 2017;10:105–115. https://doi. org/10.2147/CCID.S111019.

25. Alavi A, Farzanfar D, Lee RK, et al. The Contribution of Malodour in Quality of Life of Patients With Hidradenitis Suppurativa. *J Cutan Med Surg.* 2018;22(2):166–174. https://doi.org/10.1177/ 1203475417745826.

26. Ritz JP, Runkel N, Haier J, Buhr HJ. Extent of surgery and recurrence rate of hidradenitis suppurativa. *Int J Colorectal Dis.* 1998;13 (4):164–168. https://doi.org/10.1007/s003840050159.

27. Patil S, Apurwa A, Nadkarni N, et al. Hidradenitis suppurativa: inside and out. *Indian J Dermatol.* 2018;63(2):91–98. https://doi.org/10. 4103/ijd.IJD_412_16.

28. Kirby JS, Moore B, Leiphart P, et al. A narrative review of the definition of 'flare' in hidradenitis suppurativa. *Br J Dermatol.* 2020;182 (1):24–28. https://doi.org/10.1111/bjd.18035.

29. Gasparic J, Theut Riis P, Jemec GB. Recognizing syndromic hidradenitis suppurativa: a review of the literature. *J Eur Acad Dermatol Venereol.* 2017;31(11):1809–1816. https://doi.org/10.1111/jdv. 14464.

30. Vinkel C, Thomsen SF. Hidradenitis suppurativa: causes, features, and current treatments. *J Clin Aesthet Dermatol.* 2018;11(10):17–23.

31. Otberg N, Kang H, Alzolibani AA, et al. Folliculitis decalvans. *Dermatol Ther.* 2008;21(4):238–244. https://doi.org/10.1111/j.1529-8019.2008.00204.x.

32. Sillani C, Bin Z, Ying Z, et al. Effective treatment of folliculitis decalvans using selected antimicrobial agents. *Int J Trichology.* 2010;2 (1):20–23. https://doi.org/10.4103/0974-7753.66908.

33. Horenstein MG, Bacheler CJ. Follicular density and ratios in scarring and nonscarring alopecia. *Am J Dermatopathol.* 2013;35(8):818–826. https://doi.org/10.1097/DAD.0b013e3182827fc7.

34. Vasanth V, Chandrashekar BS. Follicular occlusion tetrad. *Indian Dermatol Online J.* 2014;5(4):491–493. https://doi.org/10.4103/ 2229-5178.142517.

35. Ingram JR. The genetics of Hidradenitis suppurativa. *Dermatol Clin.* 2016;34(1):23–28. https://doi.org/10.1016/j.det.2015.07.002.

36. Smith HS, Chao JD, Teitelbaum J. Painful hidradenitis suppurativa. *Clin J Pain.* 2010;26(5):435–444. https://doi.org/10.1097/AJP. 0b013e3181ceb80c.

4

Hidradenitis Suppurativa Differential Diagnosis and Mimickers

ELIZABETH O'BRIEN

Introduction

The average length of time from onset to diagnosis in hidradenitis suppurativa (HS) patients worldwide is 7.2 years.[1] This unfortunate delay is partly because of the nonspecific nature of many HS lesions—inflammatory papules, nodules, pustules, abscesses, and scarring—which may be confused with a variety of other cutaneous diseases. The diagnosis may also be confounded by coexistence or overlap with other inflammatory diseases presenting with similar morphology. Although there are a number of conditions that can mimic HS in their clinical appearance, HS can usually be accurately diagnosed on the basis of its chronic and recurrent history, typical anatomic locations, nonspecific bacterial culture results, and lack of systemic signs and symptoms.[2-4]

However, a high index of suspicion is sometimes needed to make an accurate diagnosis, especially in early, localized disease. It is important to note that the differential diagnosis may differ for early HS compared to late HS, and for adult HS compared to pediatric HS.[5] Overall, the differential diagnosis of HS includes both follicular and non-follicular conditions of infectious, inflammatory, and neoplastic origin.

Table 4.1 highlights the differential diagnosis for early HS lesions, and Table 4.2 the differential diagnosis for late HS lesions.

Infections

Acute lesions of HS are most often misdiagnosed as infections due to the presence of acute inflammation and significant pain.

Therefore, infectious diseases must always be considered in the differential diagnosis, especially early in the disease when there are few lesions, and during acute flares of localized HS. Bacterial culture in HS usually reveals normal flora, albeit an altered microbiome compared to normal skin.[6,7] Infections usually respond more rapidly and completely to antibiotic therapy than does HS. Cultures to rule out pathogenic or resistant bacteria such as methicillin-resistant *Staphylococcus aureus* (MRSA) and gram-negative bacteria should be considered in HS patients with unusually inflamed or painful lesions, or with systemic symptoms of infection.[8]

Superficial cutaneous infections such as bacterial folliculitis (Fig. 4.1) and furunculosis are common in the general population, may be localized to the flexures, and may be recurrent, mimicking HS; however, bacterial culture usually reveals pathogenic *Staphylococcus aureus* bacteria. The atypical HS follicular phenotype may be particularly difficult to distinguish clinically from infectious folliculitis, although the presence of numerous comedones, including double-headed comedones, and a spectrum of normal flora on culture may help indicate a diagnosis of HS.[9,10] Superficial folliculitis may also be caused by normal skin microbes, including pityrosporum (Malassezia) and demodex mites, as well as common organisms such as herpes simplex and pseudomonas aeruginosa (hot tub folliculitis). Gram-negative folliculitis may occur as a result of long-term tetracycline antibiotic therapy for acne.

Fungal folliculitis may also resemble early HS. Candidal folliculitis is common in intertriginous areas, especially in diabetics or following antibiotic therapy. Follicular dermatophyte infection (Majocchi granuloma) presents as pustules/papules, nodules, or indurated plaques usually in areas of shaving or other superficial trauma in otherwise healthy individuals. Although it traditionally involves the lower legs of women after shaving, an area not commonly affected by HS, in recent years it has been reported following pubic hair removal by shaving and waxing, and may also be transmitted through sexual contact, with organisms varying depending on the geographic locale of acquisition.[11-13] Deep dermatophytosis, presenting as dermal and subcutaneous nodules, usually in association with superficial dermatophyte infection, has been reported in immunosuppressed patients.[14,15] Widespread infections due to candida and opportunistic fungal species (such as mucor, fusarium) may occur in immunocompromised patients, manifesting as cutaneous papules, nodules, and necrotic lesions. Biopsy and tissue culture are necessary to confirm the diagnosis.

Drug-induced folliculitis is commonly seen with systemic corticosteroid therapy, lithium, and increasingly with novel chemotherapeutic agents such as epidermal growth factor receptor

TABLE
4.1
Differential Diagnosis of Early Papulopustular and Nodular Hidradenitis Suppurativa Lesions

Condition	Clinical Presentation	Differentiating Features from HS	Associated with HS
Infectious			
Bacterial folliculitis and furunculosis	Pustules, nodules, abscesses, purulent drainage	• Culture: Staphylococcus	No
Candidal folliculitis	Pustules in intertriginous areas	• KOH, culture Candida	No
Cellulitis and erysipelas	Painful localized diffuse dermal/subcutaneous redness, swelling	• Preceding trauma • Possible systemic symptoms • Tends to be unilateral	No
Gram-negative folliculitis	Pustules, papules in acne areas	• History of antibiotic therapy • Culture: gram-negative organisms	No
Herpes folliculitis	Tender vesicles, pustules	• Self-limited • Culture: Herpesvirus	No
Hot tub folliculitis	Pustules on trunk, limbs	• History of hot tub use • Culture: Pseudomonas	No
Perirectal/ischiorectal abscess	Perianal pain, swelling	• Acute onset • Culture: Aerobic or anaerobic bacteria	No
Pityrosporum folliculitis	Pustules on head, upper trunk	• Pruritic • Scraping: Malassezia, pityrosporum	No
Sexually transmitted diseases • Chancroid • Granuloma inguinale • Lymphogranuloma venereum • Noduloulcerative syphilis	Nodules, ulcers, draining abscesses, lymphadenopathy Late—possible scarring, lymphedema	• Biopsy, culture, serologies: organism-specific changes	No
Subcutaneous mycoses	Papules, nodules, abscesses, ecthyma-like lesions	• History of immunosuppression • Possible systemic symptoms • Biopsy, tissue culture: organism-specific changes	No
Sycosis barbae	Indurated plaque studded with pustules in beard area	• Contact with animals if fungal • Culture positive for bacteria (*Staphylococcus aureus*) or dermatophyte fungus (*Trichophyton verrucosum* or *Epidermophyton mentagrophytes* most commonly)	No
Inflammatory			
Acne	Papules, pustules, nodules, cysts, abscesses, scars, comedones on face and upper trunk	• Distribution on face, upper trunk, sparing flexures • Single comedones • Onset early adolescence • Usual good response to isotretinoin	Yes
Acne keloidalis nuchae	Follicular pustules, keloid scarring on nuchal scalp	• Localization to nuchal scalp • Absence of comedones	Yes
Disseminate recurrent folliculitis	Pustules, comedones, follicular scarring especially on buttocks	• Involvement of extensor trunk, limbs more than flexures	Yes
Drug-induced folliculitis	Papules, pustules on head/neck and trunk	• Corticosteroids • Lithium • EGFR inhibitors • Vemurafinib/dabrafenib	No
Frictional folliculitis	Pustules on opposing skin surfaces	• Superficial, no comedones • Culture: normal flora or Staphylococcus	No
Pseudofolliculitis	Follicular pustules, nodules, abscesses	• Presence of embedded hair • History of hair removal	No

TABLE 4.1   **Differential Diagnosis of Early Papulopustular and Nodular Hidradenitis Suppurativa Lesions—cont'd**

Condition	Clinical Presentation	Differentiating Features from HS	Associated with HS
Cysts			
Bartholin's cyst	Unilateral vulvar swelling, pain	• Solitary • Localized to posterolateral introitus	No
Epidermoid cyst	Cystic nodule, often with a visible punctum	• Typically solitary • Contains whitish keratinous debris • Not localized to intertriginous areas	Yes
Pilonidal cyst/sinus	Cystic nodule, sinus, possible drainage	• Solitary • Typical location in superior midline gluteal cleft	Yes
Steatocystoma multiplex	Cystic nodules	• Involvement of both extensor and flexural areas • Rarely inflammatory	No
Neoplastic			
Langerhans cell histiocytosis	Inflammatory papules and ulcers in inguinal, genital region	• Onset in childhood usually • Biopsy: CD1a, S-100, and Langerin (CD207) positive • Birbeck granules on EM	No

CD, Cluster of differentiation; *EGFR*, epidermal growth factor receptor; *EM*, electron microscopy; *HS*, hidradenitis suppurativa; *KOH*, potassium hydroxide; *PCR*, polymerase chain reaction.
Adapted from Saunte DM, Jemec GBE. Hidradenitis suppurativa: advances in diagnosis and treatment. *JAMA*. 2017;318(20):2019–2032.

TABLE 4.2   **Differential Diagnosis of Late Hidradenitis Suppurativa Lesions Including Scars and Sinus Tracts**

Condition	Clinical Presentation	Differentiating Features from HS	Associated with HS
Infectious			
Actinomycosis	Draining fistulae, sinus tracts	• Sites of trauma • Culture: Actinomyces • Pathology: Clumped bacteria, sulfur granules.	No
Atypical mycobacterial infection	Indurated, ulcerated plaques with exudate	• Sites of trauma • Pathology: Intracellular bacteria; AFB and PAS stain positive • Tissue culture: Organism-specific such as *M. marinum, M. kansasi, M. ulcerans* • Positive mycobacterial PCR	No
Blastomycosis	Pustules, sinus tracts, purulent drainage	• History of trauma • Favors extensor surfaces	No
Cat scratch disease	Papulopustular, suppurating lesions, +/- regional adenopathy	• History of scratch/bite • Culture: Bartonella	No
Cutaneous tuberculosis (lupus vulgaris)	Indurated plaques, gelatinous nodules, scarring	• Pathology: Intracellular bacteria, positive with AFB and PAS stains • Positive TB skin test, serology	No
Cutaneous tuberculosis (scrofuloderma)	Nodules, draining, ulcerating abscesses over lymph nodes and bone	• Painless • Presence of pulmonary TB • Positive TB skin test, serology	No
Nocardiosis	Draining fistulae, sinus tracts	• Culture: Nocardia • Pathology: Filamentous bacteria, AFB negative, Fite stain positive	No
Inflammatory			
Cutaneous Crohn's disease	Nodules, ulcers in perianal/genital region, characteristic "knife-cut" ulcers	• Absence of comedones • Pelvic MRI: Fistulae in CD may communicate with anal sphincter more commonly than in HS • Thickening of bowel wall in CD • Presence of epithelioid granulomas on pathology	Yes
Dissecting cellulitis	Pustules, nodules, sinus tracts, and scarring on scalp	• Localized to scalp	Yes

(Continued)

TABLE 4.2	Differential Diagnosis of Late Hidradenitis Suppurativa Lesions Including Scars and Sinus Tracts—cont'd		
Condition	**Clinical Presentation**	**Differentiating Features from HS**	**Associated with HS**
Folliculitis decalvans	Follicular-based pustules and scarring with tufted hair usually confined to the scalp	• Culture: *Staphylococcus aureus* • Absence of comedones	Yes
Pyoderma gangrenosum	Pustules, nodules, ulceration in sites of trauma; may heal with cribriform scarring	• Pathergy response • Often in sites of trauma • Vasculitis may be seen on pathology	Yes
Neoplasia			
Squamous cell carcinoma	Indurated nodule/plaque, ulceration	• Pathology: nests of malignant epithelial cells extending into the dermis consistent with squamous cell carcinoma	Yes
Other			
Lymphedema due to infection, obesity, neoplasia, congenital lymphedema	Scrotal, penile, vulvar lymphedema	• Absence of typical lesions of HS	Yes

AFB, Acid fast bacilli; *CD,* Crohn's disease; *HS,* Hidradenitis suppurativa; *M. kansasi, Mycobacterium kansasi; M. marinum, Mycobacterium marinum; M. ulcerans, Mycobacterium ulcerans; MRI,* magnetic resonance imaging; *PAS,* periodic Acid-Schiff; *PCR,* polymerase chain reaction; *TB,* tuberculosis.
Adapted from Saunte DM, Jemec GBE. Hidradenitis suppurativa: advances in diagnosis and treatment. *JAMA.* 2017;318(20):2019–2032.

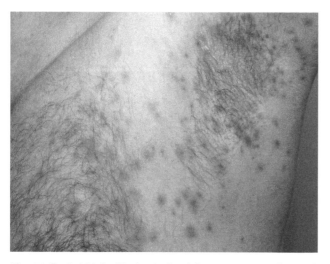

• **Fig. 4.1** Bacterial folliculitis due to *Staphylococcus aureus* affecting the axilla. (Reprinted from Jean L Bolognia MD, Julie V, Schaffer MD, Lorenzo Cerroni MD. Folliculitis and other follicular disorders. *Dermatology.* 4th ed. 2018:15–632 with permission from Elsevier.)

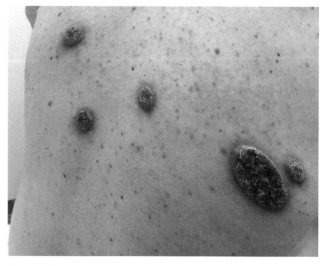

• **Fig. 4.2** Cutaneous (North American) blastomycosis presenting as inflammatory nodules and ulcerated plaques. (Courtesy Dr. Khue H. Nguyen.)

(EGFR) inhibitors, and targeted therapies such as vemurafenib and dabrafenib.[16]

Deeper cutaneous infections in typical HS locations, such as erysipelas and cellulitis,[7] and perirectal/perineal abscess are usually due to common bacteria such as *Staphylococcus aureus* and *Streptococcus*. Patients residing in certain geographic areas, travelers, and immunosuppressed patients may acquire less common infections that may resemble HS, such as nocardiosis, actinomycosis, blastomycosis (Fig. 4.2), cat scratch disease, and cutaneous tuberculosis.[17-19] All may present with inflammatory lesions suggestive of HS; however, they often occur on exposed areas of skin that are subject to trauma. History of travel, previous trauma, and diagnostic work-up including

biopsy for histopathologic examination and tissue culture should reveal the proper diagnosis.

Sexually transmitted diseases such as granuloma inguinale, lymphogranuloma venereum, and noduloulcerative syphilis may present with inflammatory or ulcerative anogenital lesions that resemble active HS (Fig. 4.3). Granuloma inguinale may present as ulcerative nodular lesions or linear fissures. The absence of other signs and symptoms of HS, a detailed history of possible exposure, and serologic screening are essential to make the correct diagnosis. The coexistence of a sexually transmitted infection in a patient with HS should also be considered and patients who have an established diagnosis of HS but present with any unusual lesions should be screened appropriately.

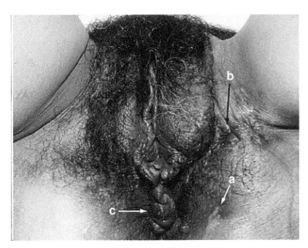

• **Fig. 4.3** Lymphogranuloma venereum presenting as draining fistulae *(arrows a, b, c)* of the vulva and perineum. (Passos, MRL. *Lymphogranuloma Venereum*: *LGV*. Elsevier: Springer Nature. 2018:159).

Inflammatory Disorders

A number of inflammatory disorders, including autoinflammatory conditions, may present with lesions similar to those seen in HS. These include both follicular disorders (such as acne, folliculitis decalvans) and non-follicular disorders (such as pyoderma gangrenosum [PG], cutaneous Crohn's disease).

Follicular Conditions

Acne vulgaris is usually distinguishable from HS by the age of onset, sparing of skin folds, gradual resolution after adolescence, and usual good response to isotretinoin.[20] However, HS can be difficult to distinguish from acne conglobata and acne fulminans because of the severity of inflammation and the widespread distribution of lesions in these conditions (Fig. 4.4). In addition, acne conglobata may

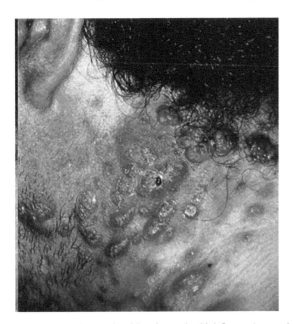

• **Fig. 4.4** Nodulocystic acne involving the neck with inflammatory nodules, abscesses, and cysts. (Andrea L. Zainglein and Diane M. Thiboutot. Chapter 36. Acne Vulgaris. In: Jean L. Bolognia, Julie V. Schaffer, Lorenzo Cerroni, eds. Dermatology. 4th ed. Elsevier; 2018:588–603.e1.)

present concomitantly with HS as part of the follicular occlusion tetrad (acne conglobata, dissecting cellulitis, HS, pilonidal sinus). Comedones are a feature of both acne and HS; however, double-headed or tombstone comedones are characteristic of HS.[10]

Severe persistent comedonal acne may be impossible to distinguish from the follicular phenotype of HS,[9,10] and the existence of both flexural and extensor involvement in an adolescent or young adult may indicate the coexistence of the two conditions. Ultrasound examination may not be helpful to distinguish acne and HS, since fistulae/tunnels may be seen in both nodulocystic acne and hidradenitis.[21] Culture of acne lesions usually reveals a predominance of cutibacterium acnes, while HS is characterized by a different spectrum of commensal bacteria including coagulase-negative staphylococci, Corynebacterium, and anaerobes, which are the most abundant organisms in HS lesions.[6,7,22] Systemic isotretinoin therapy typically has good efficacy in acne; however, response is generally poorer and less predictable in HS.[23]

Disseminate recurrent folliculitis resembles HS due to similar involvement of the buttocks and it is possible that this entity may actually be a superficial variant of HS. Similar to HS, there is a significant association with Down's syndrome patients.[24]

Folliculitis decalvans and dissecting cellulitis may both present as isolated conditions limited to the scalp or in association with HS. Thus, a focused history and careful inspection of typical HS areas of the skin are advisable in patients who present with inflammatory scalp lesions. Dissecting cellulitis may be more difficult to distinguish from HS due to the presence of deeper, tender abscesses and purulent exudate, with associated deep tunneling and significant scarring.

Dissecting cellulitis may occur with HS and acne as part of the follicular occlusion tetrad. The absence of comedones in isolated folliculitis decalvans and dissecting cellulitis is a distinguishing feature. Bacterial culture of folliculitis decalvans lesions characteristically reveal significant *Staphylococcus aureus*, and the condition is felt to possibly represent a superantigen response to the bacteria, with possibly defective host immune response.[25,26]

Frictional folliculitis is common in skin folds of overweight individuals, but comedones are typically absent. If there is secondary infection, resultant furuncle or abscess formation may resemble HS, but culture should reveal pathogenic staphylococcus. Pseudo-folliculitis due to ingrown hairs may present as inflammatory pustules and nodules in typical HS areas. Lesions may be solitary or multiple, and ultrasound may not be helpful due to the presence of hair fibers in both conditions. Surgical exploration may be necessary, with long intact hairs usually found in pseudofolliculitis.

Non-Follicular Conditions

Cutaneous Crohn's disease and PG may also mimic HS. Both Crohn's disease and HS can cause perianal abscesses and draining fistulae and have a predilection for the inguinal, perineal, and perianal folds, as well as vulvar involvement. Crohn's disease and HS frequently coexist, making clinical differentiation very difficult at times, especially when cutaneous Crohn's precedes the onset of gastrointestinal signs and symptoms.[27] Perianal skin tags, granulation tissue, and fistulae of contiguous Crohn's disease may mimic perianal fistulae and exuberant granulation tissue/pyogenic granuloma-like changes of HS (Fig. 4.5).[27,28] Metastatic Crohn's lesions, or lesions that are non-contiguous with gastrointestinal involvement, may present with edema, inflamed nodules, plaques, and ulcers. A potentially distinguishing feature is the linear shape of ulcers in cutaneous Crohn's disease, characteristically described as knife-cut ulcers (Fig. 4.6).[29-35]

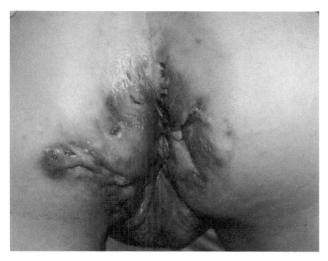

• **Fig. 4.5** Perianal cutaneous Crohn's disease contiguous with bowel involvement with inflammatory nodules, draining fistulae, and scarring resembling HS. (From Marzano A, Borghi A, Stadnicki A, et al. Cutaneous manifestations in patients with inflammatory bowel diseases: pathophysiology, clinical features, and therapy. *Inflamm Bowel Dis.* 2014;20:273–227 by permission Oxford University Press.)

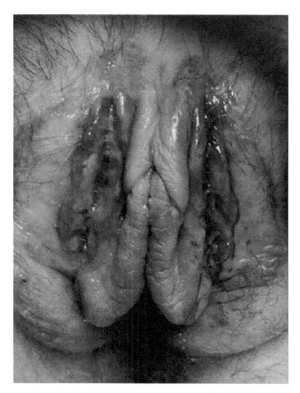

• **Fig. 4.6** "Knife cut" ulcers of metastatic cutaneous Crohn's disease involving the vulva. (Hagen JW, Swoger JM, Grandinetti LM. Cutaneous manifestations of Crohn disease. *Dermatology Clinics.* Vol 33. 2015:417–431.)

On histopathology, non-caseating granulomas are considered diagnostic of Crohn's disease. Granulomas may also be seen on histopathology of HS lesions, but are more typically foreign-body granulomas in proximity to the epidermis and hair follicles. Epithelioid granulomas, especially if located further from the epidermis and follicles, are more suggestive of Crohn's disease.[36]

Immunohistochemical staining with pankeratin may be useful to help differentiate between lesions of Crohn's and HS due to the frequent presence of keratin remnants from ruptured cysts in the skin of HS patients.[37] Perianal involvement with deep fistulae due to Crohn's or to HS can be difficult to differentiate even on magnetic resonance imaging (MRI), which is considered the gold standard for diagnosing perianal Crohn's disease.[38] Specific criteria have been proposed to facilitate the distinction between deep perianal fistulae of HS and those of Crohn's disease. A combination of three features on MRI was found to be highly specific (100% specificity) for HS: (1) Absence of rectal wall thickening, (2) bilaterality of inflammatory abnormalities, and (3) either posterior (sacral/gluteal) localization of lesions or a predominance of lesions in the perianal area. Additional potentially differentiating features include fewer fistulae and predominantly simple fistulae in HS, as well as less frequent involvement of the sphincter as compared to Crohn's. Endoanal ultrasonography has been shown to be less specific or helpful in distinguishing between HS and Crohn's disease.[39]

PG is characterized by painful inflammatory ulcers, but clinical variants may present as painful inflammatory papules, pustules, abscesses, and nodules. PG often resolves with cribriform scarring, which may also be seen in HS (Fig. 4.7). Skin biopsy in PG typically reveals a predominantly neutrophilic infiltrate, while in HS a mixed acute and chronic infiltrate is the norm; however, biopsy is not diagnostic in either condition. In addition, the two conditions may occur concomitantly in the same individual; thus atypical-appearing painful ulcerations in HS patients may warrant evaluation for PG.[40]

Sarcoidosis of the vulva may mimic early cutaneous Crohn's and HS, presenting with erythema, edema, and induration; however, a differentiating feature is that it is usually not painful.[34,35]

Miscellaneous

Cysts

An inflamed Bartholin's cyst may resemble active HS but is typically a solitary, nonrecurring lesion. Inflamed epidermoid cysts and lesions of steatocystoma multiplex may resemble abscesses and

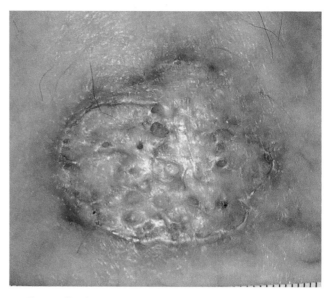

• **Fig. 4.7** Pyoderma gangrenosum healed with cribriform scarring.

cystic lesions of HS.[41] Incision and drainage of these cystic lesions reveal sebaceous or keratinous material. Pilonidal cysts are localized to the supragluteal fold and may present with inflammation and purulent drainage. Pilonidal cysts may occur as isolated lesions in association with HS, and as part of the follicular occlusion tetrad mentioned earlier. A thorough history and physical exam should be completed for patients with a pilonidal cyst to determine whether they have associated conditions.

Neoplasms

Neoplasms, including primary cutaneous tumors such as keratinocyte tumors (basal and squamous cell), may present as nodules and ulcers resembling active lesions of HS. Langerhans cell histiocytosis involving flexural areas has been reported to mimic HS both clinically, with painful ulcers, and histologically, with cystic change, keratin debris, and inflammatory infiltrate (Fig. 4.8).

Routine histopathology of Langerhans cell histiocytosis may resemble an inflammatory infiltrate; therefore, immunohistochemical staining and possible electron microscopy may be necessary for accurate diagnosis: Langerhans cells are positive for CD1a, S-100, and Langerin (CD207), and they contain Birbeck granules by electron microscopy.[42,43]

In patients undergoing malignancy screen with[18]F-fluorodeoxyglucose (FDG) positron emission tomography/computed tomography (PET/CT) imaging, HS lesions may be misinterpreted as cutaneous metastatic lesions, possibly leading to misdiagnosis and inappropriate treatment. Numerous inflammatory and infectious conditions may resemble malignant tumors on PET/CT

scans. Certain tumors in particular have been found to resemble inflammatory/infectious loci, including leukemia, lymphoma, thyroid cancer, and neuroendocrine tumors. Correlation of the clinical site and the patient's history is recommended when interpreting cutaneous and subcutaneous lesions on these scans.[44,45]

Late Hidradenitis Suppurativa Manifestations

Certain chronic infections may mimic the indurated inflammatory plaques, draining sinuses and scarring of chronic HS, particularly cutaneous tuberculosis (scrofuloderma, lupus vulgaris) (Fig. 4.9), cutaneous actinomycosis, blastomycosis, and atypical mycobacterium infection.[46,47]

Lymphedema as a complication of HS often involves the genitalia, particularly the penis and scrotum in men and the vulva in women.[48,49] Lymphedema may also result from other inflammatory, infectious, congenital, and neoplastic conditions, such as obesity, syphilis, filariasis, lymphogranuloma venereum, congenital lymphedema, and lymphatic obstruction due to surgery, malignancy, or radiotherapy (Fig. 4.10). History and lack of typical HS lesions will help inform the appropriate diagnosis.

Squamous cell carcinoma may arise de novo or as a complication of chronic HS, presenting as nodules or as ulcerated or verrucous plaques that resemble active lesions of HS (Fig. 4.11).[50-52] A high index of suspicion is important to recognize squamous cell carcinoma in longstanding HS lesions. Biopsy is essential for all persistent ulcerative or proliferative lesions, and for any HS lesions that do not respond to therapy as expected, to rule out squamous cell carcinoma.

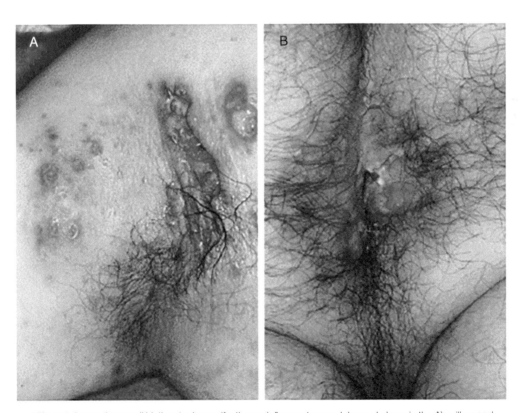

• **Fig. 4.8** Langerhans cell histiocytosis manifesting as inflammatory nodules and ulcers in the A) axillary and B) perianal regions. (Reprinted from Yasuda M, Sekiguchi A, Kanai S, et al. Langerhans cell histiocytosis masquerading as hidradenitis suppurativa. *J Dermatol.* 2016;43[6]:720 with permission from John Wiley & Sons.)

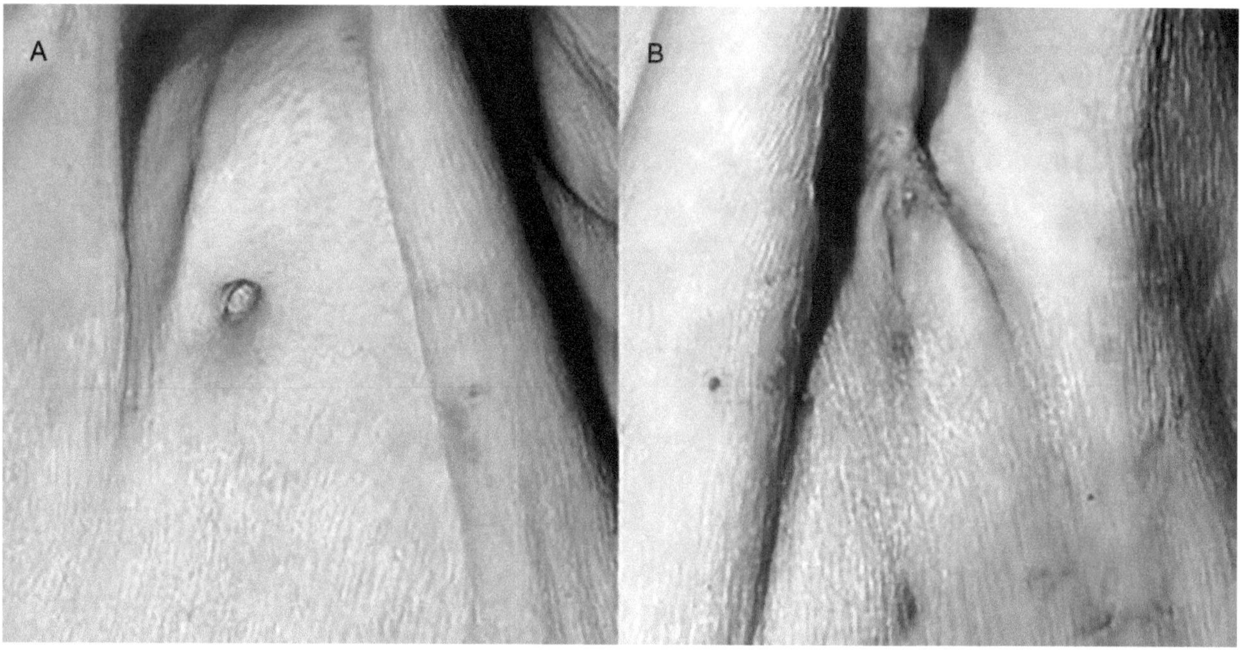

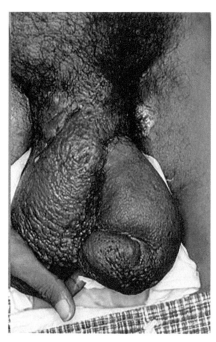

• **Fig. 4.9** Scrofuloderma (cutaneous tuberculosis) of the axilla (A right, B left) with nodules, scars, and draining sinuses. (Reprinted from Muller H, Eisendle K, Zelger B, et al. Bilateral scrofuloderma of the axilla masquerading as hidradenitis suppurativa. *Acta Derma Venereol.* 2008;88[6]:629–630.)

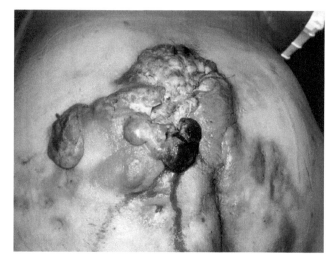

• **Fig. 4.11** A large multinodular ulcerated squamous cell carcinoma arising from chronic hidradenitis suppurativa of the buttocks. (Reprinted from Roy CF, Roy SF, Ghazawi F, et al. Cutaneous squamous cell carcinoma in Hidradenitis Suppurativa. *JCMS Case Reports.* 2019;7:1–3. Creative Commons Non Commercial CC BY-NC.)

• **Fig. 4.10** Lymphedema of the penis and scrotum resulting from chronic lymphogranuloma venereum. (from Passos, MRL. *Lymphogranuloma Venereum: LGV.* Elsevier: Springer Nature. 2018:159 with permission from Elsevier.)

Summary

In summary, the differential diagnosis for HS is broad; however, HS can usually be distinguished from other diseases based on a compatible history, the appearance of typical HS lesions and characteristic locations of involvement. There are unique sets of conditions that should be considered in the differential of HS based on whether the patient has actively inflamed nodular lesions or, in the later stage, sinus tracts and scarring. Infectious, inflammatory, neoplastic, and cystic conditions must be considered, and diagnostic tests pursued to rule out other conditions if the clinical diagnosis of HS is unclear.

References

1. Saunte DM, Boer J, Stratigos A, et al. Diagnostic delay in hidradenitis suppurativa is a global problem. *Br J Dermatol.* 2015;173(6):1546–1549.

2. Alikhan A, Lynch P, Eisen D. Hidradenitis suppurativa: a comprehensive review. *J Am Acad Dermatol.* 2009;60:539–561.

3. Micheletti RG. Natural history, presentation, and diagnosis of hidradenitis suppurativa. *Sem Cut Med Surg.* 2014;33(3S). S51–53.

4. Revuz JE, Jemec GB. Diagnosing hidradenitis suppurativa. *Dermatol Clin.* 2016;34:1–5.

5. Riis PT, Saunte DM, Sigsgaard V, et al. Clinical characteristics of pediatric hidradenitis suppurativa: a cross-sectional multicenter study of 140 patients. *Arch Dermatol Res.* 2020;312(10):715–724. https://doi.org/10.1007/s00403-020-02053-6.

6. Ring HC, Mikkelsen PR, Miller IM, et al. The bacteriology of hidradenitis: a systematic review. *Exp Dermatol.* 2015;24:727–731.

7. Ring HC, Thorsen J, Saunte D, et al. The follicular skin microbiome in patients with hidradenitis suppurativa and healthy controls. *JAMA Dermatol.* 2017;153(9):897–905.

8. Wood SC. Clinical manifestations and therapeutic management of vulvar cellulitis and abscess: Methicillin-resistant *Staphylococcus aureus*, necrotizing fasciitis, Bartholin abscess, Crohn disease of the vulva, hidradenitis suppurativa. *Clin Obstet Gynecol.* 2015;58(3):503–511.

9. Canoui-Poitrine F, Le Thuaut A, Revuz JE, et al. Identification of three hidradenitis suppurativa phenotypes: latent class analysis of a cross-sectional study. *J Invest Dermatol.* 2013;133:1506–1511.

10. Martorell A, Jfri A, Koster SBL, et al. Defining hidradenitis suppurativa phenotypes based on the elementary lesion pattern: results of a prospective study. *J Eur Acad Dermatol Venereol.* 2020;34(6):1309–1318. https://doi.org/10.1111/jdv.16183.(epub).

11. Bakardzhiev I, Chodoeva A, Tchernev G, et al. Tinea profunda of the genital area. Successful treatment of a rare skin disease. *Dermatol Ther.* 2016;29:181–183.

12. Luchsinger I, Bosshard PP, Kasper RS. Tinea genitalis: a new entity of sexually transmitted infection? Case series and review of the literature. *Sex Transm Infect.* 2015;91:493–496.

13. Gallo JG, Woods M, Graham RM, et al. A severe transmissible Majocchi's granuloma in an immunocompetent returned traveler. *Medical Mycology Case Reports.* 2017;18:5–7.

14. Okata-Kariganea U, Hatab Y, Watanabe-Okadaa E, et al. Subcutaneous abscesses caused by Trichophyton rubrum in the unilateral groin of an immunocompromised patient: a case report. *Medical Mycology Case Reports.* 2018;21:16–19.

15. Kershenovich R, Sherman S, Reiter O, et al. A unique clinicopathological manifestation of fungal infection: A case series of deep dermatophytosis in immunosuppressed patients. *Am J Clin Dermatol.* 2017;18(5):697–704.

16. MacDonald JB, MacDonald B, Golitz LE. Cutaneous adverse effects of targeted therapies. Part I: Inhibitors of the cellular membrane. *J Am Acad Dermatol.* 2015;72:203–218.

17. Nguyen N, Sink JR, Carter AJ, et al. Nocardiosis incognito: Primary cutaneous nocardiosis with extension to myositis and pleural infection. *JAAD Case Reports.* 2018;4:33–35.

18. Sadowsky LM, Mohammadi TM, Ladizinski B. Enlarging verrucous neck plaques. *International Journal of Dermatology.* 2020;59(7):e225–e227.

19. Chen Q, Chen W, Hao F. Cutaneous tuberculosis: A great imitator. *Clin Dermatol.* 2019;37:192–199.

20. Pink A, Anzengruber F, Navarini AA. Acne and hidradenitis suppurativa. *Br J Dermatol.* 2018;178(3):619–631.

21. Wortsman X, Claveria P, Valenzuela F, et al. Sonography of acne vulgaris. *J Ultrasound Med.* 2014;33(1):93–102.

22. Dreno B, Pecastaings S, Corvec S, et al. Cutibacterium acnes (Propionibacterium acnes) and acne vulgaris: a brief look at the latest updates. *J Eur Acad Dermatol Venereol.* 2018;32(Suppl. 2):5–14.

23. Alikhan A, Sayed C, Alavi A, et al. North American clinical management guidelines for hidradenitis suppurativa: a publication from the United States and Canadian Hidradenitis Suppurativa Foundations Part II: topical, intralesional, and systemic medical management. *J Am Acad Dermatol.* 2019;81:91–101.

24. Sechi A, Guglielmo A, Patrizi A, et al. Disseminate recurrent folliculitis and hidradenitis suppurativa are associated conditions; Results from a retrospective study or 131 patients with Down Syndrome and a cohort of 12,351 pediatric controls. *Dermatol Pract Concept.* 2019;9(3):187–194.

25. Powell J, Dawber R, Gatter K. Folliculitis decalvans including tufted folliculitis: clinical, histological and therapeutic findings. *Br J Dermatol.* 1999;140:328–333.

26. Otbrg N, Kang H, Azolibani A, Shapiro J. Folliculitis decalvans. *Dermatol Ther.* 2008;21:238–244.

27. Shalom G, Freud T, Yakov GB, et al. Hidradenitis suppurativa and inflammatory bowel disease: A cross-sectional study of 3,207 patients. *J Invest Dermatol.* 2016;136(8):1716–1718.

28. Marzano A, Borghi A, Stadnicki A, et al. Cutaneous manifestations in patients with inflammatory bowel diseases: pathophysiology, clinical features, and therapy. *Inflamm Bowel Dis.* 2014;20. 273–227.

29. Hagen JW, Swoger JM, Grandinetti LM. Cutaneous manifestations of Crohn disease. *Dermatol Clin.* 2015;33:417–431.

30. Company-Quiroga J, Alique-Garcia S, Martinez-Morin C. "Knife-cut" ulcers in intertriginous areas. *Eur J Dermatol.* 2019;29(1):109–110.

31. Laftah A, Bailey C, Zaheri S, et al. Vulval Crohn's disease: a clinical study of 22 patients. *J Crohns Colitis.* 2015;9(4):318–325.

32. Schneider SL, Foster K, Patek D, et al. Cutaneous manifestations of metastatic Crohn's disease. *Ped Dermatol.* 2018;35:566–574.

33. Rani U, Russell A, Tanaka S, et al. Orogenital manifestations of metastatic Crohn's disease in children: case series and review of the literature. *Urology.* 2016;92:117–121.

34. Stewart K. Challenging ulcerative vulvar conditions Hidradenitis suppurativa, Crohn disease, and aphthous ulcers. *Obstet Gynecol Clin N Am.* 2017;44:453–473.

35. Mauskar MM, Marathe K, Venkatesan A, et al. Vulvar diseases: conditions in adults and children. *J Am Acad Dermatol.* 2020;82:1287–1298.

36. Attanoos RL, Appleton MAC, Hughes LE, et al. Granulomatous hidradenitis suppurativa and cutaneous Crohn's disease. *Histopathology.* 1993;23:111–115.

37. Van der Zee H, Horvath B, Jemec GBE, et al. The association between hidradenitis suppurativa and Crohn's disease: in search of the missing pathogenic link. *J Invest Dermatol.* 2016;136:1747–1748.

38. Jorgensen AHR, Thomsen SF, Karmisholt KE, et al. Clinical microbiological, immunological and imaging characteristics of tunnels and fistulas in hidradenitis and Crohn's disease. *Exp Dermatol.* 2020;29:118–123.

39. Monnier L, Dohan A, Nedjoua A, et al. Anoperineal disease in Hidradenitis Suppurativa: MR imaging distinction from perianal Crohn's disease. *Eur Radio.* 2017;27:4100–4109.

40. Tannenbaum R, Strunk A, Garg A J. Overall and subgroup prevalence of pyoderma gangrenosum among patients with hidradenitis suppurativa: a population-based analysis in the United States. *Am Acad Dermatol.* 2019;80(6):1533–1537. https://doi.org/10.1016/j.jaad.2019.02.004.Epub2019Feb7.PMID:30738122.

41. Santana CNL, Lisboa AP, Obadia DL, et al. Steatocystoma multiplex suppurativa: case report of a rare condition. *An Bras Dermatol.* 2016;91(5supl 1):S51. S3.

42. Yasuda M, Sekiguchi A, Kanai S, et al. Langerhans cell histiocytosis masquerading as hidradenitis suppurativa. *J Dermatol.* 2016;43(6):720–721.

43. Kalen JE, Shokeen D, Mislankar M, et al. Langerhans cell histiocytosis with clinical and histologic features of hidradenitis suppurativa: brief report and review. *Am J Dermatopathol.* 2018;40(7):502–505.

44. Asamoah P, Wale DJ, Vigilanti BL, et al. Multiple hypermetabolic subcutaneous lesions from hidradenitis suppurativa mimicking metastases on ^{18}F-FDG/CT. *Clin Nucl Med.* 2018 Jan;43(1):73–74.

45. Rahman WT, Wase DJ, Viglianti BL, et al. The impact of infection and inflammation in oncologic ^{18}F-FDG PET/CT imaging. *Biomed Pharmacother.* 2019;117:109168.

46. Muller H, Eisendle K, Zelger B, et al. Bilateral scrofuloderma of the axilla masquerading as hidradenitis suppurativa. *Acta Derm Venereoluca.* 2008;88(6):629–630.

47. Ermertcan A, Ozturk F, Gencoglan G, et al. Pott's disease with scrofuloderma and psoas abscess misdiagnosed and treated as hidradenitis suppurativa. *J Dermatol Treat.* 2011;22:52–54.

48. Micieli R, Alavi A. Lymphedema in patients with hidradenitis suppurativa: a systematic review of published literature. *Int J Dermatol.* 2018;57:1471–1480.

49. Machol JA, Langenstroer P, Sanger JR. Surgical reduction of scrotal massive localized lymphedema (MLL) in obesity. *J Plast Reconstr Aesthet Surg.* 2014;67:1719–1725.

50. Chu E, Kovarik C, Lee R. Lymphedematous verrucous changes simulating squamous cell carcinoma in long-standing hidradenitis suppurativa. *Int J Dermatol.* 2013;52:808–812.

51. Roy CF, Roy SF, Ghazawi F, et al. Cutaneous squamous cell carcinoma arising in Hidradenitis suppurativa. *JCMS Case Reports.* 2019;7:1–3 [CC NC].

52. C. Dessinioti C, Plaka M, Zisimou C, et al. Advanced squamous cell carcinoma of the axillae mimicking hidradenitis suppurativa. *J Eur Acad Dermatol Venereol.* 2017;31:e386–e427.

5

Histopathology of the Pilosebaceous Unit and Interstitium of Hidradenitis Suppurativa

FARAH SUCCARIA, MICHELLE L. KERNS, AND ANGEL S. BYRD

Introduction

It is useful to consider the histological findings of hidradenitis suppurativa (HS) lesions in the context of populations at risk for HS to understand the clinical differences observed amongst these populations. HS disproportionately affects women, persons 18 to 29 years of age, and African Americans (AA). Women are more likely to have axillary and upper anterior torso involvement, while male HS patients are more likely to have moderate to severe disease and lesions in the perineal and perianal regions.[1] Considering the race discrepancy seen in HS, the histopathology of healthy skin and the pilosebaceous unit is first outlined, highlighting known differences in skin of color (Fig. 5.1). On this background of healthy skin across skin of different colors, the histology of HS

is discussed, although differences across the disease spectrum have not yet been studied systematically.

Cutaneous Structure and Cellular Composition in Healthy White and African American Skin

Epidermis

Epidermal thickness (from basal layer to stratum corneum) is location dependent and is considered to be approximately the same in White and African skin. The average epidermal thickness is 100 μm, although anatomical location determines more precise dimensions. AA skin is minimally but significantly 6μm thicker, which may result from differential expression of the dermal papillae and epidermis rete ridges.[2] The main barrier function of the skin lies in the most superficial layer of the epidermis, the stratum corneum. Not only does it protect against chemical injury and microbiologic invasion from the environment, but also maintains water and solute balance. Even though the stratum corneum is equally thick in African American and White skin, African American stratum corneum contains more cell layers (20 layers vs. 16 in Whites).[3] Also, the number of corneocyte cell layers, resistant to tape stripping and electrical resistance, were reported to be greater in African subjects presumably as a result of better intercellular cohesion.[4]

Four major resident populations make up the cells of the epidermis: keratinocytes, melanocytes, Langerhans cells, and Merkel cells. The major populations of epidermal cells are keratinocytes. These cells originate in the stem cell pool in the basal layer and undergo maturation as they migrate upward, ultimately forming the laminated stratum corneum. The human epidermis averages 50 microns in thickness, with a surface density of approximately 50,000 nucleated cells/mm^2. Under basal conditions, differentiated keratinocytes require approximately 2 weeks to exit the nucleated compartment and an additional 2 weeks to move through the stratum corneum. Markers that identify keratinocytes in normal healthy epidermis are keratin (K) K5 and K14 in basal keratinocytes, and K1, K2e, and K10 in suprabasal keratinocytes.[5]

Melanocytes are pigment producing cells located in the lower epidermis, manufacturing and secreting melanin. The main

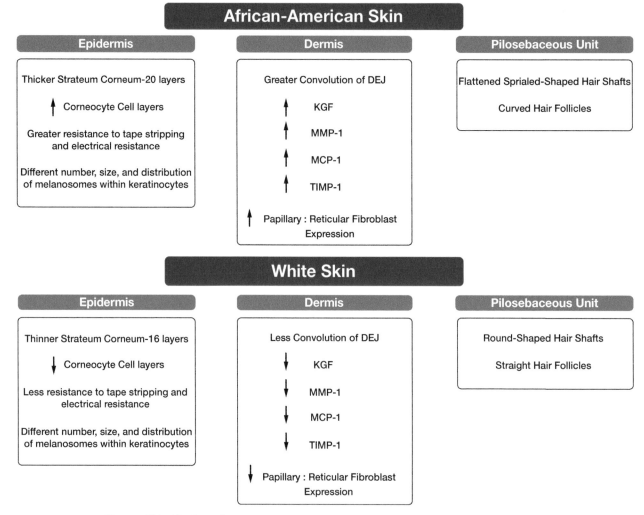

• **Fig. 5.1** Skin Histology. Comparison of histological features of white and African American skin. *DEJ*, Dermo-epidermal junction; *KGF*, keratinocyte growth factor; *MCP*, monocyte chemotactic protein; *MMP*, matrix metalloproteinase; *TIMP*, tissue inhibitor metalloproteinase protein.

function of melanin is to protect against UV radiation by absorbing and scattering the rays. Melanocytes package melanin into pigment granules called melanosomes that are transferred by excretion and phagocytosis into nearby keratinocytes. It is the greater number, larger size, increased stability and distribution of melanosomes within keratinocytes that determine differences in skin color, not the number of melanocytes. Some known markers that identify melanocytes are Melan-A, S100 (α and β subunits).[6]

Langerhans cells are the specialized immunologic cells of the skin. They traffic out of the epidermis toward regional lymph nodes, where they play a critical role in antigen presentation during the induction and regulation of skin-directed immune responses. Example of markers that identify human Langerhans cells are CD1a, CD207, and S100 (β subunit).[3]

Merkel cells are tactile cells containing neuroendocrine peptides within intracytoplasmic granules. They are also found in the basal layer of the epidermis. Each Merkel cell is in close contact with a basolaterally settled unmyelinated afferent nerve terminal (nerve plate) that has a high tactile sensitivity to light touching.[7] Markers that identify Merkel cells include cytokeratin (CK) 8, 18, 19, 20,[8] and CD56.[9]

Dermis

The dermis is predominantly composed of connective tissue, collagen, and elastic fibers. The papillary dermis (closer to the epidermis and around adnexal structures) contains mainly collagen type I and, to a lesser extent, collagen type III. The reticular dermis located underneath the papillary dermis contains thick collagen type I. In a histological study comparing the skin of White and African origins, no differences were seen in dermal collagen and elastic fiber organization.[2] However, African skin displayed a greater convolution of the dermo-epidermal junction (DEJ).

Cells found within healthy dermis include fibroblasts (CD90) and immune cells such as macrophages (CD68 and CD163), dendritic cells (CD11c, CD14, CD1c/BDCA-1, and CD303/BDCA-2), and occasional mast cells (CD11b, CD45, CD13, CD29, CD33, CD34, CD41, CD43, CD45, CD117, CD203c, mast cell tryptase). Resident leukocytes are also found in healthy skin, such as T cells and occasional B cells. The pan-T cell marker is CD3, with subsets CD4 helper T cells and C8 cytotoxic T cells. B cells are identified by CD19 and CD20, among others.

Other differences in protein expression have been reported in African skin compared to White skin, including increased keratinocyte growth factor (KGF) and monocyte chemotactic protein (MCP)-1, twofold higher ratio of papillary to reticular fibroblast expression, increased matrix metalloproteinase (MMP)-1, and tissue inhibitor metalloproteinase protein (TIMP)-1 protein expression. In an inflammatory environment, these observations make black skin more prone to pathologies or disorders such as keloids/acne keloids[10] and potentially HS.

Subcutis

The subcutaneous tissue is mainly formed of fibroblasts, lobules of adipose cells separated by collagenous septa that contain the neurovascular bundles, and macrophages.

The Pilosebaceous Unit in Healthy White and African American Skin

A key component of the clinical diagnosis of HS is the localization of symptoms to apocrine-rich areas with terminal hair follicles, such as the axillae, inguinal and anogenital regions, and perineum.[11] The oil-producing pilosebaceous unit contains a hair follicle, hair shaft, the sebaceous gland, and arrector pili muscles (Fig. 5.2). They are found all over the body except on the hands and feet.

Hair Follicle

Fully developed hair follicles have three distinct areas (see Fig. 5.2). The infundibulum extends from the follicular opening on the surface of the epidermis to where the sebaceous duct enters the follicle. Harboring a rich residential microflora and specialized innate immune defenses, the infundibulum acts as a key component of the epidermal environmental interface.[12,13] Although not well characterized in human skin, K79, LRIG1, and DLX are known transcription factors expressed within the infundibulum of the murine hair follicle.[14,15] The isthmus extends from the sebaceous duct entry to the insertion of arrector pili muscle. The inferior segment is below insertion of muscle and contains the hair follicle bulb (or matrix), the level where hair cornification starts. The layers of the hair from "inner-to-outer" are the medulla (central part of hair fiber), hair cuticle, inner root sheath (IRS), and outer root sheath (ORS). The function of the tri-layered IRS is to mold the hair by hardening filaments. The ORS forms an outer cylinder support of the hair follicle and is characterized by trichilemmal keratinization. The bulge is a special segment of the ORS near the arrector pili insertion, consisting of a major area of epithelial stem cells of the hair follicle.

The distribution of follicle density at different body sites appears to be the same in all the ethnic skin types.[16] However, there are striking racial differences in hair shaft and follicle shape. African Americans tend to have flattened spiraled hair shafts arising from a curved follicle compared to Whites.[17]

Sebaceous Glands

Sebaceous glands are found in greatest abundance on the face and scalp, although they are distributed throughout all skin sites except the palms and soles. They are composed of lobules of pale-staining cells with abundant lipid droplets in their cytoplasm. They are always associated with hair follicles, draining into the lower infundibulum, except at the following sites: tarsal plate of the eyelids (meibomian glands), buccal mucosa and vermilion border of the lip (Fordyce spots), prepuce and mucosa lateral to the penile frenulum (Tyson glands), labia minora, and female areola (Montgomery tubercles). The sebaceous gland produces and secretes sebum

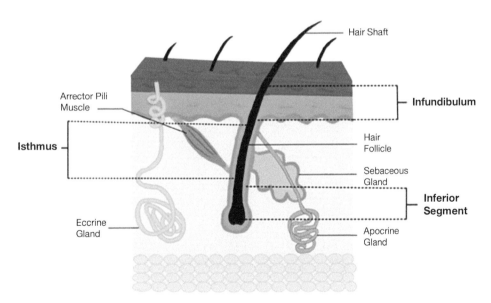

• **Fig. 5.2** Hair Follicle. The infundibulum extends from the follicular opening on the surface of the epidermis to where the sebaceous gland enters the follicle. The isthmus extends from the sebaceous duct entry to the insertion of arrector pili muscle. The inferior segment is below insertion of muscle and contains the hair follicle bulb (or matrix), the level where hair cornification starts. The layers of the hair from "inner-to-outer" are the medulla (central part of hair fiber), hair cuticle, inner root sheath (IRS), and outer root sheath (ORS). The function of the tri-layered IRS is to mold the hair by hardening filaments. The ORS forms an outer cylinder support of the hair follicle and is characterized by trichilemmal keratinization. The bulge is a special segment of the ORS near the arrector pili insertion, consisting of a major area of epithelial stem cells of the hair follicle.

into the follicular duct, a blend of lipids such as triglycerides, squalene, fatty acids, and esters of glycerol.[18] Skin lipids contribute to the barrier function, and some have antimicrobial properties. Antimicrobial lipids include free sphingoid bases derived from epidermal ceramides and fatty acids (e.g., sapienic acid) derived from sebaceous triglycerides.[19]

Apocrine Glands

The straight excretory apocrine duct opens into the infundibular portion of the hair follicle and is composed of a double layer of cuboidal epithelial cells. The coiled secretory apocrine gland is located at the junction of the dermis and subcutaneous fat. It is lined by a single layer of cells, which vary in appearance from columnar to cuboidal. This layer of cells is surrounded by a layer of myoepithelial cells. Apocrine coils appear more widely dilated than eccrine coils. The apices of the columnar cells project into the lumen of the gland and in histologic cross section appear as though they are being extruded (decapitation secretion).

Although occasionally found in an ectopic location, apocrine units of the human body are generally confined to the following sites: axillae, areolae, anogenital region, external auditory canal (ceruminous glands), and eyelids (glands of Moll). Apocrine glands do not begin to function until puberty. Apocrine secretion is mediated by adrenergic innervation and by circulating catecholamines of adrenomedullary origin. Secretions from apocrine glands produce an odor once they are metabolized by skin flora, although the precise function of this is unknown.[19] Interestingly, the scarcity of apocrine glands in the genitofemoral area in which hidradenitis emerges suggests a secondary nature of apocrine involvement.[20]

Eccrine Glands

These glands are found throughout the skin but are most concentrated in palms, soles, and forehead.[21] The eccrine glands, or merocrine glands depicting the gland's secretion, open directly onto the skin surface by a special spiral intraepidermal duct called the acrosyringium. This is formed by small polygonal cells with a central round nucleus surrounded by abundant pink cytoplasm. The straight dermal portion of the duct is composed of a double layer of cuboidal epithelial cells and is lined by an eosinophilic cuticle on its luminal side. The secretory portion of the gland is formed by an inner layer of epithelial secretory cells surrounded by a layer of flattened myoepithelial cells. The secretory cells are of two types: large, pale, glycogen-rich cells and smaller, darker-staining cells. The pale glycogen-rich cells are thought to initiate the formation of sweat. The darker cells may function similar to cells of the dermal duct, which actively reabsorb sodium, thereby modifying sweat from a basically isotonic to a hypotonic solution by the time it reaches the skin surface. These glands play a major role in thermoregulation and homeostasis.

Sweat is similar in composition to plasma, containing water and the same electrolytes, but in a more dilute concentration. Secretion of hypotonic sweat results in an adaptive response to a thermal stimulus allows greater cooling with conservation of sodium. Anatomically, the amount of sweat glands and sweat pores in African American and White skin is identical and varies with climatic changes but not with racial factors.[19]

Apoeccrine

Apoeccrine glands share some common morphological and functional characteristics with both eccrine and apocrine glands. Their long ducts open directly onto the skin surface like the eccrine sweat duct. The secretory portion of apoeccrine sweat glands consists of a pseudostratified single layer of clear and dark secretory cells surrounded by myoepithelial cells and is irregularly dilated. The dilated segment consists of an apocrine-like single layer of epithelium, but the thin segment of apoeccrine sweat glands shows eccrine sweat gland-like structures. The ratio of apoeccrine to eccrine in axillary skin for adolescent men and women is almost 1:2. However, in some persons, the apoeccrine glands represent less than 10% of the axillary sweat glands.[22] Apoeccrine sweat glands are mainly identified in the axillary and perianal locations and constitute approximately 10% to 45% of axillary sweat glands.[23]

Histological Changes in HS in Skin Structures and Across the Disease Spectrum

Clinico-Pathological Correlation

There is no single diagnostic test for HS; rather, diagnosis is based on a combination of clinical and histological features. Below is a general description of histological features seen in skin structures in HS. However, histopathology of specific HS lesions is not well described yet. Nor have there been systematic studies of histological changes as HS progresses or in specific HS phenotypes, such as HS in patients with genetic mutations.[24] The characteristic lesions of HS are inflammatory nodules, abscesses, and dermal tunnels. In early disease there are recurrent nodules and abscesses (Hurley stage 1). As the disease continues, there are persistent nodules and abscesses with dermal tunnels and scarring, separated by normal appearing skin (Hurley stage 2). As HS progresses, whole anatomic regions are affected by nodules, abscesses, extensive dermal tunnels, scarring, and double-headed comedones (Hurley stage 3). Fig. 5.3 lists the known histological features of HS and presents representative histology for established HS lesions.

Published immunohistochemical associations in HS were recently reviewed by Frew and colleagues.[25] One challenge in interpretation of histological HS studies is a lack of consensus regarding terminology to describe the location and morphology of histological specimens sampled. However, standard terminology was recently proposed to clearly define lesional, perilesional, and unaffected skin biopsies when analyzing tissue sections.[26]

Epidermis

The characteristic observation of the epidermis of established HS lesions is a thicker epidermis with more irregular rete ridges. Histologic changes of early HS may include a microscopic comedo-like area, follicular hyperkeratosis, hyperplasia of the interfollicular epithelium, and dilation of follicular infundibulum. Numerous extensions of the epidermis into the dermis of the perilesional skin resulted in isolated dermal inclusions, referred to as dermal islands. In perilesional and lesional skin, the interfollicular epidermis shows psoriasiform hyperplasia as well as follicular plugging.[27]

When there is any inflammation or injury, keratinocytes have the capacity to increase rates of proliferation and maturation. This may partly explain the thicker epidermal layer in HS, as evidenced by Ki67 expression in basal epidermal keratinocytes. Parakeratosis has also been observed in HS compared to healthy controls, likely due to the increased keratinocyte epidermal transit time.[27, 28] As it relates to the epidermis overlying HS, weak K1 and K10, as well as K16 and K17, were detected in the suprabasal layers, while K14 and K19 were positively expressed in the basal layer.[29]

EPIDERMIS	APPENDAGES
Irregular rete with epidermal extensions Hyperplasia of interfollicular epidermis and follicle Parakeratosis	Dilatation of follicular infundibulum Follicular plugging, comedo-like Reduced sebaceous glands Reduced eccrine glands Decreased PAS at infundibulum Peri-appendageal cellular infiltration

DERMIS

Mixed inflammatory infiltrate
Neutrophils (IL-17+) & NETS
Myeloid cells: macs (IL-12+, IL-23+) monos, DCs, pDCs
T cells: IL-17+
B cells, plasma cells, IgG
NK cells, mast cells
Mulit-nucleated giant cells
FB granulomas
Epidermal "dermal islands", keratin
Dermal Tunnels: epithelialized structures with biofilms
Invasive proliferative gelatinous mass (IPGM)
Tertiary lymphoid structures
Fibrosis, abscesses

A

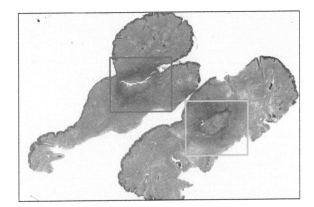

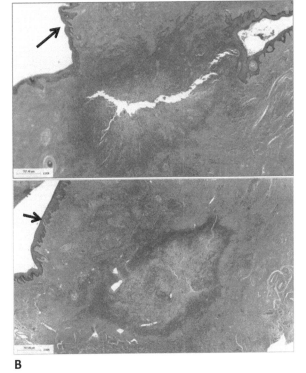

B

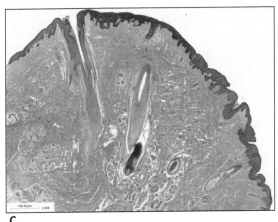

C

• **Fig. 5.3** Histological and Immunohistochemical Features of Hidradenitis Suppurativa (HS). (A) Published findings describing the histological changes in the structures and cells of the epidermis, dermis, and appendages in the skin are listed. (B) Representative histology of chronic HS is shown (5X) demonstrating the characteristic features of epidermal hyperplasia and irregular rete ridges (black arrows), epithelialized dermal sinus tract, peri-appendageal dense mixed chronic inflammatory infiltrate, surrounding fibrosis, and disorganized collagen fibers throughout the dermis (red box, 20X). Follicular cystic structure with suppurative material (blue box, 20X). (C) HS pilosebaceous unit with miniaturized sebaceous lobules with prominent dermal fibroplasia consistent with a scarring lesion (10X). DCs, Dendritic cells, Macs, macrophages, Mono, monocytes, NETs, neutrophil extracellular traps, pDCs, plasmoid dendritic cells.

Constitutive anatomical melanocyte densities may be indicative of HS lesion distributions within intertriginous areas.[30, 31] Studies have also shown many overlapping clinical and occasionally histopathologic features of Langerhans cell histiocytosis and HS.[32] However, a closer analysis and further understanding of the role of melanocytes, Langerhans cells, and Merkel cells is warranted in HS to understand the potential contributions of these cells to the disease pathogenesis and progression.

An extensive analysis of protein expression in skin compartments has shown differential expression of β-defensin-2 (HDD2), matrix metallopeptidase-1 (MMP-1), connexin-32 (GJB2), PI3 kinase (PI3), cytokeratin-16 (KRT16), matrix metallopeptidase-9 (MMP-9),

serpin-B4 (SERPINB4), serpin B3 (SERPINB3), small proline-rich protein-3 (SPRR3), calgranulin-A (S100A8), calgranulin-B (S100A9), koebnerisin (S100A7A [15]), cytokeratin-6 (KET6A), trancobalamin (TCN1), and transmembrane serine protease-11D (TMPRSS11D) have been shown in HS.[33] Of the aforementioned proteins, specific proteins have been shown to be strongly expressed compared to non-lesional and control skin: in the stratum granulosum GJB2, S100A7A(15), SERPINB4, S100A9; in the stratum spinosum S100A8 and TCN1.[33]

Antimicrobial peptide expression may be dysregulated in HS. LCN2, LL37, S100A8, S100A9, and S100A15/koebnerisin proteins were increased in lesional epidermis.[33–35] In addition, activated caspase-1 and connexin-32 proteins were strongly expressed in the stratum granulosum, and transcobalamin-1 in the stratum spinosum of HS lesions.[35]

Dermis

The hallmarks of HS lesional dermal skin are increased mixed inflammatory cellular infiltration surrounding appendages and the development of epithelialized dermal tunnels. The cellular infiltrate consists of increased numbers of resident immune cells such as T cells, B cells, macrophages, dendritic cells. A chronic lympho-plasmacytic and often granulomatous histiocytic inflammation with giant cells develops. There are abundant infiltrating neutrophils, plasma cells (CD138), NK cells (CD56), mast cells, and multinucleated giant cells. Tertiary lymphoid structures have been identified.[36] Extended elongated keratin fibers remnants of keratinocytes have been detected in the dermis of lesional skin, often engulfed by multinucleated giant cells.[27] Expression and secretion of MMP9 by monocytes has been detected.[33]

In chronic HS lesions, neutrophils are the predominant extravasated leukocyte in the dermis. Rupture and acute neutrophilic inflammation often occur with neutrophil extracellular trap (NET) formation within HS lesions, positively correlated with disease severity.[37] Interestingly, NETs detected in HS lesions were in close proximity to plasmacytoid dendritic cells (CD303), which likely contributed to the type 1 interferon signature. Additionally, plasma cells and IgG were identified in HS lesions.[37] CN2 protein was expressed in granulocytes in lesional HS.[38] Peptidylarginine deiminases (PADs) 1 to 4, enzymes were also detected via IF, which mediates citrullination within HS lesions. Therefore, neutrophils, NETs, and the innate immune system may be active contributors to the pathogenesis and immune dysregulation seen in HS lesions.[37]

Fibrosis, epidermal cysts, and abscesses have also been reported in dermal HS tissues. Of five anatomical locations, the most substantial findings were seen in the axilla and perineal anatomical regions.[39] Collagen type I and type III were predominant in normal and perilesional skin, while collagen type I was in greatest abundance in lesional skin.[40] Macrophage production of CCL18 has been reported to potentially enhance fibroblast differentiation and collagen production.[37]

Draining dermal tunnels of HS have recently been described as having three sections, types A-C, with their respective keratin expressions compared to normal skin. Infundibular-like keratinized epithelium (type A) has suprabasal expression of K1, basilar expression of K14, and absence of K16, K17, and K19.[29] Non-infundibular keratinized epithelium (type B) has K16 and K17, varying expression of K14, and non-detection of K1, K10, and K19. Non-keratinized epithelium (type C) interestingly has a robust expression of K14 in all layers, K16 and K17 in the suprabasal layers, with no detection of K1, K10, or K19.

Another study found that expression of K17 was absent in the infundibular-like keratinized epithelium of HS draining sinus tracts.[41] K17 is usually expressed in the basal layer of the epidermis, infundibulum and all of the layers of the outer root sheath. Heterozygous mutations in the keratin 17 gene give rise to two distinct disorders, pachyonychia congenita type 2 and steatocystoma multiplex, both characterized by follicular occlusion and associated with HS.[42] Murine studies have demonstrated that loss of K17 can lead to hair fragility and rupture of the hair shaft.[43] These findings suggest that follicular occlusion, a key event in early HS pathogenesis, may be secondary to abnormal expression of K17.

Regarding tissue cytokine protein expression, IL-17A positive cells were increased in perilesional lesional HS with abundant IL-17 positive neutrophils in lesional dermis.[35] IL-12 and IL-23 positive macrophages were found infiltrating papillary and reticular dermis of lesional skin.[44]

The dermal tunnels and fibrosis presumably form in attempt to control the inflammation. Recently, it has been proposed that dermal tunnels could arise from the outer root sheath of the follicle and actively contribute to inflammation.[45] Biofilms have been identified in HS tunnels by nucleic acid-fluorescence in situ hybridization (FISH) with confocal laser scanning microscopy.[46] The shiny lining of the dermal tunnels, sometimes called invasive proliferative gelatinous mass (IPGM), may contain inflammatory components[47] and also harbor biofilms which may be responsible for HS flares.

Subcutis

Fibrosis, fat necrosis, and inflammation have all been shown on histological evaluations, with the axilla and perineal having the most striking findings.[39]

Appendageal and Glandular Structures

The most distinctive feature of glandular structures in HS is peri-appendageal inflammation prominently in axillary and perineal lesions, which has been identified around hair follicles, apocrine and eccrine glands.[48] It is now considered that this peri-appendageal inflammation is more likely a secondary rather than primary event of follicular hyperkeratinization. Reduced sebaceous glands and eccrine sweat glands have also been reported in HS, particularly in perilesional regions compared to healthy controls.[28, 49]

Peri-infundibular PAS staining was reduced in established HS lesions.[50] In a recent immunohistochemical analysis of HS lesions, S100A8, S100A9, SERPINB4, and TCN1 were strongly expressed in the hair root sheath.[33] In the epidermal root sheath (follicular keratinocytes): S100A8, S100A9, SERPINB4, PI3, HBD2, and TCN1; internal root sheath: SERPINB3 and S100A7A have been reported.[51] Small proline-rich protein 3 (SPRR3), a protein of the epidermal differentiation complex, was expressed in apocrine sweat gland ducts and sebaceous glands and ducts.[33]

Conclusions

Although work has been conducted describing the histopathology of HS pathogenesis, there is a greater need for more detailed histopathologic analysis to better understand the cellular contributions and anatomic complexities. This analysis is warranted in various populations and should be correlated with specific lesion types, phenotypes, and disease severity. A more extensive determination of cellular mechanisms by broadening the analysis of cell surface markers as well as co-localization experiments would render a better understanding of the distinct cellular and immunological environment associated with HS disease progression. These analyses could help clarify the immunopathological mechanisms of the disease and its natural history, providing more targeted therapy for this debilitating disease.

The authors of this chapter would like to acknowledge the following contributors: Ginette A. Okoye (Howard University College of Medicine), Olayemi Sokumbi (Mayo Clinic), Cassandra Faye Ine Collins (University of Miami Miller School of Medicine), Susanna Adjei (Indiana University School of Medicine), Chidubem A.V. Okeke (Howard University College of Medicine), Qaren Q. Quartey (University of Maryland School of Medicine), and Sheida Naderi-Azad (University of Toronto Faculty of Medicine).

References

1. Garg A, Lavian J, Lin G, et al. Incidence of hidradenitis suppurativa in the United States: A sex- and age-adjusted population analysis. *J Am Acad Dermatol.* 2017 Jul;77(1):118–122.
2. Girardeau S, Mine S, Pageon H, et al. The Caucasian and African skin types differ morphologically and functionally in their dermal component. *Exp Dermatol.* 2009;18(8):704–711.
3. Bolognia JL, Schaffer JV, Cerroni L. *Dermatology.* Philadelphia: Elsevier; 2018.
4. Johnson LC, Corah NL. Racial differences in skin resistance. *Science.* 1963;139(3556):766–767.
5. Bergstresser PR, Taylor JR. Epidermal 'turnover time'-a new examination. *Br J Dermatol.* 1977;96(5):503–509.
6. Nordlund JJ, Sober AJ, Hansen TW. Periodic synopsis on pigmentation. *J Am Acad Dermatol.* 1985;12(2 Pt 1):359–363.
7. Morrison KM, Miesegaes GR, Lumpkin EA, et al. Mammalian Merkel cells are descended from the epidermal lineage. *Dev Biol.* 2009;336(1):76–83.
8. Moll I, Kuhn C, Moll R. Cytokeratin 20 is a general marker of cutaneous Merkel cells while certain neuronal proteins are absent. *J Invest Dermatol.* 1995;104(6):910–915.
9. Kurokawa M, Nabeshima K, Akiyama Y, et al. CD56: a useful marker for diagnosing Merkel cell carcinoma. *J Dermatol Sci.* 2003;31(3):219–224.
10. Child FJ, Fuller LC, Higgins EM, et al. A study of the spectrum of skin disease occurring in a black population in south-east London. *Br J Dermatol.* 1999;141(3):512–517.
11. Kurokawa I, Hayashi N. Japan Acne Research Society. Questionnaire surveillance of hidradenitis suppurativa in Japan. *J Dermatol.* 2015;42(7):747–749.
12. Schneider MR, Paus R. Deciphering the functions of the hair follicle infundibulum in skin physiology and disease. *Cell Tissue Res.* 2014;358(3):697–704.
13. Kabashima K, Honda T, Ginhoux F, et al. The immunological anatomy of the skin. *Nat Rev Immunol.* 2019;19(1):19–30.
14. Purba TS, Haslam IS, Poblet E, et al. Human epithelial hair follicle stem cells and their progeny: current state of knowledge, the widening gap in translational research and future challenges. *BioEssays News Rev Mol Cell Dev Biol.* 2014;36(5):513–525.
15. Veniaminova NA, Vagnozzi AN, Kopinke D, et al. Keratin 79 identifies a novel population of migratory epithelial cells that initiates hair canal morphogenesis and regeneration. *Dev Camb Engl.* 2013;140(24):4870–4880.
16. Johnston RB. 15 - Diseases of Cutaneous Appendages. In: Johnston RB, ed. *Weedon's Skin Pathology Essentials.* 2nd ed. Elsevier; 2017:299–328. [cited 2020 Sep 7] http://www.sciencedirect.com/science/article/pii/B9780702068300500153.
17. McMichael AJ. Hair and scalp disorders in ethnic populations. *Dermatol Clin.* 2003;21(4):629–644.
18. Picardo M, Ottaviani M, Camera E, et al. Sebaceous gland lipids. *Dermatoendocrinol.* 2009;1(2):68–71.
19. James WD. 1-Skin: Basic structure and function. In James WD, *Andrew's Diseases of the Skin.* 13th ed. Elsevier; 2020:1–10.
20. Jemec GBE, Hansen U. Histology of hidradenitis suppurativa. *J Am Acad Dermatol.* 1996;34(6):994–999.
21. La Ruche G, Cesarini JP. Histology and physiology of black skin. *Ann Dermatol Venereol.* 1992;119(8):567–574.
22. Sato K, Kang WH, Saga K, et al. Biology of sweat glands and their disorders. I. Normal sweat gland function. *J Am Acad Dermatol.* 1989;20(4):537–563.
23. Sato K, Leidal R, Sato F. Morphology and development of an apoeccrine sweat gland in human axillae. *Am J Physiol.* 1987;252(1 Pt 2):R166–80.
24. Jfri AH, O'Brien EA, Litvinov IV, et al. Hidradenitis suppurativa: comprehensive review of predisposing genetic mutations and changes. *J Cutan Med Surg.* 2019;23(5):519–527.
25. Frew JW, Hawkes JE, Krueger JG. A systematic review and critical evaluation of immunohistochemical associations in hidradenitis suppurativa. *F1000Research.* 2018;7:1923.
26. Frew JW, Hawkes JE, Sullivan-Whalen M, et al. Inter-relater reliability of phenotypes, and exploratory genotype- phenotype analysis in inherited hidradenitis suppurativa. *Br J Dermatol.* 2019;181(3): 566–571.
27. van der Zee HH, de Ruiter L, Boer J, et al. Alterations in leucocyte subsets and histomorphology in normal-appearing perilesional skin and early and chronic hidradenitis suppurativa lesions. *Br J Dermatol.* 2012;166(1):98–106.
28. Kamp S, Fiehn AM, Stenderup K, et al. Hidradenitis suppurativa: a disease of the absent sebaceous gland? Sebaceous gland number and volume are significantly reduced in uninvolved hair follicles from patients with hidradenitis suppurativa. *Br J Dermatol.* 2011;164(5):1017–1022.
29. Kurokawa I, Nishijima S, Kusumoto K, et al. Immunohistochemical study of cytokeratins in hidradenitis suppurativa (acne inversa). *J Int Med Res.* 2002;30(2):131–136.
30. Alaluf S, Atkins D, Barrett K, et al. Ethnic variation in melanin content and composition in photoexposed and photoprotected human skin. *Pigment Cell Res.* 2002;15(2):112–118.
31. Thingnes J, Lavelle TJ, Hovig E, et al. Understanding the melanocyte distribution in human epidermis: an agent-based computational model approach. *PloS One.* 2012;7(7), e40377.
32. Kalen JE, Shokeen D, Mislankar M, et al. Langerhans cell histiocytosis with clinical and histologic features of hidradenitis suppurativa: brief report and review. *Am J Dermatopathol.* 2018;40(7):502–505.
33. Zouboulis CC. Nogueira da Costa A, Makrantonaki E, et al. Alterations in innate immunity and epithelial cell differentiation are the molecular pillars of hidradenitis suppurativa. *J Eur Acad Dermatol Venereol.* 2020;34(4):846–861.
34. Thomi R, Schlapbach C, Yawalkar N, et al. Elevated levels of the antimicrobial peptide LL-37 in hidradenitis suppurativa are associated with a Th1/Th17 immune response. *Exp Dermatol.* 2018;27(2):172–177.
35. Lima AL, Karl I, Giner T, et al. Keratinocytes and neutrophils are important sources of proinflammatory molecules in hidradenitis suppurativa. *Br J Dermatol.* 2016;174(3):514–521.
36. Pipi E, Nayar S, Gardner DH, et al. Tertiary lymphoid structures: autoimmunity goes local. *Front Immunol.* 2018;9:1952.
37. Byrd AS, Carmona-Rivera C, O'Neil LJ, et al. Neutrophil extracellular traps, B cells, and type I interferons contribute to immune dysregulation in hidradenitis suppurativa. *Sci Transl Med.* 2019;11(508).
38. Wolk K, Wenzel J, Tsaousi A, et al. Lipocalin-2 is expressed by activated granulocytes and keratinocytes in affected skin and reflects disease activity in acne inversa/hidradenitis suppurativa. *Br J Dermatol.* 2017;177(5):1385–1393.
39. Attanoos RL, Appleton MA, Douglas-Jones AG. The pathogenesis of hidradenitis suppurativa: a closer look at apocrine and apoeccrine glands. *Br J Dermatol.* 1995;133(2):254–258.
40. Sanchez J, Le Jan S, Muller C, et al. Matrix remodelling and MMP expression/activation are associated with hidradenitis suppurativa skin inflammation. *Exp Dermatol.* 2019;28(5):593–600.
41. Kurokawa I, Nishijima S, Kusumoto K, et al. Immunohistochemical study of cytokeratins in hidradenitis suppurativa (acne inversa). *J Int Med Res.* 2002;30(2):131–136.
42. Fimmel S, Zouboulis CC. Comorbidities of hidradenitis suppurativa (acne inversa). *Dermatoendocrinol.* 2010;2(1):9–16.
43. Tong X, Coulombe PA. Keratin 17 modulates hair follicle cycling in a TNFalpha-dependent fashion. *Genes Dev.* 2006;20(10):1353–1364.
44. Schlapbach C, Hänni T, Yawalkar N, et al. Expression of the IL-23/Th17 pathway in lesions of hidradenitis suppurativa. *J Am Acad Dermatol.* 2011;65(4):790–798.
45. Frew JW, Navrazhina K, Marohn M, et al. Contribution of fibroblasts to tunnel formation and inflammation in hidradenitis suppurativa/ acne inversa. *Exp Dermatol.* 2019;28(8):886–891.

46. Ring HC, Bay L, Nilsson M, et al. Bacterial biofilm in chronic lesions of hidradenitis suppurativa. *Br J Dermatol.* 2017;176(4):993–1000.

47. Kidacki M, Cong Z, Flamm A, et al. "Invasive proliferative gelatinous mass" of hidradenitis suppurativa contains distinct inflammatory components. *Br J Dermatol.* 2019;181(1):192–193.

48. von Laffert M, Stadie V, Wohlrab J, et al. Hidradenitis suppurativa/acne inversa: bilocated epithelial hyperplasia with very different sequelae. *Br J Dermatol.* 2011;164(2):367–371.

49. Coates M, Mariottoni P, Corcoran DL, et al. The skin transcriptome in hidradenitis suppurativa uncovers an antimicrobial and sweat gland gene signature which has distinct overlap with wounded skin. *PloS One.* 2019;14(5), e0216249.

50. Danby FW, Jemec GBE, Marsch WC, et al. Preliminary findings suggest hidradenitis suppurativa may be due to defective follicular support. *Br J Dermatol.* 2013;168(5):1034–1039.

51. Buimer MG, Wobbes T, Klinkenbijl JHG, et al. Immunohistochemical analysis of steroid hormone receptors in hidradenitis suppurativa. *Am J Dermatopathol.* 2015;37(2):129–132.

6

Imaging Techniques in Hidradenitis Suppurativa and Comorbidities

XIMENA WORTSMAN AND INDERMEET KOHLI

CHAPTER OUTLINE

Introduction

The imaging support of hidradenitis suppurativa (HS) has been increasing in the last decade due to the development of high-axial-resolution devices that can detect simultaneously and with high definition abnormalities of the skin and deeper layers.[1,2] Nowadays, the spatial axial resolution, which allows the discrimination of two adjacent reflector points, is much higher on ultrasound than MRI or CT.[1] It should be kept in mind that the type of treatment in HS is decided according to the severity stage[3]; therefore, an accurate diagnosis and scoring of the severity of the HS patients' are critical for their management.[4] To date, multiple reports from different groups, countries, and racial backgrounds confirm the clinical underestimation of the severity of the disease[5–12] and the lack of good inter-rater correlations of the clinical parameters.[13–16] The objectives of using HS imaging are to detect early the disease and adequately score the severity and activity, guide percutaneous and surgical procedures, and monitor the treatment.

Essential Concepts on Imaging in Dermatology

Significant advances in HS have been made with ultrasound, which provides a significantly higher number of publications than the rest of the imaging techniques.[2,5,6,8–12,17–25] Particularly in dermatology, ultrasound has followed the validation sequence of any imaging modality and has been suggested as a standard of care for HS patients.[26] This process includes the description of the accuracy of the method, the standardization of the image acquisition process, the reference of normal patterns and values, the qualification and quantification of abnormalities, the design of the forms used for reporting the examinations, a description of the limits of the detection, and the assessment of multicentric reproducibility.[6–12,17,20–25,27–35]

Moreover, the guidelines for performing dermatologic ultrasound examinations have defined the need for adequate and updated machines as well as trained operators.[28]

The axial spatial resolution of ultrasound can vary from 100 microns at 15 MHz to 30 microns at 70 MHz, which means that ultrasonographically, it is possible to detect submillimetric changes that can be as small as 0.1 mm at 15 MHz and 0.03 mm at 70 MHz.[1,27] Furthermore, there are ultrasonographic criteria for diagnosing HS, and a sonographic scoring system of HS (SOS-HS) has been reported.[10–12]

To date, magnetic resonance imaging (MRI) has been mainly used to detect the perianal fistulous tracts and subcutaneous or more profound inflammatory signs in HS.[36–41] However, considering the commercially available devices, MRI still presents a lower axial spatial resolution than ultrasound. This resolution can go up to 500 microns using 1.5 Tesla and up to 100 microns only in experimental machines of 7 Tesla.[42,43] The latter features mean that on MRI, the abnormalities of the skin or superficial layers that measure less than 3 mm may be challenging to discriminate.[44] Moreover, to date, there are no reports on specific patterns of HS on MRI.

Regarding the discrimination between HS and Crohn's disease, the MRI characteristics rely mostly on clinical findings such as the intertriginous location and bilateral involvement of the inflammatory HS lesions.[39] Nevertheless, it should be remembered that these two conditions can be concurrent.[45] Another relevant difference between ultrasound and MRI is that ultrasonography does not usually require contrast media. In contrast, MRI frequently requires the intravenous injection of contrast media (gadolinium), which is potentially nephrotoxic and may rarely generate nephrogenic systemic fibrosis.[46–49]

Ultrasound can detect submillimeter subclinical alterations in HS and characterize the blood flow, including type (arterial or venous) and velocity of the vessels noninvasively through color Doppler.[5,6,8,10–12,50] The detection of vascularity patterns allows monitoring the degree of inflammation in HS; therefore, it can support activity level discrimination.[2,51] Furthermore, ultrasound is considered a safe and non-radiating imaging technique that is commonly used in pregnant women (Fig. 6.1).[52]

Medical infrared thermography (MIT) has also been used in HS to detect inflammation; however, it lacks anatomical details.[53,54] Nevertheless, it may be useful to detect gross data if other imaging modalities are not available.

The usefulness of other imaging modalities in HS, such as computed tomography (CT), PET-CT (positron emission tomography-CT), optical coherence tomography (OCT), or confocal microscopy (CFM), is uncertain because, to date, there are no specific reports about their clinical use in HS. CT provides a lower definition for superficial layers in comparison with MRI and ultrasound; therefore, its use is not recommended for diagnosing or monitoring HS. However, abdominal CTs can be helpful in cases with concomitant inflammatory bowel diseases. In the case of Crohn's disease or ulcerative colitis, CT may help assess the degree of bowel inflammation and rule out the presence of communicating fistulas between the abdominal cavity and wall.[55]

Regarding PET-CT, care must be taken in the interpretation of the inflammatory signs in HS patients with a concomitant history of cancer because they can be mistaken for malignant infiltration (Fig. 6.2).[56–59]

Some reviews hypothesize about the potential use of CFM or OCT to detect epidermal alterations in HS; however, there are no specific HS studies available to date in the literature.[25,60] These imaging techniques present very high axial spatial resolution, but their penetration is extremely low and goes up to 150 to 200

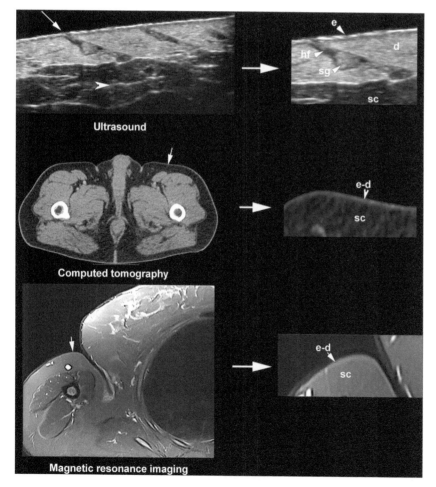

Ultrasound

Computed tomography

Magnetic resonance imaging

• **Fig. 6.1** Imaging Techniques Variable Degree of Resolution. Notice in the right part of the image a zoom of the epidermis (e), dermis (d), and subcutaneous (sc) for each imaging technique. At 70 MHz, ultrasound allows defining the cutaneous and subcutaneous layers, the hair follicles (hf), and sebaceous glands (sg). In the subcutis, it is possible to detect the fibrous bands in-between the fatty lobules (horizontal arrowhead). In contrast, in computed tomography and magnetic resonance imaging, the epidermis and dermis are fused in one thin layer, and the subcutis appear as one homogeneous layer. The arrows pointing down are marking the cutaneous layers.

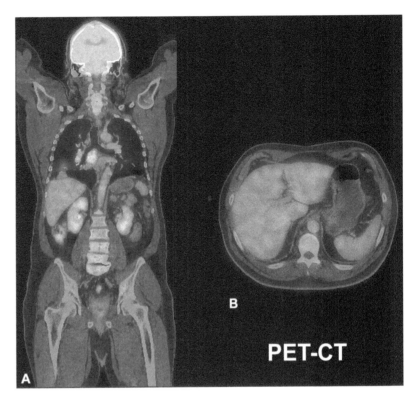

• **Fig. 6.2** Positron Emission Tomography Fused with Computed Tomography *(PET-CT)*. (A) Coronal view. (B) Transverse cross-sectional view.

microns in CFM and 1.5 to 2 mm in OCT.[61,62] This significantly limits the applications of these techniques to only the detection of epidermal or upper dermal changes. Hence, to date, neither CFM nor OCT has reported supporting the diagnosis or staging of HS.

Importantly, as in any medical procedure, all the imaging techniques need adequate machines and trained operators with proper levels of annual competence. The lack of these conditions may influence the medical decisions of requesting imaging examinations. A strong encouragement for operators' training or good coordination with the imaging facilities that already have the machines and operators can help overcome this problem.[26]

In the following sections, we will further review the details of the main indications, advantages, and disadvantages of imaging modalities in HS following a practical approach.

Basic Physics Concepts of Imaging Techniques

This section focuses on the most commonly used imaging techniques in HS.

Ultrasound

Ultrasound imaging is based on the reflection of sound waves from an interface due to differences in acoustic impedances. The transducer, also called a probe, transmits sound waves into the tissue and collects the reflected sound waves.[52,63] The color Doppler ultrasound application allows observation of blood flow in real-time.[52]

In dermatologic ultrasound examinations, multifrequency transducers are preferred. These have a wide range of operating frequencies within the same probe and users may adjust the frequency to get adequate penetration depth based on the layer being imaged. In dermatologic studies, the recommendation is to use linear or compact linear probes with higher ranges of frequencies ≥15 MHz.[28]

With improved technology, transducers with frequencies as high as 70 MHz are available for ultrasound imaging.[1,10]

The color Doppler application allows discriminating the type of vessel (arterial or venous) and the peak systolic velocity of the arterial flow (cm/s) within a user-defined area. The color Doppler maps display the vessels in different colors on the screen, but the most frequent display is the one that uses red and blue. Importantly, these colors reveal the direction of the flow and don't mean arterial and venous vessels, respectively.

In the standard configuration, the red color usually depicts flow towards the probe, and the blue color shows the flow away from the transducer. However, these settings are user-defined, and the operator may invert them. Thus, the demonstration of the spectral curve analysis of the vessels is relevant for the discrimination. The arterial flow presents a systolic and diastolic curve, and the venous flow shows a monophasic flow.

The power Doppler application is a monodirectional display of the vascularity that is usually more sensitive for detecting slow flow. Besides, several echoangio applications that subtract the tissues and present only the screen's vascularity are available in several models of ultrasound units.[50]

Magnetic Resonance Imaging

Protons within the nuclei of hydrogen atoms are essential to the formation of MRI signals and are present in fat and water molecules within the human body. These protons spin and induce a small magnetic field, resulting in a zero net magnetic field due to the random orientation. However, in the presence of a strong magnetic field, within an MRI system, there is non-zero net magnetization due to change in alignment. This net magnetization generates signals resulting in MRI images. The images are created by the excitation of individual atomic nuclei under radiofrequency (RF) and a strong magnetic field.[64,65]

RF energy is transmitted by a coil located in the site of examination of the patient. RF pulse's strength and duration determine the amount of rotation of the net magnetization from the main magnetic field's direction. Information regarding relaxation after an RF pulse composes different sequences such as T1 (longitudinal) and T2 (transverse), which help in the generation of T1 or T2 weighted images that show different features for the tissues.[64,65] The typical clinical MR systems have a magnetic field strength between 0.5 T and 3.0 T (T, tesla units).[64] Importantly, due to these potent magnets, several medical devices prevent the use of MRI, such as pacemakers and metal prostheses.[65]

Computed Tomography and Positron Emission Tomography

CT is a radiating cross-sectional technique, where the image is produced by several x-rays devices that rotate in a ring that surrounds the patient. Nowadays, fast multislice CT machines take seconds to perform the corporal segment's sweep or the whole body. CT is beneficial for detecting thoracoabdominal and bone pathologies.[66]

PET is a nuclear imaging technique that is commonly fused with CT. The fusion of techniques is called PET-CT and allows the detection of anatomical and metabolic functional abnormalities.[67] PET and PET-CT need an intravenous contrast called FDG (F-18 Fluorodeoxyglucose) which distinguishes the hypermetabolism of malignant and inflammatory conditions, named "hot spots."[67,68]

Medical Infrared Thermography

MIT is based on detecting infrared radiation emitted by an object, which is transformed into an electronic signal. The intensity of the infrared radiation generated by objects is mainly a function of its temperature; therefore, radiated energy changes represent variations in temperature within a region of interest.[69] MIT displays in colors the temperature variations. Usually, warmer temperatures are shown in bright colors (yellow to orange), while lower temperatures are shown in darker colors (red to blue). Higher temperatures are supposedly due to increased metabolism; for example, in inflammation.[53,54]

Other Potential Imaging Techniques

CFM, also called reflectance confocal microscopy (RCM) or in vivo RCM, uses near-infrared light at 830 nm. The technique generates high-resolution images utilizing intrinsic differences in cellular structures' refractive indices, primarily melanin, collagen, and keratin. This imaging technique shows a cellular resolution of the epidermis and displays the tissue in a horizontal view.[61,70] Due to limitation of penetration depth, only epidermis and superficial papillary dermis can be imaged.

OCT uses infrared light from an 830 nm superluminescence diode coupled into an optical fiber interferometer. This technique allows us to observe the epidermis and upper dermis at a high axial resolution but lower than CFM.[62,71] New applications of OCT allow detecting the dermal blood flow.[72]

Imaging of Hidradenitis Suppurativa

Ultrasound Advantages and Disadvantages in Hidradenitis Suppurativa

Among the main advantages of using ultrasound in HS are that it allows early detection of the disease, stage of severity, assessing the degree of activity, and monitoring the treatment.[2,5–12,18,20–24] The widely reported discordance between clinical and ultrasonographic evaluations supports the performance of a basal ultrasound examination in every HS patient and (not only for the pre-surgical planning, severe, or obese cases).

The limitations of ultrasound vary according to the range of frequencies of the probes; however, to date, it is impossible to detect pigments (e.g., melanin), despite the frequency.[27] The limitation of probes with a higher range of frequency up to 15 to 24 MHz includes detecting only-epidermal alterations and lesions the measure ≤ 0.1 mm.[27] The probes with a higher range of frequency up to 50 to 70 MHz present as a limitation the discrimination of abnormalities that measure ≤ 0.03 mm.[1,10]

Ultrasound, like any other medical technique or procedure, needs to follow guidelines for standardizing the performance of the examinations[28] and training of the operators.[29] Nowadays, ultrasonographic training is available under the umbrella of international scientific societies. These societies include the American Institute of Ultrasound in Medicine (AIUM; www.aium.org) and the European Federation of Societies for Ultrasound in Medicine and Biology (EFSUMB; www.efsumb.org). The literature on this topic is growing.

Other disadvantages of ultrasound include the impossibility of recording a whole corporal segment or the whole body in one view, such as in MRI. Since the sound waves' passage is stopped at the bony cortex, it is impossible to fully observe the bone medulla. Nevertheless, these limitations are not relevant to detect the soft tissue abnormalities of HS.

Definition of Early and Late Ultrasonographic Subclinical HS Lesions

Depending on the ultrasound frequency, it is possible to detect early (submillimetric) and late alterations of HS patients' dermis and subcutis.

Early Ultrasonographic Subclinical Hidradenitis Suppurativa Lesions

For detecting early subclinical and submillimetric abnormalities, it is necessary to have ultrasound devices that work with multifrequency probes that present their upper ranges ≥ 50 MHz, which may not be widely available. However, if these ultrasound machines are available, they will allow detection of the following early signs (Figs. 6.3 to 6.5)[10]:

1. Modification of the axis of the hair follicle from straight (slightly oblique) to curved
2. Thickening of the hair follicles and tracts
3. Ballooning of the hair follicles
4. Donor Sign: Dilated hair follicles that donate their keratinous content to fluid collections and tunnels.
5. Sword Sign: Fragments of hair tracts going from the cavity of a dilated hair follicle to the surrounding dermis.
6. Bridge Sign: Communications between adjacent and curved hair follicles. These connections may be conformed by single or multiple bridges between neighboring hair follicles.
7. Two types of fragmentations of the keratin are multifragment and cylindrical. Multifragment is the presence of multiple small fragments of hyperechoic linear fragments within the dilated hair follicles, fluid collections, or tunnels. The cylindrical type is composed of hypoechoic thick bands within the same structures that sometimes may show hyperechoic borders.[10]

The signs significantly associated with the disease's severity are the presence of "bridge" and "sword" signs and the cylindrical type

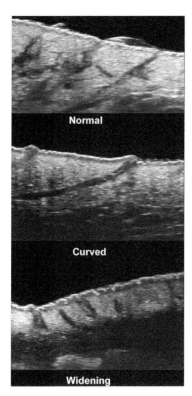

• **Fig. 6.3** Ultrasonographic early modifications of the hair follicles' shape and width in hidradenitis suppurativa (HS) at 70 MHz (submillimetric changes). Top, normal straight oblique axis and thin morphology. Notice the curved shape and the widening of the hair follicles. There is also thickening and undulation of the epidermis, which is more notorious in the bottom part.

of keratin fragmentation.[10] Thus, tunnels and fibrotic changes are more frequent in these cases.[10] The rest of the ultrasonographic signs may explain the initial formation of the primary clinical lesions.[10]

Late Ultrasonographic Subclinical Hidradenitis Suppurativa Lesions

To detect late subclinical HS lesions, it is necessary to scan the patients with color Doppler ultrasound devices working with multifrequency probes that present an upper range of 15 to 24 MHz.[a] These devices are widely available and allow detection of subclinical lesions, scoring the severity of the disease, and the evaluation of the degree of inflammatory activity, besides other anatomical details.

These key ultrasonographic signs are (Fig. 6.6)[b]:
1. Dilation of hair follicles
2. Increased thickness and decreased echogenicity of the dermis
3. Pseudocysts (i.e., round or oval-shaped anechoic or hypoechoic dermal and/or hypodermal nodule <1 cm)
4. Fluid collections (i.e., anechoic or hypoechoic sac-like dermal and/or hypodermal structures ≥1 cm connected to the base of dilated hair follicles)
5. Tunnels, also called fistulous tracts (i.e., anechoic or hypoechoic band-like dermal or hypodermal structures connected

[a]References: 2, 5, 6, 8, 11, 12, 18, 20, 21, 23, 24.
[b]References: 2, 5, 6, 8, 11, 20, 21, 23, 24.

to the bottom of dilated hair follicles), which can be communicated between them or not.

Ultrasound Diagnostic Criteria of Hidradenitis Suppurativa

The diagnostic criteria of HS are the presence of three or more key lesions.[11] The translation of clinical lesions such as nodules, abscesses, or fistulas into pseudocysts, fluid collections, or tunnels may be inexact because imaging lesions are three-dimensional anatomical structures that may not correlate with the palpable lesions. For example, an inflammatory nodule may appear as a tunnel on ultrasound.

Ultrasound Staging of Hidradenitis Suppurativa

The sonographic staging of HS may be used separately or associated with a clinical scoring system. The ultrasonographic staging, called SOS-HS,[11] which means sonographic scoring of HS and reminds the acronym of help, defines three levels of severity that try to parallel with the Hurley clinical classification. These levels of severity are characterized as follows and shown in Table 6.1.[11]

Ultrasound Classification of Hidradenitis Suppurativa Tunnels

The level of subcutaneous edema and fibrosis surrounding the fistulous tracts may support the discrimination of good and bad responders to the medical treatment.[22] Thus, fibrosis's high presence surrounding the tunnels may imply a lower response to systemic medical therapy.[22,32]

The surrounding subcutaneous **edema** to the tunnels can be categorized as[22]:

0-absent
1-diffuse hyperechogenicity of the subcutis surrounding the tunnels
2-diffuse hyperechogenicity of the subcutis and anechoic or hypoechoic fluid in between the fatty lobules

The **fibrosis** surrounding the tunnels can be categorized as[22]:

0-absent
1-Thin hypoechoic laminar band surrounding the tunnel
2-Thick hypoechoic laminar band surrounding the tunnel that may conform a "halo sign" in transverse view (cross-sectional view)

The tunnels' main classification is based on the degree of edema, and fibrosis is shown in Table 6.2 (Fig. 6.7).[22] There is another **classification of the tunnels according to the layer of involvement** that divides the tunnels into four types: dermal fistula (Type A), dermo-epidermal fistula (Type B), complex fistula (Type C), and subcutaneous fistula (Type D). Fistulas Type A and B tend to show a complete resolution after 6 months of different medical therapies in up to 95% and 65% of cases, respectively. Conversely, fistulas Type C and D have been reported to present no significant response after a medical intervention.[32] Moreover, ultrasonography has been demonstrated to predict early fistulization in comparison with the Hurley staging.[73]

Protocol for Scanning and Reporting Hidradenitis Suppurativa Patients

The ideal situation is to perform a bilateral scan of all the usually affected areas, following the guidelines for performing

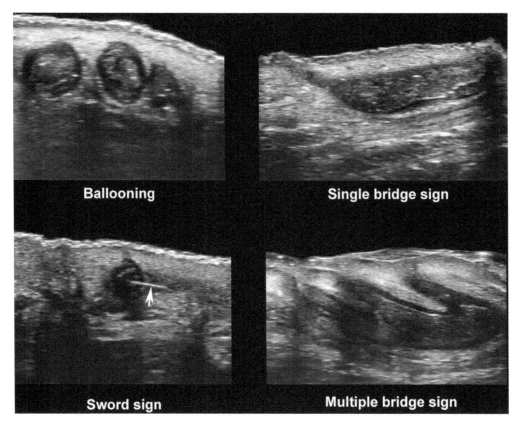

• **Fig. 6.4** Ultrasound Early Signs of Hidradenitis Suppurativa at 70 MHz of Frequency. The sword and bridge signs are associated with a higher degree of severity. The arrow points to the extrusion of the fragment of a hair tract outside the ballooned hair follicle.

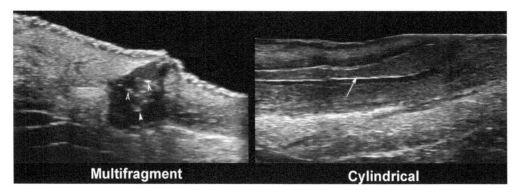

• **Fig. 6.5** Ultrasonographic types of Keratin Fragmentation in Hidradenitis Suppurativa at 70 MHz. Notice the multiple small fragments *(arrowheads)* within the ballooned hair follicle in the multifragment type and the thick hypoechoic dermal band *(arrow)* with hyperechoic borders in the cylindrical type.

dermatologic ultrasound examinations.[28] This scanning includes the use of a standardized protocol with grayscale, color Doppler, and spectral curve analysis.[50] The scanning of the axillary regions should include the proximal third and inner parts of the arms. The groin regions' scanning must include the pubic region, both sides of the perineal region, and the proximal part of the thighs' inner aspects.

The images should be kept in a digital storage system and not in the machine's memory to warranty access to the previous examinations. The memory of any imaging device is limited; therefore, it is not recommended to only rely on the capacity of storage of these devices. After the examination, a formal report should be made to register the abnormalities properly. The reports include the number, type, and size of the lesions in mm or cm obtained from at least two perpendicular axes, the description of the characteristics and degree of hypervascularity, and fibrosis in the lesional areas.[11,33] The report of the ultrasonographic staging such as SOS-HS and the tunnels' classification are encouraged.

Ultrasound Assessment of Hidradenitis Suppurativa Activity

The activity of HS may be defined by the presence and size of the key ultrasonographic lesions and also by the type and degree of vascularity on color or power Doppler.[21,22,24]

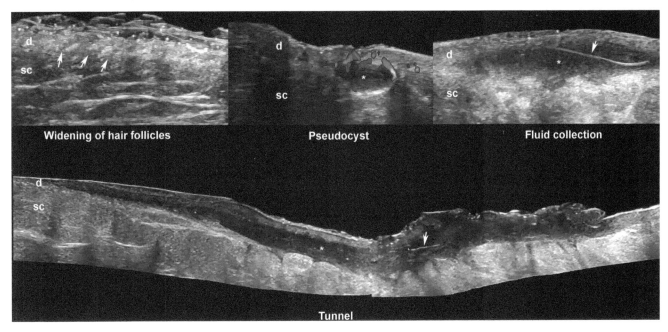

• **Fig. 6.6** Ultrasound key lesions *(*)* in HS at 18 MHz (grayscale, except the pseudocyst demonstrated on color Doppler). Notice the widening of the hair follicles *(arrows pointing up)* and the hair tract fragments within the fluid collection and the tunnel *(arrows pointing down).d*, Dermis, *sc*, subcutis.

TABLE 6.1	Ultrasound Staging of Severity—SOS-HS Classification of HS
Stage	Description
I	Single fluid collection and dermal changes (hypoechoic or anechoic pseudocystic nodules, widening of the hair follicles, alterations in the dermal thickness or echogenicity) affecting a single body segment (e.g., axilla, groin, breast, buttock) (uni- or bilateral) without fistulous tracts
II	Two to four fluid collections or a single fistulous tract with dermal changes affecting up to two body segments (uni- or bilateral)
III	Five or more fluid collections or two or more fistulous tracts with dermal changes or involvement of three or more body segments (uni- or bilateral)

SOS-HS, Sonographic scoring system of hidradenitis suppurativa.

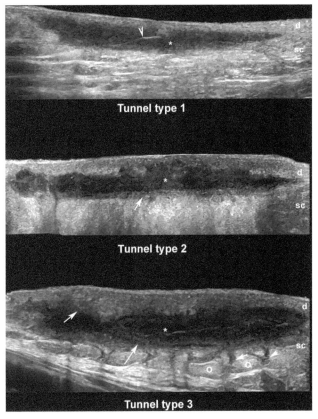

TABLE 6.2	Ultrasound Classification of Hidradenitis Suppurativa Tunnels
Type	Definition
1	Low fibrotic scarring (grades 0-1) with high or low edema (grades 0-2)
2	High fibrotic scarring (grade 2) with low edema (grades 0-1)
3	High fibrotic scarring (grade 2) with high edema (grade 2)

• **Fig. 6.7** Ultrasonographic types of fistulous tracts *(*)* at 18 MHz. There is a variable degree of inflammatory and fibrotic changes in the periphery of these tracts *(arrows pointing up)*. Enlargement of the fatty lobules *(o)* and thickening of the septa *(arrows pointing left)* of the subcutaneous tissue are present in type 3. In type 1, there is a hair tract fragment *(arrowhead)*. *d*, Dermis; *sc*, subcutis.

Thus, the degree of vascularity can be classified as (Figs. 6.8 and 6.9)[22]:

0-lack of hypervascularity
2-peripheral hypervascularity
3-peripheral and internal hypervascularity

The measurement of the vessels' maximum thickness and the peak systolic velocity of the arterial vessels can also support the therapy's monitoring.[22]

The power Doppler intensity has been reported as a valid biomarker in HS.[74] It has shown a significant correlation with pain scores, abscesses, nodule counts, International HS Severity Scoring System score, and the number of draining tunnels. Additionally, a significant correlation between power Doppler and dermal CD3 + and CD11c+ cell counts has been found.[60,74,75]

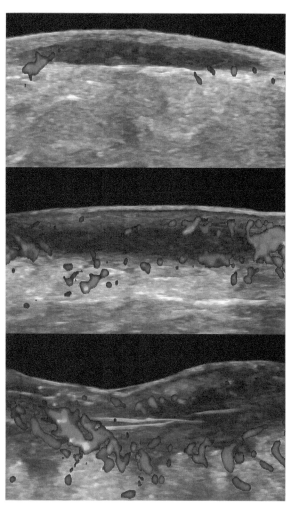

• **Fig. 6.9** Variable degree of activity in tunnels on color doppler ultrasound. Top, low, and bottom, high. There are fragments of hair tracts within the tunnel at the bottom part.

Ultrasound-Guided Surgical Planning and Monitoring of HS Treatment

According to recent reports, preoperative ultrasonography improves surgical margin delimitation and can lower recurrence rates at 24 weeks in HS patients.[7,76]

Additionally, the ultrasound monitoring of systemic therapies and percutaneous localized treatments has also been described.[77–81] These reports include the follow-up of antibiotics such as clindamycin and rifampicin,[82] some biological drugs such as adalimumab and secukinumab,[79,81] as well as the guidance of the injection of intralesional steroids[83] and the monitoring of photodynamic therapy.[77,78] The clinical and ultrasonographic correlation of the cases is of paramount importance for accurate staging and HS monitoring (Figs. 6.10 and 6.11).

Magnetic Resonance Imaging of Hidradenitis Suppurativa

Description of Lesions, Main Advantages, and Disadvantages

The MRI images show signs of superficial edema of the dermis and subcutis, fluid collections, and tortuous bands that correspond to the tunnels.[36–41,84,85] These areas appear as hypointense

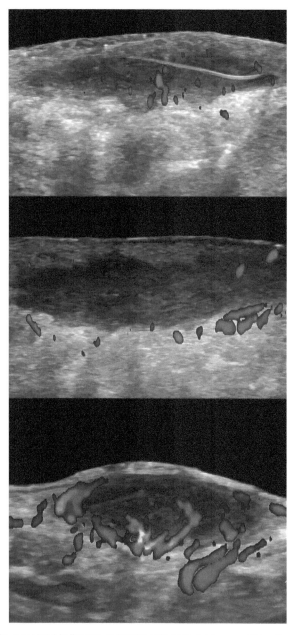

• **Fig. 6.8** Variable Degree of Activity of Fluid Collections on Color Doppler Ultrasound. Top, low, and bottom, high.

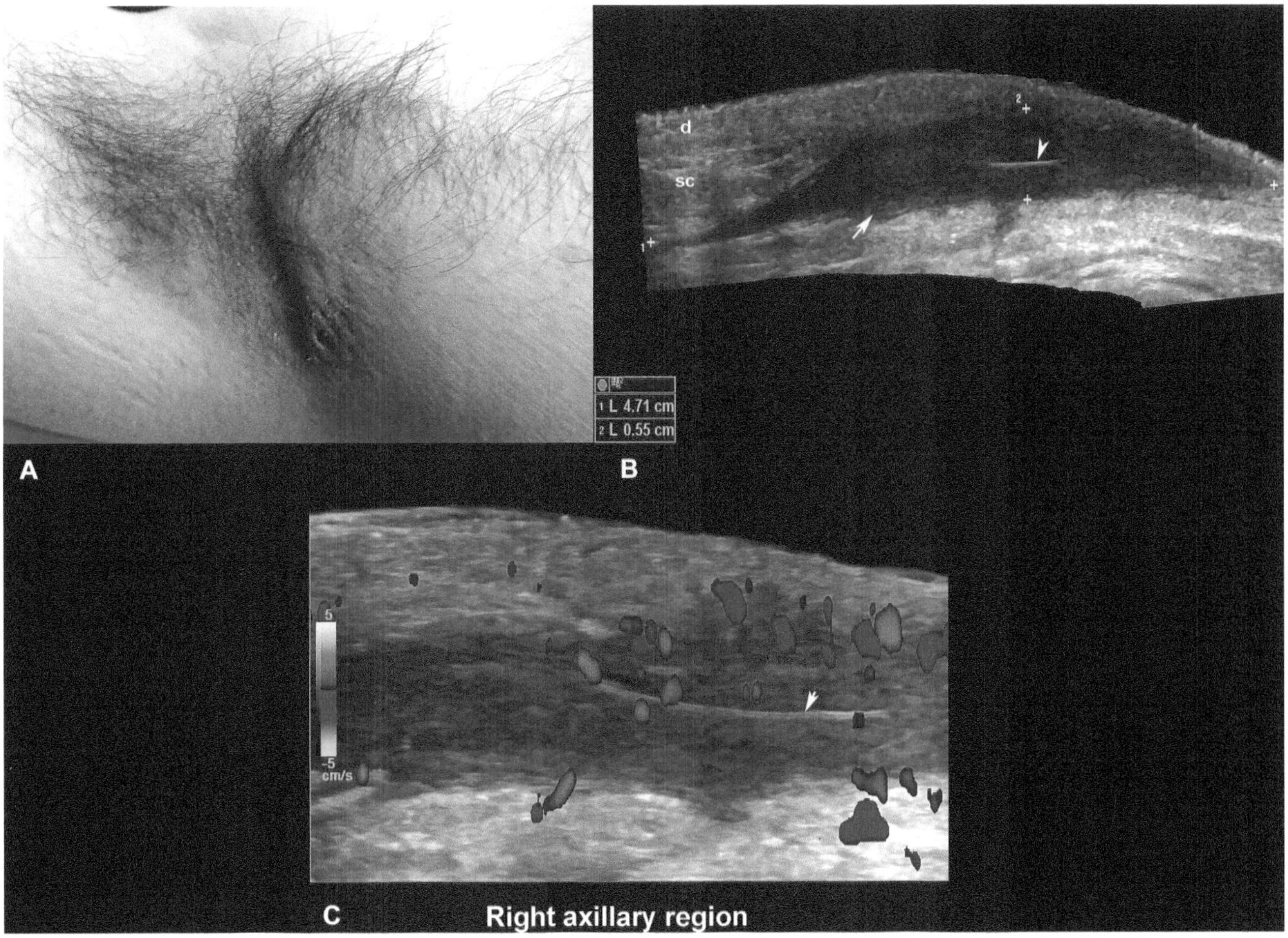

• **Fig. 6.10** Clinical and Ultrasound Correlation of Hidradenitis Suppurativa. (A) Clinical image of a patient staged as Hurley II. (B and C) Ultrasound images (B, grayscale and C, color Doppler) demonstrate hypoechoic dermal and subcutaneous tunnel type 2 measuring 4.71 cm (long) × 0.55 cm (thickness). Ultrasound staging was SOS-HS II. Notice the hypoechoic fibrotic laminar band surrounding the tunnel's deep part *(arrow pointing up)* in part (B). There are hyperechoic bilaminar fragments of hair tracts *(arrowheads pointing down)* within the tunnel in parts (B) and (C). Besides, there is active inflammation with internal and peripheral dermal and subcutaneous hypervascularity. Additionally, there is a fragment of a hair tract within the tunnel in part C. *d*, Dermis; *sc*, subcutis.

on T1 weighted images and hyperintense on T2 weighted images and sagittal short tau inversion recovery (STIR) sequences. Enhancement of the rim of the collections and tunnels after the injection of contrast (gadolinium) is also commonly found (Fig. 6.12).[36–41,84–86]

It should be kept in mind that MRI cannot discriminate well the border between the dermis and the subcutis; therefore, the alterations of these layers appear as one superficial area of abnormalities and increased thickness. Also, on MRI, it is not possible to detect the widening of the hair follicles or the connections between the dilated hair follicles and the fluid collections or tunnels. Furthermore, the areas of communications of the tunnels may be challenging to observe because they are tortuous and thin, which could leave them under the detection threshold.

MRI may help distinguish HS's tunnels from the ones originated by Crohn's disease[39]; however, this discrimination can be challenging because these conditions may be concomitant. According to a report, in Crohn's disease, the tunnels and fluid collections tend to involve the anal sphincter complex and respect the perineal, gluteal, and inguinal areas.[39]

As stated in the literature, the use of MRI has been concentrated in HS's presurgical planning, particularly in patients with multiple

anoperineal tunnels and extensive inflammation.[36–41,84–86] MRIs' main advantages include the broad anatomical view that could show several corporal segments and the data's standard registration, which allows monitoring cases under similar protocols.

The major disadvantages of MRI include the lower axial resolution compared with ultrasound that may prevent identifying superficial alterations that measure ≤3 to 5 mm, the lack of definition for detecting alterations in the hair follicles, and the dermis. The discrimination of fluid collections and tunnels, as well as signs of fibrosis, may also be challenging to diagnose in cases with a high degree of inflammation.[2]

Medical Infrared Thermography of Hidradenitis Suppurativa

Description of Lesions, Main Advantages, and Disadvantages

This imaging technique can identify variations of the skin temperature in HS and display them on a map. So far, there are few reports on MIT's use in HS, but this technique may support the mapping of inflammatory areas or rule out inflammation, such as in cases

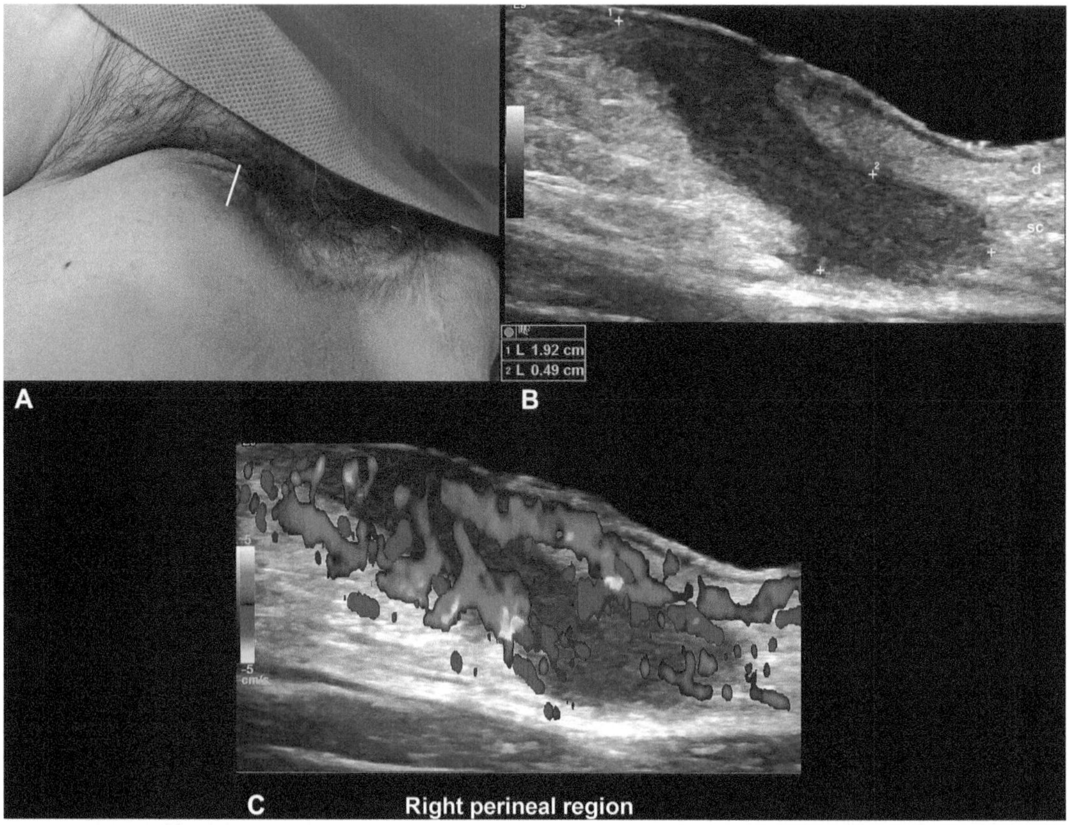

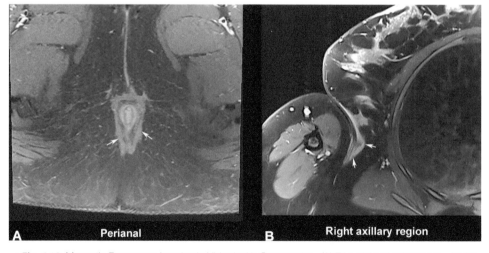

• **Fig. 6.11** Clinical and Ultrasonographic Correlation in Hidradenitis Suppurativa Showing Discordance of the Staging. (A) Clinical image of a patient with a history of surgery in the right perineal region staged as Hurley I. (B and C) Ultrasound images (B, grayscale and C, color Doppler) show a hypoechoic dermal and subcutaneous tunnel running from the perineal area to the inner part f the thigh (axis is shown as a white line in A). Ultrasound staging was SOS-HS II, and there were prominent signs of activity with dermal and subcutaneous hypervascularity within and at the periphery of the tunnel. *d*, Dermis; *sc*, subcutis.

• **Fig. 6.12** Magnetic Resonance Imaging in Hidradenitis Suppurativa. (A) T1 weighted axial image with fat suppression of the perianal region shows hyperintensity of the dermis and upper subcutis *(arrows)* surrounding the external sphincter suggestive of inflammation. (B) T2 weighted STIR axial image of the right axillary region shows hyperintensity of the dermis and upper subcutis *(arrows)* compatible with inflammatory changes.

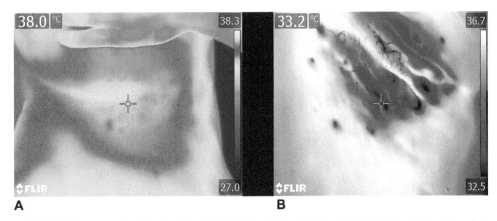

• **Fig. 6.13** Thermography in HS (courtesy Prof. Christos Zouboulis). (A) Submammary inflammation with the temperature reaching 38.0–38.3°C at the center of the lesion. (B) Differentiation between draining tunnels and inactive scars through thermography. The low temperature (33.2°C) of the lesions indicates the presence of inactive scars.

with prominent scarring (Fig. 6.13). Additionally, MIT can also provide a gross confirmation of the excision of the affected tissues after surgery.[53,54]

Concomitant use of MIT, color Doppler ultrasound, and MRI have been reported, which might provide more anatomical details.[87,88] To date, MIT's use is still in the research phase, and there are no specific patterns of involvement reported for HS except for the usual intertriginous location of the inflammation.[53,54,87,88] Among the advantages are the low cost and presumably faster training of the operators, in comparison with ultrasound or MRI.[53,54] The disadvantages include the lack of anatomical details that prevent the discrimination of the exact causes of inflammation.

Use of Other Imaging Modalities in Hidradenitis Suppurativa

PET-CT and CT

PET is a nuclear imaging method mostly used in the staging of malignancies.[56,57] Nevertheless, PET-CT can present false positives or false negatives.[56,57] Among the causes of false positives are inflammatory conditions such as HS.[59] Therefore, care must be taken to interpret abnormalities in the usual sites affected by HS in patients that present a concurrent history of malignancy. The false negatives are commonly related to the size of the lesions because PET-CT cannot discriminate well alterations that measure ≤8 mm.[56,57] CT alone is rarely used in the diagnosis, staging, or monitoring of HS; however, it may be helpful in cases with concomitant inflammatory bowel diseases. Nevertheless, neither CT nor PET-CT can discriminate dermal from subcutis alterations; therefore, they do not provide specific signs for HS.

Imaging of Hidradenitis Suppurativa Related Diseases

Several conditions that affect other body regions have been associated with HS, including the follicular occlusion tetrad composed

by HS, pilonidal cyst, acne conglobata, and dissecting cellulitis of the scalp (DCS).[89] These conditions share similar imaging findings on ultrasound and seem to be variants of the same entity.[51,90]

Pilonidal Cyst or Sinus

This epithelial structure, usually located in the intergluteal region, has been studied on ultrasound and MRI.[51,91] On ultrasound, it has been demonstrated that its morphology is similar to the fluid collections and tunnels of HS; therefore, it is compatible with a localized variant of HS.[51] They present as sac-like or band-like dermal and subcutaneous hypoechoic structures, connected to widened hair follicles. Pilonidal cysts or sinus usually contain hyperechoic bilaminar fragments of hair tracts and hypoechoic keratin. On color Doppler, there is a variable degree of vascularity within or at the periphery of the structure, according to the degree of inflammation (Fig. 6.14).[51] On MRI, they show as hyperintense structures in T2 weighted and STIR sequences and present a rim enhancement after the injection of gadolinium.[91]

Dissecting Cellulitis of the Scalp

Also known as perifolliculitis capitis abscedens et suffodiens, this condition has been studied on ultrasound.[90] Its ultrasonographic characteristics are similar to the typical alterations produced by HS; therefore, it is believed that DCS is another variant of presentation of HS.[90] Thus, in the dermis and subcutis of the scalp, there are hypoechoic pseudocysts, fluid collections, and tunnels that contain a variable amount of hyperechoic laminar fragments of hair tracts (Fig. 6.15).[90]

Acne Conglobata and Acne Keloidalis Nuchae

These severe forms of acne presentation share ultrasonographic similarities with HS that include the presence of widening of the hair follicles, pseudocysts, fluid collections, and tunnels.[92] These alterations differ from the ultrasound features of acne

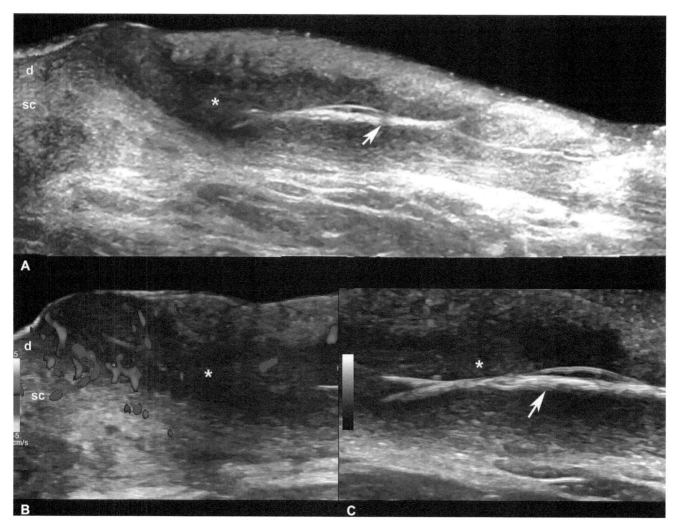

• **Fig. 6.14** Pilonidal Sinus. (A to C) Ultrasound images (longitudinal views; intergluteal region; [A and C] grayscale; A with color filter; B, color Doppler) show hypoechoic dermal and subcutaneous band-like structure (*). There are hyperechoic fragments of hair tracts (arrows) within the lesion. On color Doppler, there is hypervascularity in the periphery and some vessels within the structure. d, Dermis; sc, subcutis.

vulgaris[93] in their severity and the prominent presence of laminar hypoechoic areas suggestive of scarring that can displace the epidermis upward.

Imaging of Comorbidities of Hidradenitis Suppurativa

Carotid Atherosclerosis

Ultrasound allows the measuring of the thickness of the intima of the carotid arteries besides the detection of atheromatous plaques.[94] It has been reported that ultrasonographically HS patients present an increased prevalence of subclinical atherosclerosis;

therefore, these cases present a higher cardiovascular risk, which can be stratified on ultrasound.[94–97]

Fatty Liver

The ultrasonographic examination of HS patients has revealed a high prevalence of the non-alcoholic fatty liver disease, which generates a fibrotic liver at its late stage.[98,99]

On ultrasound, early stages of liver involvement generate steatohepatitis that appears as an increase in the liver's size and echogenicity. At the end-fibrotic stages, the liver shows a significant decrease in size and echogenicity.[100] Elastography, an ultrasound application that supports the detection and measurement of the stiffness of the tissues, may support the detection of liver fibrosis.[101]

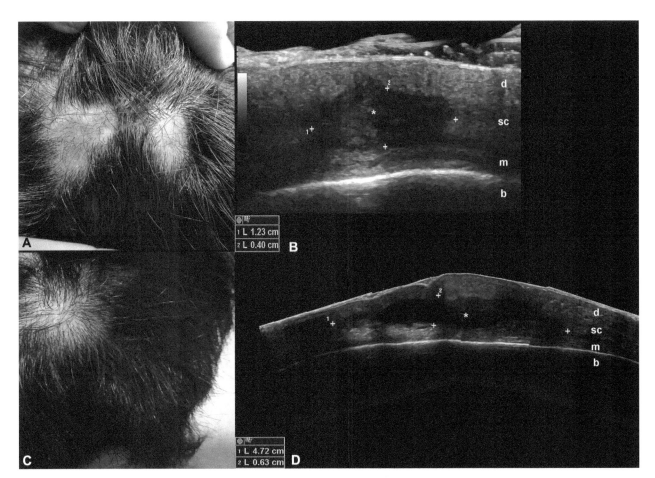

• **Fig. 6.15** Dissecting Cellulitis of the Scalp. (A) Clinical image and (B) Grayscale ultrasound of the same case. Notice the hypoechoic fluid dermal and subcutaneous collection (*) that measures 1.23 cm (transverse) ×0.4 cm (thickness). (C) Clinical and (D) grayscale ultrasound demonstrate in a second case the presence of anechoic dermal and subcutaneous tunnel (*) that measures 4.72 cm (longitudinal) ×0.63 cm (thickness). *b*, bony margin of the scalp; *d*, dermis; *m*, musculoaponeurotic layer; *sc*, subcutis.

Polycystic Ovaries

Ultrasound is the first-choice technique for detecting polycystic ovaries.[102] The Rotterdam ultrasonographic criteria include the presence of 12 or more follicles, measuring between 2 and 9 mm, and an ovarian volume >10 cm.[102] Nevertheless, these criteria should be added to other clinical and laboratory criteria. The presence of polycystic ovaries has been reported as one of the prevalent comorbidities of HS.[103,104]

Osteoarticular Pathologies

Some osteoarticular pathologies can be concomitant with HS.[105,106] Among these are the signs of synovitis, that are part of SAPHO (synovitis, acne, pustulosis, hyperostosis, osteitis) syndrome and can be detected by ultrasound and MRI, being more sensitive to ultrasound.[107] These signs are similar to those observed in other inflammatory articular diseases and seem not to be associated with bony erosions.[108]

MRI better show the signs of osteitis, also part of the SAPHO syndrome, and the accompanying signs of axial spondyloarthritis.[109–111]

Crohn´s Disease and Ulcerative Colitis

Ultrasound, CT, MRI, as well as computed tomography enterography (CTE) and magnetic resonance imaging enterography (MRIE) can be used for supporting the diagnosis and activity in inflammatory bowel diseases.[55,112–117] The selection of the technique will depend on adequate equipment and trained operators.

Conclusion

Nowadays, ultrasound is the only validated and first-choice technique for supporting early diagnosis, the staging of severity, grading of activity, presurgical planning, guided-ultrasound procedures, and monitoring of the treatment in HS. If necessary, MRI could be used for presurgical planning of perianal HS, and MIT may be used to confirm or rule out relevant degrees of inflammation. Other imaging techniques are currently in the research phase and without substantial evidence for their use in HS. Knowledge of each imaging technique's characteristics, main use, advantages, and disadvantages is necessary to make a proper selection (Table 6.3). The presence of adequate machines, standardized protocols, and trained operators is relevant for all imaging techniques.

TABLE 6.3	Summary of Main Indications, Advantages, and Disadvantages of Imaging Techniques	
Type	**Main Use, Advantages, and Disadvantages**
Ultrasound	
Main Use	HS: diagnosis, staging, assessment of activity, presurgical planning, and monitoring of treatment at all corporal sites
	Comorbidities: detection of carotid atherosclerosis, fatty liver, polycystic ovaries, synovitis, evaluation of Crohn's disease and ulcerative colitis
Advantages	Non-radiating, safe, no need for intravenous contrast
Disadvantages	Detection of alterations ≥0.1 mm at 15–24 MHz and ≥0.03 at 70 MHz
MRI	
Main Use	HS: pre-surgical planning of perianal fistulas
	Comorbidities: detection of synovitis, osteitis and axial spondyloarthritis, evaluation of Crohn's disease and ulcerative colitis (MRI enterography)
Advantages	A wide view of the corporal segments
Disadvantages	Require injection of contrast media (gadolinium), potential risk of nephrotoxicity and nephrogenic fibrosis, high cost, lower axial resolution than ultrasound
	Detection of alterations ≥3–5 mm
CT	
Main Use	Comorbidities: evaluation of Crohn's disease and ulcerative colitis (CT or CT enterography)
Advantages	A wide view of the corporal segments
Disadvantages	Radiating technique, it may require an injection of contrast media with potential nephrotoxicity, lower axial resolution than ultrasound
	Detection of alterations ≥5 mm
PET-CT	
Main Use	Staging of concomitant malignancy
Advantages	Functional imaging
Disadvantages	It may provide false positives in HS due to the hypermetabolism of inflammation, lower axial resolution than ultrasound and MRI
	Detection of alterations ≥8 mm
Medical Infrared Thermography	
Main Use	HS: assessment of sites with inflammation through the detection of high regional temperatures
Advantages	Faster training of operators, lower cost of the devices in comparison with ultrasound, MRI, CT, and PET-CT
Disadvantages	Lack of detailed anatomical data

HS, Hidradenitis suppurativa; *MRI*, magnetic resonance imaging; *PET-CT*, positron emission tomography-computed tomography.

References

1. Wortsman X, Carreño L, Ferreira-Wortsman C, et al. Ultrasound characteristics of the hair follicles and tracts, sebaceous glands, montgomery glands, apocrine glands, and arrector pili muscles. *J Ultrasound Med.* 2019;38(8):1995–2004. https://doi.org/10.1002/jum.14888.
2. Wortsman X. Imaging of hidradenitis suppurativa. *Dermatol Clin.* 2016;34(1):59–68. https://doi.org/10.1016/j.det.2015.08.003.
3. Saunte DML, Jemec GBE. Hidradenitis suppurativa: advances in diagnosis and treatment. *J Am Med Assoc.* 2017;318(20):2019–2032. https://doi.org/10.1001/jama.2017.16691.
4. Wortsman X. Diagnosis and treatment of hidradenitis suppurativa. *JAMA.* 2018;319(15):1617–1618. https://doi.org/10.1001/jama.2018.0814.
5. Lacarrubba F, Dini V, Napolitano M, et al. Ultrasonography in the pathway to an optimal standard of care of hidradenitis suppurativa: the Italian Ultrasound Working Group experience. *J Eur Acad Dermatology Venereol.* 2019;33(S6):10–14. https://doi.org/10.1111/jdv.15847.
6. Loo CH, Tan WC, Tang JJ, et al. The clinical, biochemical, and ultrasonographic characteristics of patients with hidradenitis suppurativa in Northern Peninsular Malaysia: a multicenter study. *Int J Dermatol.* 2018;57(12):1454–1463. https://doi.org/10.1111/ijd.14210.
7. Marasca C, Marasca D, Megna M, et al. Ultrasound: an indispensable tool to evaluate the outcome of surgical approaches in patients affected by hidradenitis suppurativa. *J Eur Acad Dermatology Venereol.* 2020;34(8):e413–e414.
8. Nazzaro G, Passoni E, Guanziroli E, et al. Comparison of clinical and sonographic scores in a cohort of 140 patients with hidradenitis suppurativa from an Italian referral centre: a retrospective observational study. *Eur J Dermatology.* 2018;28(6):845–847. https://doi.org/10.1684/ejd.2018.3430.
9. Oranges T, Vitali S, Benincasa B, et al. Advanced evaluation of hidradenitis suppurativa with ultra-high frequency ultrasound: a promising tool for the diagnosis and monitoring of disease progression. *Ski Res Technol.* 2020;26(4):513–519. https://doi.org/10.1111/srt.12823.
10. Wortsman X, Calderon P, Castro A. Seventy-mhz ultrasound detection of early signs linked to the severity, patterns of keratin fragmentation, and mechanisms of generation of collections and tunnels in hidradenitis suppurativa. *J Ultrasound Med.* 2020;39(5):845–857. https://doi.org/10.1002/jum.15164.
11. Wortsman X, Moreno C, Soto R, et al. Ultrasound in-depth characterization and staging of hidradenitis suppurativa. *Dermatologic Surg.* 2013;39(12):1835–1842. https://doi.org/10.1111/dsu.12329.
12. Wortsman X, Rodriguez C, Lobos C, et al. Ultrasound diagnosis and staging in pediatric hidradenitis suppurativa. *Pediatr Dermatol.* 2016;33(4):e260–e264. https://doi.org/10.1111/pde.12895.
13. Kirby JS, Butt M, King T. Severity and area score for hidradenitis (SASH): a novel outcome measurement for hidradenitis suppurativa. *Br J Dermatol.* 2020;182(4):940–948. https://doi.org/10.1111/bjd.18244.
14. Lipsker D, Severac F, Freysz M, et al. The ABC of hidradenitis suppurativa: a validated glossary on how to name lesions. *Dermatology.* 2016;232(2):137–142. https://doi.org/10.1159/000443878.
15. Ovadja ZN, Schuit MM, van der Horst CMAM, et al. Inter- and intrarater reliability of Hurley staging for hidradenitis suppurativa. *Br J Dermatol.* 2019;181(2):344–349. https://doi.org/10.1111/bjd.17588.
16. Thorlacius L, Garg A, Riis PT, et al. Inter-rater agreement and reliability of outcome measurement instruments and staging systems used in hidradenitis suppurativa. *Br J Dermatol.* 2019;181(3):483–491. https://doi.org/10.1111/bjd.17716.

17. Elkin K, Daveluy S, Avanaki K. Hidradenitis suppurativa: current understanding, diagnostic and surgical challenges, and developments in ultrasound application. *Ski Res Technol*. 2020;26(1): 11–19. https://doi.org/10.1111/srt.12759.

18. Kelekis NL, Efstathopoulos E, Balanika A, et al. Ultrasound aids in diagnosis and severity assessment of hidradenitis suppurativa. *Br J Dermatol*. 2010;162(6):1400–1402. https://doi.org/10.1111/j.1365-2133.2010.09710.x.

19. Lyons A, Zubair R, Kohli I, et al. Preoperative Ultrasound for evaluation of hidradenitis suppurativa. *Dermatol Surg*. 2019;45(2):294–296. https://doi.org/10.1097/DSS.0000000000001696.

20. Martorell A, Alfageme Roldán F, Vilarrasa Rull E, et al. Ultrasound as a diagnostic and management tool in hidradenitis suppurativa patients: a multicentre study. *J Eur Acad Dermatology Venereol*. 2019;33(11):2137–2142. https://doi.org/10.1111/jdv.15710.

21. Nazzaro G, Passoni E, Calzari P, et al. Color Doppler as a tool for correlating vascularization and pain in hidradenitis suppurativa lesions. *Ski Res Technol Technol*. 2019;25(6):830–834. https://doi.org/10.1111/srt.12729.

22. Wortsman X, Castro A, Figueroa A. Color Doppler ultrasound assessment of morphology and types of fistulous tracts in hidradenitis suppurativa (HS). *J Am Acad Dermatol*. 2016;75(4):760–767. https://doi.org/10.1016/j.jaad.2016.05.009.

23. Wortsman X, Jemec GBE. Real-time compound imaging ultrasound of hidradenitis suppurativa. *Dermatologic Surg*. 2007;33(11): 1340–1342. https://doi.org/10.1111/j.1524-4725.2007.33286.x.

24. Caposiena Caro RD, Solivetti FM, Bianchi L. Power doppler ultrasound assessment of vascularization in hidradenitis suppurativa lesions. *J Eur Acad Dermatology Venereol*. 2018;32(8):1360–1367. https://doi.org/10.1111/jdv.14745.

25. Elkin K, Daveluy S, Avanaki K. Review of imaging technologies used in Hidradenitis Suppurativa. *Ski Res Technol*. 2020;26(1):3–10. https://doi.org/10.1111/srt.12772.

26. Wortsman X. Color Doppler ultrasound: a standard of care in hidradenitis suppurativa. *J Eur Acad Dermatology Venereol*. 2020;34(10): e616–e617. https://doi.org/10.1111/jdv.16496.

27. Wortsman X, Wortsman J. Clinical usefulness of variable-frequency ultrasound in localized lesions of the skin. *J Am Acad Dermatol*. 2010;62(2):247–256. https://doi.org/10.1016/j.jaad.2009.06.016.

28. Wortsman X, Alfageme F, Roustan G, et al. Guidelines for performing dermatologic ultrasound examinations by the dermus group. *J Ultrasound Med*. 2016;35(3):577–580. https://doi.org/10.7863/ultra.15.06046.

29. Wortsman X, Alfageme F, Roustan G, et al. Proposal for an assessment training program in dermatologic ultrasound by the DERMUS Group. *J Ultrasound Med*. 2016;35(11):2305–2309. https://doi.org/10.7863/ultra.15.10068.

30. Wortsman X, Wortsman J. Ultrasound accuracy in the diagnosis of skin and soft-tissue lesions. *AJR Am J Roentgenol*. 2015;204(2): W220. https://doi.org/10.2214/AJR.14.13366.

31. Martorell A, Jfri A, Koster SBL, et al. Defining hidradenitis suppurativa phenotypes based on the elementary lesion pattern: results of a prospective study. *J Eur Acad Dermatology Venereol*. 2020;34 (6):1309–1318. https://doi.org/10.1111/jdv.16183.

32. Martorell A, Giovanardi G, Gomez-Palencia P, et al. Defining fistular patterns in hidradenitis suppurativa: impact on the management. *Dermatologic Surg*. 2019;45(10):1237–1244. https://doi.org/10.1097/DSS.0000000000001916.

33. Martorell A, Wortsman X, Alfageme F, et al. Ultrasound evaluation as a complementary test in hidradenitis suppurativa: proposal of a standardized report. *Dermatologic Surg*. 2017;43(8):1065–1073. https://doi.org/10.1097/DSS.0000000000001147.

34. Napolitano M, Calzavara-Pinton PG, Zanca A, et al. Comparison of clinical and ultrasound scores in patients with hidradenitis suppurativa: results from an Italian ultrasound working group. *J Eur Acad Dermatology Venereol*. 2019;33(2):e84–e87. https://doi.org/10.1111/jdv.15235.

35. Nazzaro G, Passoni E, Calzari P, Marzano AV. Ultrasonographic assessment of fibrosis in hidradenitis suppurativa fistulae helps in addressing treatment. *Ski Res Technol*. 2020;26(3):445–446. https://doi.org/10.1111/srt.12805.

36. Griffin N, Williams AB, Anderson S, et al. Hidradenitis suppurativa: MRI features in anogenital disease. *Dis Colon Rectum*. 2014;57 (6):762–771. https://doi.org/10.1097/DCR.0000000000000131.

37. Jhaveri KS, Thipphavong S, Guo L, et al. MR imaging of perianal fistulas. *Radiol Clin North Am*. 2018;56(5):775–789. https://doi.org/10.1016/j.rcl.2018.04.005.

38. Kelly AM, Cronin P. MRI features of hidradenitis suppurativa and review of the literature. *Am J Roentgenol*. 2005;185(5):1201–1204. https://doi.org/10.2214/AJR.04.1233.

39. Monnier L, Dohan A, Amara N, et al. Anoperineal disease in hidradenitis suppurativa: MR imaging distinction from perianal Crohn's disease. *Eur Radiol*. 2017;27(10):4100–4109. https://doi.org/10.1007/s00330-017-4776-1.

40. Virgilio E, Bocchetti T, Balducci G. Utility of MRI in the diagnosis and post-treatment evaluation of anogenital hidradenitis suppurativa. *Dermatol Surg*. 2015;41(4):865–866. https://doi.org/10.1097/DSS.0000000000000379.

41. Takiyama H, Kazama S, Tanoue Y, et al. Efficacy of magnetic resonance imaging in the diagnosis of perianal hidradenitis suppurativa, complicated by anal fistulae: A report of two cases and review of the literature. *Int J Surg Case Rep*. 2015;15:107–111. https://doi.org/10.1016/j.ijscr.2015.08.028.

42. Edlow BL, Mareyam A, Horn A, et al. 7 Tesla MRI of the ex vivo human brain at 100 micron resolution. *Sci data*. 2019;6 (1):244. https://doi.org/10.1038/s41597-019-0254-8.

43. Ladd ME, Bachert P, Meyerspeer M, et al. Pros and cons of ultra-high-field MRI/MRS for human application. *Prog Nucl Magn Reson Spectrosc*. 2018;109:1–50. https://doi.org/10.1016/j.pnmrs.2018.06.001.

44. Al-Qattan MM, Al-Namla A, Al-Thunayan A, et al. Magnetic resonance imaging in the diagnosis of glomus tumours of the hand. *J Hand Surg Am*. 2005;30(5):535–540. https://doi.org/10.1016/j.jhsb.2005.06.009.

45. Phan K, Tatian A, Woods J, et al. Prevalence of inflammatory bowel disease (IBD) in hidradenitis suppurativa (HS): systematic review and adjusted meta-analysis. *Int J Dermatol*. 2020;59(2):221–228. https://doi.org/10.1111/ijd.14697.

46. Hasebroock KM, Serkova NJ. Toxicity of MRI and CT contrast agents. *Expert Opin Drug Metab Toxicol*. 2009;5(4):403–416. https://doi.org/10.1517/17425250902873796.

47. Takahashi EA, Kallmes DF, Mara KC, et al. Nephrotoxicity of gadolinium-based contrast in the setting of renal artery intervention: Retrospective analysis with 10-year follow-up. *Diagnostic Interv Radiol*. 2018;24(6):378–384. https://doi.org/10.5152/dir.2018.18172.

48. Van Der Molen AJ. Nephrogenic systemic fibrosis and the role of gadolinium contrast media. *J Med Imaging Radiat Oncol*. 2008;52 (4):339–350. https://doi.org/10.1111/j.1440-1673.2008.01965.x.

49. Garcia J, Liu SZ, Louie AY. Biological effects of MRI contrast agents: gadolinium retention, potential mechanisms and a role for phosphorus. *Philos Trans R Soc A Math Phys Eng Sci*. 2017;375 (2107). https://doi.org/10.1098/rsta.2017.0180.

50. Wortsman X. *Atlas of Dermatologic Ultrasound. First Edit*. New York, NY: Springer International Publishing; 2018. https://doi.org/10.1007/978-3-319-89614-4.

51. Wortsman X, Castro A, Morales C, et al. Sonographic comparison of morphologic characteristics between pilonidal cysts and hidradenitis suppurativa. *J Ultrasound Med*. 2017;36(12):2403–2418. https://doi.org/10.1002/jum.14282.

52. Ihnatsenka B, Boezaart AP. Ultrasound: basic understanding and learning the language. *Int J Shoulder Surg*. 2010;4(3):55–62. https://doi.org/10.4103/0973-6042.76960.

53. Polidori G, Renard Y, Lorimier S, et al. Medical infrared thermography assistance in the surgical treatment of axillary hidradenitis suppurativa: a case report. *Int J Surg Case Rep*. 2017;34:56–59. https://doi.org/10.1016/j.ijscr.2017.03.015.

54. Zouboulis CC, Nogueira Da Costa A, GBE Jemec, et al. Long-wave medical infrared thermography: a clinical biomarker of inflammation in hidradenitis suppurativa/acne inversa. *Dermatology.* 2019;235(2):144–149. https://doi.org/10.1159/000495982.

55. Gandhi NS, Dillman JR, Grand DJ, et al. Computed tomography and magnetic resonance enterography protocols and techniques: survey of the society of abdominal radiology crohn's disease disease-focused panel. *Abdom Radiol.* 2020;45(4):1011–1017. https://doi.org/10.1007/s00261-020-02407-8.

56. Long NM, Smith CS. Causes and imaging features of false positives and false negatives on 18F-PET/CT in oncologic imaging. *Insights Imaging.* 2011;2(6):679–698. https://doi.org/10.1007/s13244-010-0062-3.

57. Nijhuis AAG, Dieng M, Khanna N, et al. False-positive results and incidental findings with annual CT or PET/CT surveillance in asymptomatic patients with resected stage III melanoma. *Ann Surg Oncol.* 2019;26(6). https://doi.org/10.1245/s10434-019-07311-0. 1960-1868.

58. Simpson RC, Dyer MJS, Entwisle J, et al. Positron emission tomography features of hidradenitis suppurativa. *Br J Radiol.* 2011;84 (1004):e164–e165. https://doi.org/10.1259/bjr/74184796.

59. Asamoah P, Wale DJ, Viglianti BL, et al. Multiple hypermetabolic subcutaneous lesions from hidradenitis suppurativa mimicking metastases on 18F-FDG PET/CT. *Clin Nucl Med.* 2018;43 (1):73–74. https://doi.org/10.1097/RLU.0000000000001911.

60. Grand D, Navrazhina K, Frew JW. A scoping review of non-invasive imaging modalities in dermatological disease: potential novel biomarkers in hidradenitis suppurativa. *Front Med.* 2019;6(6):253. https://doi.org/10.3389/fmed.2019.00253.

61. Levine A, Markowitz O. Introduction to reflectance confocal microscopy and its use in clinical practice. *JAAD Case Reports.* 2018;4 (10):1014–1023. https://doi.org/10.1016/j.jdcr.2018.09.019.

62. Popescu DP, Choo-Smith LP, Flueraru C, et al. Optical coherence tomography: Fundamental principles, instrumental designs and biomedical applications. *Biophys Rev.* 2011;3(3):155–169. https://doi.org/10.1007/s12551-011-0054-7.

63. Jakowski JD. The basics of sonography and ultrasound terminology. *Pathol Case Rev.* 2013;18(1):5–11. https://doi.org/10.1097/PCR.0b013e318281c8a0.

64. Pooley RA. Fundamental physics of MR imaging. *Radiographics.* 2005;25(4):1087–1099. https://doi.org/10.1148/rg.254055027.

65. Sands MJ, Levitin A. Basics of magnetic resonance imaging. *Semin Vasc Surg.* 2004;17(2):66–82. https://doi.org/10.1053/j.semvascsurg.2004.03.011.

66. Salmon E, Bernard Ir C, Hustinx R. Pitfalls and limitations of PET/CT in brain imaging. *Semin Nucl Med.* 2015;45(6):541–551. https://doi.org/10.1053/j.semnuclmed.2015.03.008.

67. Anand SS, Singh H, Dash AK. Clinical applications of PET and PET-CT. *Med J Armed Forces India.* 2009;65(4):353–358. https://doi.org/10.1016/S0377-1237(09)80099-3.

68. Basu S, Kwee TC, Surti S, et al. Fundamentals of PET and PET/CT imaging. *Ann N Y Acad Sci.* 2011;1228(1):1–18. https://doi.org/10.1111/j.1749-6632.2011.06077.x.

69. Harrap MJM, De Ibarra NH, Whitney HM, et al. Reporting of thermography parameters in biology: a systematic review of thermal imaging literature. *R Soc Open Sci.* 2018;5(12). https://doi.org/10.1098/rsos.181281.

70. Que SKT, Grant-Kels JM, Longo C, et al. Basics of confocal microscopy and the complexity of diagnosing skin tumors: new imaging tools in clinical practice, diagnostic workflows, cost-estimate, and new trends. *Dermatol Clin.* 2016;34(4):367–375. https://doi.org/10.1016/j.det.2016.05.001.

71. Welzel J, Lankenau E, Birngruber R, et al. Optical coherence tomography of the human skin. *J Am Acad Dermatol.* 1997;37 (6):958–963. https://doi.org/10.1016/S0190-9622(97)70072-0.

72. Themstrup L, Welzel J, Ciardo S, et al. Validation of Dynamic optical coherence tomography for non-invasive, in vivo microcirculation imaging of the skin. *Microvasc Res.* 2016;107:97–105. https://doi.org/10.1016/j.mvr.2016.05.004.

73. Costa IMC, Pompeu CB, Mauad EBS, et al. High-frequency ultrasound as a non-invasive tool in predicting early hidradenitis suppurativa fistulization in comparison with the Hurley system. *Ski Res Technol.* 2020. https://doi.org/10.1111/srt.12954.

74. Grand D, Frew JW, Navrazhina K, et al. Doppler ultrasound-based noninvasive biomarkers in hidradenitis suppurativa: evaluation of analytical and clinical validity. *Br J Dermatol.* 2021;184(4):688–6963. https://doi.org/10.1111/bjd.19343.

75. Wortsman X. Strong validation of ultrasound as an imaging biomarker in hidradenitis suppurativa. *Br J Dermatol.* 2021;184 (4):591–592. https://doi.org/10.1111/bjd.19433.

76. Cuenca-Barrales C, Salvador-Rodríguez L, Arias-Santiago S, et al. Pre-operative ultrasound planning in the surgical management of patients with hidradenitis suppurativa. *J Eur Acad Dermatology Venereol.* 2020;34(10):2362–2367. https://doi.org/10.1111/jdv.16435.

77. Agut-Busquet E, Romaní J, Gilaberte Y, et al. Photodynamic therapy with intralesional methylene blue and a 635 nm light-emitting diode lamp in hidradenitis suppurativa: a retrospective follow-up study in 7 patients and a review of the literature. *Photochem Photobiol Sci.* 2016;15(8):1020–1028. https://doi.org/10.1039/c6pp00082g.

78. Álvarez P, García-Martínez FJ, Poveda I, et al. Intralesional triamcinolone for fistulous tracts in hidradenitis suppurativa: an uncontrolled prospective trial with clinical and ultrasonographic follow-up. *Dermatology.* 2020;236(1):46–51. https://doi.org/10.1159/000499934.

79. Kanni T, Argyropoulou M, Spyridopoulos T, et al. MABp1 targeting IL-1α for moderate to severe hidradenitis suppurativa not eligible for adalimumab: a randomized study. *J Invest Dermatol.* 2018;138(4):795–801. https://doi.org/10.1016/j.jid.2017.10.030.

80. Nazzaro G, Zerboni R, Passoni E, et al. High-frequency ultrasound in hidradenitis suppurativa as rationale for permanent hair laser removal. *Ski Res Technol.* 2019;25(4):587–588. https://doi.org/10.1111/srt.12671.

81. Prussick L, Rothstein B, Joshipura D, et al. Open-label, investigator-initiated, single-site exploratory trial evaluating secukinumab, an anti-interleukin-17A monoclonal antibody, for patients with moderate-to-severe hidradenitis suppurativa. *Br J Dermatol.* 2019;181(3):609–611. https://doi.org/10.1111/bjd.17822.

82. Caposiena Caro RD, Cannizzaro MV, Botti E, et al. Clindamycin versus clindamycin plus rifampicin in hidradenitis suppurativa treatment: clinical and ultrasound observations. *J Am Acad Dermatol.* 2019;80 (5):1314–1321. https://doi.org/10.1016/j.jaad.2018.11.035.

83. Salvador-Rodriguez L, Arias-Santiago S, Molina-Leyva A. Ultrasound-assisted intralesional corticosteroid infiltrations for patients with hidradenitis suppurativa. *Sci Rep.* 2020;10(1):13363. https://doi.org/10.1038/s41598-020-70176-x.

84. Balcı S, Onur MR, Karaosmanoğlu AD, et al. Mri evaluation of anal and perianal diseases. *Diagnostic Interv Radiol.* 2019;25(1):21–27. https://doi.org/10.5152/dir.2018.17499.

85. Scholtes VC, Ardon CB, van Straalen KR, et al. Characterization of perianal fistulas in patients with hidradenitis suppurativa. *J Eur Acad Dermatology Venereol.* 2019;33(9):e337–e338. https://doi.org/10.1111/jdv.15629.

86. Poh F, Wong SK. Imaging of hidradenitis suppurativa and its complications. *Case Rep Radiol.* 2014;2014:1–5. https://doi.org/10.1155/2014/294753.

87. Derruau S, Renard Y, Pron H, et al. Combining magnetic resonance imaging (MRI) and medical infrared thermography (MIT) in the pre- and peri-operating management of severe hidradenitis suppurativa (HS). *Photodiagnosis Photodyn Ther.* 2018;23:9–11. https://doi.org/10.1016/j.pdpdt.2018.05.007.

88. Nazzaro G, Moltrasio C, Marzano AV. Infrared thermography and color Doppler: two combined tools for assessing inflammation in hidradenitis suppurativa. *Ski Res Technol.* 2020;26(1):140–141. https://doi.org/10.1111/srt.12750.

89. Vasanth V, Chandrashekar B. Follicular occlusion tetrad. *Indian Dermatol Online J.* 2014;5(4):491. https://doi.org/10.4103/2229-5178.142517.

90. Cataldo-Cerda K, Wortsman X. Dissecting cellulitis of the scalp early diagnosed by color doppler ultrasound. *Int J Trichology.* 2017;9(4):147–148. https://doi.org/10.4103/ijt.ijt_2_17.

91. Taylor SA, Halligan S, Bartram CI. Pilonidal sinus disease: MR imaging distinction from fistula in ano. *Radiology.* 2003;226 (3):662–667. https://doi.org/10.1148/radiol.2263011758.

92. Wortsman X, Wortsman J, Matsuoka L, et al. Sonography in pathologies of scalp and hair. *Br J Radiol.* 2012;85(1013):647–655. https://doi.org/10.1259/bjr/22636640.

93. Wortsman X, Claveria P, Valenzuela F, et al. Sonography of acne vulgaris. *J Ultrasound Med.* 2014;33(1):93–102. https://doi.org/10.7863/ultra.33.1.93.

94. Pascual JC, González I, Corona D, et al. Assessment of subclinical atherosclerosis in hidradenitis suppurativa. *J Eur Acad Dermatology Venereol.* 2017;31(7):1229–1238. https://doi.org/10.1111/jdv.14076.

95. González-López MA, Lacalle M, Mata C, et al. Carotid ultrasound is useful for the cardiovascular risk stratification in patients with hidradenitis suppurativa. *PLoS One.* 2018;13(1). https://doi.org/10.1371/journal.pone.0190568.

96. González-López MA, Hernández JL, Lacalle M, et al. Increased prevalence of subclinical atherosclerosis in patients with hidradenitis suppurativa (HS). *J Am Acad Dermatol.* 2016;75(2):329–335. https://doi.org/10.1016/j.jaad.2016.03.025.

97. González I, Pascual JC, Corona D, et al. European Heart Systemic Coronary Risk Evaluation may underestimate cardiovascular risk after assessing cardiovascular disease with carotid ultrasound in hidradenitis suppurativa. *Br J Dermatol.* 2018;178(1):e22–e23. https://doi.org/10.1111/bjd.15776.

98. Damiani G, Leone S, Fajgenbaum K, et al. Nonalcoholic fatty liver disease prevalence in an Italian cohort of patients with hidradenitis suppurativa: a multi-center retrospective analysis. *World J Hepatol.* 2019;11(4):391–401. https://doi.org/10.4254/wjh.v11.i4.391.

99. Durán-Vian C, Arias-Loste MT, Hernández JL, et al. High prevalence of non-alcoholic fatty liver disease among hidradenitis suppurativa patients independent of classic metabolic risk factors. *J Eur Acad Dermatology Venereol.* 2019;33(11):2131–2136. https://doi.org/10.1111/jdv.15764.

100. Ozturk A, Grajo JR, Gee MS, et al. Quantitative hepatic fat quantification in non-alcoholic fatty liver disease using ultrasound-based techniques: a review of literature and their diagnostic performance. *Ultrasound Med Biol.* 2018;44(12):2461–2475. https://doi.org/10.1016/j.ultrasmedbio.2018.07.019.

101. Ferraioli G. Review of liver elastography guidelines. *J Ultrasound Med.* 2019;38(1):9–14. https://doi.org/10.1002/jum.14856.

102. Lujan ME, Jarrett BY, Brooks ED, et al. Updated ultrasound criteria for polycystic ovary syndrome: Reliable thresholds for elevated follicle population and ovarian volume. *Hum Reprod.* 2013;28 (5):1361–1368. https://doi.org/10.1093/humrep/det062.

103. Bachanek M, Abdalla N, Cendrowski K, Sawicki W. Value of ultrasonography in the diagnosis of polycystic ovary syndrome – literature review. *J Ultrason.* 2015;15(63):410–422. https://doi.org/10.15557/JoU.2015.0038.

104. Garg A, Neuren E, Strunk A. Hidradenitis suppurativa is associated with polycystic ovary syndrome: a population-based analysis in the United States. *J Invest Dermatol.* 2018;138(6):1288–1292. https://doi.org/10.1016/j.jid.2018.01.009.

105. Fimmel S, Zouboulis C. Comorbidities of hidradenitis suppurativa (acne inversa). *Dermatoendocrinol.* 2010;2(1):9–16. https://doi.org/10.4161/derm.2.1.12490.

106. Tzellos T, Zouboulis CC. Review of comorbidities of hidradenitis suppurativa: implications for daily clinical practice. *Dermatol Ther (Heidelb).* 2020;10(1):63–71. https://doi.org/10.1007/s13555-020-00354-2.

107. Soscia E, Scarpa R, Cimmino MA, et al. Magnetic resonance imaging of nail unit in psoriatic arthritis. *J Rheumatol Suppl.* 2009;83:42–45. https://doi.org/10.3899/jrheum.090222.

108. Fauconier M, Reguiai Z, Barbe C, et al. Association between hidradenitis suppurativa and spondyloarthritis. *Jt Bone Spine.* 2018;85 (5):593–597. https://doi.org/10.1016/j.jbspin.2017.09.005.

109. Coates LC, Hodgson R, Conaghan PG, et al. MRI and ultrasonography for diagnosis and monitoring of psoriatic arthritis. *Best Pract Res Clin Rheumatol.* 2012;26(6):805–822. https://doi.org/10.1016/j.berh.2012.09.004.

110. Crowley EL, O'Toole A, Gooderham MJ. Hidradenitis suppurativa with SAPHO syndrome maintained effectively with adalimumab, methotrexate, and intralesional corticosteroid injections. *SAGE Open Med Case Rep.* 2018;6. https://doi.org/10.1177/2050313x18778723. 2050313X1877872.

111. Krajewska-Włodarczyk M, Owczarczyk-Saczonek A, Placek W, et al. Ultrasound assessment of changes in nails in psoriasis and psoriatic arthritis. *Biomed Res Int.* 2018;2018:8251097. https://doi.org/10.1155/2018/8251097.

112. Allocca M, Danese S, Laurent V, et al. Use of cross-sectional imaging for tight monitoring of inflammatory bowel diseases. *Clin Gastroenterol Hepatol.* 2020;18(6):1309–1323.e4. https://doi.org/10.1016/j.cgh.2019.11.052.

113. Calabrese E, Maaser C, Zorzi F, et al. Bowel ultrasonography in the management of Crohn's disease. A review with recommendations of an international panel of experts. *Inflamm Bowel Dis.* 2016;22 (5):1168–1183. https://doi.org/10.1097/MIB.0000000000000706.

114. Krzesiek E, Nienartowicz E, Iwańczak B. Value of magnetic resonance enterography in diagnosis and treatment follow up in Crohn's disease in children. *Adv Med Sci.* 2020;65(1):214–222. https://doi.org/10.1016/j.advms.2020.01.005.

115. Lee S, Choi YH, Cho YJ, et al. Quantitative evaluation of Crohn's disease using dynamic contrast-enhanced MRI in children and young adults. *Eur Radiol.* 2020;30(6):3168–3177. https://doi.org/10.1007/s00330-020-06684-1.

116. Lu C, Merrill C, Medellin A, et al. Bowel ultrasound state of the art: grayscale and doppler ultrasound, contrast enhancement, and elastography in Crohn disease. *J Ultrasound Med.* 2019;38(2):271–288. https://doi.org/10.1002/jum.14920.

117. Wright EK, Novak KL, Lu C, et al. Transperineal ultrasonography in perianal Crohn disease: A valuable imaging modality. *Can J Gastroenterol Hepatol.* 2015;29(8):445–447. https://doi.org/10.1155/2015/120123.

7

Clinical Evaluation

MONICA ROSALES SANTILLAN, MARTINA L. PORTER, AND ALEXA B. KIMBALL

CHAPTER OUTLINE

Overview of Patient Population with HS Prior to Initiating Therapy

Hidradenitis suppurativa is a clinical diagnosis based on history, physical exams, patterns of recurrence, types of lesions, and scarring. No diagnostic test is currently available and biopsy results are relatively non-specific compared to clinical patterns. Once the diagnosis has been made, an assessment of severity and comorbidities should follow, as they will affect treatment choices.

Obtaining History Related to HS Onset and Family History

Onset of Hidradenitis Suppurativa Symptoms

Patients may develop signs and symptoms of hidradenitis suppurativa (HS) throughout most of the life span, with most reports ranging from 15 to 60 years old. Women, who make up 70% of the HS population, tend to present in their 20s and 30s, reporting symptoms that started years earlier.[1,2] There may also be smaller peak that occurs in the post-menopausal population. HS is more common in African Americans and Caucasians and may

occur less frequently in Asian populations.[2,3] Since the majority of HS epidemiology studies are from North America and Europe, the current HS racial demographics may not be fully representative of the actual prevalence of HS.

There is, on average, a 7-year gap between symptoms and receiving a diagnosis.[4] The delay in diagnosis may be due to multiple factors ranging from reluctance to disclose their symptoms/signs to misdiagnosis, such as folliculitis. Additionally, patients can have gradual development of HS symptoms prior to deciding to seek care.

Initial HS symptoms include the development of multiple recurrent papules or nodules in one or more locations.[1] Inflammatory nodules may evolve into abscesses, fistulas, and/or sinus tracts. Pocketed scarring and sinus tracts are classic features and very helpful in distinguishing this disease from folliculitis, which also tends to present with smaller, more superficial lesions. Some patients may not present with these classic features early in their HS disease or if they have only mild disease, which can lead to delay in diagnosis if a thorough patient history is not obtained. While obtaining history, clinicians should ask patients to describe their lesions and whether they have noted changes over months to years. It is often helpful to provide examples to the patient of what HS lesions look like and the locations where they tend to appear. Patients often have historical pictures they can provide as well.

A thorough history of timeline of events prior to and after HS symptom onset can also be contributory. Changes to patient's diet, medications, weight gain, stress, tobacco use, menses onset, pregnancy, and menopause onset as relevant may aid in determining triggers.[5-7] For example, in women, flares due to hormonal fluctuation are common.[7]

Family History of Hidradenitis Suppurativa Symptoms/Diagnosis

Hidradenitis suppurativa has autosomal dominant, albeit complicated, inheritance pattern with one-third of patients reporting a family member with HS-like symptoms.[8,9] Furthermore, patients with early-onset HS disease are more likely to have a family history of HS compared to patients with normal-onset HS, which is defined at onset of puberty or later. Although some genes have been identified, they do not explain the majority of cases.[9] If available, the family member's affected HS lesion location(s), flare triggers, and treatment history may be useful: for a patient with extensive disease and a family history of chronic HS lesions with prominent scarring, early initiation of systemic therapy should be discussed.

The Physical Exam

Pertinent Locations

Hidradenitis suppurativa is predominant, but not exclusive to apocrine gland-bearing regions. Commonly affected areas include the axillae, inframammary area, lower abdomen, inguinal region, perineum, and gluteal region.[1] Patients will describe having multiple papules that evolve into nodules, abscesses, and/or fistulas. Scarring is a prominent feature of moderate-to-severe HS, which may appear as pocketed, cribriform scars, and/or interconnected scars.

On initial exam, the physician should examine all locations where HS may appear to keep note of lesion progression, which is common. Patients may report not having any active lesions in an area, but still present with HS lesions, such as non-draining fistulas. This should be noted on exam to have a consistent Hurley staging and Physician's Global Assessment.[10,11] Both of these assessments are described in further detail later on in this chapter.

When examining the patient, the physician can assist the patient in positioning them to examine symmetrically affected areas, such as both axillae, at the same time to minimize pain and discomfort. This technique minimizes the amount of time a patient has to be in an uncomfortable position due to limited mobility from scarring. Additionally, patients should be given the choice to remove their wound dressing. If the patient prefers keeping the dressing on, then the clinician should make note of it and ask the patient to describe any active lesions they have at the site.

When the axillae and groin are affected, patients may describe having limited mobility due to pain and scarring. Fig. 7.1 demonstrates the classic tunneling scars with overlying fibrosis and post-inflammatory hyperpigmentation seen with hidradenitis suppurativa in the axilla. Another commonly affected area is the inframammary region. Fig. 7.2 demonstrates inframammary region affected with abscesses and papules with overlying erythema in a female patient (see Fig. 7.2A) and male patient (see Fig. 7.2B), respectively. The groin region is also affected in HS and female patients tend to present with isolated groin disease when they have limited disease extent. Fig. 7.3 shows a few inflammatory nodules with surrounding scarring tracts in a female patient.

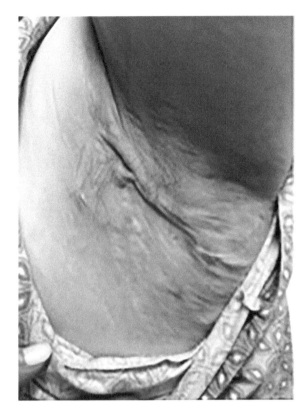

• **Fig. 7.1** Left axilla: There is prominent cribriform scarring with overlying post-inflammatory hyperpigmentation and linear fibrotic scarring on a female patient with hidradenitis suppurativa.

Lesion Count

Lesion count assessment consists of assessing the number of nodules, abscesses, and/or fistulas present. Papules are not generally formally included in the assessment. Although papules may occur as a new early lesion, most HS lesions are large and deep (>1 cm) such that a papule-predominant presentation may prompt evaluation for another condition such as folliculitis. When counting lesions, the clinician should determine whether the lesions are interconnected, which may be part of the same underlying process. When documenting lesions, the clinician should categorize the lesion for fully assessing disease severity. While there is currently no standardized HS lesional terminology, there are available validated terminologies that can be used.[12]

When assessing the patient, the clinician should fully visualize all the affected areas, including regions where the patient may not have any active lesions. There may still be background disease that should be noted. The physical exam may be difficult for some patients due to lesion tenderness. Additionally, patients will often have wound dressings over their lesions that are removed for the physical exam. The clinician can allow the patient to remove their own dressings to avoid any unnecessary pain in the process. New wound dressings can be offered following the physical exam.

Lesion Description

Lesion characteristics are also used for determining disease severity. On exam, fistulas may drain spontaneously or on palpation. If a patient's fistulas no longer drain on a subsequent exam, then the disease severity score may change. HS nodule assessment also will affect the disease severity score based on tenderness presence on

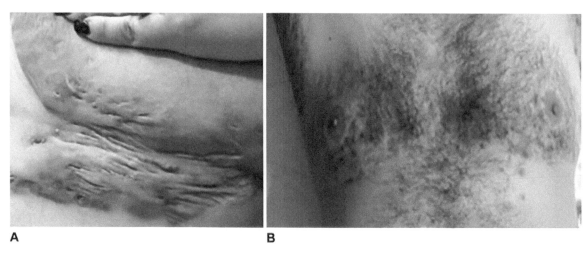

A   **B**

• **Fig. 7.2** (A) (Picture on left) There are abscesses with overlying erythema and scarring tracts on the left inframammary area in a female patient. (B) (Picture on right) There are multiple scattered inflammatory papules with overlying hyperpigmentation on both inframammary regions in a male patient.

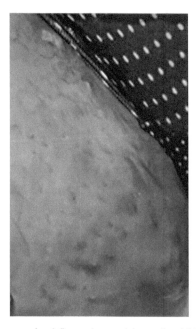

• **Fig. 7.3** There are a few inflammatory nodules on the right inguinal region with scattered scarring with overlying hyperpigmentation that extends to the right inner thigh in a female patient.

palpation. Patients may report tenderness even without palpation; therefore, clinicians should minimize lesion palpation for the patient unless required for scoring in a clinical trial or other disease assessment. Scarring and post-inflammatory hyperpigmentation should also be assessed to monitor for signs of improvement over-time and with HS treatment.

Documenting Other Pertinent Features on Skin Exam

Other medical conditions that have higher prevalence in patients with HS compared to the general population include metabolic syndrome.[13] On exam, patients may appear overweight and have skin findings, such as acanthosis nigricans, which supports metabolic dysregulation. In female patients, polycystic ovarian syndrome (PCOS) is another comorbidity seen in HS.[14] Features on physical exam include darkened hairs on the face, peri-areolar area, and groin region.

Hidradenitis Suppurativa Disease Assessment

Detailed discussion of clinical assessment tools can be found in Chapter 13, "Disease Evaluation and Outcome Measures."

Hurley Staging

The Hurley staging system was developed initially for clinical staging prior to undergoing surgery. This staging system is now commonly used in the clinical and research setting for staging overall disease severity. Physicians use this to determine whether a patient may require systemic therapies for their disease. Different but overlapping treatment algorithms have been associated with each Stage in the literature, including follow-up visit planning and lab monitoring.[15] Patients with more severe disease will require frequent clinic visits for monitoring, specifically in the first 4 to 6 months of starting a systemic therapy, such as adalimumab or infliximab, to monitor progress.

While disease activity may improve, the Hurley stage may remain unchanged due to the permanence of scarring and sinus tracts. If treatment has been optimized and the patient continues to have rare HS flares, then clinicians can start to focus on surgical options for scar and sinus tract management. The Hurley staging system is excellent for initial evaluation in helping determine the appropriate aggressiveness of the therapy, but should also be used with other dynamic assessments, such as the physician's global assessment and Dermatology Life Quality Index (DLQI) which are discussed in the next sections.[10,11,16]

Hidradenitis Suppurativa Physician's Global Assessment

The hidradenitis suppurativa physician's global assessment (HS-PGA) as initially used to evaluate the efficacy of adalimumab in patients with moderate-to-severe HS disease in a parallel randomized trial.[11] This assessment consists of different stages with a score from 0 to 5 This includes clear (score: 0), minimal (score: 1), mild (score: 2), moderate (score: 3), severe (score: 4), and very severe (score: 5). This scoring system is calculated based on the lesion count and description. The clinician assesses the number of abscesses, draining fistulas, inflammatory nodules, and non-inflammatory nodules. Clinical improvement based on the HS PGA score is defined as improvement in the score by a minimum of 2 grade points to a score of clear, minimal, or mild. This scoring system is highly useful for adjusting a patient's treatment based on their physical exam findings.

Dermatology Life Quality Index Assessment

The DLQI assesses the patient's perspective of their disease.[16] It is rapidly performed, designed for clinical use, and allows patients to further define treatment success for their chronic disease. The DLQI includes questions inquiring about symptoms and impact on personal relationships, leisure, daily activities, treatment, and occupation.[16] Patients may have higher scores for questions related to pain, personal relationships, and occupation. Lesion pain with associated limited mobility leads to missing work, social events, and relationship commitments.

Pain Assessment

While pain is assessed in the DLQI assessment, clinicians can also monitor patient's pain secondary to their HS at every visit.[17] Patients will often have recurrent pain that worsens during HS flares. The numeric rating scale (NRS) for pain of 0 to 10, with 0 being no pain to 10 being the worst pain experienced, can be used to track treatment progress and determine if management should be adjusted. The visual analogue scale (VAS) for pain is another scale that uses defines two extreme endpoints of no pain to worse pain possible. The distance from no pain to where the patient marks their pain determined the pain severity level.

Other Important Considerations Regarding Therapeutic Choices

Hidradenitis Suppurativa Flare Triggers

There are multiple known triggers for HS flares. These include menses, androgen-containing oral contraceptives (OCPs), dairy intake, stress, heat, sweating, friction, and pregnancy.[5-7,18]

Female predominance in HS has led to multiple theories and studies evaluating potential roles of hormones. In our experience, those who present with peri-menstrual flares often have their disease limited in location with the groin and thighs predominantly affected. These patients often respond well to anti-androgen therapy, such as spironolactone.[19] The disease course improves after menopause for most women with this type of disease, but some may have persistent disease.

Another identified flare trigger in our population is androgen-containing OCPs that do not have opposing estrogen.[5] OCPs can also be discussed with a patient's obstetrician-gynecologist (OB/GYN) to determine which one is the best option for them. Hormonal modulation is discussed in the next section.

Pregnancy often leads to HS flares, a finding that also supports the role of hormones in this chronic disease.[7] Patients will often report worsening of their HS during and particularly after

pregnancy. While treatment options are limited during pregnancy, treatment can be switched to other similar therapies to avoid HS flares. Certolizumab is often used in place of adalimumab during pregnancy because it is not transported across the placenta. Clinicians will want to collaborate with patients' OB/GYNs to discuss treatment options during pregnancy. HS considerations in women is further discussed in Chapter 31, "Hidradenitis Suppurativa in Women."

Diet continues to be a popular topic in HS patient support groups. Often, patients will present for initial evaluation and report changing their diet. Approaches include eliminating food they consider promoting inflammatory processes such as dairy, carbohydrates, or nightshades. Extrapolating from acne, it is possible that dairy (especially androgenic whey proteins found in skim milk and some protein powders and bars) can trigger HS flares and elimination seems reasonable to try. To date, there is insufficient evidence for other food categories. Weight loss appears to beneficial for the preponderance of patients, although large skin folds can foster continued problems.

Heat, sweating, and friction are well-described triggers for HS flares. Heat and sweating exacerbate the affected HS lesions due to their location, including the axillae, inflamed region, and groin region. Friction also can irritate the lesions and prevent them from healing due to constant movement of the affected areas. During evaluation, the clinician should discuss with the patient what types of dressings they have tried. Wound dressings are constantly being developed to manage frequent lesion drainage and prevent friction. Weight loss also may help decrease friction in the affected HS areas.

Another trigger commonly shared by patients at initial and follow-up visits is stress. They describe having treatment improvement but then developing HS flares due to a stressful event. Clinicians may wish to discuss with patient how frequently this occurs to be able to adjust the treatment regimen. A short course of antibiotic can be provided with refills as well. This will help shorten the duration of the patient's HS flare.

Hormonal Modulation

Birth control choice can be very important in patients with HS. Some patients describe gradually developing HS lesions after starting a new birth control: high-androgen containing OCPs and androgen-only birth control, even in the intrauterine device (IUD) form, can trigger and worsen HS.[5] Clinicians should inquire of any potential contraindications to a type of birth control, such as having migraines with auras or long-term smoking. Additionally, birth control compliance should be discussed with patients to determine which birth control would be the best option for the patient.

Low-androgen OCPs, such as ethinyl estradiol-drospirenone and ethinyl estradiol-desogestrel, can benefit females who have perimenstrual flares with limited disease. This type of OCP can be used with spironolactone or by itself to prevent flares in this patient group.[19] Copper-containing IUDs do not contain hormones and can also be a birth control option for patients.

Following discussion with patients about birth control, clinicians may determine whether changing birth control is recommended and also whether the patient plans on becoming pregnant in the near future. Patients may have an IUD or birth control implant that they prefer to remove at a later point. If this is the case, the clinician can provide the patient with a list of optimal birth control options once the patient chooses to change birth control.

Obtaining Information of Other Medical Problems

A thorough medical history should be obtained prior to initiating systemic management. This includes inquiring about history of malignancy and, depending on the agents, central nervous system disorders and cardiac disease.[20,21] Since some immunomodulating therapies used for HS can increase risk of infection, clinicians should also ask about history of hepatitis infection and any opportunistic infections, such as tuberculosis.

The risk of developing malignancy while on systemic therapy will vary by agent, but if a treatment with immunomodulating effect is being contemplated, clinicians should determine a patient's baseline risk. Annual skin exams are generally recommended in these circumstances with special attention to the perianal area in men, where squamous cell carcinomas (SCCs) have been reported to develop.

Infection, including hepatitis B reactivation and tuberculosis, may occur while on biologic therapies. Clinicians should obtain information about any past treatment patients underwent if they have a history of these infections. Infectious disease may be consulted regarding infection management options prior to treatment initiation. Baseline labs for these infections are discussed in the last section of this chapter.

Another demographic that is common and associated with HS is the smoking population.[22] Some studies have suggested that patients who smoke are less responsive to therapy; however, evidence about whether smoking is associated with the pathogenesis of this skin disease is still non-definitive.

Socioeconomic Factors

Patients with hidradenitis suppurativa are affected by lower socioeconomic status than age and gender-matched controls in studies performed in the United States and in the Netherlands.[23,24] This status can affect management options, effective follow-up, and lead to a negative cycle of events including decreased work productivity, short- and long-term disability, and increased work absenteeism, all of which can result in cumulative life course impairment.

Clinicians should work closely with their patients to address factors that may be leading to inability to go to work. One of the most common factors associated with HS is pain associated with a patient's lesions. Patient may miss work due to inability to complete tasks without experiencing recurrent pain, and aggressive medical management is often essential to get pain under control.

Impact of Disease on Patient's Quality of Life

Assessing Socioeconomic Factors During Visits

HS is a chronic disease that can impact a patient's quality of life. Pain and drainage secondary to HS are often reported as reasons patients miss work. In clinical management, socioeconomic status should be assessed for its potential impact on patient care. Inquiry about the patient's occupation and the daily tasks they perform may yield important information about patients who miss work due to experiencing HS lesion pain and drainage, especially while doing physical work.

There are various healthcare resources for optimizing care in patients with low socioeconomic status, including offering free counseling services for weight loss, diet, and smoking cessation. Additionally, the physician can provide different online sources for patients to find low-cost wound dressings and medication discounts. When discussing management options with the patient, low health literacy should be taken into account with low socioeconomic status. The physician may provide an HS overview handout with simplified explanations and go over it with the patient during the initial visit.

Physicians can offer short-term treatment regimens in addition to maintenance therapy for patients to optimize their quality of life. In addition to medical management, physicians may be requested to provide letters of medical necessity on behalf of their patients to adjust their work tasks to lower the risk of HS-related pain and/or drainage. Requested changes may include changing the patient's work desk to a standing work desk if the patient reports HS-related pain secondary to HS lesion in the groin and buttocks region. Additionally, patients may benefit from having their work tasks spaced out if they include physical work, to prevent constant HS lesion-related pain.

Disability Secondary to Hidradenitis Suppurativa Disease

Patients may also seek disability status due to the effects of their disease. In a 2018 U.S. cohort study comparing patients with HS ($n = 1204$) to those without ($n = 6020$), patients with HS had statistically significant more disability-related costs and days missed from work compared to the control group.[25]

Physicians can collaborate with the patient's primary care doctor, who, in our practice, is usually the provider who corresponds with the patient when applying for disability. As mentioned in the previous section optimizing the patient's medical care can assist them in being able to improve their ability to go to work. Physicians can adjust a patient's medication regimen while the primary care doctor can determine whether the patient requires pain medication as well. It may take weeks to months to optimize the patient's medication regimen. Once this is achieved, the patient's pain medication can be gradually tapered.

Determining Management Options

Treatments Based on Hidradenitis Suppurativa Disease Level of Severity

The Hurley staging system and HS PGA scoring system can be used in combination for determining treatment options. The HS PGA scoring system is good for assessing the patient's current disease severity.

Patients with mild HS disease may only require topical treatment with maintenance or short-term antibiotic courses. Topical treatment options include clindamycin and clobetasol. Antibiotics used for maintenance include doxycycline, minocycline, and amoxicillin. Short-course antibiotic options includes Augmentin, which may used with a prednisone taper. Additionally, spironolactone is often used for patients with mild HS disease located predominantly in the groin region, which was discussed earlier in this chapter. Spironolactone can be used for females with perimenstrual HS flares. If pursuing this option, the clinician should make sure the patient is on some form of contraception due to the potential birth-defects associated with spironolactone. Low-androgen containing OCPs can also be used for patients with peri-menstrual flares.

Patients with moderate HS disease may be started on maintenance antibiotics with short-term intermittent prednisone taper based on HS flare frequency. Based on the Hurley staging, patients can also be transitioned to biologic therapy. Adalimumab is currently considered the first-line biologic for moderate-to-severe HS disease.[11] However, if patients do not respond to this biologic, the 40 mg/wk dosing can sometimes be increased off-label to 80 mg/wk. Patients should be aware that it can take a few months to determine treatment efficacy for each dose change. If patients report having HS flares that are uncontrolled with their current therapy, they can be offered intralesional kenalog injections at the affected lesion sites.

Patients with severe HS disease should be assessed for starting systemic therapy. Therapies to consider include adalimumab, infliximab, methotrexate, tofacitinib, and acitretin, among others. Adalimumab will generally be the first treatment choice followed by infliximab if adalimumab is not effective. Infliximab, can be increased to 10 mg/kg every 4 to 6 weeks if needed. Methotrexate is another treatment option for patients with persistent HS disease. Other biologics that are currently being studied for HS includes secukinumab and guselkumab. There are currently three clinical trials for secukinumab. Guselkumab is currently being studied in one clinical trial and two open-label studies for HS. Cases reported in the literature for secukinumab or guselkumab used dosing similar to psoriasis and demonstrated improvement.[26,27] Methotrexate has been shown to be more effective as monotherapy compared to being used with other systemic therapies for HS. Tofacitinib has been shown to work for some patients, but there is less long-term and large cohort evidence for supporting its use. Patients who have been unresponsive to common HS systemic therapies may respond to tofacitinib after several months. Acitretin is another systemic therapy option that is primarily used for patients with comedonal pattern to their HS disease.

Treatment Options Based on Patient's Comorbidities

Inflammatory bowel disease has been reported in patients with HS as a comorbidity. Patients who have Crohn's disease, for example, may be on infliximab or adalimumab for their condition at the time of initial HS evaluation. Since these biologics can also help their HS disease, they can be continued on this regimen and potentially have the dose and frequency increased if their disease does not improve. Another comorbidity to consider is PCOS. Patients may be placed on metformin, which may help their HS. Spironolactone is also used for hirsutism related to PCOS. Patients can be started at a low dose with gradual dose increase based on response.

Patient Co-Management with Other Specialties

Management of patients with HS often involves continued communication between the clinician and the patient's other providers. Multi-disciplinary care team may include surgical specialists, OB/GYNs, gastroenterologists, and primary care doctors. If a patient's treatment regimen is being changed, the clinician should notify the patient's other providers when this change may affect their other comorbidities.

Patient Follow-Up and Lab Monitoring

Treatment Initiation and Baseline Labs

Prior to starting biologic therapy, patients should obtain baseline labs. This includes complete blood count with differential, complete metabolic panel, tuberculosis test, hepatitis B and C panels, and HIV screening test (in patient populations determined to have baseline risk). For patients who will be starting spironolactone, potassium levels should be checked if they have risk factors for hyperkalemia, such as a cardiac comorbidity. Adalimumab serum trough levels and anti-drug antibodies detection are available for monitoring. However, these levels are not typically used in the routine clinical setting.

Abnormal Labs in Hidradenitis Suppurativa

Hidradenitis suppurativa presents with an inflammatory chronic state that can be seen in monitoring labs. Patients will often have elevated white blood cell (WBC) count, elevated platelet count, and/or low hemoglobin lab values on baseline labs. These lab results are all inflammatory markers that are also seen in other inflammatory chronic diseases. One way to evaluate infection versus chronic elevation is by comparing the patient's baseline and general WBC trends with the current WBC count. If there is a clinically significant increase in WBC count, then it may be important to further evaluate the patient for an underlying infection. Trending elevated platelet counts and low hemoglobin lab values also support the general pattern that accompanies elevated WBC count. If patient has other risk factors that could contribute to an elevated platelet count or low hemoglobin, these factors should be further evaluated.

Follow-Up Based on Current Treatment Regimen and Response

Patients should have follow-up visits based on their disease severity and current treatment regimen. Patients on systemic therapies should be seen more frequently to assess treatment response. At systemic therapy initiation, patients can be seen every 3 to 4 months followed by every 6 months after treatment response. Patients on maintenance therapy with stable disease can be seen every 6 months or sooner if needed for HS flares.

Monitoring According to Treatment Regimen and Comorbidities

Patients on systemic therapies require lab monitoring. It is recommended that patients undergo tuberculosis screening annually after starting immunosuppressive therapies. They should also be monitored for any signs of infection or malignancy for further evaluation. The clinician can perform an annual full-body skin exam for patients on biologic therapy for skin cancer screening, including evaluating for squamous cell cancer in severely affected HS lesions. Clinicians should continue collaborating with the patient's other providers for the patient's comorbidities. This includes notifying them of any pertinent treatment changes, such as changing the infliximab dose in a patient with Crohn's disease. Multidisciplinary care can optimize the patient's care by including everyone's input, including that of the HS clinician (dermatologist), patient, and other providers (i.e., patient's primary care doctor).

Since HS is a chronic skin condition, clinicians have the opportunity to develop a great rapport with their patients and ultimately become part of the patient's primary medical care follow-up.

Conclusion

HS has variable patient presentation, including age of onset and disease severity. Taking medical history is a major component of clinical evaluation and can help determine risk factors for flare, comorbidities, and inform treatment planning. The physical exam, in addition to the DLQI and pain assessments, provides a baseline assessment that ideally is reassessed at every visit in a standardized manner to evaluate treatment efficacy. Socioeconomic status and health literacy should be integrated into management planning and discussion in order for patients to receive optimal care. The dermatologist also can play an important role, providing management input for their patients in interdisciplinary team HS care. Follow-up depends on treatment choice, disease severity, and lab monitoring. HS management is a rewarding experience for clinicians, as it allows them to develop plans that greatly aid patients while developing long-term rapport.

References

1. Jemec GB. Clinical practice: hidradenitis suppurativa. N Engl J Med. 2012;366(2):158–164. https://doi:10.1056/NEJMcp1014163.
2. Garg A, Kirby JS, Lavian J, et al. Sex- and age-adjusted population analysis of prevalence estimates for hidradenitis suppurativa in the United States. JAMA Dermatol. 2017;153(8):760–764. https://doi:10.1001/jamadermatol.2017.0201.
3. Vaidya T, Vangipuram R, Alikhan A. Examining the race-specific prevalence of hidradenitis suppurativa at a large academic center; results from a retrospective chart review. Dermatol Online J. 2017;23(6). 13030/qt9xc0n0z1.
4. Saunte DM, Boer J, Stratigos A, et al. Diagnostic delay in hidradenitis suppurativa is a global problem. Br J Dermatol. 2015;173(6):1546–1549. https://doi:10.1111/bjd.14038.
5. Karagiannidis I, Nikolakis G, Sabat R, et al. Hidradenitis suppurativa/acne inversa: an endocrine skin disorder? Rev Endocr Metab Disord. 2016;17(3):335–341. https://doi:10.1007/s11154-016-9366-z.
6. Rils PT, Ring HC, Themstrup L, et al. The role of androgens and estrogens in hidradenitis suppurativa- a systematic review. Acta Dermatovenerol Croat. 2016;24:239–249.
7. Vossen AR, van Straalen KR, Prens EP, et al. Menses and pregnancy affect symptoms in hidradenitis suppurativa: a cross-sectional study. J Am Acad Dermatol. 2017;76:155–156. https://doi:10.1016/j.jaad.2016.07.024.
8. Ingram JR. The genetics of hidradenitis suppurativa. Dermatol Clin. 2016;34(1):23–28. https:doi:https://doi.org/10.1016/j.det.2015.07.002.
9. Pink AE, Simpson MA, Desai N, et al. Mutations in the γ-secretase genes NCSTN, PSENEN, and PSEN1 underlie rare forms of hidradenitis suppurativa (acne inversa). J Invest Dermatol. 2012;132 (10):2459–2461. https://doi:10.1038/jid.2012.162.
10. Hurley HJ. Axillary hyperhidrosis, apocrine bromhidrosis, hidradenitis suppurativa and familial benign pemphigus. Surgical approach. In: Roenigk RH, Roenigk Jr JJ, eds. Dermatol Surgery, Principles and Practice. 2nd ed. New York: Marcel Dekker; 1989:623–646.
11. Kimball AB, Kerdel F, Adams D, et al. Adalimumab for the treatment of moderate to severe Hidradenitis suppurativa: a parallel randomized trial. Ann Intern Med. 2012;157(12):846–855. https://doi:10.7326/0003-4819-157-12-201212180-00004.
12. Lipsker D, Severac F, Freysz M, et al. The ABC of hidradenitis suppurativa: a validated glossary on how to name lesions. Dermatology. 2016;232(2):137–142. https://doi:10.1159/000443878.
13. Ergun T. Hidradenitis suppurativa and the metabolic syndrome. Clin Dermatol. 2018;36(1):41–47. https://doi:10.1016/j.clindermatol.2017.09.007.
14. Shlyankevich J, Chen AJ, Kim GE, et al. Hidradenitis suppurativa is a systemic disease with substantial comorbidity burden: a chart-verified case-control analysis. J Am Acad Dermatol. 2014;71(6):1144–1150. https://doi:10.1016/j.jaad.2014.09.012.
15. Charrow A, Savage KT, Flood K, et al. Hidradenitis suppurativa for the dermatologic hospitalist. Cutis. 2019;104(5):276–280.
16. Alavi A, Anooshirvani N, Kim WB, et al. Quality-of-life impairment in patients with hidradenitis suppurativa: a Canadian study. Am J Clin Dermatol. 2015;16(1):61–65. https://doi:10.1007/s40257-014-0105-5.
17. Matusiak L, Sczech J, Kaaz K, et al. Clinical characteristics of pruritus and pain in patients with hidradenitis suppurativa. Acta Derm Venereol. 2018;98(2):191–194. https://doi:10.2340/00015555-2815.
18. Danby FW. Diet in the prevention of hidradenitis suppurativa (acne inversa). J Am Acad Dermatol. 2015;73(5 Suppl 1):S52–S54. https://doi:10.1016/j.jaad.2015.07.042.
19. Golbari NM, Porter ML, Kimball AB. Antiandrogen therapy with spironolactone for the treatment of hidradenitis suppurativa. J Am Acad Dermatol. 2019;8(1):114–119. https://doi:10.1016/j.jaad.2018.06.063.
20. AbbVie. Humira (adalimumab). [cited 2020 May 13]. https://www.accessdata.fda.gov/drugsatfda_docs/label/2011/125057s0276lbl.pdf.
21. Inc JB. Remicade (Infliximab). 2013. [cited 2020 May 13]. Available from: https://www.accessdata.fda.gov/drugatfda_docs/label/2018/103772s5385lbl.pdf.
22. Micheletti R. Tobacco smoking and hidradenitis suppurativa: associated disease and an important modifiable risk factor. Br J Dermatol. 2018;178(3):587–588.
23. Deckers IE, Janse IC, van der Zee, et al. Hidradenitis suppurativa (HS) is associated with low socioeconomic status (SES): a cross-sectional reference study. J Am Acad Dermatol, 2016;75(4):755–759.e1. https://doi:10.1016/j.jaad.2016.04.067.
24. Wertenteil S, Strunk A, Garg A. Association of low socioeconomic status with hidradenitis suppurativa in the United States. JAMA Dermatol. 2018;154(9):1086–1088. https://doi:10.1001/jamadermatol.2018.2117.
25. Tzellos T, Yang H, Mu F, et al. Impact of hidradenitis suppurativa on work loss, indirect costs and income. Br J Dermatol. 2019;181(11): 147–154. https://pubmed.ncbi.nlm.nih.gov/30120887/ https://doi.org/10.1111/bjd.17101
26. Marasca C, Megna M, Balato A, et al. Secukinumab and hidradenitis suppurativa: friends or foes? JAAD Case Rep. 2019;5(2):184–187. https://doi:10.1016/j.jdcr.2018.12.002.
27. Casseres RG, Kahn JS, Her MJ, et al. Guselkumab in the treatment of hidradenitis suppurativa: a retrospective chart review. J Am Acad Dermatol. 2019;81(1):265–267. https://doi:10.1016/j.jaad.2018.12.017.

8

Comorbidities and Systemic Associations

NEETA MALVIYA AND AMIT GARG

CHAPTER OUTLINE

Introduction

HS represents a prime candidate to bridge diseases of the integument and comorbid systemic disease, as a chronic inflammatory disease of the pilosebaceous unit characterized by inflammatory nodules, suppuration and abscess formation resulting in pain and disfigurement.[1] In addition to its locally destructive course, HS has gained recognition for its association with individual comorbid diseases[2] as well as all-cause mortality.[3] Indeed, patients with HS have been observed to have a higher global comorbidity burden than both healthy patients and patients with psoriasis.[2] Systemic disease states with Charlson Comorbidity Indices similar to HS include systemic lupus erythematosus,[4] dermatomyositis,[5] and ankylosing spondylitis.[6]

The chronic inflammatory state in HS may represent shared pathways yet to be characterized, which link HS to comorbid conditions. At present, biomarker expression in tissue and serum of HS patients appears complex and its description likely remains incomplete. Cytokine expression profiles in lesional skin have demonstrated increased levels of tumor necrosis factor (TNF), interleukin (IL)-1β, IL-6, IL-8, IL-10, IL-12, IL-17, and IL-23.[7-12] The serum of HS patients has also shown elevated levels of C-reactive protein, TNF, IL-17, and IL-6.[13-16]

Comorbid conditions observed to be associated with HS range across almost every organ system, from the skin to the gastrointestinal tract to the cardiovascular system (Fig. 8.1). HS symptoms may be the first to prompt patients to seek healthcare, providing an opportunity for comorbidity screening and the interdisciplinary management of HS patients with the goal of supporting overall health and clinical outcomes. Therefore, awareness of comorbid associations by physicians treating HS patients is highly relevant. This chapter includes an evidence-based summary of comorbid associations in HS. It is important to note that comorbidities in HS is a dynamic content area for which further evidence-based updates in the coming years may be necessary.

Associated Inflammatory Skin Diseases

Pyoderma Gangrenosum

Pyoderma gangrenosum (PG) is a neutrophilic dermatosis characterized by painful ulcerations with undermined and violaceous borders. This rare disorder can greatly impact quality of life and can cause significant morbidity in afflicted patients.[17,18] Both HS and PG exhibit intense neutrophilic predominant inflammation and have overlap in treatment modalities, including anti-TNF agents.[19,20] The cytokines IL-8 and IL-17, which are involved in promoting tissue neutrophilia, are overexpressed in both disorders.[21,22]

The prevalence of PG among patients with HS has ranged from 0.2% to 0.4% as compared to only 0.01% in patients without a diagnosis of HS. This represents prevalence of PG 18 times higher

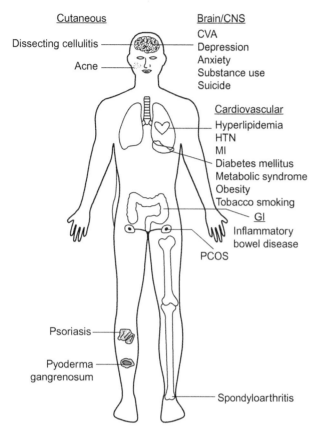

• **Fig. 8.1** Diagram of human body with organ systems highlighted and list of comorbidities associated with hidradenitis suppurativa. *CNS*, central nervous system; *CVA*, Cerebrovascular accident; *GI*, gastrointestinal; *HTN*, hypertension; *MI*, myocardial infarction; *PCOS*, polycystic ovarian syndrome.

in HS patients.[23,24] In addition, patients who have concomitant HS and Crohn's disease (CD) are more than 21 times as likely to have PG as compared to HS patients without comorbid CD.[23] The development of PG in HS patients typically occurs 2 to 19 years after HS diagnosis.[25,26] This may implicate ongoing immune dysregulation in HS patients which ultimately contributes to the development of PG. This is an area needing further investigation.

Psoriasis

Psoriasis is another chronic inflammatory disease of the skin with similar inflammatory mediators as HS, including TNF, IL-12, IL-23, IL-17.[6] Both diseases have also shown response to a similar profile of targeted therapies, including TNF-alpha, IL-17, and IL-12/23 inhibitors.[27-29] While the two disease phenotypes are vastly different, the overlap in inflammatory pathways may be due to a link between HS and psoriasis.

Evidence for the association between HS and psoriasis has been somewhat inconsistent in the literature. In a cross-sectional study with 68,836 psoriasis patients, the prevalence of HS was found to be significantly increased in the psoriasis group (0.3%) as compared to controls (0.2%).[30] A statistically significant association between HS and psoriasis was found in a multivariate analysis adjusting for smoking, obesity, healthcare utilization, and Charlson Comorbidity index.[30]

However, another large population-based study found no statistically significant difference in psoriasis prevalence. The prevalence of psoriasis among HS patients was 1.0%, whereas that among controls was 0.9%.[31] Additional studies are needed to confirm this association.

Associated Disorders of Follicular Occlusion

Acne Vulgaris and Acne Conglobata

Both acne vulgaris and HS are chronic inflammatory disorders involving the pilosebaceous unit. Acne conglobata refers to a more severe inflammatory variant which results in tender inflammatory nodules, and in some cases double comedones and sinus tract formation, which is also appreciated in HS. For this reason, HS is often also referred to as acne inversa. The prevalence of acne vulgaris/conglobata in patients with HS ranges from 4.5% to 15.2%, which is significantly higher than the prevalence noted in patients without HS (0.9% to 6.2%).[31-34] The odds of a patient with HS developing acne vulgaris/conglabata is up to 5 times higher than an individual without HS. While acne vulgaris and acne conglobata can often be treated with isotretinoin, there is limited therapeutic benefit of this medication as a monotherapy in HS.[35] A modified treatment approach should therefore be used in patients with both diseases.

Pilonidal Disease

Pilonidal disease is a chronic inflammatory disorder of the pilosebaceous unit resulting in abscesses, cysts, and/or sinus formation in the sacral region. There is considerable overlap in the clinical manifestations of this disorder with HS, perhaps pointing to common inflammatory pathways which likely contribute to their association with one another.

The prevalence of pilonidal disease in HS patients ranges from 1.4% to 2.3%, compared to 0.1% to 0.3% in non-HS patients. HS patients have 5 times the odds of developing pilonidal disease compared to non-HS patients.[33,34,36] There is some evidence to suggest that HS patients with more severe disease are more likely to have pilonidal disease compared to HS patients with milder disease.[32]

Dissecting Cellulitis of the Scalp

Dissecting cellulitis of the scalp (DCS) is a chronic inflammatory disorder of the pilosebaceous unit and is part of the follicular occlusion tetrad along with HS, acne conglobata, and pilonidal disease. DCS is characterized by pustules, abscesses, inflammatory nodules, and significant tunnel formation on the scalp that ultimately results in scarring of affected areas. Overlap among these four entities in the follicular occlusion tetrad may be the result of a common pathogenesis, for which the exact trigger remains to be elucidated. Hyperplasia and overactivity of the pilosebaceous unit is noted first, then followed by follicular occlusion, development of double-ended comedones, and bacterial colonization. Subsequent rupture of occluded follicles results in an inflammation response with suppuration and eventual tunneling with scarring.[37] This shared underlying proposed mechanism may be the basis for the association between HS and DCS. Some consider DCS to be a manifestation of HS involving the scalp.

The prevalence of DCS in patients with HS is 9.2%, compared to that of 0.7% in non-HS patients representing a 13-fold higher prevalence in HS patients.[33]

Associated Cardiovascular Disorders

Major Adverse Cardiovascular Events

Major adverse cardiovascular events (MACE) are the sum composite of myocardial infarction (MI), cerebrovascular accident (CVA), and cardiovascular mortality. This definition may vary to include heart failure, percutaneous coronary intervention, coronary artery bypass grafting, and all-cause mortality.[38] Both psoriasis and HS are inflammatory skin disorders that have been linked to a higher risk of MACE.[39-41] The association between HS and MACE is thought to be the result of an increased systemic inflammatory burden consisting of elevated circulating TNF and IL-6 that contribute to thrombosis, endothelial injury, and atherosclerosis.[15,42-45] HS patients have been observed to have a 23% increased risk of incident MI and a similar increase in risk for the development of CVA when compared to non-HS patients.[39] This is an adjusted risk that accounts for covariates related to MI and CVA; examples include obesity, hypertension, diabetes mellitus, and tobacco smoking.[39] The risk of cardiovascular-related death is higher in HS patients compared to that in severe psoriasis patients, which may point to a higher systemic inflammatory burden in HS patients, more severe involvement with disease covariates, or less robust control of these covariates.[40]

Hypertension

The importance of hypertension as a comorbidity lies in the damage it causes to the cardiovascular system with consequent impact on the heart, kidneys, and brain. In one study, the prevalence of hypertension among HS patients was 34%, compared to only 3% in non-HS patients.[46] After adjustments for age, sex, and smoking status, patients with HS were found to be twice as likely to have hypertension. However, not all studies have confirmed this association.[47] Most adult patients have their vitals screened at the start of the primary medical visit, and as such it is important to ensure HS patients are linked to a primary care provider for this type of screening, as well as many others.

Tobacco Smoking

Nicotine has been shown to induce infundibular epithelial hyperplasia and hyperkeratosis, alter the cutaneous microbiome, stimulate release of TNF by keratinocytes and Th17 cells, disturb polymorphic neutrophil granulocyte chemotaxis, and immunomodulate macrophage function.[48-52]

One study described "relaxation" and the "alleviation of negative feelings" as major motivators to smoke.[53] The high prevalence of anxiety and depression in this HS patient population may also contribute to tobacco use.

The prevalence of tobacco smoking in HS patients has been observed to be as high as 80%.[54-60] HS patients have four times greater odds of being active tobacco smokers and six times greater odds of having ever smoked.[61] In one study of 4 million tobacco smokers in the United States, a temporal relationship between smoking and the development of HS was established, suggesting that tobacco smoking could be a risk factor for HS.[54] While evidence supporting smoking cessation as a means to improve disease course is limited, reducing or eliminating tobacco exposures has proved beneficial for overall health.

Associated Metabolic Disorders

Metabolic Syndrome

Metabolic syndrome is an aggregation of multiple factors that contribute to an elevated risk of cardiovascular disease. There are multiple definitions for metabolic syndrome, with the primary components being truncal obesity, hypertension, dyslipidemia, and insulin resistance.[62] HS, like other chronic inflammatory diseases, has been linked to an increased prevalence of metabolic syndrome. The biological link between HS and metabolic syndrome may be explained by the downstream systemic effects of adipose tissue secretion of pro-inflammatory mediators in obesity, along with insulin resistance in the setting of chronic inflammation.[63-66]

In five studies, the prevalence of metabolic syndrome among HS patients ranges from 10.4% to 50.6%, compared to 7.1% to 30.2% among controls.[47,59,67-69] Pooled adjusted odds of metabolic syndrome among HS patients range from 1.8 to 2.2 times that of controls.[70,71]

Obesity

Obesity is defined as a body-mass index greater than 30 kg/m^2 and it is a significant risk factor in the development of comorbidities such as hypertension, type II diabetes, and coronary artery disease. While HS can affect people regardless of their BMI, it is predominantly seen in those who are overweight or obese. The connection between obesity and HS may be related to a higher systemic inflammatory burden from adipose tissue and/or from local factors such increased friction in intertriginous areas.

The prevalence of obesity among HS cohorts may be as high as 88%.[32,47,58,59,67,72] In a meta-analysis of 8 studies, HS patients were observed to have a 3.5-fold higher odds of being obese compared to patients without HS.[61]

The relationship between obesity and HS should not further stigmatize patients who are afflicted with HS. Given the negative impact of the condition on physical functioning, the authors acknowledge that HS may contribute to weight gain. There are also other risk factors likely to contribute to the development of HS. Indeed, there are numerous non-obese patients who also develop disease. Accordingly, it is essential that clinicians do not ascribe development of HS to obesity alone. We suggest approaching the topic of obesity in HS with the utmost sensitivity, only after establishing a patient-doctor relationship based on principles of empathy, trust, and overall health advocacy.

Type II Diabetes Mellitus

Type II diabetes mellitus results from insulin resistance over time and is linked to being overweight or obese. The association between diabetes and HS is thought to be multifactorial. A contributing factor may be TNF dysregulation, which leads to systemic insulin resistance by means of inhibiting the insulin receptor tyrosine kinase in muscle and fat, thereby preventing glucose uptake by these cells.[73]

The prevalence of diabetes mellitus among HS patients ranges from 7% to 24%.[31,59,68,74] Pooled odds ratios from several studies revealed that HS patients had 1.7 to 2.8 times the odds of having diabetes compared to patients without HS.[75,76] This risk is independent of covariates, including obesity, which potentially implicates shared underlying pathways between HS and diabetes.

Hyperlipidemia

Hyperlipidemia (HLD) is an umbrella term that encompasses a wide range of disorders resulting in elevated lipid levels in the blood and a doubled risk for cardiovascular disease. It is one of the components of the metabolic syndrome and has been consistently observed to be associated with HS.

The prevalence of dyslipidemia among HS patients ranges from 3.3% to 45.3%, as compared with 1.6 to 18.7% among controls.[24,31,33,46] In a meta-analysis of nine studies comprising

6174 HS patients, odds of hypertriglyceridemia and low HDL among HS patients were 1.7 (95% CI 1.1–2.5, $P = .009$) and 2.5 (95% CI 1.5–4.2, $P < .001$) times that of controls, respectively.[60]

Associated Endocrine Diseases

Polycystic Ovarian Syndrome

Polycystic ovarian syndrome (PCOS) is characterized by hyperandrogenism, ovulatory dysfunction, and polycystic ovaries seen on ultrasound. Both PCOS and HS have in common a similar demographic composition, link to obesity and metabolic syndrome, and response to anti-androgen therapy. However, increased androgen levels have not been reliably appreciated in HS.

The prevalence of PCOS among women with HS is as high as 9.0%.[77] Across studies, women with HS had 1.2 to 13.4 times the odds of having PCOS compared to controls.[31,33,71,77,78]

Associated Gastrointestinal Diseases

Inflammatory Bowel Disease

Similar to HS, inflammatory bowel disease (IBD), including ulcerative colitis (UC) and CD, is characterized by chronic, recurrent inflammation involving epithelia, which is inhabited by commensal flora. HS and CD are further characterized by suppuration and granulomatous inflammation, which may eventuate in fistula and sinus tract formation. Dysbiosis has been implicated as a cause of IBD as well as a cause of HS, which may also help to explain the link between IBD and HS.[79] These diseases may also share overlapping cytokine signatures, including IL-23/Th-17 and TNF, with response to corresponding targeted therapies.

There are a number of population-based studies that have evaluated the association between HS and IBD. In the largest study, the prevalence of CD among over 50,000 HS patients was 2%, compared to 0.6% among non-HS patients.[80] Adjusted odds of having CD among HS patients were three times that of controls.[80] In three other studies, prevalence of CD among HS patients ranged from 0.2% to 0.8%.[24,59,81] Among HS patients, the adjusted odds of having CD was 1.2 to 2.0 times that of controls.[24,59,81] The prevalence of UC among HS patients ranges from 0.3% to 1.3%. In adjusted analyses from three population-based studies, HS patients had 1.3 to 1.8 times the odds of UC compared to controls.[24,59,81]

Associated Musculoskeletal Diseases

Spondyloarthritis and HS appear to share key inflammatory mediators including TNF, IL-1, and IL-17, suggesting there may be a biological link between these two conditions.[8,82,83]

In a recent large cohort study, patients with HS had an increased risk for developing ankylosing spondylitis (incidence rate, 0.60 vs. 0.36 per 1000; HR, 1.65 [95% CI, 1.15–2.35]), psoriatic arthritis (incidence rate, 0.84 vs. 0.58 per 1000; HR, 1.44 [95% CI, 1.08–1.93]), and rheumatoid arthritis (incidence rate, 4.54 vs. 3.86 per 1000; HR, 1.16 [95% CI, 1.03–1.31]) compared to controls.[84]

In other studies, the prevalence of spondyloarthritis among HS patients ranged from 0.3% to 28% as compared with 0.2% to 2.6% among controls. The adjusted odds of spondyloarthritis among HS patients ranged from 1.5 to 9.4 times that of controls.[24,85]

Associated Psychiatric Diseases

Depression

Major depressive disorders are the number one cause of disability in the United States and worldwide, and it has significant impact on employment, school, and interpersonal relationships.[86] The connection between depression and HS may be linked to the significant disease-specific impact of HS on quality of life. However, there is also evidence to support a potential link via an increased immune system activation, as has been observed in cytokine-induced sickness behavior in which a high level of pro-inflammatory cytokines results in depression and loss of energy.[87]

The prevalence of depression among HS patients was calculated to be 21% from pooled data in a 2019 meta-analysis of 28 studies and analysis of case-control studies. HS patients had twice the likelihood of having depression compared to controls.[88] The prevalence of depression may be greater among patients with higher Hurley stages.[89]

Generalized Anxiety Disorder

Fear and unpredictability of pain, odor and discharge, as well as concern about the ability to participate in daily activities can lead to excessive worry among HS patients that may result in chronic functional impairment.

In a 2018 meta-analysis of 10 studies, the prevalence of Generalized Anxiety Disorder (GAD) among HS patients was approximately 5%.[90] Several retrospective clinical and administrative database studies have also described a higher prevalence and likelihood of anxiety among HS patients compared to controls.[33,91,92]

Substance Use Disorder

HS patients experience chronic pain and have significant physical, emotional and psychological disease impact which may increase risk for substance use disorder (SUD).

In a cross-sectional study of over 32,000 HS patients, the prevalence of SUD was 4.0%, which was significantly higher compared to 2.0% in controls.[93] The most common forms of SUD were alcohol (48% of SUD cases) opioids (33% of SUD cases).[93] HS patients had a 50% greater increase in risk of SUD compared to controls.[93] In a separate retrospective cohort study involving over 20,000 HS patients, the 1-year incidence of chronic opioid use (COU) among opioid-naïve HS patients was 0.3%, double that of controls.[94] In adjusted analysis, HS patients had a 50% greater risk of developing COU compared to the general population.[94] Given the significant impact of HS and the related risks of substance use, heightened awareness of potential abuses should be maintained with use of screening tools and referral as appropriate.

Completed Suicide

Data from European national registries indicate a higher incidence of completed suicide among HS patients. In Finland, the incidence of suicide was 4.4% among HS patients, with odds of suicide almost three times higher than in the general population.[72] In Denmark, HS patients were observed to have a suicide incidence of 0.3 per 1000 person-years, which translated to an adjusted risk of 2.4 times that of the general population.[92]

Associated Genetic Diseases

Down Syndrome

Expression of amyloid precursor protein (APP) is increased in Down syndrome (DS). In the epidermis, APP plays a role in stimulating keratinocyte adhesion, migration, and proliferation. In this way, DS patients may be prone to keratinocyte hyperproliferation and follicular plugging.

In a cross-sectional study of nearly 12,000 DS patients, the prevalence of HS was 2.1%, compared to 0.3% in controls. Patients with DS had five times the risk of HS (adjusted odds ratio 5.24 [95% CI 4.62–5.94]) compared to patients without DS.[95] Over 80% of DS patients had their HS diagnosed by age 29 years.[95] In a retrospective single-center study, the prevalence of HS among DS patients was 24%, compared to 0.5% among controls.[96]

Associated Inflammatory Syndromes

HS may be a component of rare genetic inflammatory syndromes, including pyoderma gangrenosum, acne and hidradenitis suppurativa (PASH) syndrome; pyoderma gangrenosum, acne vulgaris, hidradenitis suppurativa and ankylosing spondylitis (PASS) syndrome; pyogenic arthritis, PG, acne vulgaris, and hidradenitis suppurativa (PAPASH) syndrome; and psoriatic arthritis, pyoderma gangrenosum, acne, and hidradenitis suppurativa (PsAPASH) syndrome. These disorders arise from a disruption of the inflammasome and result in over-expression of IL-1 and TNF and a neutrophil predominant inflammation. A mutation in the PSTPIP1 gene is observed in PASH and PAPASH. For the other syndromes in this group, including PASS and PsAPASH, a specific mutation has not yet been identified. These HS-related syndromes underscore the importance of evaluating the constellation of symptoms and comorbid conditions which afflict HS patients.

Emerging Comorbidities

There have also been a number of additional observations of comorbid conditions in HS; examples include anemia,[97] nonalcoholic fatty liver disease,[98] obstructive sleep apnea,[99] thyroid disease,[100] and lymphomas.[23] However, at present, the quantity and/or quality of data does not support routine screening of HS patients for these disorders unless suggestive signs or symptoms in an individual patient are present to warrant further investigation.

Conclusion

There are a number of comorbid conditions that can afflict patients with HS and contribute to poor health and impaired quality of life, beyond the significant impact of the disease itself. The discussion in this chapter is intended to support health advocacy efforts along with comprehensive care strategies for HS patients. Based on evidence, the authors suggest interdisciplinary screening for comorbidities discussed herein. Dermatologists may examine the skin for cutaneous associations and consider streamlined approaches for management of HS and any associated skin conditions. Dermatologists may also perform a simple review of systems or screening laboratory tests for other comorbidities. However, given the large comorbidity burden among HS patients, dermatologists may best advocate for optimizing overall health by ensuring HS patients are linked to primary care. Primary care doctors should be prompted to screen for comorbid conditions that do not already fall within standards of care based on age and other risk factors.

While there have been significant advances in our understanding of HS comorbidities in recent years, several knowledge gaps still exist; examples include risk of squamous cell carcinoma and the influence of HS on pregnancy course and outcomes. There is also a need to identify which comorbid conditions afflict children and adolescents with HS. Additionally, little is known about disparate disease and comorbid outcomes across demographic groups. Study of health disparities is particularly important in HS, which disproportionately affects women and Black patients in the United States.[101] With identification of novel immune targets and the development of advanced therapeutic agents that effectively address inflammation in HS, there will be opportunity to also understand whether treatment of HS allows for better control of comorbid conditions or reduces risk of developing comorbid disease.

References

1. Hoffman LK, Ghias MH, Garg A, et al. Major gaps in understanding and treatment of hidradenitis suppurativa. *Semin Cutan Med Surg.* 2017;36(2):86–92.
2. Reddy S, Strunk A, Garg A. Comparative overall comorbidity burden among patients with hidradenitis suppurativa. *JAMA Dermatol.* 2019;155(7):797–802.
3. Reddy S, Strunk A, Garg A. All-cause mortality among patients with hidradenitis suppurativa: A population-based cohort study in the United States. *J Am Acad Dermatol.* 2019;81(4):937–942.
4. Lalani S, Pope J, de Leon F, et al. Clinical features and prognosis of late-onset systemic lupus erythematosus: results from the 1000 faces of lupus study. *J Rheumatol.* 2010;37(1):38–44.
5. Linos E, Fiorentino D, Lingala B, et al. Atherosclerotic cardiovascular disease and dermatomyositis: an analysis of the Nationwide inpatient sample survey. *Arthritis Res Ther.* 2013;15(1):R7.
6. Durcan L, Wilson F, Conway R, et al. Increased body mass index in ankylosing spondylitis is associated with greater burden of symptoms and poor perceptions of the benefits of exercise. *J Rheumatol.* 2012;39(12):2310–2314.
7. Schlapbach C, Hänni T, Yawalkar N, Hunger RE. Expression of the IL-23/Th17 pathway in lesions of hidradenitis suppurativa. *J Am Acad Dermatol.* 2011;65(4):790–798.
8. van der Zee HH, de Ruiter L, van den Broecke DG, et al. Elevated levels of tumour necrosis factor (TNF)-α, interleukin (IL)-1β and IL-10 in hidradenitis suppurativa skin: a rationale for targeting TNF-α and IL-1β. *Br J Dermatol.* 2011;164(6):1292–1298.
9. Bechara FG, Sand M, Skrygan M, et al. Acne inversa: evaluating antimicrobial peptides and proteins. *Ann Dermatol.* 2012;24(4):393–397.
10. Kelly G, Hughes R, McGarry T, et al. Dysregulated cytokine expression in lesional and nonlesional skin in hidradenitis suppurativa. *Br J Dermatol.* 2015;173(6):1431–1439.
11. Wolk K, Warszawska K, Hoeflich C, et al. Deficiency of IL-22 contributes to a chronic inflammatory disease: pathogenetic mechanisms in acne inversa. *J Immunol.* 2011;186(2):1228–1239.
12. Hotz C, Boniotto M, Guguin A, et al. Intrinsic defect in keratinocyte function leads to inflammation in hidradenitis suppurativa. *J Invest Dermatol.* 2016;136(9):1768–1780.
13. Matusiak L, Bieniek A, Szepietowski JC. Increased serum tumour necrosis factor-alpha in hidradenitis suppurativa patients: is there a basis for treatment with anti-tumour necrosis factor-alpha agents? *Acta Derm Venereol.* 2009;89(6):601–603.
14. Matusiak Ł, Szczęch J, Bieniek A, et al. Increased interleukin (IL)-17 serum levels in patients with hidradenitis suppurativa: Implications

for treatment with anti-IL-17 agents. *J Am Acad Dermatol.* 2017; 76(4):670–675.

15. Xu H, Xiao X, He Y, et al. Increased serum interleukin-6 levels in patients with hidradenitis suppurativa. *Postepy dermatologii i alergologii.* 2017;34(1):82–84.

16. Jiménez-Gallo D, de la Varga-Martínez R, Ossorio-García L, et al. The clinical significance of increased serum proinflammatory cytokines, C-reactive protein, and erythrocyte sedimentation rate in patients with hidradenitis suppurativa. *Mediators Inflamm.* 2017;2017:2450401.

17. Gerard AJ, Feldman SR, Strowd L. Quality of life of patients with pyoderma gangrenosum and hidradenitis suppurativa. *J Cutan Med Surg.* 2015;19(4):391–396.

18. Xu A, Balgobind A, Strunk A, et al. Prevalence estimates for pyoderma gangrenosum in the United States: an age- and sex-adjusted population analysis. *J Am Acad Dermatol.* 2020;83(2):425–429.

19. Blanco R, Martínez-Taboada VM, Villa I, et al. Long-term successful adalimumab therapy in severe hidradenitis suppurativa. *Arch Dermatol.* 2009;145(5):580–584.

20. Brooklyn TN, Dunnill M, Shetty A, et al. Infliximab for the treatment of pyoderma gangrenosum: a randomised, double blind, placebo controlled trial. *Gut.* 2006;55(4):505–509.

21. Frew JW, Hawkes JE, Krueger JG. A systematic review and critical evaluation of inflammatory cytokine associations in hidradenitis suppurativa. *F1000Research.* 2018;7:1930.

22. Marzano A, Fanoni D, Antiga E, et al. Expression of cytokines, chemokines and other effector molecules in two prototypic autoinflammatory skin diseases, pyoderma gangrenosum and S weet's syndrome. *Clini Exp Immunol.* 2014;178(1):48–56.

23. Tannenbaum R, Strunk A, Garg A. Overall and subgroup prevalence of pyoderma gangrenosum among patients with hidradenitis suppurativa: A population-based analysis in the United States. *J Am Acad Dermat.* 2019;80(6):1533–1537.

24. Lee JH, Kwon HS, Jung HM, et al. Prevalence and comorbidities associated with hidradenitis suppurativa in Korea: a nationwide population-based study. *J Eur Acad Dermatol Venereol.* 2018; 32(10):1784–1790.

25. Vural S, Gundogdu M, Kundakci N, Ruzicka T. Familial Mediterranean fever patients with hidradenitis suppurativa. *Int J Dermatol.* 2017;56(6):660–663.

26. Hsiao JL, Antaya RJ, Berger T, et al. Hidradenitis suppurativa and concomitant pyoderma gangrenosum: a case series and literature review. *Arch Dermatol.* 2010;146(11):1265–1270.

27. Maarouf M, Clark AK, Lee DE, Shi VY. Targeted treatments for hidradenitis suppurativa: a review of the current literature and ongoing clinical trials. *J Dermatol Treat.* 2018;29(5):441–449.

28. Thorlacius L, Theut Riis P, Jemec G. Severe hidradenitis suppurativa responding to treatment with secukinumab: a case report. *Br J Dermatol.* 2018;179(1):182–185.

29. Prussick L, Rothstein B, Joshipura D, et al. Open-label, investigator-initiated, single-site exploratory trial evaluating secukinumab, an anti-interleukin-17A monoclonal antibody, for patients with moderate-to-severe hidradenitis suppurativa. *Br J Dermatol.* 2019;181(3):609–611.

30. Kridin K, Shani M, Schonmann Y, et al. Psoriasis and hidradenitis suppurativa: a large-scale population-based study. *J Am Acad Dermatol.* 2018;S0190–9622(18). 32962–1.

31. Ingram JR, Jenkins-Jones S, Knipe DW, et al. Population-based clinical practice research datalink study using algorithm modelling to identify the true burden of hidradenitis suppurativa. *Br J Dermatol.* 2018;178(4):917–924.

32. Wertenteil S, Strunk A, Garg A. Overall and subgroup prevalence of acne vulgaris among patients with hidradenitis suppurativa. *J Am Acad Dermatol.* 2019;80(5):1308–1313.

33. Kimball AB, Sundaram M, Gauthier G, et al. The Comorbidity Burden of Hidradenitis Suppurativa in the United States: A claims data analysis. *Dermatol Ther.* 2018;8(4):557–569.

34. Yang JH, Moon J, Kye YC, et al. Demographic and clinical features of hidradenitis suppurativa in Korea. *J of Dermatol.* 2018;45(12): 1389–1395.

35. Boer J, van Gemert MJ. Long-term results of isotretinoin in the treatment of 68 patients with hidradenitis suppurativa. *J Am Acad Dermatol.* 1999;40(1):73–76.

36. Ingram JR, Jenkins-Jones S, Knipe D, et al. Population-based Clinical Practice Research Datalink study using algorithm modelling to identify the true burden of hidradenitis suppurativa. *Br J Dermatol.* 2018;178(4):917–924.

37. Chicarilli ZN. Follicular occlusion triad: hidradenitis suppurativa, acne conglobata, and dissecting cellulitis of the scalp. *Ann Plas Surg.* 1987;18(3):230–237.

38. Tsai I-T, Wang C-P, Lu Y-C, et al. The burden of major adverse cardiac events in patients with coronary artery disease. *BMC Cardiovasc Disord.* 2017;17(1):1.

39. Reddy S, Strunk A, Jemec GB, Garg A. Incidence of myocardial infarction and cerebrovascular accident in patients with hidradenitis suppurativa. *JAMA Dermatol.* 2020;156(1):65–71.

40. Egeberg A, Gislason GH, Hansen PR. Risk of major adverse cardiovascular events and all-cause mortality in patients with hidradenitis suppurativa. *JAMA Dermatol.* 2016;152(4):429–434.

41. Armstrong EJ, Harskamp CT, Armstrong AW. Psoriasis and major adverse cardiovascular events: a systematic review and meta-analysis of observational studies. *J Am Heart Assoc.* 2013;2(2):e000062.

42. Riis PT, Søeby K, Saunte DM, Jemec GB. Patients with hidradenitis suppurativa carry a higher systemic inflammatory load than other dermatological patients. *Arch Dermatol Res.* 2015;307(10): 885–889.

43. Libby P. Inflammation in atherosclerosis. *Nature.* 2002;420(6917): 868–874.

44. Hansson GK. Inflammation, atherosclerosis, and coronary artery disease. *N Engl J Med.* 2005;352(16):1685–1695.

45. Kimball AB, Okun MM, Williams DA, et al. Two phase 3 trials of Adalimumab for hidradenitis suppurativa. *N Engl J Med.* 2016; 375(5):422–434.

46. Shlyankevich J, Chen AJ, Kim GE, Kimball AB. Hidradenitis suppurativa is a systemic disease with substantial comorbidity burden: a chart-verified case-control analysis. *J Am Acad Dermatol.* 2014;71 (6):1144–1150.

47. Gold DA, Reeder VJ, Mahan MG, Hamzavi IH. The prevalence of metabolic syndrome in patients with hidradenitis suppurativa. *J Am Acad Dermatol.* 2014;70(4):699–703.

48. Ralf Paus L, Kurzen H, Kurokawa I, et al. What causes hidradenitis suppurativa? *Exp Dermatol.* 2008;17(5):455–456.

49. Durmaz R, Tekerekoğlu MS, Kalcioğlu T, Ozturan O. Nasal carriage of methicillin-resistant *Staphylococcus aureus* among smokers and cigarette factory workers. *New Microbiol.* 2001;24(2):143–147.

50. Jeong SH, Park JH, Kim JN, et al. Up-regulation of TNF-alpha secretion by cigarette smoke is mediated by Egr-1 in HaCaT human keratinocytes. *Exp Dermatol.* 2010;19(8):e206–e212.

51. Torii K, Saito C, Furuhashi T, et al. Tobacco smoke is related to Th17 generation with clinical implications for psoriasis patients. *Exp Dermatol.* 2011;20(4):371–373.

52. Mortaz E, Adcock IM, Ito K, et al. Cigarette smoke induces CXCL8 production by human neutrophils via activation of TLR9 receptor. *Eur Respir J.* 2010;36(5):1143–1154.

53. Deilhes F, Rouquet R, Gall Y, et al. Profile of smoking dependency in hidradenitis suppurativa patients and smoking cessation outcomes. *J Eur Acad Dermatol Venereol.* 2020.

54. Garg A, Papagermanos V, Midura M, Strunk A. Incidence of hidradenitis suppurativa among tobacco smokers: a population-based retrospective analysis in the USA. *Br J Dermatol.* 2018;178(3): 709–714.

55. König A, Lehmann C, Rompel R, Happle R. Cigarette smoking as a triggering factor of hidradenitis suppurativa. *Dermatol.* 1999; 198(3):261–264.

56. Revuz JE, Canoui-Poitrine F, Wolkenstein P, et al. Prevalence and factors associated with hidradenitis suppurativa: results from two case-control studies. *J Am Acad Dermatol.* 2008;59(4):596–601.

57. Akdogan N, Alli N, Uysal PI, et al. Visfatin and insulin levels and cigarette smoking are independent risk factors for hidradenitis suppurativa: a case–control study. *Arch Dermatol Res.* 2018;310(10): 785–793.

58. Theut Riis P, Pedersen O, Sigsgaard V, et al. Prevalence of patients with self-reported hidradenitis suppurativa in a cohort of Danish blood donors: a cross-sectional study. *Br J Dermatol.* 2019;180(4): 774–781.

59. Shalom G, Freud T, Harman-Boehm I, et al. Hidradenitis suppurativa and metabolic syndrome: a comparative cross-sectional study of 3207 patients. *Br J Dermatol.* 2015;173(2):464–470.

60. Schmitt JV, Bombonatto G, Martin M, Miot HA. Risk factors for hidradenitis suppurativa: a pilot study. *An Bras Dermatol.* 2012; 87(6):936–938.

61. Tzellos T, Zouboulis C, Gulliver W, et al. Cardiovascular disease risk factors in patients with hidradenitis suppurativa: a systematic review and meta-analysis of observational studies. *Br J Dermatol.* 2015;173(5):1142–1155.

62. Kassi E, Pervanidou P, Kaltsas G, Chrousos G. Metabolic syndrome: definitions and controversies. *BMC Med.* 2011;9(1):48.

63. de Winter K, van der Zee HH, Prens EP. Is mechanical stress an important pathogenic factor in hidradenitis suppurativa? *Exp Dermatol.* 2012;21(3):176–177.

64. Hotamisligil GS. Inflammation and metabolic disorders. *Nature.* 2006;444(7121):860–867.

65. Riis PT, Søeby K, Saunte D, Jemec G. Patients with hidradenitis suppurativa carry a higher systemic inflammatory load than other dermatological patients. *Arch Dermatol Res.* 2015;307(10):885–889.

66. Goossens GH. The role of adipose tissue dysfunction in the pathogenesis of obesity-related insulin resistance. *Physiology Behav.* 2008;94(2):206–218.

67. Sabat R, Chanwangpong A, Schneider-Burrus S, et al. Increased prevalence of metabolic syndrome in patients with acne inversa. *PloS one.* 2012;7(2), e31810.

68. Miller IM, Ellervik C, Vinding GR, et al. Association of metabolic syndrome and hidradenitis suppurativa. *JAMA Dermatol.* 2014;150 (12):1273–1280.

69. Loo CH, Tan WC, Tang JJ, et al. The clinical, biochemical, and ultrasonographic characteristics of patients with hidradenitis suppurativa in Northern Peninsular Malaysia: a multicenter study. *Int J Dermatol.* 2018;57(12):1454–1463.

70. Rodríguez-Zuñiga MJM, García-Perdomo HA, Ortega-Loayza AG. Association between hidradenitis suppurativa and metabolic syndrome: a systematic review and meta-analysis. *Actas Dermosifiliogr.* 2019;110(4):279–288.

71. Phan K, Charlton O, Smith SD. Hidradenitis suppurativa and diabetes mellitus: updated systematic review and adjusted meta-analysis. *Clin Exp Dermatol.* 2019;44(4):e126–e132.

72. Tiri H, Huilaja L, Jokelainen J, et al. Women with hidradenitis suppurativa have an elevated risk of suicide. *J Invest Dermatol.* 2018; 138(12):2672–2674.

73. Hotamisligil GS, Budavari A, Murray D, Spiegelman BM. Reduced tyrosine kinase activity of the insulin receptor in obesity-diabetes. Central role of tumor necrosis factor-alpha. *J Clinical Invest.* 1994;94(4):1543–1549.

74. Garg A, Birabaharan M, Strunk A. Prevalence of type 2 diabetes mellitus among patients with hidradenitis suppurativa in the United States. *J Am Acad Dermatol.* 2018;79(1):71–76.

75. Bui T-L, Silva-Hirschberg C, Torres J, Armstrong AW. Hidradenitis suppurativa and diabetes mellitus: A systematic review and meta-analysis. *J Am Acad Dermatol.* 2018;78(2):395–402.

76. Phan K, Charlton O, Smith S. Hidradenitis suppurativa and diabetes mellitus: updated systematic review and adjusted meta-analysis. *Clinical and experimental dermatology.* 2019;44(4):e126–e132.

77. Garg A, Neuren E, Strunk A. Hidradenitis suppurativa is associated with polycystic ovary syndrome: a population-based analysis in the United States. *J Invest Dermatol.* 2018;138(6):1288–1292.

78. Phan K, Charlton O, Smith SD. Hidradenitis suppurativa and polycystic ovarian syndrome: Systematic review and meta-analysis. *Australas J Dermatol.* 2020;61(1):e28–e33.

79. van der Zee HH, Horvath B, Jemec GB, Prens EP. The association between hidradenitis suppurativa and Crohn's disease: in search of the missing pathogenic link. *J Invest Dermatol.* 2016;136(9): 1747–1748.

80. Garg A, Hundal J, Strunk A. Overall and subgroup prevalence of Crohn disease among patients with hidradenitis suppurativa: a population-based analysis in the United States. *JAMA Dermatol.* 2018;154(7):814–818.

81. Egeberg A, Jemec GBE, Kimball AB, et al. Prevalence and risk of inflammatory bowel disease in patients with hidradenitis suppurativa. *J Invest Dermatol.* 2017;137(5):1060–1064.

82. Monnet D, Kadi A, Izac B, et al. Association between the IL-1 family gene cluster and spondyloarthritis. *Ann Rheum Dis.* 2012;71 (6):885–890.

83. Dougados M, Baeten D. *Spondyloarthritis Lancet.* 2011;377(9783): 2127–2137.

84. Schneeweiss MC, Kim SC, Schneeweiss S, et al. Risk of inflammatory arthritis after a new diagnosis of hidradenitis suppurativa. *JAMA dermatology.* 2020;156(3):342–345.

85. Fauconier M, Reguiai Z, Barbe C, et al. Association between hidradenitis suppurativa and spondyloarthritis. *Joint Bone Spine.* 2018; 85(5):593–597.

86. James SL, Abate D, Abate KH, et al. Global, regional, and national incidence, prevalence, and years lived with disability for 354 diseases and injuries for 195 countries and territories, 1990–2017: a systematic analysis for the Global Burden of Disease Study 2017. *Lancet.* 2018;392(10159):1789–1858.

87. Lee C-H, Giuliani F. The role of inflammation in depression and fatigue. *Front Immunol.* 2019;10:1696.

88. Jalenques I, Ciortianu L, Pereira B, et al. The prevalence and odds of anxiety and depression in children and adults with hidradenitis suppurativa: systematic review and meta-analyses. *J Am Acad Dermatol.* 2020;83(2):542–553.

89. Onderdijk AJ, van der Zee HH, Esmann S, et al. Depression in patients with hidradenitis suppurativa. *J Eur Acad Dermatol Venereol.* 2013;27(4):473–478.

90. Machado MO, Stergiopoulos V, Maes M, et al. Depression and anxiety in adults with hidradenitis suppurativa: a systematic review and meta-analysis. *JAMA Dermatol.* 2019;155(8):939–945.

91. Huilaja L, Tiri H, Jokelainen J, et al. Patients with Hidradenitis suppurativa have a high psychiatric disease burden: a Finnish nationwide registry study. *J Invest Dermatol.* 2018;138(1):46–51.

92. Thorlacius L, Cohen AD, Gislason GH, et al. Increased suicide risk in patients with hidradenitis suppurativa. *J Invest Dermatol.* 2018;138(1):52–57.

93. Garg A, Papagermanos V, Midura M, et al. Opioid, alcohol, and cannabis misuse among patients with hidradenitis suppurativa: a population-based analysis in the United States. *J Am Acad Dermatol.* 2018;79(3):495–500. e491.

94. Reddy S, Orenstein LAV, Strunk A, Garg A. Incidence of long-term opioid use among opioid-naive patients with hidradenitis suppurativa in the United States. *JAMA Dermatol.* 2019;155(11):1284–1290.

95. Garg A, Strunk A, Midura M, et al. Prevalence of hidradenitis suppurativa among patients with Down syndrome: a population-based cross-sectional analysis. *Br J Dermatol.* 2018;178(3):697–703.

96. Sechi A, Guglielmo A, Patrizi A, et al. Disseminate recurrent folliculitis and hidradenitis suppurativa are associated conditions: results from a retrospective study of 131 patients with Down syndrome and a cohort of 12,351 pediatric controls. *Dermatol Pract Concept.* 2019;9(3):187–194.

97. Soliman YS, Chaitowitz M, Hoffman LK, et al. Identifying anaemia in a cohort of patients with hidradenitis suppurativa. *J Eur Acad Dermatol Venereol.* 2020;34(1):e5–e8.
98. Durán-Vian C, Arias-Loste MT, Hernández JL, et al. High prevalence of non-alcoholic fatty liver disease among hidradenitis suppurativa patients independent of classic metabolic risk factors. *J Eur Acad Dermatol Venereol.* 2019;33(11):2131–2136.
99. Wertenteil S, Strunk A, Garg A. Incidence of obstructive sleep apnoea in patients with hidradenitis suppurativa: a retrospective population-based cohort analysis. *Br J Dermatol.* 2018;179(6):1398–1399.
100. González-López MA, Hernández JL, Vilanova I, et al. Thyroid autoimmunity in patients with hidradenitis suppurativa: a case-control study. *Clin Exp Dermatol.* 2017;42(6):642–644.
101. Garg A, Kirby JS, Lavian J, et al. Sex- and age-adjusted population analysis of prevalence estimates for hidradenitis suppurativa in the United States. *JAMA Dermatol.* 2017;153(8):760–764.

9

Disease Complications

MARIA ALESHIN AND JENNIFER HSIAO

CHAPTER OUTLINE

Introduction

Over time, repeated episodes of hidradenitis suppurativa (HS) disease flares can lead to a number of debilitating cutaneous, systemic, as well as psychological and social complications. Given the progressive course of this disease, early diagnosis and initiation of appropriate treatment is critical to limiting the development of serious complications.

Cutaneous Complications

The typical skin lesions associated with HS include tender subcutaneous nodules and sterile abscesses; however, long term, poorly controlled disease can lead to cutaneous complications including sinus tracts, fistulas, lymphedema, scarring/contractures, and squamous cell carcinomas (SCC).

Sinus Tracts

Sinus tracts are advanced HS lesions that manifest as subcutaneous tunnels that often drain malodorous discharge and can coalesce to form large areas of honeycombing under the skin (Fig. 9.1).[1] The development of sinus tracts may result from the connection of multiple ruptured follicles over time.[2] The presence or absence of, as well as the extent of, sinus tract formation is used to help determine the severity of disease. Patients with at least one sinus tract are automatically staged Hurley Stage II disease, whereas the presence of multiple interconnected sinus tracts are staged Hurley Stage III disease. However, not all sinus tracts can be visualized or detected by manual palpation, suggesting that a subset of patients may be incorrectly classified as having lower stage disease and undertreated as a result. Ultrasound imaging can help detect subclinical lesions

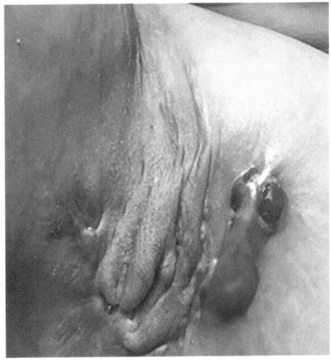

• **Fig. 9.1** Sinus tracts in the right axilla. (Photo credit: Jennifer Hsiao MD.)

and be used as a tool to more accurately stage patients and aid in management.[2]

Although biologics have been reported to help aid in the closure of some sinus tracts,[3] most patients require surgical intervention for definitive treatment. If extensive surgery of the perineal/perianal area is being considered, preoperative magnetic resonance imaging (MRI) is recommended to rule out the presence of anal fistulas. Wide surgical excision provides a low rate of recurrence, however, extensive surgery often requires general anesthesia and can be associated with postoperative pain and contractures.[4] Deroofing is a tissue-sparing technique that can be utilized in cases where wide excision may result in significant complications and/or burden.

Fistulas

A fistula is defined as an abnormal connection between two epithelial-lined surfaces and can occur as a complication after surgery, infection, or from chronic inflammatory conditions such as inflammatory bowel disease and HS. Anal and urethrocutaneous fistulas can occur in patients with chronic, poorly controlled anogenital HS. An anal fistula is an abnormal tract between the perianal skin and the anal canal, whereas a urethrocutaneous fistula is an abnormal tract between the skin and the urethra.

Anal fistulas should be suspected in any patient with HS that has persistent perianal pain and draining of purulent or bloody discharge from a sinus opening near the anal orifice.[5] If an anal fistula is suspected, an MRI of the anogenital region should be obtained to confirm the diagnosis. For example, if Crohn's disease is on the differential, further imaging may be needed to characterize the type of fistula as this could determine treatment.

Anal fistulas are often resistant to medical therapy and require surgical intervention. A multidisciplinary approach involving a colorectal surgeon is recommended. Various surgical techniques have been described depending on the complexity and extent of the fistula. See Chapter 23 for a discussion on operating room-based surgical procedures. Simple inter-sphincteric or low trans-sphincteric anal fistulas can be managed with a fistulotomy or fistulectomy.[6] A fistulotomy (similar to de-roofing of a sinus tract) involves "laying open" the fistula tract. A probe is inserted into the tract and an incision is made over the entire length of the fistula. The tract is then curetted to prevent recurrence and allowed to heal by secondary intent. During a fistulectomy, the entire fistulous tract is cut out. More complex anal fistulas, including trans-sphincteric or supra-sphincteric fistulas, have increased risk of fecal incontinence with surgical intervention.[6] A modified seton procedure, which involves dissecting out the fistula tract while preserving the anal sphincter muscle, has been used to manage patients with HS with complex anal fistulas. This procedure, in conjunction with excision of remaining HS affected tissue, has been used to successfully manage complex anogenital HS disease with anal fistulas.[6]

Urethrocutaneous fistulas are much rarer complications of HS, with fewer than ten cases reported in the literature.[7,8] A urethrocutaneous fistula should be suspected if a patient has difficulty passing urine or experiences leaking of urine during micturition. An ascending urethrogram should be obtained if a urethrocutaneous fistula is suspected. Once diagnosis is confirmed, a multidisciplinary treatment approach involving a urologist is recommended.

Lymphedema

Lymphedema is characterized by soft tissue swelling that occurs when lymph fluid is unable to drain due to blockade or destruction of local lymphatics. It commonly occurs on the arms and legs, but can affect every part of the body, including the genitals (Fig. 9.2). Genital lymphedema is a rare and debilitating complication of long-standing HS and can lead to recurrent infections, ulceration, increased risk of malignancy, as well as significant psychosocial morbidity.[9-11]

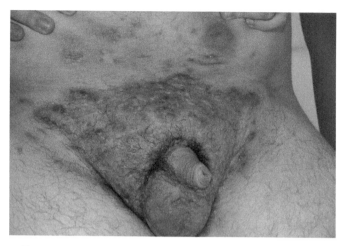

• **Fig. 9.2** Lymphedema of pubic and inguinal regions associated with HS. (Reprinted from, Musumeci ML, Scilletta A, Sorci F, et al. Genital lymphedema associated with hidradenitis suppurativa unresponsive to adalimumab treatment. *JAAD Case Rep.* 2019;5[4]:326–328 with permission from Elsevier.)

A systematic review of 27 patients with HS found that men have a higher incidence of lymphedema than women, with the scrotum (59%) and penis (44%) most frequently affected, followed by the labia majora (15%), perineum (11%), groin (11%), buttocks (7%), and rarely the abdomen (4%). Interestingly, all cases only involved the lower part of the body. Over 20% of patients had more than 2 locations affected.[9] Typically, lymphedema is thought to occur in patients with long-standing HS; however, rapid progression of lymphedema occurring after 3 to 4 years from disease onset has been reported, suggesting that lymphedema may not only be a complication of chronic HS, but also of aggressive HS.[12]

Clinically, lymphedema presents with swelling of the skin, frequently with overlying induration characterized by a "woody appearance." A severe variant of scrotal lymphedema, scrotal elephantiasis, has been described in patients with filariasis, following inguinal node irradiation or surgical lymphatic destruction, and rarely in patients with HS.[13,14] Scrotal elephantiasis is characterized by massive scrotal swelling with gross genital deformation, oftentimes presenting with obscuration of the penis.[15]

Lymphatic obstruction can also cause lymphangiectasias (dilated superficial lymphatic channels) which manifests as clear vesicles on an indurated plaque and is common on scrotal skin or the labia majora in HS patients with genital lymphedema.[9,16] Verrucous papules, plaques, and nodules can also be present. Providers should have a low threshold to biopsy these polypoid lesions as they can mimic verrucous carcinoma and SCC.[9]

Lymphedema is often managed with physical compression; however, this is not practical for managing lymphedema of the anogenital area, given the technical limitations associated with adequately compressing this area. Patients also often have insufficient response to medical therapy including oral antibiotics, oral corticosteroids, acitretin, and biologic therapy.[9,10,16-18] Surgical intervention is often required with removal of the affected tissue and superficial lymphatics, followed by various methods to cover the surgical defects. Split-thickness skin grafts are most often used, followed by skin flaps, and lastly healing by secondary intention.[9,11] Overall, patients have favorable responses to surgical intervention with adverse events (including penile edema, wound breakdown, and cellulitis) reported in 14% of patients.[9] Carbon dioxide (CO_2) laser excision with secondary-intention healing has also been reported in the literature to successfully treat genital HS lesions with associated lymphedema.[18]

Scarring, Contractures, and Mobility Limitations

Scarring is a common complication seen in patients with HS. Recurrent episodes of inflammation followed by wound healing lead to scar formation, which can cause significant physical symptoms and limitations as well as psychological symptoms in patients with HS.[19]

Inflammatory HS lesions typically heal with different types of scars, including atrophic and hypertrophic scars. Atrophic scars present as shallow, indented, dyspigmented papules, and plaques, while hypertrophic scars present as firm plaques or rope-like bands that can involve entire anatomic locations in severe cases. Keloids can also occur in HS patients prone to keloid formation (see Fig. 9.3).[20-22]

Scar formation is not only disfiguring and painful but can also lead to limb contractures and reduced mobility, especially in the groin and axillae.[1,22] Scarring in the anogenital area can predispose to stricture formation of the urethra, anus, and rectum. A stricture is an abnormal narrowing of a body passage which can occur secondary to scar tissue. Patients with strictures can present with difficulty or pain with defecation and/or urination.[1] A thorough history and physical exam is necessary to assess for physical deformity and functional limitations related to scarring, contractures, and strictures, especially in patients with chronic, severe disease.[22]

Scarring can have a profound emotional impact on patients with HS. Patients may feel embarrassed about the appearance of visible scars and feel compelled to hide them by wearing long-sleeved clothing and may limit certain activities such as swimming. The pursuit of new intimate relationships is also seen as a great burden in patients with scarring secondary to HS.[23]

In order to prevent the physical and psychological complications associated with scarring in HS patients, early and aggressive treatment is needed. Once scarring and contractures form, medical management is often insufficient. Although intralesional triamcinolone injections may help flatten some hypertrophic scars, definitive treatment often requires surgical intervention. Fractional CO_2 lasers have also shown efficacy in the treatment of many different types of scars, including HS-related scarring.[24,25] Patients who are prone to developing keloids may require additional adjunct treatments, including a trial of biologic therapy and or/ intralesional triamcinolone injections.[20]

Cutaneous Squamous Cell Carcinoma

SCC is a rare, yet serious complication of chronic HS, with studies showing a prevalence rate ranging from <1% to 4.6%.[26,27] Although HS is three times more common in women,[26] SCC much more commonly occurs in men, which may be attributed to the higher burden of disease men experience in the perianal/perineal area. HS-associated SCC typically presents in the gluteal and perianal region (Fig. 9.4), though cases involving the perineal, vulvar, groin, thighs, and sacrum have been described.[26,28] Interestingly, SCC of the axillary area is rarely seen, which suggests regional factors may play a role in the formation of SCC.

HS-associated SCC can be referred to as a Marjolin ulcer, a cutaneous malignancy that arises in chronically inflamed wounds or scarred tissue.[29] A review of 85 cases of SCC arising in patients with HS found the average age at time of diagnosis of SCC was 52 years. The latency period between onset of HS and SCC

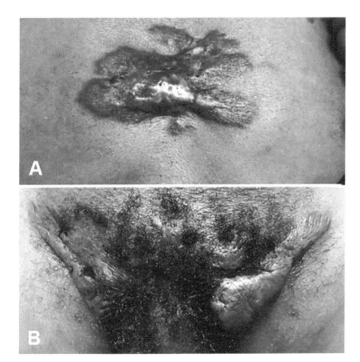

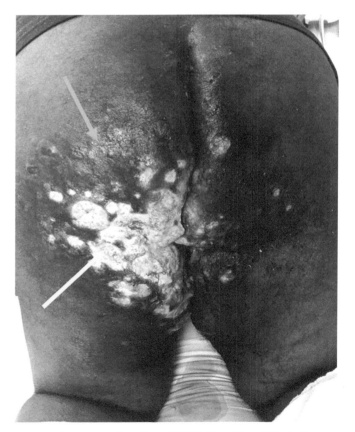

• **Fig. 9.3** Keloids in the mid chest (A) and bilateral inguinal region (B). (Reprinted from, Jfri A, O'Brien E, Alavi A, Goldberg SR. Association of hidradenitis suppurativa and keloid formation: A therapeutic challenge. *JAAD Case Rep.* 2019:675–678 with permission from Elsevier.)

• **Fig. 9.4** Squamous cell carcinoma (SCC) in the setting of hidradenitis suppurativa, blue arrow shows chronic scarring, yellow arrow shows indurated nodules and ulcerations consistent with SCC. (Reprinted from Giesey R, Delost GR, Honaker J, Korman NJ, Metastatic squamous cell carcinoma in a patient treated with adalimumab for hidradenitis suppurativa. *JAAD Case Rep.* 2017;3[6]:489–491, with permission from Elsevier.)

development was 26 years.[26] However, a case developing after only 3 years of active HS has been reported in the literature.[30]

Chronic inflammation and scarring in HS lesions predispose to SCC formation. Other possible contributing risk factors include tobacco exposure and human papillomavirus (HPV) infection. In a retrospective review of 80 cases of SCC complicating HS, 80% of patients reported tobacco use.[31] Similarly, a study by Lavogiez et al. found that a significant number (10 out of 13) of patients with HS that were heavy smokers (>30 pack-year history) developed SCC.[32] HPV is a known risk factor for the development of anogenital SCC, independent of HS. It has been hypothesized that a similar association may exist for HS-related SCC. Lavogiez et al. found HPV in all eight cases of SCC-related HS, with seven of eight cases identified as high-risk HPV. In contrast, no cases of HPV were detected by Kohorst et al. looking at 12 patients with HS-related SCC.[33] Importantly, many of the biologic agents used to treat HS, such as tumor necrosis factor (TNF) alpha inhibitors, may also increase patient risk for reactivating latent infections, such as HPV. Further studies are needed to better elucidate a possible relationship between HPV and HS-related SCC.

Clinically, any nonhealing, ulcerative, or indurated lesion forming within a chronic wound or scar should raise suspicion for an SCC. SCC in chronic HS can also present with localized pain, which can make it challenging to distinguish from an inflammatory lesion of HS. Therefore, a low threshold for biopsy of any suspicious lesion is recommended.[26] Multiple biopsies are often needed to diagnose SCC; therefore, if clinical suspicion is high, a repeat biopsy is recommended. A case reported in 1964 described a case of SCC that was missed with the initial 7 biopsies.[34]

Although histologically the majority of SCCs arising in HS patients are characterized as well- or moderately-differentiated, these SCCs tend to be more aggressive and have an increased risk of metastasis and mortality.[31] Patients can present with nodal metastasis at time of SCC diagnosis,[32,33] and mortality rates up to 50% to 60% have been reported,[27,28,33] suggesting early detection and aggressive intervention are required.

Once a diagnosis of a SCC is made, a multidisciplinary treatment approach including medical and surgical oncology is recommended. Prior to surgery, imaging with MRI or positron emission tomography (PET) scans may be helpful in establishing the extent of disease. A large and deep surgical excision with a minimum margin of 2 cm is recommended. Sentinel lymph node evaluation should be considered given the high prevalence of lymph node metastasis at time of diagnosis. Furthermore, adjuvant radiotherapy under the care of a radiation oncologist should be considered in select cases.[31] Despite aggressive surgical intervention, recurrence rates of these SCCs are high, necessitating close surveillance.[33]

Systemic Complications

The chronic, inflammatory nature of HS can predispose to multiple systemic complications including anemia, systemic amyloidosis/nephrotic syndrome, serious infection/sepsis, and chronic pain. As with cutaneous complications, early recognition and management of HS is needed to prevent these complications (Table 9.1).

Anemia

Anemia of chronic inflammation is a known complication of various chronic inflammatory conditions such as inflammatory bowel disease and rheumatoid arthritis. HS is also a chronic inflammatory condition; however, studies investigating anemia in HS patients are limited and at times conflicting, suggesting additional investigational studies are needed. The first report examining anemia in HS patients was published in 1968 by Tennant et al. who described the occurrence of severe anemia (hemoglobin [Hgb] <10.0g/100cc) in 10 out of 42 (24%) patients with severe HS with another 10 patients having milder anemia.[35] In 2016, a large Danish population-based study did not find an increased prevalence of anemia in HS patients compared to controls, but did detect a significant negative correlation between Sartorius score and hemoglobin level.[36]

A retrospective analysis conducted in the United States on 1431 patients with HS found that HS patients were 2.2 times more likely to be anemic compared to controls. When evaluating genders individually, male HS patients were found to be 5.61 times (and female patients 1.86 times) more likely to be anemic compared to controls. There was a negative correlation between hemoglobin and erythrocyte sedimentation rate (ESR), an acute phase reactant, meaning that patients with increased ESR were likely to have more severe anemia. Not surprisingly, both male and female patients with more severe disease (Hurley stage III) had significantly lower hemoglobin levels compared to patients with milder disease (Hurley stage I).[37] This suggests that at least one component of anemia seen in HS patients may be attributable to inflammation.

It is important to remember that causes of anemia may be multi-factorial and HS patients may also have a component of iron-deficiency anemia.[38] Soliman et al. investigated 661 patients with HS and found that 12.9% of male and 17.8% of female HS patients had microcytic anemia (compared to 8.8% of male and 4.8% of female control patients).[38] Thus, iron deficiency may be an underrecognized component of anemia in HS patients. The etiology of iron-deficiency anemia in HS is unclear but may be related to persistent drainage from HS lesions, menstrual loss in women of child-bearing age,[22,39] gastrointestinal (GI) blood loss from HS associated Crohn's disease, as well as blood loss from peptic ulcers in patients taking chronic nonsteroidal anti-inflammatory drugs (NSAIDs) for pain management.[22]

Patients with clinical signs or symptoms of anemia including fatigue, weakness, pallor, dizziness, lightheadedness, shortness of breath, and tachycardia, should undergo a thorough work-up to determine the cause of anemia. If GI-related causes of anemia are suspected, a multidisciplinary approach including the patient's primary care provider and gastroenterologist is recommended for further work-up and treatment.

Treatment of anemia of chronic inflammation requires managing the underlying inflammation associated with HS. If there is evidence of concurrent iron-deficiency anemia, iron supplementation should be considered. When selecting potential therapies for HS, caution should be used with treatments such as dapsone, which may worsen anemia.

Systemic Amyloidosis and Nephrotic Syndrome

Systemic amyloid A (AA) amyloidosis is a complication that can occur secondary to chronic inflammatory diseases such as rheumatoid arthritis, juvenile idiopathic arthritis, inflammatory bowel disease, and chronic infections. It is characterized by the extracellular tissue deposition of fibrils originating from fragments of serum amyloid A (SAA), an acute phase reactant produced by the liver. Although any organ can be affected, the kidneys are most often involved. Renal complications occur when SAA is deposited in the glomeruli, initially manifesting as asymptomatic proteinuria.

TABLE 9.1 Summary of HS Complications

Cutaneous Complications	Description	Management
Sinus tracts	• Subcutaneous tunneling wounds that can drain pus • Associated with moderate to severe HS • May be subclinical and require ultrasound imaging for detection	• Surgical excision or deroofing procedure
Anal and urethrocutaneous fistulas	• Anal fistula—abnormal tract between perianal skin and anal canal • Suspect in patient with perianal pain and persistent drainage or discharge • Urethrocutaneous fistula—abnormal tract between skin and urethra • Suspect in patient with difficulty passing urine or leaking of urine during micturition	• Surgical treatment based on complexity/extent of fistulas • Fistulotomy, fistulectomy, modified seton procedure • Multidisciplinary treatment approach with urology
Lymphedema	• Presents with swelling of the skin with overlying induration and "woody appearance" • Can see overlying verrucous papules, plaques, nodules • Lymphangiectasias (dilated superficial lymphatic channels) present with clear vesicles on an indurated plaque • Scrotal elephantiasis—massive scrotal swelling with gross genital deformation	• Surgical intervention with removal of affected tissue and superficial lymphatic channels • Carbon dioxide laser excision with marsupialization • Low threshold to biopsy polypoid lesions as they can mimic SCC
Scarring, limb contractures and mobility limitations	• Caused by recurrent episodes of inflammation followed by wound healing • Atrophic scars – shallow, indented, dyspigmented papules and plaques • Hypertrophic scars – fibrotic rope-like bands • Limb contractures can develop and impair mobility • Scarring in the anogenital area can predispose to strictures of the urethra, anus, and rectum	• Intralesional triamcinolone • Surgical excision
Cutaneous SCC	• More common in men and in gluteal/perianal skin • Risk factors: chronic inflammation and scarring, smoking, HPV infection • Histologically, most HS-related SCCs are well or moderately differentiated; however, clinically, these SCCs are more aggressive and have increased risk of metastasis and mortality • Recurrence rates are high despite aggressive surgical intervention	• Imaging with MRI or PET scan prior to surgery to establish extent of disease • Large and deep surgical excision with minimum 2-cm margins • Sentinel lymph node should be considered • Adjuvant radiotherapy can be considered in select cases

Systemic Complications	Description	Management
Anemia	• HS patients are more likely to be anemic compared to general population • Anemia felt to be related to chronic inflammation, however patients may also have a component of iron-deficiency anemia • If patients have any signs/symptoms of anemia—should undergo thorough work-up to determine cause of anemia	• Treat underlying inflammation associated with HS • Consider iron supplementation if iron-deficiency anemia present
Systemic amyloidosis and nephrotic syndrome	• Systemic amyloidosis is characterized by extracellular tissue deposition of fibrils from fragments of serum amyloid A • Any organ can be affected; kidneys most often involved • Renal complications include asymptomatic proteinuria, nephrotic syndrome, and kidney failure • Nephrotic syndrome: proteinuria, low serum albumin, hyperlipidemia, and edema	• Treat underlying inflammation associated with HS

(Continued)

TABLE 9.1 Summary of HS Complications—cont'd

Cutaneous Complications	Description	Management
Serious infection/sepsis	• Secondary infections of HS lesions may progress to include cellulitis, epidural abscesses, osteomyelitis, septicemia, and, rarely, sepsis	• Management depends on infectious complication
Chronic pain	• Pain can be secondary to inflammatory nature of lesions, +/- secondary infection, as well as scarring/contractures • Almost all patients will experience pain during their disease with nearly two-thirds describing pain as being moderate or higher	• See Chapter 19

Psychological and Social Complications	Description	Management
Depression/anxiety/suicide risk	• One in 4 adults with HS have depression • One in 5 adults with HS have anxiety • Patients with HS have higher prevalence of suicide	• Appropriate screening • Multidisciplinary treatment approach involving psychology/psychiatry
Stigma/Social Isolation	• Due to fear of stigma associated with their disease, HS patients may socially isolate themselves from others	• Support groups
Decreased relationship satisfaction/sexual dysfunction	• HS patients often face challenges dating and may experience difficulty engaging in sexual activity • Higher prevalence of erectile dysfunction in men and sexual dysfunction in women	• Support groups • Treat underlying inflammation associated with HS • Multidisciplinary treatment approach
Work productivity and activity impairment	• HS patients have higher rates of unemployment, higher risk of leaving the workforce, lower annual income, and decreased work productivity • Three quarters of patients report impairment in activities of daily living	• Treat underlying inflammation associated with HS • Multidisciplinary treatment approach

HPV, Human papilloma virus; HS, hidradenitis suppurativa; MRI, magnetic resonance imaging; PET, positron emission tomography; SCC, squamous cell carcinoma.

If left untreated, nephrotic syndrome and ultimately renal failure can occur.

Patients with HS can develop systemic AA amyloidosis; however, it is extremely rare, with only 10 cases reported in the literature to date. It tends to develop in patients that have long-standing, poorly controlled disease, and is often refractory to multiple conventional treatments.[22]

Systemic AA amyloidosis in HS patients most often presents with asymptomatic proteinuria or nephrotic syndrome. Nephrotic syndrome is characterized by a constellation of clinical and laboratory findings of renal disease, including large amounts of protein in the urine, serum hypoalbuminemia, hyperlipidemia, and significant edema. Aside from swelling (most commonly of the lower extremities), patients with nephrotic syndrome can also present with symptoms of weight gain, fatigue, foamy urine, and loss of appetite.

Physicians should consider work-up for systemic AA amyloidosis in HS patients with long-standing and severe disease. Some suggest screening in patients with moderate-to-severe HS with clinical duration greater than 3 years.[40] Given the kidneys are the first organ affected by AA amyloidosis, checking for microalbuminuria and serum albumin may be useful for early detection.[41] Serum creatinine may be normal in a subset of patients with kidney involvement, therefore, screening with creatinine alone may not be sufficient. If the patient history, physical examination, and laboratory findings are suggestive of AA amyloidosis, a biopsy is recommended for definitive diagnosis (most often renal biopsy), which will show glomerular, perivascular, or interstitial deposits of amyloid.[42]

Early recognition and prompt treatment of systemic amyloidosis is needed to stop the long-term deposition of amyloid and prevent related complications including renal failure and death. If there is evidence of renal involvement, a multidisciplinary treatment approach involving a nephrologist is recommended. As systemic amyloidosis is known to occur secondary to a chronic inflammatory state, the goal of therapy is to treat the underlying inflammation associated with HS. Successful treatment has been described using infliximab in two patients with severe HS complicated by systemic amyloidosis with renal involvement. Both had significant reduction in HS activity and proteinuria following treatment with infliximab.[43,44] Surgical therapy for HS has also been proposed for severe cases refractory to aggressive medical therapy.[41]

Serious Infection and Sepsis

Cultures taken from early HS lesions are often sterile, suggesting that HS is primarily an inflammatory disease of the follicular epithelium. However, lesions can become colonized and infected by bacteria,[1] resulting in serious secondary infections including cellulitis, epidural abscesses, osteomyelitis, and septicemia.[1,45] Sepsis is an extremely rare life-threatening complication that can be a consequence of infected HS lesions and may occur in the setting of immunosuppression from medications used to treat HS, or from an infected ulcerative SCC.[46,47]

Based on data collected from a 2002-2012 National Inpatient Sample of over 87,000,000 US hospitalizations, hospitalized patients with HS have a higher prevalence of serious infections as well as antibiotic-resistant infections, septicemia, and skin infections compared to patients without HS. Hospitalized HS patients that had a serious infection had significantly increased mortality compared to HS patients without infection.[48] Further studies are needed to better characterize the types of infections seen in HS patients as well as potential risk factors for infection.

Chronic Pain

Pain is a nearly universal symptom experienced by patients with HS and is known to have a negative impact on quality of life.[49] When compared to other common skin diseases such as leg ulcers, blistering disorders, atopic dermatitis, and psoriasis, patients with HS have a significantly higher odds ratio of experiencing pain/discomfort associated with their disease.[50]

HS-related pain may arise from the inflammatory nature of typical lesions as well as their location in intertriginous areas. Secondary infections can further exacerbate pain and long-standing disease can lead to significant scarring and contractures which can cause discomfort and pain with movement.[22]

Two types of HS-related pain have been described: acute and chronic. Acute pain is thought to arise from acute inflammatory nodules/abscesses and presents as nociceptive pain characterized by burning, stinging, shooting, and stabbing sensations. Chronic pain is associated with chronic inflammation, scarring/contractures, and friction from clothing, and presents as stimulus-dependent, neuropathic pain that is characterized by gnawing, aching, tenderness and throbbing.[51]

Almost all patients with HS will experience pain at some point during their disease, with over three quarters of patients reporting pain within the past week alone.[52] Furthermore, nearly two-thirds of patients report their pain as moderate or higher, with almost 5% describing their recent pain to be the worst possible.[53]

Patients' pain should be assessed at every visit with particular attention paid to the severity and timing of the pain, as well as the quality of the pain. Pain management begins with adequately treating the underlying inflammation associated with HS. Chronic pain has been shown to be improved following initiation of adalimumab in patients with moderate to severe HS.[54] See Chapter 19 for a comprehensive discussion about pain management.

Mortality Rate and Mortality Associations

A recent study conducted by Reddy et al. suggests that HS may confer an independent risk of all-cause mortality; however, the mechanism by which this occurs is still unclear.[55] Interestingly, other chronic inflammatory diseases such as psoriasis and rheumatoid arthritis have also been independently associated with increased mortality risk.

A recent retrospective cohort study looking at the 5-year mortality rate among over 13,000 patients with HS compared to control individuals, found that patients with HS had a 77% increase in 5-year mortality risk compared with control individuals after adjustment for age, sex, and race. After additionally adjusting for body mass index (BMI), smoking status, and comorbidity burden, the increase in mortality risk was attenuated to 14%. This suggests that mortality in HS may also in part be attributable to tobacco smoking and comorbid conditions.[55] Chronic inflammation associated with the underlying disease state is thought to predispose to accelerated atherosclerosis and increased cardiovascular mortality.[55]

Psychological and Social Complications

HS greatly impacts the quality of life and can have profound negative psychological and social implications.

Depression, Anxiety, and Suicidality

Based on a recent systematic review of 39 studies, approximately one in four adults with HS were found to have concurrent depression (26.5% compared to 6.6% in patients without HS) and one in five adults with HS were found to have concurrent anxiety (18.1% vs. 7.1% in controls). Studies have also found a higher prevalence of suicide in patients with HS compared to controls: 0.8% vs. 0.3% in a U.S. study and 0.14% vs. 0.07% in a Danish study.[56]

The reason why patients with HS have higher rates of depression, anxiety and/or suicidality is likely multifactorial and may include reduced quality of life secondary to chronic pain, impaired sexual health, limitations in social and professional life, as well as a chronic inflammatory state.[21] A pro-inflammatory state may contribute to depression through the psychological effects of circulating cytokines as well as through cytokines' direct effects on the microglia.[57] Treatment of underlying inflammation in HS patients may help reduce their pain scores as well as their depressive symptoms.[58] Interestingly, surgical intervention has also been found to significantly improve depressive and anxiety symptoms among HS patients.[56] Given the high association between HS and psychological disorders, screening for these comorbidities is imperative and a multidisciplinary treatment approach is recommended.

Stigma/Social Isolation

Patients with HS often feel shame and embarrassment regarding the appearance and associated drainage and odor of their lesions. Due to fear of being stigmatized by others, patients may socially isolate themselves.[59] Support groups, such as Hope for HS (https://www.hs-foundation.org/support/), not only connect individuals living with HS, but also help spread awareness of the disease. More detailed information on HS support groups can be found in Chapter 33.

Decreased Relationship Satisfaction and Sexual Health

The World Health Organization defines sexual health as a "state of physical, mental, and social well-being in relation to sexuality." Chronic diseases like HS can negatively affect sexual health and have a significant effect on patient quality of life. Sexual dysfunction (SD), which appears to be present in around half of HS patients, may be caused by either organic or psychological factors (or both) and can involve any element of the sexual response. Not surprisingly, sexual distress, which refers to the emotional impact that sexual difficulties have on an individual, is higher in patients with HS and correlates with both SD in women and erectile dysfunction in men.[60] Intimate relations are even more burdensome for patients who are dating or are in new relationships, as patients are embarrassed by the appearance of their skin lesions and find it challenging to talk about their condition with their partners.[23]

Work Productivity and Activity Impairment

HS can have a negative effect on patients' work productivity as well as affect activities of routine life. Patients with HS have higher rates of unemployment[61] and higher risk of leaving the workforce if they are employed.[62] One study in the US database found that HS patients have a lower annual income ($54,925 vs. $62,357) and lower income growth ($324 less per year) when compared to patients without HS.[62] Patients also report frequently missing work as well as loss of work productivity secondary to their HS.[61] HS can significantly affect patients' activities of daily living, with nearly three quarters of patients with HS reporting daily activity impairment.[61] Further discussion regarding the impact of HS on sexual health and work productivity can be found in Chapter 21.

Summary

Due to the chronic inflammatory nature of HS, with associated painful abscesses and nodules occurring in sensitive intertriginous areas, a number of cutaneous, systemic, psychological, and social complications may result as a consequence of long-standing, poorly controlled disease. Early recognition and aggressive treatment are necessary to help prevent and manage complications of this challenging disease.

References

1. Alikhan A, Lynch PJ, Eisen DB. Hidradenitis suppurativa: A comprehensive review. *J Am Acad Dermatol.* 2009;60(4):539–561. https://doi.org/10.1016/j.jaad.2008.11.911.
2. Elkin K, Daveluy S, Avanaki K. Hidradenitis suppurativa: Current understanding, diagnostic and surgical challenges, and developments in ultrasound application. *Skin Res Technol.* 2020;26(1):11–19. https://doi.org/10.1111/srt.12759.
3. Elkjaer M, Dinesen L, Benazzato L, et al. Efficacy of Infliximab treatment in patients with severe Fistulizing Hidradenitis Suppurativa. *J Crohns Colitis.* 2008;2(3):241–245. https://doi.org/10.1016/j.crohns.2008.02.002.
4. Dahmen RA, Gkalpakiotis S, Mardesicova L, et al. Deroofing followed by thorough sinus tract excision: a modified surgical approach for hidradenitis suppurativa. *J Dtsch Dermatol Ges.* 2019;17(7):698–702. https://doi.org/10.1111/ddg.13875.
5. Scholtes VC, Ardon CB, van Straalen KR, et al. Characterization of perianal fistulas in patients with hidradenitis suppurativa. *J Eur Acad Dermatol Venereol.* 2019;33(9):e337–e338. https://doi.org/10.1111/jdv.15629.
6. Tokunaga Y, Sasaki H. Clinical role of modified seton procedure and coring out for treatment of complex anal fistulas associated with hidradenitis suppurativa. *Int Surg.* 2015;100(6):974–978. https://doi.org/10.9738/INTSURG-D-14-00237.1.
7. Gronau E, Pannek J. Urethral fistula caused by acne inversa (hidradenitis suppurativa): A case report. *Int Urol Nephrol.* 2002;34(3):375–378. https://doi.org/10.1023/A:1024419200996.
8. Gys B, De Hous N, Hubens G. Fistula-tract Laser Closure (FiLaC™) for complex urethroperineal fistula. *Acta Chirurgica Belgica.* 2018;118(6):398–401. https://doi.org/10.1080/00015458.2018.1515337.
9. Micieli R, Alavi A. Lymphedema in patients with hidradenitis suppurativa: a systematic review of published literature. *Int J Dermatol.* 2018;57(12):1471–1480. https://doi.org/10.1111/ijd.14173.
10. Musumeci ML, Scilletta A, Sorci F, et al. Genital lymphedema associated with hidradenitis suppurativa unresponsive to adalimumab treatment. *JAAD Case Reports.* 2019;5(4):326–328. https://doi.org/10.1016/j.jdcr.2019.01.019.
11. Pacheco YD, García-Duque O, Fernández-Palacios J. Penile and scrotal lymphedema associated with hidradenitis suppurativa: Case report and review of surgical options. *Cir Cir.* 2018;86(1):84–88. https://doi.org/10.24875/CIRU.M18000007.
12. Caposiena Caro RD, Cannizzaro MV, Mazzeo M, et al. Letter to the editor regarding "Lymphedema in patients with hidradenitis suppurativa: a systematic review of published literature". *Inter J Dermatol.* 2019;58(4):E92–E93. https://doi.org/10.1111/ijd.14342.
13. Good LM, Francis SO, High WA. Scrotal elephantiasis secondary to hidradenitis suppurativa. *J Am Acad Dermatol.* 2011;64(5):993–994. https://doi.org/10.1016/j.jaad.2009.08.011.
14. Konety BR, Cooper T, Flood HD, et al. Scrotal elephantiasis associated with hidradenitis suppurativa. *Plast Reconstr Surg.* 1996;97(6):1243–1245. https://doi.org/10.1097/00006534-199605000-00023.

15. Brotherhood HL, Metcalfe M, Goldenberg L, et al. A surgical challenge: Idiopathic scrotal elephantiasis. *Can Urol Assoc J.* 2014;8(7–8): E500–E507. https://doi.org/10.5489/cuaj.1739.

16. Moosbrugger EA, Mutasim DF. Hidradenitis suppurativa complicated by severe lymphedema and lymphangiectasias. *J Am Acad Dermatol.* 2011;64(6):1223–1224. https://doi.org/10.1016/j.jaad.2009. 10.045.

17. De Vasconcelos PT, Décio-Ferreira J, Filipe PL. Scrotal elephantiasis secondary to recalcitrant hidradenitis suppurativa. *Indian J Dermatol Venereol Leprol.* 2015;81(5):524–525. https://doi.org/10.4103/ 0378-6323.158656.

18. Hazen PG, Daoud S. Scrotal hidradenitis suppurativa with secondary lymphedema and lymphangiomata: Successful management with carbon dioxide laser excision and marsupialization. *Dermatol Surg.* 2015;41(3):431–432. https://doi.org/10.1097/DSS. 0000000000000302.

19. Kirby Joslyn S. Qualitative study shows disease damage matters to patients with hidradenitis suppurativa. *J Am Acad Dermatol.* 2016;74(6):1269–1270. https://doi.org/10.1016/j.jaad.2016.01.001.

20. Jfri A, O'Brien E, Alavi A, et al. Association of hidradenitis suppurativa and keloid formation: A therapeutic challenge. *JAAD Case Reports.* 2019;5(8):675–678. https://doi.org/10.1016/j.jdcr.2019. 06.001.

21. Sabat R, Jemec GBE, Matusiak Ł, et al. Hidradenitis suppurativa. *Nat Rev Dis Primers.* 2020;6(1):18. https://doi.org/10.1038/s41572-020-0149-1.

22. Yuan JT, Naik HB. Complications of hidradenitis suppurativa. *Semin Cutan Med Surg.* 2017;36(2):79–85. https://doi.org/10.12788/j. sder.2017.022.

23. Esmann S, Jemec GBE. Psychosocial impact of hidradenitis suppurativa: A qualitative study. *Acta Dermato-Venereologica.* 2011;91(3):328–332. https://doi.org/10.2340/00015555-1082.

24. Krakowski AC, Admani S, Uebelhoer NS, et al. Residual scarring from hidradenitis suppurativa: Fractionated CO_2 laser as a novel and noninvasive approach. *Pediat.* 2014;133(1):e248–e251. https://doi.org/10.1542/peds.2012-3356.

25. Nicholson CL, Hamzavi I, Ozog DM. Rapid healing of chronic ulcerations and improvement in range of motion after fractional carbon dioxide (CO2) treatment after CO2 excision of hidradenitis suppurativa axillary lesions: A case report. *JAAD Case Reports.* 2016;2(1): 4–6. https://doi.org/10.1016/j.jdcr.2015.11.001.

26. Chapman S, Delgadillo D, Barber C, et al. Cutaneous squamous cell carcinoma complicating hidradenitis suppurativa: A review of the prevalence, pathogenesis, and treatment of this dreaded complication. *Acta Dermatovenerol Alp Pannonica Adriat.* 2018;27(1):25–28. https://doi.org/10.15570/actaapa.2018.5.

27. Constantinou C, Widom K, Desantis J, et al. Hidradenitis suppurativa complicated by squamous cell carcinoma. *The American Surgeon.* 2008;74(12):1177–1181.

28. Huang C, Lai Z, He M, et al. Successful surgical treatment for squamous cell carcinoma arising from hidradenitis suppurativa A case report and literature review. *Medicine (Baltimore).* 2017;96(3), e5857. https://doi.org/10.1097/MD.0000000000005857.

29. Chong AJ, Klein MB. Marjolin's ulcer. *N Engl J Med.* 2005;352(10), e9. https://doi.org/10.1056/NEJMicm040020.

30. Zachary LS, Robson MC, Rachmaninoff N. Squamous cell carcinoma occurring in hidradenitis suppurativa. *Ann Plast Surg.* 1987; 18(1):71–73. https://doi.org/10.1097/00000637-198701000-00015.

31. Jourabchi N, Fischer AH, Cimino-Mathews A, et al. Squamous cell carcinoma complicating a chronic lesion of hidradenitis suppurativa: a case report and review of the literature. *Int Wound J.* 2017; 14(2):435–438. https://doi.org/10.1111/iwj.12671.

32. Lavogiez C, Delaporte E, Darras-Vercambre S, et al. Clinicopathological study of 13 cases of squamous cell carcinoma complicating hidradenitis suppurativa. *Dermatol.* 2010;220(2):147–153.

33. Kohorst JJ, Shah KK, Hallemeier CL, et al. Squamous cell carcinoma in perineal, perianal, and gluteal hidradenitis suppurativa: Experience in 12 patients. *Dermatol Surg.* 2019;45(4):519–526. https://doi.org/ 10.1097/DSS.0000000000001713.

34. Donsky HJ, Mendelson CG. Squamous cell carcinoma as a complication of hidradenitis suppurativa. *Arch Dermatol.* 1964;90(5):488–491. https://doi.org/10.1001/archderm.1964.01600050036008.

35. Tennant F, Bergeron JR, Stone OJ, et al. Anemia associated with hidradenitis suppurativae. *JAMA Dermatol.* 1968;92(2):138–140. https://jamanetwork.com/journals/jamadermatology/article-abstract/ 530690.

36. Miller IM, Johansen ME, Mogensen UB. Is hidradenitis suppurativa associated with anaemia?: A population-based and hospital-based cross-sectional study from Denmark. *J Eur Acad Dermatol Venereol.* 2016;30(8):1366–1372. https://doi.org/10.1111/jdv.13326.

37. Soliman YS, Chaitowitz M, Hoffman LK, et al. Identifying anaemia in a cohort of patients with hidradenitis suppurativa. *J Eur Acad Dermatol Venereol.* 2020;34(1):e5–e8. https://doi.org/10.1111/jdv. 15837. Blackwell Publishing Ltd.

38. Soliman Y, Hoffman L, Chaitowitz M, et al. Identifying and characterizing anemia in patients with hidradenitis suppurativa. *J Am Acad Dermatol.* 2018;79(3):AB155. https://doi.org/10.1016/j.jaad.2018. 05.640.

39. Braunberger TL, Lowes MA, Hamzavi IH. Hemoglobin as an indicator of disease activity in severe hidradenitis suppurativa. *Intern J Dermatol.* 2019;58(9):1090–1091. https://doi.org/10.1111/ ijd.14170.

40. Iannone M, Oranges T, Chiricozzi A, et al. Potential role of serum amyloid A in hidradenitis suppurativa. *JAAD Case Reports.* 2019;5(5): 406–409. https://doi.org/10.1016/j.jdcr.2019.02.026.

41. Utrera-Busquets M, Romero-Maté A, Castaño A, et al. Severe hidradenitis suppurativa complicated by renal AA amyloidosis. *Clinical and Experimental Dermatology.* 2016;41(3):287–289. https://doi.org/10. 1111/ced.12731.

42. Ilgen U, Çelebi ZK, Kuzu I, et al. Renal amyloidosis secondary to hidradenitis suppurativa. *Clini Kidney J.* 2013;6(6):667–668. https://www.ncbi.nlm.nih.gov/pmc/articles/PMC4438379/.

43. Montes-Romero JA, Callejas-Rubio JL, Sánchez-Cano D, et al. Amyloidosis secondary to hidradenitis suppurativa. Exceptional response to infliximab. *Eur J Intern Med.* 2008;19(6):e32–e33. https://doi. org/10.1016/j.ejim.2007.11.014.

44. Özer İ, Karaçin C, Adışen E, et al. Two diseases one remedy? Systemic amyloidosis secondary to hidradenitis suppurativa: Treatment with infliximab. *Dermatol Therapy.* 2017;30(2). https://doi.org/10.1111/ dth.12445.

45. Margesson LJ, Danby FW. Hidradenitis suppurativa. *Best Pract Res Clin Obstet Gynaecol.* 2014;28(7):1013–1027.

46. Verdelli A, Antiga E, Bonciani D, et al. A fatal case of hidradenitis suppurativa associated with sepsis and squamous cell carcinoma. *Int J Dermatol.* 2016;55(1):e52–e53.

47. Vossen MG, Gattringer KB, Khalifeh N, et al. Gemella morbillorum bacteremia after anti-tumor necrosis factor alpha as acne inversa therapy. *J Clin Microbiol.* 2012;50(3):1109–1112. https://doi.org/10. 1128/JCM.06161-11.

48. Lee HH, Patel KR, Singam V, et al. Associations of cutaneous and extracutaneous infections with hidradenitis suppurativa in U.S. children and adults. *Br J Dermatol.* 2020;182(2):327–334. https://doi. org/10.1111/bjd.18093.

49. Patel ZS, Hoffman LK, Buse DC, et al. Pain, psychological comorbidities, disability, and impaired qualify of life in hidradenitis suppurativa. *Curr Pain and Headache Rep.* 2017;21(12):49.

50. Balieva F, Kupfer J, Lien L, et al. The burden of common skin diseases assessed with the EQ5D™: a European multicentre study in 13 countries. *Br J Dermatol.* 2017;176(5):1170–1178. https://doi.org/ 10.1111/bjd.15280.

51. Horváth B, Janse IC, Sibbald GR. Pain management in patients with hidradenitis suppurativa. *J Am Acad Dermat.* 2015;73(5):S47–S51. https://doi.org/10.1016/j.jaad.2015.07.046.

52. Matusiak Ł, Szczęch J, Kaaz K, et al. Clinical characteristics of pruritus and pain in patients with hidradenitis suppurativa. *Acta*

Dermato-Venereologica. 2018;98(2):191–194. https://doi.org/10.2340/00015555-2815.

53. Garg A, Neuren E, Cha D, et al. Evaluating patients' unmet needs in hidradenitis suppurativa: Results from the global survey of impact and healthcare needs (VOICE) project. *J Am Acad Dermatol.* 2020;82(2):366–376. https://doi.org/10.1016/j.jaad.2019.06.1301.

54. Kimball AB, Sundaram M, Shields AL, et al. Adalimumab alleviates skin pain in patients with moderate-to-severe hidradenitis suppurativa: Secondary efficacy results from the PIONEER I and PIONEER II randomized controlled trials. *J Am Acad Dermat.* 2018;79(6):1141–1143. https://doi.org/10.1016/j.jaad.2018.05.015.

55. Reddy S, Strunk A, Garg A. All-cause mortality among patients with hidradenitis suppurativa: A population-based cohort study in the United States. *J Am Acad Dermatol.* 2019;81(4):937–942.

56. Patel KR, Lee HH, Rastogi S, et al. Association between hidradenitis suppurativa, depression, anxiety, and suicidality: A systematic review and meta-analysis. *J Am Acad Dermatol.* 2020;83(3):737–744.

57. Farzanfar D, Dowlati Y, French LE, et al. Inflammation: a contributor to depressive comorbidity in inflammatory skin disease. *Skin Pharmacol Physiol.* 2018;31(5):246–251.

58. Scheinfeld N, Sundaram M, Teixeira H, et al. Original reduction in pain scores and improvement in depressive symptoms in patients with hidradenitis suppurativa treated with adalimumab in a phase 2, randomized, placebo-controlled trial. *Dermatol Online J.* 2016;22(3):13030.

59. Kirby JS, Leiphart P. Standing up together to the shame and stigma associated with hidradenitis suppurativa. *Br J Dermatol.* 2020;182(2):267–268.

60. Cuenca-Barrales C, Molina-Leyva A. Risk factors of sexual dysfunction in patients with hidradenitis suppurativa: A cross-sectional study. *Dermatolog.* 2020;236(1):37–45.

61. Yao Y, Jørgensen AHR, Thomsen SF. Work productivity and activity impairment in patients with hidradenitis suppurativa: a cross-sectional study. *Int J Dermatol.* 2020;59(3):333–340.

62. Tzellos T, Yang H, Mu F, et al. Impact of hidradenitis suppurativa on work loss, indirect costs and income. *Br J Dermatol.* 2019;181(1):147–154.

Pathogenesis

10

Follicular Occlusion and Inflammation

JOHN W. FREW

CHAPTER OUTLINE

Introduction

The pathogenic model of hidradenitis suppurativa (HS) may be in the midst of a paradigm shift, balancing the initial model of a disorder of (primary) follicular occlusion[1] with consideration as an autoinflammatory keratinization disease (AiKD).[2] There is observational, experimental, and therapeutic evidence to support the concept of HS as a primarily inflammatory disorder[1] and/or a disorder of autoimmunity[3] (in contrast to that primarily of follicular occlusion); however, the lack of reliable disease models[4,5] has limited experimental/mechanistic evidence to support or refute one pathogenic model over another (Fig. 10.1). Continual re-evaluation and integration of current clinical, histological, and molecular data into our pathogenic model of HS is essential in order to advance our understanding of the disease.[6] Challenging existing paradigms[1] through observation, hypothesis, and experimentation (while maintaining an open mind) is a core component of the scientific process,[7] and is essential to enable accurate identification of novel therapeutic targets and treatment strategies.[8,9] It is also vital to the understanding of differential treatment response in different individuals and exploring the potential role of variations in inflammatory endotypes (disease subtypes defined by a distinct functional or pathological mechanism) in the disease,[8] in a similar way to how this has been identified in atopic dermatitis.[8] This review aims to synthesize existing knowledge from clinical observation, classical histology, as well as modern molecular biology techniques to evaluate the evidence for HS as either a disorder of follicular occlusion or an AiKD.

The Evolving Pathogenic Paradigm(s) of Hidradenitis Suppurativa

Historically, HS has been proposed to be a disorder of apocrine gland inflammation,[10,11] although multiple independent histological studies have demonstrated that inflammatory involvement of apocrine glands is a secondary phenomenon,[12-14] and that the primary inflammatory driver of the disease exists adjacent to keratinocytes of the follicular infundibulum and interfollicular epidermis.[12,15,16] It is now widely accepted that the primary driver of disease activity centers upon the follicular infundibulum.[15,16] Additionally, other disorders such as pilonidal sinus disease[17] and dissecting cellulitis of the scalp[18] share many clinical, histological, and inflammatory features with HS[17-19] and are beginning to be considered as uni-localized variants of disease.[20] Melnik's seminal 2013 paper[21] began to shift the pathogenic paradigm of HS away from an apocrine-gland based inflammatory or infectious disorder, to a disorder of follicular occlusion and proposed dysregulated Notch signaling[21,22] as the unifying feature of HS pathogenesis.

Emerging evidence as to the role of the inflammasome,[23-26] complement,[27-31] and IL-1 isoforms[32-35] has led to the suggestion of HS as an AiKD.[2] Evidence of systemic inflammation,[36,37] activation of B cells,[3,38] and plasma cells[3,39,40] have raised the possibility of HS having an autoimmune or antibody-mediated component.[38] However, follicular occlusion is still considered the "primem movens" of HS[1] preceding the inflammatory drive of disease.

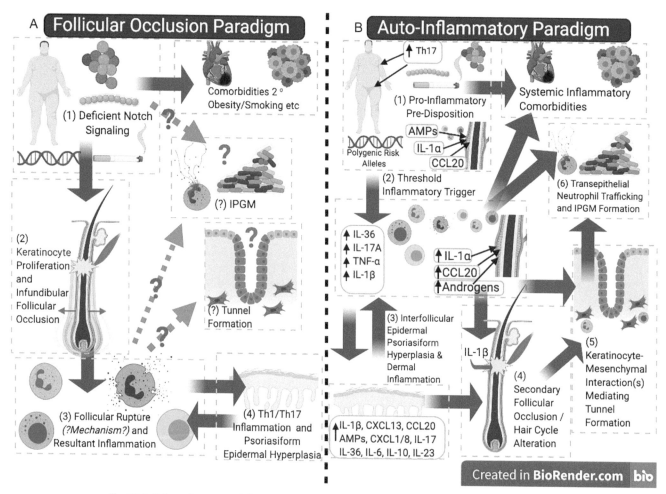

• **Fig. 10.1** Schematic representation and comparison of the follicular occlusion paradigm and the autoinflammatory paradigm in the pathogenesis of hidradenitis suppurativa. (A) In the follicular occlusion paradigm, deficient Notch signaling may directly result in infundibular keratinocyte proliferation and follicular occlusion, leading to follicular dilatation, rupture, and resultant inflammation. One deficiency of this paradigm is the lack of hypothesized mechanisms by which rupture occurs and why deep follicular rupture occurs preferentially to expulsion of the comedone. The resultant Th1/Th17 inflammatory axis then results in the observed inflammatory profile of disease; however, no clear mechanism is hypothesized for how tunnels form and how the infiltrative proliferative gelatinous mass (IPGM) results. (B) The autoinflammatory paradigm places inflammation as the primary driver of disease, with subclinical inflammation developing as a result of disparate contributing factors on a background of pro-inflammatory disposition of specific anatomical sites (axilla, groin, etc.). Dermal inflammatory infiltrates then drives secondary follicular occlusion with resultant tunnel formation, a result of keratinocyte-mesenchymal interactions mimicking outer-root sheath keratinocyte downgrowth in follicular development and early anagen. Chemokine gradients in epithelialized tunnels then drive neutrophil trafficking to the lumen and formation of the IPGM. AMP: Anti-Microbial Peptides; TNF: Tumor Necrosis Factor; IL: Interleukin.

The Problem(s) with Animal and Ex-Vivo Models in Hidradenitis Suppurativa

The development of animal models in HS dates from the identification of gamma secretase associated polymorphisms in familial HS.[4] Gamma secretase and Notch-1 null mice were incompatible with life[4] due to the vital role of notch signaling in body segment development; however, post-natal knockdown of Notch-1 results in hyperproliferative epidermis, hair loss, and epidermal cyst formation in adult mice.[4,5] Combined Notch-1 and Notch-2 knockdown results in an atopic-dermatitis-like epidermal disorder and a rapidly fatal myeloproliferative disorder in adult mice.[4] When interpreting these results through the follicular occlusion paradigm, it is reasonable to assume that epidermal cyst formation is consistent with the proposed initial steps in HS pathogenesis; however, the lack of

inflammation, cyst rupture or tunnel development argue against Notch-1 knockdown being a high fidelity animal model for HS.[4]

One possible explanation for the lack of comparable dermal inflammation and tunnel formation in Notch-1 knockdown murine models may be the difference in dermal thickness between human and murine skin and the differential localization of the follicular unit in the dermis (human) and subcutis (murine). In order to overcome these potential issues, a murine xenotransplantation model was developed involving direct transplantation of lesional HS tissue to immunosuppressed mice.[5] The most recent model developed involves a transwell ex-vivo model,[5] which overcomes the structural and morphological issues of dermal thickness and follicular insertion of murine models and has relatively less infection risk than xenotransplantation models. However, given the overlapping limitations of existing models, only translational studies of interventions in human subjects give the greatest fidelity in both mechanistic and clinically relevant responses to pharmacological interventions in HS in order to explore the pathogenic mechanisms of disease.

Follicular Occlusion: Comedones are Clinically and Experimentally a Product of Inflammation, Rather Than a Cause

Histological studies illustrate the prominent roles of comedogenesis, follicular hyperkeratosis, and comedogenesis in HS tissues.[12,15,16] However, in each instance, the coexistence of perifollicular inflammation is comparably prominent.[12,15,16] Clinically, comedones (both open and closed), as well as typical double-sided comedones,[42] are present in diseased areas, inflamed tissues, and also in scarred, non-inflamed tissues.[15,16,41-43] They are also present in areas not exposed to flexural occlusion.[44]

Von Laffert et al.[15,16] report comedones as more common in end stage fibrotic and scarred lesions and independent of the follicular unit.[15,16] These comedones are more likely to be those of the double-ended variety which were once considered to be pathognomonic of HS.[42] From these clinical observations, it can be concluded that comedones are associated with HS; however, the establishment of causation requires mechanistic evidence. Such mechanistic evidence is available thanks to investigations into comedogenesis in acne research.[45-49] Recent findings have identified subclinical inflammation as preceding comedogenesis in acne prone skin,[45] disrupting the longstanding assumption that follicular occlusion is the primary initiating factor in acne.[48] The molecular mechanisms of comedogenesis involve follicular keratinocytes, producing a number of pro-inflammatory mediators[45,46,48-51] (including antimicrobial peptides, microbial associated proteins including lipotechoic acid, CCL20, and IL-1α). Ex-vivo studies of the follicular infundibum[52] isolated in vitro are able to recapitulate the formation of comedones with addition of IL-1α and prevent formation with the addition of IL-1RA.[52] It is acknowledged that the in vitro studies performed are based on highly sebaceous follicular units which have distinct differences from apocrine bearing skin[53]; however, the similarities in immunological milieu between sebaceous and apocrine skin in Th17 associated mediators[8,53] (central to inflammation in HS)[54] raise the theoretical possibility of these mechanisms being shared between body sites. Reproduction of these experiments using follicular infundibular from apocrine gland bearing regions would hopefully be definitive in confirming or refuting these findings.

Therefore, it can be concluded that molecular and ex-vivo evidence suggests comedone formation is possible secondary to subclinical inflammation, rather than inflammation being the result of comedone formation and follicular rupture.[1] The precise mechanisms that have been demonstrated in human skin, however, require validation in apocrine gland bearing skin given the unique immunological milieu of these sites. These results may explain the diffuse scattering of comedones seen in HS prone areas, the presence of comedones in extra-flexural sites, and the presence of comedones in previously inflamed ("burnt out") tissue or sites distant from a follicular unit. It also raises the additional question of what differentiates conditions in which subclinical inflammation and diffuse flexural comedone formation (such as Dowling-Degos disease[55,56]) exist, from highly inflammatory HS lesions. Direct molecular comparisons of these conditions may further inform the differences in subclinical inflammation that leads to the

development of one condition over another (or the coexistence of both conditions at different timepoints).

Skin Fold Occlusion is Associated with Microbiome Alterations and Subsequent Pro-Inflammatory Keratinocyte Responses

On a microscopic level, follicular occlusion in HS refers to occlusion of the follicle at the infundibulum.[1,12,15,16] However, from a clinical viewpoint, "follicular occlusion" may refer to the anatomical sites of predilection in HS: namely axillary, inguinal, and submammary folds.[1] These areas are subjected to friction, skin-to-skin contact, and well-documented alterations in moisture, pH, and microbiological colonization[57,58] (Fig. 10.2A and B). In the setting of obesity, the posterior neck folds, abdominal pannus, gluteal cleft and inner thighs, and other anatomical sites can undergo similar microbiological milieu alterations secondary to heat, moisture, and pH changes.[59]

The follicular infundibulum is an immunologically active, microbially colonized site,[60-62] involved in the development of immune tolerance to commensal organisms.[60-62] This differs substantially from other portions of the follicle (such as the bulb), which are considered immunologically privileged sites.[63] Infundibular keratinocytes produce CCL20 and antimicrobial peptides under normal physiological conditions.[60] Increasing moisture decreases the pH of the stratum corneum[58,59] and pH reductions are known to promote the colonization and activity of porphyromonas sp (a well-documented microbiont-associated with HS).[64-65] Other bacterial species including Staphylococcus aureus[66] Propionibacterium acnes,[67] yeasts,[68] and their associated proteins (including lipoteichoic acid) are able to induce the release of preformed IL-1α in keratinocytes.[69] Indirect evidence for the role of yeasts in inflammatory activity in HS[70] is demonstrated in recent observational studies of anti-Saccharomyces cerevisae antibodies in severe HS,[71] which can also cross-react to other fungal and bacterial species.[70] While the precise mechanisms of specific microbiological species and/or strains in HS are ill-defined, their functional role in producing an aberrant pro-inflammatory response (either directly or indirectly via keratinocytes) is consistent with observational studies identifying these microbionts in both early and advanced disease.[65,66]

Genetic Variants in HS May Act via EGFR-Associated Pathways Linking Follicles, Th17 Mediated Inflammation, and Drug-Induced Disease

Chapter 12 summarizes the published literature on genetics and epigenetics of HS. The role of inherited mutations in Notch signaling as the pathogenic mechanism in HS has come under scrutiny,[72,73] with the existing genetic and molecular evidence suggesting a more complex interplay between genetics and infundibular keratinocyte-derived inflammation (see Fig. 10.2C).

The first documented mutation in familial HS was in Nicastrin, a component of the gamma secretase complex (GSC), identified in 2010 in an East-Asian kindred.[74] Mutations in the GSC are also associated with familial Alzheimer's disease[75] and cardiomyopathy,[76] although no common variants with HS are known. Since then, a small minority of patients with familial and spontaneous

INITIATING FACTORS IN HIDRADENITIS SUPPURATIVA

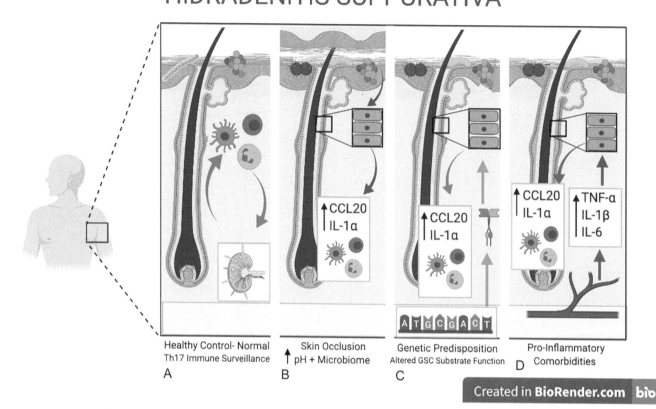

• **Fig. 10.2** Potential Initiating Factors in Hidradenitis Suppurativa. (A) Normal control skin from hidradenitis suppurativa-associated cutaneous sites (e.g., axilla) have healthy skin-associated microbionts (including within the follicular infundibulum), which are continuously monitored by circulating immune cells in homeostasis (to and from the lymph node). (B-D) Known predisposing factors increase the inflammatory drive of infundibular keratinocytes (purple rectangular cells) via varied mechanisms, including skin occlusion, predisposing genetic mutations, and pro-inflammatory comorbidities such as obesity and insulin resistance. (B) Skin occlusion alters the microbiological composition of the skin (red and yellow microbionts) via increases in cutaneous pH. These microbionts increase the production of CCL20 and IL-1α by infundibular keratinocytes. (C) Genetic mutations in the gamma secretase complex are known to affect Notch signaling but also substrates, including EGF receptors, which are active in the follicular infundibulum. Dysregulation of EGFR signaling is known to increase CCL20 and IL-1α production by infundibular keratinocytes. (D) Metabolic comorbidities produce increased levels of circulating TNF-α, IL-1β, and IL-6. These mediators stimulate CCL20 and IL-1α production.

HS have been identified with GSC mutations.[77] This suggests that other identified loci may contribute to genetic predisposition to HS, although this will only be elucidated with the results of genome wide association studies in HS. The precise mechanism of action of GSC mutations in the pathogenesis of HS is unclear.[72] The GSC complex cleaves over 70 different substrates involved in cell cycle and inflammation including EGFR, IL-1, TNF-α, complement regulatory protein CD46, and Notch.[72] Melnik's seminal 2013 paper[21] proposed Notch signaling as the unifying motif in HS pathogenesis via associations with keratinocyte proliferation, smoking, and sequence variants in GSC.[21-22] The molecular evidence for Notch being associated with keratinocyte hyperproliferation is well established[78,79]; however, dysregulated Notch signaling is also associated with other inflammatory skin disorders including psoriasis, atopic dermatitis, and alopecia areata.[73] Notch dysregulation may be an epiphenomenon secondary to keratinocyte

proliferation (as it is present in multiple other inflammatory dermatoses) rather than the primary cause of HS.[73]

In-silico evidence[72] has identified HS-specific GSC substrates ERbb4 and Tie1[72] as differentially expressed substrates that distinguish the transcriptome of HS from familial Alzheimer's disease and other inflammatory skin diseases.[72] ErbB4 and Tie1 are components of the EGFR pathway (active in the follicular infundibulum)[51] and are associated with SOX9 and Wnt signaling linked with hair cycle progression, IL-17A production[51,80] (through shared downstream Act1 activity), and epithelial cell fate,[80] all mechanisms identified in transcriptomic analysis of HS tissues.[40,113]

In vitro studies have demonstrated diverse pro-inflammatory results of Nicastrin knockdown including IL-36a production,[81] alterations in EGFR signaling,[82] as well as increased sensitivity to interferon mediated pro-inflammatory pathways.[83] Recently, mutations in POFUT1 have been identified in cases of

Dowling-Degos Disease associated with HS.[84,85] POFUT-1 is a fucosyltransferase which is active upon multiple substrates including Notch and EGFR[86] and is important for post-translational modification of receptors.[86] Therefore, abnormal activity of the EGFR pathway is linked with infundibular keratinocyte differentiation[51] and Th17 inflammatory pathways.[80] The link to clinical disease activity is supported by reports of HS associated with use of EGFR antagonists in oncology.[87] Therefore, dysregulation of EGFR associated pathways secondary to GSC mutations may explain both the infundibular localization of HS, the involvement of the Th17 immune axis, and cases of HS-like features in the setting of EGFR antagonism.

Disease Initiation is Associated with Systemic Subclinical Inflammation and Dysregulated Infundibular Keratinocytes

The site of initial inflammation in HS is centered upon the infundibulum of the hair follicle.[15,16] Given the active immunologic role of the follicular infundibulum,[51] a degree of baseline inflammatory activity around the follicle is considered normal. Understanding of the initiating factors associated with the excessive and self-perpetuating peri-follicular inflammation in HS remains incomplete (see Fig. 10.2D). Epidemiological and clinical observations suggest that a number of systemic disorders (including insulin resistance, hormonal dysregulation, and obesity) may be associated with HS[88] and contribute to a pro-inflammatory state. In other inflammatory disorders such as psoriasis,[89] rheumatoid arthritis[90] and atherosclerosis,[91] these factors have been found to be associated. However, the causation between disease and systemic inflammation is still a topic of contention[89] and is in need of further mechanistic enquiry.

Regardless of the direction of causation between HS comorbidities and inflammation, guidelines[92,93] and limited clinical evidence[94,95] suggest benefits to weight loss, smoking cessation, and dietary counseling as an integral part of HS management.[92,93] The mechanisms of these pro-inflammatory cascades are complex and incompletely understood.[96-98] Smoking, via polycyclic aromatic hydrocarbons, can directly alter follicular keratinocyte differentiation resulting in comedogenesis.[99] It can also produce widespread methylation changes and systemic increases in IL-6, C-Reactive Protein (CRP), fibrinogen, and multiple members of the NF-κB family.[98] Adipose tissue can produce pro-inflammatory signatures including IL-6, IL-1β, and TNF-α in the setting of chronic nutrient excess.[96,97] Additionally, adipokines can mediate both inflammation and the development of insulin resistance,[100] which is also associated with HS.[88] Keratinocytes in the infra-infundibulum of the follicle express Type 1 5-hydroxy-testosterone[101]; modulating infundibular keratinocyte differentiation programs both directly as well as via fibroblast activation and fibroblast-keratinocyte interactions,[102] contributing to androgen-induced follicular changes.[102]

Overall, these associations suggest that a systemic pro-inflammatory state and localized infundibular keratinocyte dysregulation are potential predisposing factors to clinical disease. There are contradictory reports[103] pertaining to the benefit of withdrawing these predisposing factors (e.g., cessation of smoking/weight loss) during established disease. These findings only appear contradictory if one holds the assumption that the initiating and perpetuating factors of clinical disease in HS are one and the same. As other authors have suggested,[104] there may be unique factors contributing to each state (initiation of disease and perpetuation of disease), and our lack of data regarding early (subclinical) disease has not allowed us to appreciate this fact.[104]

Inflammation in Hidradenitis Suppurativa: Evidence from Existing Studies

The inflammatory signature of established HS has been well characterized in multiple histological[54,110] and molecular studies.[54,111-114] Similarities and parallels with psoriasis[54] have been observed in lesional and perilesional HS tissue,[54] with lesional nodules demonstrating mixed inflammatory infiltrates comprising of T cell, dendritic cells, plasma cells, neutrophils, and monocytes.[110] Chronic longstanding disease also demonstrates B cell infiltrates,[3,39] NETosis,[3] and development of epithelialized tunnels.[115] An issue with understanding the characteristics of inflammation in HS is that the majority of specimens isolated for studies are from those with severe, longstanding disease.[3,39,40] Hence, we have limited insight into the initiating events in early and/or mild HS. Additionally, until recently, there were no standardized, defined biopsy sites for investigational studies.[116] Given that HS is morphologically diverse, it would be erroneous to assume that a biopsy from one portion of tissue is representative of all the different epidermal (and deep dermal) morphologies present across the spectrum of HS.[116] Therefore, studies which do not define the severity, treatments, sites, and lesion types of biopsies should be interpreted with caution.[110,111]

The common inflammatory signatures identified by qRT-PCR studies in HS lesional tissue include TNF-α, IL-1α, IL-1β, IL-6, IL-17A, IL-17F, IL-32, IL-36α, IL-36g, and IL-10.[111] Additional chemokines include CCL3, CCL5, CCL27, and BLC.[111] Non-lesional tissue also demonstrates upregulated levels of many of these cytokines,[53,111] although variation does exist due to previous lack of standardized biopsy sites and combination of both partially treated as well as untreated specimens.[111] Transcriptomic studies demonstrate strong B-cell signatures with IgG1 and IgG3 immunoglobulins and aspects of the complement cascade highly upregulated.[40] Additionally, signals of keratinocyte hyperplasia (Keratin 6, Keratin 16) are also seen with keratinocyte derived factors being elevated in lesional and perilesional tissue compared with unaffected and control skin.[110] Variation in cytokine levels do occur (between lesional, perilesional, and non-lesional tissue) in terms of type and degree of inflammation, although reliable characterization of inflammation matched with disease morphology (e.g., nodules vs. tunnels) is yet to be undertaken. Scarred tissue demonstrates decreased inflammatory profiles compared to non-scared areas,[111] and the presence of occult dermal tunnels can also induce highly inflammatory profiles in normal-appearing skin.[111] The use of clinical ultrasound has been suggested as a method of confirming or excluding the presence of tunnels prior to biopsy.[116]

Analysis of serum has identified IL-1β, IL-6, IL-8, IL-10, IL-12p70, IL-17, and TNF-α as upregulated in multiple studies;[111] however, conflicting results exist between serum levels of IL-10, IL-17, and IFN-y, which may be secondary to the severity of included participants and the methods of cytokine analysis.[111] The majority of data regarding serum inflammation is based on patients with Hurley stage 2 and 3 disease,[111] with the changes in serum inflammatory markers in early and mild disease unclear.

In terms of establishing mechanism—it has been assumed, based on observational studies, that perilesional inflammation is of the same character (albeit less intense) as nearby lesional inflammation.[111,112,117] Therefore, given the known feedback mechanisms between IL-1 and IL-17[118] leading to self-perpetuating feed-forward inflammation, it is reasonable to assume that lesional tissue inflammatory characteristics may be replicated by adding pro-inflammatory cytokines to ex-vivo perilesional tissue. This experiment (conducted by Vossen et al.[117]) was unable to replicate the lesional HS inflammatory profile, suggesting that IL-1α and/or IL-1β are not the sole triggers necessary to induce development of lesions in HS.[117,119] Other possibilities are that a combination of multiple inflammatory mediators are required; or as-yet-unknown predisposing factors are involved in inducing active inflammatory nodules on a background of perilesional subclinical inflammation.[119] This raises the prospect that the process of inflammation in HS is more complex than initially thought. The underlying assumption thus far in HS research is that perilesional tissue represents the same inflammatory profile as lesional tissue, differing only in the degree, intensity, and more superficial location of inflammation.[119] However, an alternative hypothesis that the inflammatory characteristics of perilesional tissue are distinct from lesional tissue[119] remains to be thoroughly investigated.

TH17 Feed-Forward Inflammation is Prominent in Established Disease

The Th17 axis is strongly implicated in established self-perpetuating clinical disease[54]; however, the mechanisms leading to Th17 feed-forward self-amplification in HS are still unclear. It is assumed to be similar to the activation of the Th17 axis in psoriasis, with the predisposition of the axillae and other areas of apocrine gland-rich skin to a Th17 immune response as demonstrated experimentally.[53] There is well-documented evidence (largely from the psoriasis literature) regarding positive feedback loops ("feed-forward mechanisms") between IL-1β, IL-6, and TNF-α by IL-17, leading to further IL-1β, IL-6, and TNF-α production as well as downstream activation of acute phase reactants, neutrophilic, and complement mediated inflammatory responses.[105-108] This is perpetuated through leucocyte-keratinocyte interactions,[102,109] amplifying antimicrobial peptide and chemokine production (including CXCL1 and CXCL8),[108] leading to additional inflammatory cell recruitment adjacent to IL-17-activated epidermal keratinocytes (Fig. 10.3A). Such inflammatory cell localization has been seen surrounding intrafollicular and interfollicular sites adjacent to epidermal keratinocytes in early histological specimens of HS,[12,15,16] with evidence of early psoriasiform hyperplasia suggestive of IL-17-induced epidermal changes. Despite the majority of translational work focusing upon IL-17A (given the body of pre-existing work based in psoriasis), significant elevations of other IL-17 isoforms including IL-17C and IL-17F are seen in HS tissue[32,108] and may be significant contributors to disease activity which are not targeted by anti-IL-17A therapies alone.

The Role of B Cells, Despite their Dominance, Remains Unclear

Longstanding and severe disease may have a unique inflammatory profile compared to milder or less established forms of HS. Histological and transcriptomic studies[40,113] identify a high level of B-cell and plasma cell signatures, complement (specifically C5a) activation, and extensive tissue remodeling via matrix metalloproteinases (MMPs), with subsequent destruction of follicular and glandular structures in the dermis.[40,113] The role and

characteristics of B cells in mild-moderate HS is unclear. The presence of B cells[3,39] and plasma cells in skin and blood[3,39] suggests the possibility that some component of severe or longstanding HS may be an autoimmune or antibody-mediated disorder. However, no product to date has been identified as an autoimmune target for the disease.[38] B cells are present in other chronic inflammatory disorders without known autoimmune targets including psoriasis and atopic dermatitis.[38] In these conditions, they are thought to be bystanders (secondary to combined B cell and T cell chemoattractants such as CXCL13 or CCL20) or secondary amplifiers of T-cell mediated inflammation[38] (see Fig. 10.3A). Byrd et al.[3] demonstrated that antibodies to citrullinated peptides contribute to the development of neutrophil extracellular traps (NETs) in advanced disease with parallels to B cell and NETs in rheumatoid arthritis.[3] Case reports of rituximab ameliorating HS disease activity are known,[38] but overall, the role of B cells as bystanders, amplifiers of existing inflammation, or central pathogenic players is unclear and requires further investigation.[38]

The Evidence and Proposed Mechanisms for Follicular Rupture

Follicular rupture is proposed as the primary mechanism that follicular occlusion leads to diffuse dermal inflammation in HS.[1] The histological evidence for follicular rupture is largely based on observational studies demonstrating the coexistence of dense perifollicular and intrafollicular inflammation and discontinuities in follicular epithelium in affected tissues[12,15,16] (see Fig. 10.3B). Longstanding disease often has a noticeable absence of follicular and adnexal structures replaced with dense inflammatory infiltrates and scarring[120] consistent with the known profound dermal inflammation, but the mechanisms and process of follicular rupture are poorly understood. Danby et al.[121] documented PAS staining of the basement membrane zone (BMZ) in lesional HS tissues and identified decreased staining compared to healthy controls.[121] The authors proposed that defects or thinning of the BMZ may predispose the follicle in HS to rupture, with subsequent spillage of intrafollicular contents into the dermis, stimulating the inflammatory cascade.[1] The authors point to reduction in PAS staining to support this claim. In examination of the histological images, the PAS positive material measures approximately 60 μm in diameter, which would be consistent with the thickness and morphology of the fibroreticular lamina that exists surrounding the basal lamina.[122] The thinner dense staining (<10 μm diameter) would be consistent with the basal lamina (which appears intact).[122] Other studies have not identified a reduction in desmosomal or hemidesmosomal components by IHC in HS specimens[123] suggesting conflicting evidence using different methodologies. Whilst the presence of epithelial discontinuities in HS follicles is not disputed, the elevated levels of matrix metalloproteinases (MMP2, MMP3) and inflammatory cells[124] may be implicated in the reduction of the thickness of the fibroreticular lamina. Therefore, further IHC staining and electron microscopy studies are needed to definitively establish the role of BMZ dysfunction in the rupture of the hair follicle in HS.

The mechanisms of follicular rupture in HS remain obscure. Occluded follicles in other conditions (such as epidermal inclusion cysts[125]) is proof of the potential size intrafollicular collections may progress to prior to rupture. However, the early presence of inflammation in HS lesions may suggest an inflammation-related mechanism which is well documented to disassemble the BMZ as part of

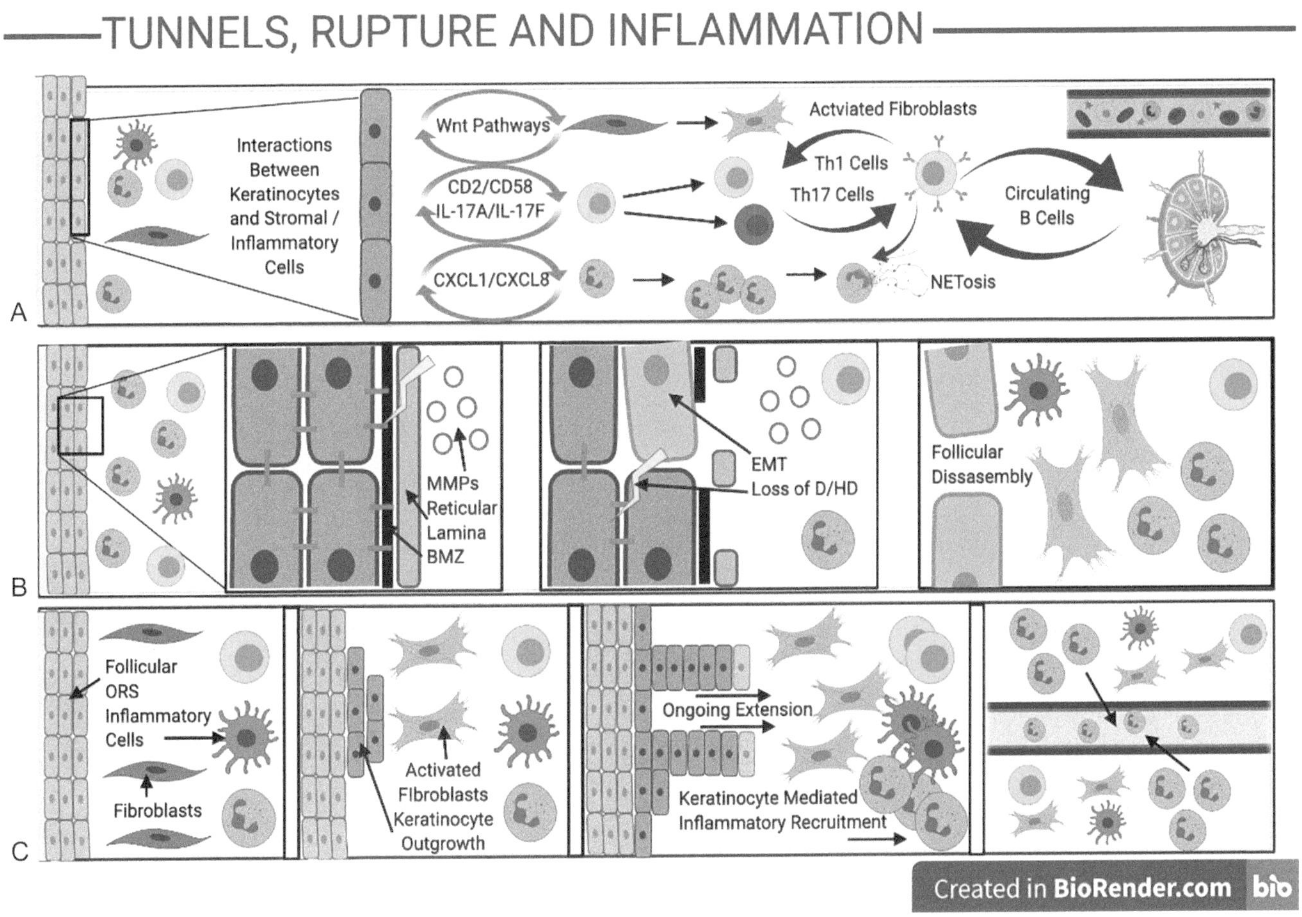

TUNNELS, RUPTURE AND INFLAMMATION

• **Fig. 10.3** Proposed mechanisms of tunnel formation, follicular rupture, and perpetuation of inflammation in hidradenitis suppurativa. (A) Mechanisms of inflammatory amplification. Activated keratinocytes interact with inflammatory and stromal cells via various pathways to result in activated fibroblasts, Th1 and Th17 cells and infiltration of dendritic cells and neutrophils. Circulating B cells, activated by the high interferon-mediated milieu, interact with multiple cell types to amplify existing inflammatory loops, as well as recirculating in the lymphatic and vascular system, contributing to systemic inflammation. (B) Mechanisms of follicular rupture. The inflammatory infiltrate is associated with high levels of matrix metalloproteinases *(MMPs)* which degrade the reticular lamina. Keratinocyte-leucocyte crosstalk activated epithelial-mesenchyme-transition *(EMT)* mechanisms, leading to degradation of the basement membrane zone *(BMZ)*, loss of desmosomes and hemidesmosomes *(D/HD)*, and keratinocytes expressing mesenchymal cell surface markers (yellow keratinocytes). Eventually, the follicular wall is disassembled and replaced by mesenchymal cells and dense inflammatory infiltrates. (C) Development of tunnels. Inflammation adjacent to the follicular outer root sheath *(ORS)* activates fibroblasts, with stromal-keratinocyte feedback resulting in keratinocyte outgrowth from the follicular wall. The ongoing keratinocyte outgrowth results in keratinocyte-mediated inflammatory cell recruitment further amplifying the stromally mediated keratinocyte outgrowth in a positive feedback loop. The inflammatory cells are attracted to the keratinocyte chemokine (CXCL1/CXCL8) gradient resulting in migration into the lumen of the tunnels.

the wound healing process. Epithelial-mesenchymal transition (EMT) pathways[109] are part of the normal wound healing response and have been identified in transcriptomic analysis of HS tissues.[126] EMT allows keratinocytes to detach from the surrounding epidermis, become motile and express fibroblast surface proteins and migrate to sites requiring re-epithelialisation.[109] It may also explain the presence of keratin staining cells in the dermis of HS sections[110] (via keratinocytes undergoing EMT but still expressing keratin proteins), the destruction of follicular and adnexal structures in advanced disease,[120] and the development of dermal tunnels.[109] Similar inductions in EMT-associated signaling pathways are seen in malignancy and wound healing and contribute to the metastatic potential of cancer and longstanding wounds.[109,127]

Hence, the concept of follicular rupture may be more appropriately described as a process of "follicular disassembly," induced by the chronic inflammatory changes via EMT and aberrant extracellular remodeling wound healing programs.[127]

Dermal Tunnels are Active Inflammatory Organs

Dermal tunnels in HS are unique structures comprised of stratified squamous epithelia which recapitulate the structure of the overlying epidermis.[128] This is in contrast to other tunnel-like structures in chronic inflammatory conditions, such as fistulizing Crohn's disease, which do not recapitulate mucosal structures with the same degree of fidelity.[129] These tunnels are comprised of keratinocytes, melanocytes, and Langerhans cells[128] that express pro-inflammatory mediators and are a second source of keratinocyte-derived inflammatory chemokines and cytokines in the dermis. Tunnels rarely extend into the subcutaneous tissues or fistulize with other hollow organs (except in the context of coexistent inflammatory bowel disease), suggesting an association with signaling from the dermis.[109]

The Development of Dermal Tunnels is Orchestrated by Dermal Inflammation

The precise mechanisms leading to tunnel formation are unclear; however, it is hypothesized that these tunnels derive from the aberrant keratinocyte outgrowth from the outer root sheath of the follicle[60,109] (see Fig. 10.3C). The development of tunnels may parallel the development of the hair follicle and early anagen keratinocyte downgrowth during the hair cycle,[130,131] which are mediated via PDGFα derived signaling from the dermal condensate.[131] PDGFα-mediated signaling has also been identified in transcriptomic data from HS-associated fibroblasts.[109] Given that these fibroblast-derived signals are secondary to inflammation-mediated epigenetic modifications,[109] it is plausible to assume that the development of tunnels is an inflammation-driven process. However, once these tunnels are established, the CXCL1/8 gradient established across the epithelia[108] (including tunnels) results in transepithelial neutrophil trafficking and NET formation in tunnel lumen.[3] This results in development of the infiltrative proliferative gelatinous mass (IPGM)[132] and biofilm formation in HS tunnels.[133] This in turn drives further inflammatory recruitment surrounding these established tunnels, leading to the ongoing cycle of severe intractable inflammation and drainage. Therefore, rather than an end-stage phenomenon, dermal tunnels are an inflammation-driven process resulting in the development of active inflammatory organs contributing to the perpetuation of dermal inflammation in established disease.

Conclusions

The available histological and molecular evidence suggest inflammation is a central component to the pathogenesis of HS. The current pathogenic paradigm of follicular occlusion as the *"primem movens"* in HS pathogenesis relegates inflammation as a secondary phenomenon. The same evidence used to support the primary follicular occlusion paradigm is valid in supporting the concept of HS as a primarily inflammatory disorder with follicular occlusion, a secondary event. Placing inflammation as the primary driver of disease provides a scaffold for testable hypotheses regarding polygenic risk loci for the development of HS; drug-induced causes of HS; the development of dermal tunnels and the infiltrative proliferative gelatinous mass (IPGM: Infiltrative Proliferative Gelatinous Mass), which are currently poorly integrated into the follicular occlusion model of HS. Removing follicular occlusion as the primary driver of HS recalibrates the focus of therapy to addressing the inflammatory nature of the disease. Whilst follicular occlusion is associated with HS, the evidence suggests that occlusion does not exclusively occur prior to inflammation.

What is required is a move towards clinical or pathological biomarkers of disease activity. Furthermore, there may not be one

"ideal" target for HS given the heterogeneity of disease and a reliable patient classification (both clinically and molecularly) is mandatory. Further ex-vivo and translational work into the inflammatory profiles of different disease tissues (keratinocytes, fibroblasts, leukocytes), morphologies (nodules, tunnels, comedones, ulcerations), and presentations (classic, syndromic, atypical) should be encouraged to work towards functional inflammatory profiles (endotypes) of disease in order to direct targeted therapy in HS for more successful outcomes. Realigning the pathogenic paradigm of HS with the molecular evidence is the first step to enable exploration of novel interventions and therapeutics for this debilitating disease.

References

1. Vossen ARJV, van der Zee HH, Prens EP. Hidradenitis suppurativa: A systematic review integrating inflammatory pathways into a cohesive pathogenic model. *Front Immunol.* 2018;9:2965.
2. Akiyama M, Takeichi T, McGrath JA, Sugiura K. Autoinflammatory keratinization diseases. *J Allerg Clin Immunol.* 2017;140:1545–1547.
3. Byrd AS, Carmona-Rivera C, O'Neil LJ, et al. Neutrophil extracellular traps, B cells, and type I interferons contribute to immune dysregulation in hidradenitis suppurativa. *Science Transl Med.* 2019;11 (508). eaav5908.
4. Van der zee HH, Laman JD, Prens EP. Can animal skin diseases or current transgenic mice serve as a model for Hidradenitis Suppurativa? *Dermatol.* 2012;225(1):9–13.
5. Frew JW, Piguet V. Ex-Vivo models and interpretation of mechanistic studies in Hidradenitis suppurativa. *J Invest Dermatol.* 2020; 140(7):1323–1326.
6. Frew JW. Commentary: Hidradenitis suppurativa: A systematic review integrating inflammatory pathways into a cohesive pathogenic model. *Front Immunol.* 2019;25(10):302.
7. Schwartz MA. The importance of indifference in scientific research. *J Cell Sci.* 2015;128(15):2745–2746.
8. Czarnowicki T, He H, Krueger JG, Guttman-Yassky E. Atopic dermatitis enodytpes and implications for targeted therapeutics. *J Allerg Clin Immunol.* 2019;143(1):1–11.
9. Frew JW, Marzano A, Wolk K, et al. Identifying novel therapeutic targets in hidradenitis suppurativa. *J Invest Dermatol.* 202;141 (2):316–324.
10. Shelley WB, Cahn MM. The pathogenesis of hidradenitis suppurativa in man; experimental and histologic observations. *AMA Arch Derm.* 1955;72(6):562–565.
11. Lever WF. Hidradenitis suppurativa. *Arch Derm Syphilol.* 1947;55 (5):713.
12. Jemec GB, Hansen U. Histology of hidradenitis suppurativa. *J Am Acad Dermatol.* 1996;34(6):994–999.
13. Attanoos RL, Appleton MA, Douglas-Jones AG. The pathogenesis of hidradenitis suppurativa: a closer look at the apocrine and apoeccrine glands. *Br J Dermatol.* 1995;133(2):254–258.
14. Zouboulis CC. Nogueira de Costa A, Fimmel S, Zouboulis KC. Apocrine glands are bystanders in hidradenitis suppurativa and their involvement in gender specific. *J Eur Acad Dermatol Venereol.* 2020;34(7):1555–1563.
15. Von von Laffert M, Stadie V, Wohlrab J, Marsch WC. Hidradenitis suppurativa/acne inversa: bilocated epithelial hyperplasia with very different sequelae. *Br J Dermatol.* 2011;164(2):367–371.
16. von Laffert M, Helmbold P, Wohlrab J, et al. Hidradenitis suppurativa (acne inversa): early inflammatory events at terminal follicles and at interfollicular epidermis. *Exp Dermatol.* 2010;19 (6):533–537.
17. Benhadou F, van der Zee HH, Pascual JC, et al. Pilonidal sinus disease: AN intergluteal localization of hidradenitis suppurativa/acne inversa: a cross sectional study among 2465 patient. *Br J Dermatol.* 2019;181(6):1198–1206.

18. Matard B, Cavelier-Balloy B, Reygagne P. Epidermal psoriasiform hyperplasia, an unrecognized sign of folliculitis decalvans: A histological study of 26 patients. *J Cutan Pathol.* 2017;44(4):352–357.

19. Wortsman X, Castro A, Morales C, et al. Sonographic Comparison of morphologic characteristics between pilonidal cysts and hidradenitis suppurativa. *J Ultrasound Med.* 2017;36(12):2403–2418.

20. Von Laffert M, Stadie V, Ulrich J, et al. Morphology of pilonidal sinus disease: some evidence of its being a unlocalized type of hidradenitis suppurativa. *Dermatol.* 2011;223(4):349–355.

21. Melnik BC, Plewig G. Impaired Notch signalling: the unifying mechanism explaining the pathogenesis of hidradenitis suppurativa (acne inversa). *Br J Dermatol.* 2013;168(4):876–878.

22. Melnik BC, Plewig G. Impaired Notch-MKP-1 signalling in hidradenitis suppurativa: an approach to pathogenesis by evidence from translational biology. *Exp Dermatol.* 2013;22(3):172–177.

23. Frings VG, Sennefelder H, Presser D, et al. Altered NOX expression does not seem to account for epidermal NLRP3 inflammasome activation in hidradenitis suppurativa. *Br J Dermatol.* 2019;181(2):391–392.

24. Shah A, Alhusayen R, Amini-Nik S. The critical role of macrophages in the pathogenesis of hidradenitis suppurativa. *Inflamm Res.* 2017;66(11):931–945.

25. Lima AL, Karl I, Giner T, et al. Keratinocytes and neutrophils are important sources of proinflammatory molecules in hidradenitis suppurativa. *Br J Dermatol.* 2016;174(3):514–521.

26. Marzano AV, Borghi A, Meroni PL, Cugno M. Pyoderma gangrenosum and its syndromic forms: evidence for a link with autoinflammation. *Br J Dermatol.* 2016;175(5):882–891.

27. Ghias MH, Hyde MJ, Tomalin LE, et al. Role of the Complement pathway in inflammatory skin diseases: a focus on hidradenitis suppurativa. *J Invest Dermatol.* 2020;140(3). 531–536.e1.

28. Grand D, Navrazhina K, Frew JW. Integrating complement into the molecular pathogenesis of Hidradenitis Suppurativa. *Exp Dermatol.* 2020;29(1):86–92.

29. Kanni T, Zenker O, Habel M, et al. Complement activation in hidradenitis suppurativa: a new pathway of pathogenesis? *Br J Dermatol.* 2018;179(2):413–419.

30. Kanni T, Zenker O, Habel M, et al. *Br J Dermatol.* 2018;179(2):413–419.

31. Giamarellos-Bourboulis EJ, Argyropoulou M, Kanni T, et al. Clinical efficacy of complement C5a inhibition by IFX-1 in hidradenitis suppurativa: an open-label single-arm trial in patients not eligible for adalimumab. *Br J Dermatol.* 2020;183(1):176–178.

32. Witte-Handel E, Wolk K, Tsausi A, et al. The IL-1 pathway is hyperactive in hidradenitis suppurativa and contributed to skin infiltration and destruction. *J Invest Dermatol.* 2019;139(6):1294–1305.

33. Wolk K, Warszawska K, Hoeflich C, et al. Deficiency of IL-22 contribute to a chronic inflammatory disease: pathogenetic mechanisms in acne inversa. *J Immunol.* 2011;186(2):1228–1239.

34. Tzanetakou V, Kanni T, Giatrakou S, et al. Safety and efficacy of anakinra in severe hidradenitis suppurativa: a randomized clinical trial. *JAMA Dermatol.* 2016;152(1):52–59.

35. Gottlieb A, Natsis NE, Kerdel F, et al. A phase II open-label study og Bermekimab in patients with hidradenitis suppurativa shows resolution of inflammatory lesions and pain. *J Invest Dermatol.* 2020;140(8):1538–1545.

36. Jimenez-Gallo D, de la Varga-Martinez R, Ossorio-Garcia L, et al. The clinical significance of increased serum proinflammatory cytokines, c-reactive protein, and erythrocyte sedimentation rate in patients with hidradenitis suppurativa. *Mediators Inflamm.* 2017;2450401.

37. Kanni T, Tzanetakou V, Savva A, et al. Compartmentalized cytokine responses in hidradenitis suppurativa. *PLoS One.* 2015;10(6):e0130522.

38. Frew JW, Grand D, Navrazhina K, et al. Beyond antibodies: B cells in Hidradenitis Suppurativa: bystanders, contributors or therapeutic targets? *Exp Dermato.* 29(5):509–515.

39. Musilova J, Moran B, Sweeney CM, et al. Enrichment of plasma cells in the peripheral blood and skin of patients with hidradenitis suppurativa. *J Invest Dermatol.* 2020;1091–1094.

40. Hoffman LK, Tomalin LE, Schultz G, et al. Integrating the skin and blood transcriptomes and serum proteome in hidradenitis suppurativa reveals complement dysregulation and a plasma cell signature. *PLoS One.* 2018;13(9):e0203672.

41. Lacarubba F, Dall'Oglio F, Musumeci ML, et al. Secondary comedones in a case of acne congolobata correlate with double-ended pseudocomedones in hidradenitis suppurativa. *Acta Derma Venereol.* 2017;97(8):969–970.

42. Boer J, Jemec GB. Mechanical stress and the development of pseudo-comedones and tunnels in Hidradenitis Suppurativa/Acne inversa. *Exp Dermatol.* 2016;25(5):396–397.

43. Lacarrubba F, Musumeci ML, Nasca MRW, et al. Double-ended Pseudocomedones in hidradenitis suppurativa: clinical, dermoscopic, and histopathological correlation. *Actw Derm Venerol.* 2017;97(6):763–764.

44. Higgins R, Pink A, Hunger R, et al. Generalized comedones, acne, and hidradenitis suppurativa in a patient with an *FGFR2* missense mutation. *Front Med (Lausanne).* 2017;4:16.

45. Fontao F, von Engelbrechten M, Seilaz C, et al. Microcomedones in non-lesional acne prone skin new orientations on comedogenesis and its prevention. *J Eur Acad Dermatol Venereol.* 2020;34(2):357–364.

46. Capitanio B, Lora V, Ludovici M, et al. Modulation of sebum oxidation and interleukin-1α levels associates with clinical improvement of mild comedonal acne. *J Eur Acad Dermatol Venereol.* 2014;28(12):1792–1797.

47. Saurat JH. Strategic targets in acne: the comedone switch in question. *Dermatol.* 2015;231(2):105–111.

48. Antiga E, Verdelli A, Bonciani D, et al. Acne: a new model of immune-mediated chronic inflammatory skin disease. *G Ital Dermatol Venereol.* 2015;150(2):247–254.

49. Ingham E, Eady A, Goodwin CE, et al. Pro-inflammatory levels of interleukin-1α-like bioactivity are present in the majority of open comedones in acne vulgaris. *J Invest Dermatol.* 1992;98(6):895–901.

50. Jeremy AHT, Holland DB, Roberts SG, et al. Inflammatory events are involved in acne lesion initiation. *J Invest Dermatol.* 2003;121(1):20–27.

51. Schneider MR, Paus R. Deciphering the functions of the hair follicle infundibulum in skin physiology and disease. *Cell Tissue Res.* 2014;358(3):697–704.

52. Guy R, Green MR, Kealey T. Modeling acne in vitro. *J Invest Dermatol.* 1996;106(1):176–182.

53. Jenei A, Dajnoki Z, Medgyesi B, et al. Apocrine gland–rich skin has a non-inflammatory IL-17–related immune milieu, that turns to inflammatory IL-17–mediated disease in hidradenitis suppurativa. *J Invest Dermatol.* 2019;139(4):964–968.

54. Melnik BC, John SM, Chen W, et al. T helper 17 cell/regulatory T-cell imbalance in hidradenitis suppurativa.acne inversa: the link to hair follicle dissection, obesity, smoking and autoimmune comorbidities. *Br J Dermatol.* 2018;179(2):260–272.

55. Agut-Busquet E, Gonzalez-villanueva I. Romani de Gabriel J, et al. Dowling-Degos disease and hidradenitis suppurativa. epidemiological and clinical study of 15 patients and review of the literature. *Acta Derm Venereol.* 2019;99(10):917–918.

56. Gonzales-Villanueva I, Guiterrez M, Hispan P, et al. Novel POFUT1 mutation association with hidradenitis suppurativa-Dowling-Degos disease firm up a role for Notch signaling in the pathogenesis of this disorder. *Br J Dermatol.* 2018;178(4):984–986.

57. Grice EA, Segre JA. The skin microbiome. *Nat Rev Microbiol.* 2011;9(4):244–253.

58. Grice EA, Kong HH, Conlan S, et al. Topographical and temporal diversity of the human skin microbiome. *Sci.* 2009;324(5931):1190–1192.

59. Grice EA. The skin microbiome: potential for novel diagnostic and therapeutic approach to cutaneous disease. *Semin Cutan Med Surg.* 2014;33(2):98–103.

60. Schneider MR, Paus R. Deciphering the functions of the hair follicle infundibulum in skin physiology and disease. *Cell Tissue Res.* 2014;358(3):697–704.

61. Polak-Witka K, Rudnicka L, Bume-Peytavi U, et al. The role of the microbiome in scalp hair follicle biology and disease. *Exp Dermatol.* 2020;29(3):286–294.

62. Scharschmidt TC, Vasquez KS, Pauli ML, et al. Commensal microbes and hair follicle morphogenesis coordinately drive treg migration into neonatal skin cell host. *Microbe.* 2017;21(4):467–477.

63. Paus R, Bulfone-Paus S, Bertolini M. Hair follicle immune privilege revisited: the key to alopecia areata management. *J Investig Dermatol Symp Proc.* 2018;19(1):S12–S17.

64. Ring HC, Thorsen J, Saunte DM, et al. The follicular skin microbiome in patients with hidradenitis suppurativa and healthy controls. *JAMA Dermatol.* 2017;153(9):897–905.

65. Ring HC, Sigsgaard V, Thorsen J, et al. The microbiome of tunnels in hidradenitis suppurativa. *J Eur Acad Dermatol Venereol.* 2019;33(9):1775–1780.

66. Brauweiler AM, Goleva E, Leung DYM. Staphylococcus aureus lipoteichoic acid damaged the epidermal barrier through an IL-1 mediated pathway. *J Invest Dermatol.* 2019;139(8):1753–1761.e4.

67. Qin M, Pirouz A, Kim MH, et al. Propionibacterium acnes induces IL-1β secretion via the NLRP3 inflammasome in human monocytes. *J Invest Dermatol.* 2014;134(2):381–388.

68. Altmeier S, Toska A, Sparber F, et al. IL-1 coordinates the neutrophil response to *C. albicans* in the oral mucosa. *PLoS Pathog.* 2016;12(9):e1005882.

69. Sanmiguel JC, Olaru F, Li J, et al. Interleukin-1 regulated keratinocyte expression of T cell targeting chemokines through interleukin-1 receptor associated kinase (IRAK-1) dependent and independent pathways. *Cell Signal.* 2009;21(5):685–694.

70. Frew JW. ASCA antibodies in Hidradenitis Suppurativa: more than a gut feeling. *J Allergy Clin Immunol.* 2020;146(2):458.

71. Assan F, Gottlieb J, Tubach F, et al. Anti-*Saccharomyces cerevisiae* IgG and IgA antibodies are associated with systemic inflammation and advanced disease in hidradenitis suppurativa. *J Allerg Clin Immunol.* 2020;146:452–455.

72. Frew JW, Navrazhina K. In silico analysis of gamma-secretase-complex mutations in hidradenitis suppurativa demonstrates disease-specific substrate recognition and cleavage alterations. *Front Med.* 2019;6:206.

73. Frew JW, Navrazhina K. No evidence that impaired notch signalling differentiates hidradenitis suppurativa from other inflammatory skin diseases. *Br J Dermatol.* 2020;182:1042–1043.

74. Wang B, Yang W, Wen W, et al. Gamma-secretase gene mutations in familial acne inversa. *Sci.* 2010;330(6007):1065.

75. Hung COY, Livesey FJ. Altered y-secretase processing of APP disrupts lysosome and autphagosome function in monogenic Alzheimers disease. *Cell Rep.* 2018;25(13):3647–3660.

76. Urbanek K, Cabral-da-Silva MC, Ide-Iwata N, et al. Inhibition of notch1-dependent cardiomyogenesis leads to dilated cardiomyopathy in the neonatal heart. *Circ Res.* 2010;107(3):429–441.

77. Duchatelet S, Miskintye S, Delage M, Ungeheuer MN, et al. Low prevalence of gamma-secretase complex gene mutations in a large cohort of predominantly Caucasian patients with Hidradenitis Suppurativa. *J Invest Dermatol.* 2020;140(10):2085–2088.

78. Xiao X, He Y, Li C, et al. Nicastrin mutations in familial acne inversa impact keratinocyte proliferation and differentiation through the Notch and Phosphoinositide 3-kinase/AKT signalingpathways. *Br J Dermatol.* 2016;174(3):522–532.

79. He Y, Li C, Xu H, et al. AKT-dependent hyperproliferation of keratinocytes in familial hidradenitis suppurariga with a NCSTN mutation: a potential role of defective miR-100-5p. *Br J Dermatol.* 2020;182(2):500–502.

80. McGeachy MJ, Cua DJ, Gaffen SL. The IL-17 family of cytokines in health and disease. *Immunity.* 2019;50:892–906.

81. Yang J, Wang L, Zhang X, et al. Keratin05-Cre driven deletion of NCSTN in acne inversa like mouse model leads to markedly increasd IL36q and SPRR2 expression. *Front Med.* 2020;14(3):305–317.

82. He Y, Xu H, LI C, et al. Nicastrin/miR-30a-3p/RAB31 axis regulates keratinocyte differentiation by impairing EGFR signaling in familial. *Acne Inversa J Invest Dermatol.* 2019;139(1):124–134.

83. Cao L, Morales-Heil DJ, Roberson EDO. Nicastrin haploinsufficiencty alters expression of type 1 interferon stimulated genes: the relationship to familial hidradenitis suppurativa. *Clin Exp Dermatol.* 2019;44(4):e118–e125.

84. Gonzalez-Villanueva I, Guiterrez M, HIspan P, et al. Novel POFUT1 mutation associated with hidradenitis suppurativa-Dowling-Degos disease firm up a role for Notch signaling in the pathogenesis of this disorder. *Br J Dermatol.* 2018;178(4):984–986.

85. Jfri AH, O'Brien E, Litvinov I, et al. Hidradenitis Suppurativa: comprehensive review of predisposing genetic mutations and changes. *J Cutan Med Surg.* 2019;23(5):519–527.

86. Liu Y, Yen H, Chen CY, et al. Sialylation and fucosylation of epidermal growth factor receptor suppresses its dimerization and activation in lung cancer cells. *PNAS.* 2011;108(28):11322–11373.

87. Frew JW, Vekic DA, Woods JA, et al. Drug-associated Hidradenitis Suppurativa: a systematic review of case reports. *J Am Acad Dermatol.* 2018;78(1):217–219.

88. Porter ML, Kimball AB. Comorbidities of hidradenitis suppurativa. *Semin Cutan Med Surg.* 2017;36(2):55–57.

89. Gisondi P, Bellinato F, Girolomi G, et al. Pathogenesis of chronic plaque psoriasis and its intersection with cardiometabolic comorbidities. *Front Pharmacol.* 2020;11:117.

90. Romano S, Salustri E, Ruscitti P, et al. Cardiovascular and metabolic comorbidities in rheumatoid arthritis. *Curr Rheumatol Rep.* 2018;20(12):81.

91. Raggi OP, Genest J, Giles JT, et al. Role of inflammation in the pathogenesis of atherosclerosis and therapeutic interventions. *Atherosclerosis.* 2018;276:98–108.

92. Alikhan A, Sayed C, Alavi A, et al. North American clinical management guidelines for Hidradenitis Suppurativa: A publication from the United States and Canadian Hidradenitis Suppurativa Foundations: Part II Topical, intralesional and systemic medical management. *J Am Acad Dermatol.* 2019;81(1):91–101.

93. Zouboulis CC, Desai N, Emtestam L, et al. European S1 Guideline for the treatment of hidradenitis suppurativa/acne inversal. *J Eur Acad Dermatol Venereol.* 2015;29(4):619–644.

94. SImonart T. Hidradenitis Suppurativa and smoking. *J Am Acad Dermatol.* 2010;62(1):149–150.

95. Gallagher C, Kirthi S, Burke T, et al. Remission of hidradenitis suppurativa after bariatric surgery. *JAAD Case Rep.* 2017;3(5):436–437.

96. Reily SM, Saltiel AR. Adapting to obesity with adipose tissue inflammation. *Nat Rev Endocrinol.* 2017;13:633–643.

97. Deng T, Lyon CJ, Bergin S, et al. Obesity, inflammation and cancer. *Annual Reviw Pathol.* 2016;11:421–449.

98. Gonçalves RB, Coletta RD, Silvério KG, et al. Impact of smoking on inflammation: overview of molecular mechanisms. *Inflamm Res.* 2011;60(5):409–424.

99. Patterson AT, Tian FT, Elston DM, et al. Occluded cigarette smoke exposure causgin localized chloracne-like comedones. *Dermatol.* 2015;231:322–325.

100. Kwon H, Pessin JE. Adipokines mediate inflammation and insulin resistance. *Front Endocrinol.* 2013;4:71.

101. Guy R, Kealey T. Modelling the infundibulum in acne. *Dermatol.* 1998;196(1):32–37.

102. Kumtomrut C, Yamauchi T, Koike S, et al. Androgens modularte keratinocyte differentiation indirectly through enhancing growth factor production from dermal fibroblasts. *J Dermatol Sci.* 2019;93(3):150–158.

103. Sivanand A, Gulliver WP, Josan CK, et al. Weight loss and dietary interventions for hidradenitis suppurativa: a systematic review. *J Cutan Med Surg.* 2020;24(1):64–72.

104. Hoffman LK, Ghias MH, Lowes MA. Pathophysiology of Hidradenitis Suppurativa. *Semin Cutan Med Surg.* 2017;36(2):47–54.

105. Ogura H, Murakami M, Okuyama Y, et al. Interleukin-17 promotes autoimmunity by triggering a positive-feedback loop via interleukin-6 induction. *Immunity.* 2008;29:628–636.

106. Veldhoen M. Interleukin 17 is a chief orchestrator of immunity. *Nat Immunol.* 2017;18:612–621.

107. Ramirez-Carrozzi V, Sambandam A, Luis E, et al. IL-17C regulates the innate immune functions of epithelial cells in an autocrine manner. *Nat Immunol.* 2011;12:1159–1166.

108. Navrazhina K, Frew JW, Krueger JG. Interleukin 17C is elevated in lesional tissue of hidradenitis suppurativa. *Br J Dermatol.* 2020; 182(4):1045–1047.

109. Frew JW, Navrazhina K, Marohn M, et al. Contribution of fibroblasts to tunnel formation and inflammation in hidradenitis suppurativa/ acne inversa. *Exp Dermatol.* 2019;28(8):886–891.

110. Frew JW, Hawkes JE, Krueger JG. A systematic review and critical evaluation of immunohistochemical associations in Hidradenitis Suppurativa. *F100Res.* 2018;7:1923.

111. Frew JW, Hawkes JE, Krueger JG. A systematic review and critical evaluation of inflammatory cytokine associations in Hidradenitis Suppurativa. *F100Res.* 2018;7:1930.

112. Vossen ARJV, Ardon CB, van der Zee HH, et al. The anti-inflamamtory potency of biologics targeting tumour necrosis factor-alpha, intereukin (IL)-17A, IL-12/23 and CD20 in hidradenitis suppurativa: an ex vivo study. *Br J Dermatol.* 2019;181(2): 314–323.

113. Zouboulis CC, Nogueira da Costa A, Makrantonaki E, et al. Alterations in innate immunity and epithelial cell differentiation are the molecular pillars of hidradenitis suppurativa. *J Eur Acad Dermatol Venereol.* 2020;34(4):846–861.

114. Shanmugan VK, Jones D, McNish S, et al. Transcriptome patterns in hidradenitis suppurativa: support for the role of antimicrobial peptides and interferon pathways in disease pathogenesis. *Clin Exp Dermatol.* 2019;44(8):882–892.

115. Kurzen H, Jung EG, Hartschuh W, et al. Forms of epithelial differentiation of draining sinus in acne inversa (hidradenitis suppurativa). *Br J Dermatol.* 1999;141(2):231–239.

116. Frew JW, Navrazhina K, Byrd AS, et al. Defining lesional, perilesional and unaffected skin in hidradenitis suppurativa: proposed recommendations for clinical trials and translational research studies. *Br J Dermatol.* 2019;181(6):1339–1341.

117. Vossen ARJV, van Straalen KR, Florencia EF, et al. Lesional inflammatory profile in hidradenitis suppurativa is not solely driven by IL-1. *J Invest Dermatol.* 2020;140(7):1463–1466.

118. Krueger JG, Brunner PM. Interluekin-17 alters the biology of many cell types involved in the genesis of psoriasis, systemic inflammation and associated comorbidities. *Exp Dermatol.* 2018;27(2):115–123.

119. Frew JW, PIguet V. Ex Vivo models and interpretation of mechanistic studies in hidradenitis suppurativa. *J Invest Dermatol.* 2020; 140(7):1323–1326.

120. Rongioletti F. Ch4: histopathology. In: MIcali G, ed. *Hidradenitis Suppurativa: A Diagnostic Atlas.* 1st ed. New York: Wiley; 2017.

121. Danby FW, Jemec GB, Marsch WCh, et al. Preliminary findings suggest hidradenitis suppurativa may be due to defective follicular support. *Br J Dermatol.* 2013;168(5):1034–1039.

122. Chuang YH, Dean D, Allen J, et al. Comparison between the expression of basement membrane zone antigens of human interfollicular epidermis and anagen hair follicle using indirect immunofluorescence. *Br J Dermatol.* 2003;149(2):274–281.

123. Kurzen H, Jung EG, Hartschuh W, et al. Forms of epithelial differentiation of draining sinus in acne inversa (Hidradenitis suppurativa). *Br J Dermatol.* 1999;141(2):231–239.

124. Mozeika E, Pilmane M, Nürnberg BM, et al. Tumour necrosis factor-alpha and matrix metalloproteinase-2 are expressed strongly in hidradenitis suppurativa. *Acta Derm Venereol.* 2013;93(3): 301–304.

125. Hoang VT, Trinh CT, Nguyen CH, et al. Overview of epidermoid cyst. *Eur J Radiol Open.* 2019;6:291–301.

126. Gauntner TD. Hormonal, stem cell and Notch signaling as possible mechanisms of disease in Hidradenitis Suppurativa: a systems-level transcriptomic analysis. *Br J Dermatol.* 2018;180(1):203–204.

127. Coates M, Mariottoni P, Cocoran DL, et al. The skin transcriptome in hidradenitis suppurativa uncovers an antimicrobial and sweat gland gene signature which has distinct overall with wounded skin. *PLoS One.* 2019;14(5), e0216249.

128. Navrazhina K, Frew JW, Sullivan-Whelan M, et al. Epithelialized dermal tunnels drive "Feed-Forward" inflammation and transepithelial neutrophil migration in hidradenitis suppurativa. *Sci Trans Med.* 2020; [In Press].

129. Scharl M, Rogler G. Pathophysiology of fistula formation in Crohn's disease. *World J Gastrointest Pathophys.* 2014;5(3):205–212.

130. Oh JW, Kloepper J, Langan EA, et al. A guide to studying human hair follicle cycling in vivo. *J Invest Dermatol.* 2016;136(1):34–44.

131. Ge Y, Fuchs E. Stretching the limits: from homeostasis to stem cell plasticity in wound healing and cancer. *Nat Rev Genet.* 2018;19:311–325.

132. Kidacki M, Cong Z, Flamm A, et al. Invasive proliferative gelatinous mass of hidradenitis suppurativa contains distinct inflammatory components. *Br J Dermatol.* 2019;181(1):192–193.

133. Ring HC, Bay L, Nilsson M, et al. Bacterial biofilm in chronic lesions of hidradenitis suppurativa. *Br J Dermatol.* 2017;l176 (4):993–1000.

11

Microbiota Perturbations in Hidradenitis Suppurativa

HALEY B. NAIK

CHAPTER OUTLINE

Introduction

Hidradenitis suppurativa (HS) is a disabling chronic inflammatory disease with significant comorbidities that affects an estimated 1% of the Western population.[1] A poor understanding of HS biology has limited the development of uniformly effective treatments. The characteristic lesions of HS in conjunction with disease improvement with broad spectrum antibiotic therapy have implicated bacteria in HS pathogenesis[2-4] and suggested novel areas for consideration of therapeutic development.

Role of Bacteria in Hidradenitis Suppurativa Biology

HS is characterized by painful recurrent abscesses, malodorous purulent drainage, dermal tunnel formation, and disfiguring scarring involving intertriginous body sites including the axillae, breasts, groin, and buttocks.[2-4] The clinical characteristics of HS lesions have implicated bacteria in HS biology, which has guided the variably successful use of broad-spectrum antibiotics for HS. Despite its clinical presentation, however, HS is not thought to be an infectious disease for several reasons. First, bacterial organisms common to all HS lesions have not been identified and proven

to be pathogenic. Second, HS is not reproducible upon inoculation of an unaffected susceptible host. Third, HS responds to immunomodulatory therapy, including tumor necrosis factor (TNF) inhibitors and intralesional steroids, which would presumably worsen an infectious condition.[5] Disease response to immunomodulatory therapies suggests an important role for immune dysregulation in HS pathogenesis.

Limited studies have implicated dysregulated immune responses in HS, including elevations in TNF,[6-9] interleukin (IL)-1β,[8] IL-12/23,[10-12] and IL-17,[13] and activation of the JAK pathway.[14,15] Furthermore, TNF inhibitor adalimumab is currently the only US Food and Drug Administration-approved drug for HS,[6-9,16] thus underscoring the important role of TNF in HS-related inflammation. Initial studies have also suggested a role for humoral immunity in HS pathogenesis.[17] These findings have collectively guided the study of novel interventional treatments and the clinical use of biologic agents for HS.

Taken together, these observations suggest that chronic dysregulated immune responses to abnormal and pathogenic microbial colonization of the mucocutaneous surfaces, also known as *microbial perturbations* or *dysbiosis*, may result in persistent tissue inflammation in HS.

Bacteriology of Hidradenitis Suppurativa

Until the last decade, culture-based approaches were the standard for characterizing microbial diversity on the skin and at other body sites. Conventional culture-based methods for characterizing microbes are limited, however, because less than 1% of bacterial species are cultivatable under standard laboratory conditions. Fastidious growth requirements of some bacteria make isolation and cultivation difficult. This is underscored by the fact that historically, skin microbial research focused on investigation of a small number of cultivatable microbial species that were associated with common skin disorders. Resultantly, differential recovery of skin microbes using culture-based approaches can lead to misinterpretation of the true relative abundance of bacterial species in a given sample.

Although the presence of abscesses and malodorous drainage has implicated microorganisms in HS pathogenesis, no consistent organism has been cultivated from HS lesions using conventional culture-based methods. Polymicrobial flora, including coagulase-negative *Staphylococci*, mixed anaerobes, *Staphylococcus aureus*, and *Corynebacterium* species,[18-22] have been identified in only approximately 50% of HS lesions using conventional culture-based methods. These findings have largely guided the use of broad spectrum topical and systemic antimicrobial therapy—including antiseptic washes and antibiotics—as first-line management for HS management.

Although antibiotic therapy can be effective for HS management, treatment strategies that rely on repeated and lengthy antibiotic courses may induce antibiotic-resistant bacterial species. In a single center study, antibiotic therapy with topical clindamycin, oral ciprofloxacin, and trimethoprim/sulfamethoxazole were associated with cultivation of antibiotic resistant organisms.[23] These data caution antibiotic stewardship in the management of HS.

Biofilm in Hidradenitis Suppurativa

Biofilm is an architectural colony of microorganisms within a matrix of extracellular polymeric substance which they produce. Within biofilm, microbial cells adhere to one another and to a static surface, thereby sheltering themselves from clearance by host defenses and antibiotics.[24] Biofilms are thought to play an important role in the maintenance of chronic HS dermal tunnels (also called sinus tracts) and have also been hypothesized to play a role in development of acute HS lesions.

In a single study examining chronic HS lesions, biofilms were more commonly observed in lesional rather than perilesional skin, and specifically in sinus tracts and in the follicular infundulum.[25] Active bacteria were noted in sinus tracts, which were associated with lymphocytic infiltration and giant cell reactions. In a subsequent study, biofilms were found in a minority of acutely inflamed hair follicles.[26] These data together suggest that biofilms may play an important role in maintaining chronic HS lesions.

Skin Microbiota Alterations in Hidradenitis Suppurativa

In recent years, advances in high-throughput, culture-free, sequence-based genomic technologies have facilitated more comprehensive assessment of the diverse and uncultivatable microorganisms on the skin and mucosal surfaces of HS patients.[27] Sequencing of the 16S ribosomal RNA gene, which is highly conserved in prokaryotes, has facilitated unbiased phylogenetic categorization of bacteria. Shotgun metagenomic sequencing consists of shearing the entire genomes of all microbes in a given sample, and then sequencing and assembling the fragments into a continuous sequence based on a reference or by forming larger contigs. This method allows not only for phylotyping but can also reveal functional information about microbial communities.

The health of microbial ecosystems is thought to be related to microbial diversity. Examining differences in microbial diversity can provide insights into microbial shifts within samples. Bacterial diversity can be measured by richness (the number of different species in a sample) and evenness (the extent to which species are evenly distributed). Alpha diversity is a measure of species richness within a sample, while beta diversity is a measure of differences in species composition across samples. The Shannon and Simpson diversity indices are mathematical measures that account for both the abundance and evenness of species in a given sample.

Skin Microbiota Perturbations in Hidradenitis Suppurativa Lesional Skin

Cross-sectional studies examining skin microbiota in HS have reported perturbations in skin commensal and anaerobic bacteria using 16S rRNA biomarker sequencing. These studies have focused primarily on microbial alterations observed at HS lesional sites, and concur in their reports of decreased relative abundances of skin commensal bacteria, specifically *Cutibacterium acnes* (previously *Propionobacterium acnes*), and increased relative abundances of mixed anaerobic bacteria at HS lesional sites as compared with both nonlesional HS skin and healthy control skin.[28,29]

Although increased relative abundances of anaerobic bacteria have been reported in HS lesions as compared with nonlesional HS skin and healthy control skin, the specific identified anaerobic organisms driving microbial perturbations has varied between studies, including *Prevotella*, *Porphyromonas*, and *Peptoniphilus* phyla, and *Clostridiales* order.[28-31] In addition to variations in their assessment of bacterial composition and the taxa primarily driving diversity in HS lesional skin, HS nonlesional skin, and healthy control skin, these studies also differ in their assessment of differences in bacterial diversity as measured by community richness and evenness.[28-31] One study reported increased evenness and richness of lesional skin as compared with healthy control skin, another reported increased evenness and richness in nonlesional skin as compared with lesional and normal skin, and the third reported no difference in evenness and richness across all three groups.[28-31] This observed variation may be attributable to methodological differences in sample collection and processing, underscoring the importance of a standardized approach to human microbiome studies to ensure the reproducibility of results. Uniform practices for skin preparation, exposure and clinical metadata collection, and sample acquisition and processing, are critical to ensure that observed microbiota perturbations can be attributed to the exposure under investigation, rather than to unanticipated confounders.[32]

Increased bacterial diversity has been linked specifically to severe HS lesions and there is a positive association between relative abundance of anaerobic bacteria and disease severity; however, limited overlap is observed in the microbial drivers reported across studies.[28,30] In one study, worsening HS severity positively correlated with increased relative abundances of mixed gram-negative and gram-positive anaerobes, including *Prevotella*, *Porphyromonas* and *Peptoniphilus*, and *Clostridiales* order. In contrast, the relative abundances of major skin commensals, including commensal staphylococci, *Cutibacterium* spp., and *Corynebacterium* spp., inversely correlated with disease severity. There was higher within group variation in bacterial composition in severe HS as compared with mild and moderate HS.[32] Similarly, a second study found that severe HS lesions were associated with increased bacterial diversity, but in contrast, the most abundant organisms identified in severe HS patients (Hurley stage 3) were *Fusobacterium*, *Parvimonas*, *Streptococcus*, and *Clostridiales* order bacteria.[30]

A single study has examined the microbial composition within HS tunnels and demonstrated an abundance of anaerobic bacteria, including *Prevotella*, *Porphyromonas*, and *Peptoniphilus* spp., and skin commensals including *Corynebacterium* spp. and *Staphylococcus* spp., within these structures.[33]

Skin Microbiota Perturbations in Hidradenitis Suppurativa Nonlesional Skin

Two studies have examined the skin microbiota of unaffected but clinically relevant skinfolds in HS patients compared with healthy controls. An initial study reported decreased relative abundance of commensal bacteria on unaffected skin as compared with healthy control skin, similar to observations made in HS lesional skin.[32] Additionally, gram-negative and gram-positive anaerobic bacteria predominated in unaffected HS skin as compared with healthy control skin, and bacterial diversity as measured by the Shannon diversity index was increased in unaffected HS skin as compared with healthy control skin.

In a second larger study designed specifically to understand skin microbiota shifts in unaffected HS skinfolds, decreased mean abundances of skin commensal bacteria, including coagulase negative *Staphylococci* and *Cutibacterium acnes,* in the skin folds of HS patients, and increased mean abundances of anaerobic bacteria in the inguinal and gluteal cleft folds of HS patients, were found using conventional culture-based methods.[34] The mean abundance of *Corynebacterium* spp. abundances correlated with more severe disease, while *Cutibacterium* spp. abundances inversely correlated with severe disease.

Using 16S rRNA biomarker sequencing, this study also observed greater bacterial evenness and found decreased relative abundance of *Staphylococci* and increased relative abundances of anaerobic bacteria in unaffected HS skinfolds as compared with healthy control skin.[34] Over 60% of HS samples were associated with anaerobic bacteria, including *Prevotella, Porphyromonas,* and *Peptoniphilus asaccharolyticus*—all of which have been individually associated with microbial shifts at HS lesional sites in prior studies.[28-31] While anaerobic bacteria previously identified in HS lesions were significantly more abundant in unaffected HS skinfolds, only *S. aureus* was associated with HS clinical severity.

Taken together, these findings suggest that even in the absence of clinical lesions, HS skin has a distinct microbiome.

Gut Microbiome Alterations in Hidradenitis Suppurativa

HS has been associated with inflammatory bowel disease, a condition linked to perturbations in the gut microbiota.[35-39] Additionally, HS patients anecdotally report variation in disease activity in response to dietary modifications. These data suggest that gut dysbiosis may be associated with HS. A single small case-control series of three patients and three controls has used 16S rRNA sequencing to examine the gut microbiome in HS patients and found that alpha diversity was increased in age- and sex-matched healthy controls as compared with HS patients.[40] HS gut samples were also notable for reduced relative abundance of *Firmicutes* compared with healthy controls. *Bilophila* and *Holdemania* genera were more abundant and *Lachnobacterium* and *Veillonella* genera were less abundant in HS patients as compared with healthy controls. These findings are consistent with previous studies that report decreased gut microbiota diversity in inflammatory bowel disease (IBD) and obesity and increased relative abundance of microbes associated with metabolic dysfunction.[41,42] Although these data are limited by small sample size, and the investigators did not control for tobacco smoking which is known to alter the gut microbiota, these preliminary data suggest that gut dysbiosis may be associated with

HS.[43] Larger controlled studies from diverse populations are needed to confirm these findings and their generalizability across the HS patient population.

Relevance to Therapy

The causal relationship between microbial perturbations and HS has yet to be clarified. Whether microbiome perturbations are drivers of disease or secondary to disease-associated patterns has not been elucidated.[44] In other inflammatory diseases associated with microbiota shifts, previous proof-of-concept studies using high-resolution approaches have provided insights into the role of microbial perturbations and have led to development of novel therapeutic approaches. In atopic dermatitis, for example, relative abundance of *S. aureus* has been associated with disease flare,[45] *S. aureus* has been shown to elicit inflammation and exacerbate eczema, and *S. aureus*-targeted treatment has been shown to reduce skin inflammation.[46] These findings have led to the development of novel therapeutic strategies aimed at repopulating skin commensal bacteria.[47] In inflammatory bowel disease, high-resolution approaches have provided insights into microbial shifts relevant to disease progression[45,48] that have led to novel treatment approaches, including fecal microbiota transplants aimed at repopulating gut commensals.[49,50]

Conclusion and Future Directions

Cross-sectional data from the skin and gut of HS patients have demonstrated microbial shifts that may have clinical relevance in HS. Longitudinal studies are needed to examine how microbiota perturbations shift over the course of waxing and waning disease and if these shifts portend disease development and progression. A deeper understanding of microbial drivers and microbial products that may have a role in immune dysregulation in HS may potentially lead to novel microbe-based interventions. Identification of microbiota clusters, or even specific microbial species, that may serve as biomarkers for disease prognosis or predictors of treatment response may potentially inform clinical practice. Finally, a deeper understanding of the functional impact of specific abundant or unique microbes in HS will be important to advance novel microbiota-based therapies.

References

1. Ingram JR, Jenkins-Jones S, Knipe DW, et al. Population-based clinical practice research datalink study using algorithm modelling to identify the true burden of hidradenitis suppurativa. *Br J Dermatol.* 2018;178:917–924.
2. Jemec GB. Hidradenitis suppurativa. *Plast Reconst Surg.* 1987;80:754–755.
3. von der Werth JM, Williams HC. The natural history of hidradenitis suppurativa. *J Eur Acad Dermatol Venereol.* 2000;14:389–392.
4. McMichael A, Curtis AR, Guzman-Sanchez D, Kelly AP. *Dermatology.* 3rd ed. Cambridge, Massachusetts: Elsevier; 2012.
5. Naik HB, Nassif A, Ramesh MS, et al. Are Bacteria Infectious pathogens in hidradenitis suppurativa? Debate at the symposium for hidradenitis suppurativa advances meeting, November 2017. *J Invest Dermatol.* 2019;139:13–16.

6. Jemec GB. Predicting response to anti-TNF-alpha treatment in Hidradenitis suppurativa. *Br J Dermatol.* 2013;168:233.

7. Sbidian E, Hotz C, Seneschal J, et al. Anti-TNFalpha therapy for hidradenitis suppurativa. Results from a national cohort study between 2000 and 2013. *Br J Dermatol.* 2016;174(3):667–670.

8. van der Zee HH, de Ruiter L, van den Broecke DG, et al. Elevated levels of tumour necrosis factor (TNF)-alpha, interleukin (IL)-1beta and IL-10 in hidradenitis suppurativa skin: a rationale for targeting TNF-alpha and IL-1beta. *Br J Dermatol.* 2011;164: 1292–1298.

9. van Rappard DC, Limpens J, Mekkes JR. The off-label treatment of severe hidradenitis suppurativa with TNF-alpha inhibitors: a systematic review. *J Dermatolog Treat.* 2013;24:392–404.

10. Baerveldt EM, Kappen JH, Thio HB, et al. Successful long-term triple disease control by ustekinumab in a patient with Behcet's disease, psoriasis and hidradenitis suppurativa. *Ann Rheum Dis.* 2013;72: 626–627.

11. Gulliver WP, Jemec GB, Baker KA. Experience with ustekinumab for the treatment of moderate to severe hidradenitis suppurativa. *J Eur Acad Dermatol Venereol.* 2012;26:911–914.

12. Santos-Perez MI, Garcia-Rodicio S, Del Olmo-Revuelto MA, Pozo-Roman T. Ustekinumab for hidradenitis suppurativa: a case report. *Actas dermo-sifiliograficas.* 2014;105:720–722.

13. Jorgensen AR, Yao Y, Thomsen SF. Therapeutic Response to Secukinumab in a 36-year-old woman with Hidradenitis Suppurativa. *Case Rep Dermatol Med.* 2018;2018:8685136.

14. Savage KT, Santillan MR, Flood KS, et al. Tofacitinib shows benefit in conjunction with other therapies in recalcitrant hidradenitis suppurativa patients. *JAAD Case Rep.* 2020;6:99–102.

15. Lyons AB, Shabeeb N, Nicholson CL, et al. Emerging medical treatments for hidradenitis suppurativa. *J Am Acad Dermatol.* 2020;83:554–562.

16. Kimball AB, Okun MM, Williams DA, et al. Two phase 3 trials of Adalimumab for hidradenitis suppurativa. *N Engl J Med.* 2016;375:422–434.

17. Hoffman LK, Tomalin LE, Schultz G, et al. Integrating the skin and blood transcriptomes and serum proteome in hidradenitis suppurativa reveals complement dysregulation and a plasma cell signature. *PloS one.* 2018;13:e0203672.

18. Jemec GB. Hidradenitis suppurativa. *J Cutan Med Surg.* 2003;7: 47–56.

19. Brook I, Frazier EH. Aerobic and anaerobic microbiology of axillary hidradenitis suppurativa. *J Med Microbiol.* 1999;48:103–105.

20. Leach RD, Eykyn SJ, Phillips I, et al. Anaerobic axillary abscess. *Br Med J.* 1979;2:5–7.

21. Gener G, Canoui-Poitrine F, Revuz JE, et al. Combination therapy with clindamycin and rifampicin for hidradenitis suppurativa: a series of 116 consecutive patients. *Dermatology.* 2009;219:148–154.

22. Join-Lambert O, Coignard H, Jais JP, et al. Efficacy of rifampin-moxifloxacin-metronidazole combination therapy in hidradenitis suppurativa. *Dermatol.* 2011;222:49–58.

23. Fischer AH, Haskin A, Okoye GA. Patterns of antimicrobial resistance in lesions of hidradenitis suppurativa. *J Am Acad Dermatol.* 2017;76:309–313. e2.

24. Costerton W, Veeh R, Shirtliff M, et al. The application of biofilm science to the study and control of chronic bacterial infections. *J Clin Invest.* 2003;112:1466–1477.

25. Ring HC, Bay L, Nilsson M, et al. Bacterial biofilm in chronic lesions of hidradenitis suppurativa. *Br J Dermatol.* 2017;176:993–1000.

26. Okoye GA, Vlassova N, Olowoyeye O, et al. Bacterial biofilm in acute lesions of hidradenitis suppurativa. *Br J Dermatol.* 2017;176:241–243.

27. Turnbaugh PJ, Ley RE, Hamady M, et al. The human microbiome project. *Nature.* 2007;449:804–810.

28. Naik HB, Jo JH, Paul M, Kong HH. Skin microbiota perturbations are distinct and disease severity-dependent in hidradenitis suppurativa. *J Invest Dermatol.* 2020;140(4):922–925.

29. Schneider AM, Cook LC, Zhan X, et al. Loss of skin microbial diversity and alteration of bacterial metabolic function in hidradenitis suppurativa. *J Invest Dermatol.* 2020;140:716–720.

30. Guet-Revillet H, Jais JP, Ungeheuer MN, et al. The microbiological landscape of anaerobic infections in hidradenitis suppurativa: a prospective metagenomic study. *Clin Infect Dis.* 2017;65: 282–291.

31. Ring HC, Thorsen J, Saunte DM, et al. The follicular skin microbiome in patients with hidradenitis suppurativa and healthy controls. *JAMA Dermatol.* 2017;153:897–905.

32. Naik HB, Jo JH, Paul M, Kong HH. Skin microbiota perturbations are distinct and disease severity-dependent in hidradenitis suppurativa. *J Invest Dermatol.* 2020;140:922–925. e3.

33. Ring HC, Sigsgaard V, Thorsen J, et al. The microbiome of tunnels in hidradenitis suppurativa patients. *J Eur Acad Dermatol Venereol.* 2019;33(9):1775–1780.

34. Riverain-Gillet E, Guet-Revillet H, Jais JP, et al. The surface microbiome of clinically unaffected skinfolds in hidradenitis suppurativa: a cross-sectional culture-based and 16S rRNA gene amplicon sequencing study in 60 patients. *J Invest Dermatol.* 2020;140: 1847–1855.

35. Garg A, Hundal J, Strunk A. Overall and subgroup prevalence of Crohn disease among patients with hidradenitis suppurativa: a population-based analysis in the United States. *JAMA Dermatol.* 2018;154:814–818.

36. Lee JH, Kwon HS, Jung HM, et al. Prevalence and comorbidities associated with hidradenitis suppurativa in Korea: a nationwide population-based study. *J Eur Acad Dermatol Venereol.* 2018;32:1784–1790.

37. Egeberg A, Jemec GBE, Kimball AB, et al. Prevalence and risk of inflammatory bowel disease in patients with hidradenitis suppurativa. *J Invest Dermatol.* 2017;137:1060–1064.

38. Cices A, Ibler E, Majewski S, et al. Hidradenitis suppurativa association at the time of, or subsequent to, diagnosis of inflammatory bowel disease in a large U.S. patient population. *J Eur Acad Dermatol Venereol.* 2017;31:e311–e2.

39. Shalom G, Freud T, Ben Yakov G, et al. Hidradenitis suppurativa and inflammatory bowel disease: a cross-sectional study of 3,207 patients. *J Invest Dermatol.* 2016;136:1716–1718.

40. Kam S, Collard M, Lam J, Alani RM. Gut Microbiome perturbations in patients with hidradenitis suppurativa: a case series. *J Invest Dermatol.* 2021;141:225–228.

41. Alam MT, Amos GCA, Murphy ARJ, et al. Microbial imbalance in inflammatory bowel disease patients at different taxonomic levels. *Gut Pathog.* 2020;12:1.

42. Devkota S, Chang EB. Interactions between diet, bile acid metabolism, gut microbiota, and inflammatory bowel diseases. *Dig Dis.* 2015;33:351–356.

43. Savin Z, Kivity S, Yonath H, Yehuda S. Smoking and the intestinal microbiome. *Arch Microbiol.* 2018;200:677–684.

44. Naik HBNA, Ramesh MS, Schultz G, et al. Are bacteria infectious pathogens in hidradenitis suppurativa (HS)? Debate at the symposium for hidradenitis suppurativa advances meeting (November 2017). *J Invest Dermatol.* 2019;139:13–16.

45. Kong HH, Oh J, Deming C, et al. Temporal shifts in the skin microbiome associated with disease flares and treatment in children with atopic dermatitis. *Genome research.* 2012;22:850–859.

46. Kobayashi T, Glatz M, Horiuchi K, et al. Dysbiosis and *Staphylococcus aureus* colonization drives inflammation in atopic dermatitis. *Immunity.* 2015;42:756–766.

47. Myles IA, Earland NJ, Anderson ED, et al. First-in-human topical microbiome transplantation with Roseomonas mucosa for atopic dermatitis. *JCI Insight.* 2018;3:e120608.

48. Kaur N, Chen CC, Luther J, Kao JY. Intestinal dysbiosis in inflammatory bowel disease. *Gut Microbes.* 2011;2:211–216.

49. Moayyedi P, Surette MG, Kim PT, et al. Fecal microbiota transplantation induces remission in patients with active ulcerative colitis in a randomized controlled trial. *Gastroenterology*. 2015;149:102–109. e6.

50. Targeted Microbiome Transplant in Atopic Dermatitis. National Institutes of Health; 2015. http://grantome.com/grant/NIH/U19-AI117673-01-8604. Accessed January 15, 2017.

12

Genetics and Epigenetics of Hidradenitis Suppurativa

BRIDGET MYERS, NICHOLAS BROWNSTONE, AND WILSON LIAO

CHAPTER OUTLINE

Introduction

Hidradenitis suppurativa (HS) is an inflammatory condition characterized by painful and sometimes purulent nodules, abscesses, and sinus tracts located in intertriginous regions.[1] Lesions may progress to form hypertrophic scars or dermal tunnels. HS patients are regarded as having one of the worst qualities of life among the major dermatologic conditions. Comorbidities include obesity, asthma, acne, diabetes, dyslipidemia, hypertension, thyroid disease, rheumatoid arthritis, depression, psoriasis, and polycystic ovarian syndrome.[2]

The hypothesized pathogenesis of HS is multifaceted. On a cellular level, it is characterized by follicular hyperkeratosis which leads to a deleterious pathway involving follicular occlusion, dilation, inflammation, and rupture. The etiology involves a complex interplay between a dysregulated immune system and genetic, environmental, and microbiological factors.[3]

Given the morbid nature of this disease, its etiology is of great interest to both patients and clinicians alike. The question "to what extent is HS caused by genetic factors?" was recently identified as

one of the top 10 most important uncertainties in a Priority Setting Partnership, in which patients and clinicians agreed on mutually important HS research questions.[4] While poor quality of life greatly affects these patients, they are more often worried about passing this condition on to their offspring.

Many features of HS support a genetic basis. Thirty to 42% of HS patients report a family history of HS.[5] Family history of HS is significantly higher in early onset HS, which is also associated with more widespread involvement.[6] There is an increased incidence of HS in monogenic disorders such as Dowling-Degos disease,[7–10] Down syndrome,[11–14] and keratitis, ichthyosis, and deafness syndrome,[15,16] among others. Different HS phenotypes (axillary–submammary, follicular, and gluteal) show preferences in regard to sex predominance, age of onset, lesion type, location affected, and disease severity suggesting genetic heterogeneity.[17(p53)] HS is also associated with many inflammatory diseases that have known polygenic etiologies, such as inflammatory bowel disease.[18]

This chapter provides a general overview of the HS genetics and epigenetics literature. First, a review of HS investigational genetic studies is presented, describing mutations reported to be associated with HS susceptibility, phenotype, or treatment response (Table 12.1). These studies are discussed according to study design: family linkage analyses, genome-wide association studies (GWAS), or target candidate gene studies. Genetic findings in syndromic HS— HS presenting as part of or along with a medical syndrome—are reviewed as well (Table 12.2). Early work on HS epigenetics and microRNAs is discussed next. The chapter concludes by discussing the biological and clinical relevance of these findings as well as areas for future study.

Methods

A literature search of PubMed and Embase databases was conducted for the terms "hidradenitis suppurativa" or "acne inversa" and "genes" or "genetics" or "genomics" or "mutations" or "epigenetics" or "DNA methylation." Our search was limited to English-language articles and/or those published prior to January 20, 2020. For review, the authors manually identified the relevant articles discussing the genetics of HS specifically. Duplicate articles were excluded. In total, we identified 42 primary research studies analyzing the genetics of HS patients and two analyzing the epigenetics of HS. An additional 48 studies related to HS, its genetic basis, and the biology or functional significance of implicated genes were also included.

Family-Based Linkage Analysis

To date, six linkage analysis studies have been performed in HS patients.[19–24] Linkage analysis is an unbiased, systematic method of identifying the chromosomal location of a heritable condition's susceptibility genes. To perform linkage analysis, genome-wide or local chromosomal markers are tested in pedigrees to examine for segregation of these markers within a disease of interest. Loci exhibiting the strongest evidence of linkage, surpassing a predefined significance value of a logarithm of odds (LOD) score of 3 or greater, localize susceptibility genes to chromosome segments inhabited by those markers.[25] The first seminal genome-wide linkage analysis (GWLA) study, performed by Gao et al. in 2006, was the first to identify a 76 Mb susceptibility locus at chromosome 1p21.1–1q25.3, with a maximum LOD score of 3.26 at marker D1S2624, in a large four-generation Han Chinese family demonstrating autosomal dominant HS (n = nine affected and six unaffected family members).[19] This region includes the *NCSTN* (nicastrin) gene, with subsequent exome sequencing of three of these family members identifying a splice site mutation in *NCSTN* later confirmed in remaining family members. Following this, researchers sequenced *NCSTN* in another HS family (n = five affected and eight unaffected family members), identifying a splice site and frameshift mutation in *NCSTN*.[21] Along with this work by Liu et al., 30 different mutations in *NCSTN* have been identified in HS and determined to be likely pathogenic (see Table 12.1).

In 2010, Wang et al. collected samples from six Han Chinese families exhibiting autosomal dominant HS, performing a combined linkage analysis in two HS families. They identified a 5.5 Mb susceptibility locus at chromosome 19q13 spanning 200 genes. Sequencing revealed two unique frameshift mutations in *PSENEN* (presenilin enhancer 2), resulting in a premature termination codon in family 1 and a delayed termination codon in family 2. Since *PSENEN* is one of four γ-secretase subunits, the researchers went on to sequence the remaining γ-secretase subunits in three other HS families, finding a single *PSEN1* (presenilin 1) truncating mutation and three different *NCSTN* mutations (splicing, nonsense, and frameshift). The researchers observed reduced mRNA transcripts for all mutant alleles, suggesting the later substantiated involvement of γ-secretase haploinsufficiency in a subset of familial HS.[20]

HS family-based linkage analyses have also been done in multigenerational African American,[22] Iranian,[23] and Japanese[24] families demonstrating autosomal dominant HS, together identifying one nonsynonymous[24] and two nonsense[22,23] *NCSTN* mutations.

Genome Wide Association Studies

As of yet, only one GWAS has been published in the HS literature. This study by Liu et al. (2019) was not looking to identify HS susceptibility genes, but rather genes associated with HS response to adalimumab, a tumor necrosis factor (TNF) inhibitor that is FDA-approved to treat moderate to severe HS. Researchers performed a GWAS in adalimumab-treated subjects from the most extensive HS clinical trials to date (PIONEER I and II) (n = 307). In their analysis, five single-nucleotide polymorphisms, all located within gene *BCL2*, significantly associated with a positive adalimumab response and high *BCL2* gene expression and protein abundance in hair follicles. The minor allele frequencies of these variants are low in Caucasian populations, at 0.04, but are somewhat common in Asian and African populations, at 0.12 and 0.27, respectively.

BCL-2, an anti-apoptotic regulatory protein, is involved in preventing cellular death and maintaining skin homeostasis in outer root sheath cells of hair follicles.[26] TNF knockdown in human outer root sheath cells by Liu et al. resulted in significantly reduced *BCL2* mRNA expression (P = .000171), suggesting that a pathway involving BCL-2 may play a role in adalimumab response in HS patients.[27]

γ-Secretase Target Candidate Gene Studies

To date, 22 target candidate gene studies have been done identifying mutations in two of the four γ-secretase subunits, *NCSTN* and *PSENEN,* in pure HS (see Table 12.1), as compared to HS presenting as part of or along with a medical syndrome. γ-secretase is an intramembranous complex capable of cleaving an excess of 30 type-1 transmembrane proteins, including amyloid precursor protein (APP), Notch, N-cadherin, and E-cadherin. The complex is composed of four hydrophobic proteins: presenilin, presenilin enhancer-2, nicastrin, and anterior pharynx defective encoded by *PSEN1/PSEN 2, PSENEN, NCSTN,* and *APH1A/APH1B,* respectively.[28]

Pink et al. in 2011 reported the first *PSENEN* mutation in Caucasian individuals by studying 53 individuals of seven multigenerational British families with HS as an autosomal dominant trait. Sequencing revealed a heterozygous single nucleotide insertion in *PSENEN* (c.66_67insG) predicted to cause a frameshift and altered protein product (p.Phe23ValfsX98). The mutation was absent in unaffected family members and 200 control chromosomes of European ancestry.[29] Since this work by Pink et al., a total of 15 *PSENEN* mutations, including frameshift, nonsense, splicing, and missense mutations, have been reported in HS literature. In their review, Tricarico et al. recognized that *PSENEN* mutations result in one of three phenotypes: (1) HS, (2) Dowling-Degos disease, or (3) HS and Dowling-Degos disease, with Dowling-Degos disease involving reticulate hyperpigmentation in flexural areas. Of the 15 *PSENEN* mutations that they identified, only four are regarded as likely pathogenic in pure HS phenotype and seven are regarded as likely pathogenic in HS and Dowling-Degos disease phenotype.[30]

With regard to nicastrin, more than 30 unique likely pathogenic *NCSTN* mutations have been identified to date in 16 target candidate gene studies in HS patients of many different ethnicities, including Chinese, Japanese, French, British, and others. They have also been found in HS patients with both familial and sporadic disease. *NCSTN* mutations identified in these studies include 2 frameshift, 5 splice site, 7 missense, and 10 truncating mutations (see Table 12.1). These mutations have been linked to haploinsufficiency[31] and altered protein product.[32] Many have been predicted to lead to loss of function, loss of transmembrane domain, modulation of substrate recruitment sites, reduced synthesis of additional ligand binding sites, and alteration of post-translational modifications and disulfide bonds.[30] Examining the distribution of *NCSTN* sequence variants in HS patients, researchers have not been able to identify a strong predilection pertaining to specific protein domains or components. Four of seven identified missense variants are located adjacent to or within the Lid protein domain, a vital binding site for nicastrin, including the singular missense variant associated with a decrease in Notch, a signaling molecule implicated in HS pathogenesis.[17,33,34]

Other Target Candidate Gene Studies

Several target candidate gene studies in patients with HS have found pathogenic mutations in genes beyond the γ-secretase complex; however, they are much less represented in HS literature. In 2019, a study by Savva et al. found 238 single nucleotide polymorphisms (SNPs) in *TNF*'s promoter region to be associated with HS predisposition.[35] Giatrakos et al. studied the impact of *IL12Rb1* haplotypes on HS, finding that SNPs in *IL12RB1* did not convey genetic predisposition to HS, but rather correlated with HS severity and age of onset.[36] Agut-Busquet et al. studied *MYD88* (myeloid differentiation primary response protein) in HS patients, a gene encoding a cytosolic adapter protein central in innate and adaptive immune response. Analyzing the DNA of 101 HS patients, researchers identified an association between SNPs in *MYD88* and predisposition to severe HS (Hurley stage III disease). A study by Giamarellos-Bourboulis et al. found that a copy number of *DEFB*, a cluster of nine ββ–defensin genes, of six or more associated with a 6.72 odds ratio (OR) of developing HS ($P < .0001$). β–defensin is a pro-inflammatory mediator, and deposits of ββ–defensin-2 and -3 have been found in HS lesional skin.[37] Finally, in a study of 53 Japanese HS patients, researchers Shibuya et al. found that 51% had the wet ear wax phenotype, which is significantly higher than the 12% who have it in the general Japanese population. When they excluded gluteal HS, only looking at apocrine gland-bearing subtype HS, the proportion with wet ear wax was even higher at 68%. This suggests that the SNP in the gene *ABCC11* which confers wet ear wax phenotype could be a predisposing factor to apocrine gland-bearing HS.[38]

Genetic Studies in Syndromic Hidradenitis Suppurativa

Several genetic mutations have been linked to syndromic HS in which HS presents as part of or along with a medical syndrome. Medical syndromes with HS as one of their characteristic manifestations include pyoderma gangrenosum, acne, HS (PASH) syndrome, pyogenic arthritis, pyoderma gangrenosum, acne, HS (PAPASH) syndrome, and follicular occlusion triad, which presents with HS, acne conglobata, and dissecting cellulitis (see Table 12.2).

Genetic analysis of unrelated PASH patients led to the identification of CCTG microsatellite motif repetition within the promoter region of *PSTPIP1* (proline-serine-threonine phosphatase-interacting protein 1).[39] Presumed pathogenic variants of *PSTPIP1* in PASH patients have been identified in three other studies as well. In two of these studies, mutations in *NLRP3* (nod-like receptor family pyrin domain containing 3), *IL1RN* (interleukin 1 receptor antagonist), *MEFV* (Mediterranean fever), *NOD2* (nucleotide-binding oligomerization domain-containing protein 2), *PSMB8* (proteasome subunit beta type 8), and *NCSTN* were also identified.[40,41] A *PSTPIP1* missense mutation has been seen in an individual with PASH syndrome in addition to pyogenic arthritis, known as PAPASH syndrome.[42] Genetic profiling of a follicular occlusion triad patient revealed a missense mutation in gene *KRT17* (keratin 17).[43]

Other cases of syndromic HS in HS genetics literature include HS presenting as a comorbid condition in individuals with Down syndrome, keratitis-ichthyosis-deafness (KID), familial Mediterranean fever (FMF), nevus comedonicus syndrome, and Dent disease 2 (see Table 12.2). Ten cases of patients with both Down

syndrome and HS have been reported.[11-14] In one of these articles, Blok et al. propose a hypothesis that gene alterations in Down syndrome predispose patients to develop HS, as APP is increased in trisomy 21 and/or greatly expressed in human epidermis. Furthermore, Notch and APP are competitive substrates for γ-secretase, thus an increase in APP may result in reduced Notch-signaling, a suspected pathogenic feature in a subset of HS.[14,44(p1)]

Another study by Higgins et al. performed whole exome sequencing on an individual with a severe presentation of HS, with features resembling Nevus comedonicus syndrome. Genetic analysis revealed a rare missense mutation in *FGFR2* (fibroblast growth factor receptor 2) predicted to be detrimental.[45] Two patients with both KID and follicular occlusion triad have been genetically analyzed, identifying a missense mutation in gene *GJB2* and/or transversion mutation in gene *G12R*, both affecting the connexin-26 protein.[15,16] Reports of individuals with HS and Dent disease 2 suggest that gene *OCRL1* (inositol polyphosphate 5-phosphatase) mutations, resulting in significantly reduced inositol polyphosphate 5-phosphatase activity, could be predisposing to HS. Diminished OCRL1 protein results in increased phosphoinositol-4,5-bisphosphonate within the plasma membrane, which has been seen to facilitate staphylococcal aggression in fibroblasts.[46] Therefore, an increased susceptibility to cutaneous staphylococcal infections may be the link between Dent disease 2 and HS.[47] Two cases of HS and Darier's disease occurring together have been reported, with authors postulating that a potential connection between the two may arise from an interaction between notch homolog1 and the sarcoplasmic reticulum calcium transport ATPase (SERCA2). SERCA2 is encoded by *ATP2A2*, the gene mutated in Darier's disease.[48]

Seven unique *PSENEN* mutations have been identified in patients with both HS and Dowling-Degos disease, including one missense, one transversion, two missense, and three splice site mutations.[8-10] A novel *POFUT1* (protein O-Fucosyltransferase 1) mutation has also been identified in a single case of comorbid Dowling-Degos disease and HS,[7] with knockdown *POFUT1* experiments in human keratinocytes showing reduced Notch expression.[49]

A retrospective review of 119 complex HS patients, defined as having Hurley stage III disease and/or additional inflammatory symptoms, found that 38% had a pathogenic *MEFV* variant. For complex HS patients, the OR of harboring a pathogenic *MEFV* variant was determined to be 2.80 (95% confidence interval 1.31 to 5.97, $P < .001$). *MEFV* encodes pyrin, a protein involved in inflammasome function, with wild-type mutations resulting in gain-of-function and unregulated inflammasome formation.[50]

Finally, a case of HS and pachyonychia congenita, a rare dermatosis affecting the nails, skin, oral mucosa, larynx, teeth, and hair, was reported by Pedraz et al. and associated with a missense mutation in *KRT6A*, encoding keratin 6 protein.[51]

Epigenetic Studies

Another important aspect of HS pathogenesis is at the epigenetic level. Epigenetic changes have no effect on the DNA code but alter gene expression by a variety of mechanisms. In 2017, Hessam et al. investigated the global DNA methylation and hydroxymethylation status in lesional HS, perilesional HS, and healthy skin samples. They noted significantly diminished abundance of DNA hydroxymethylation in lesional HS and perilesional HS skin samples

TABLE 12.1 Mutations Associated With Hidradenitis Suppurativa Identified Through Family Linkage Analyses, One Genome-Wide Association Study, and Target Candidate Gene Studies

Study	Gene	Protein	Function	Identified Mutation(s)	Ethnicity	Familial/sporadic
Genome-Wide Linkage Analysis/Unbiased Linkage Analysis Studies						
Gao et al., 2006[19]	Susceptibility locus 1p211–1q25.3				Han Chinese	Familial
Wang et al., 2010[20]	NCSTN PSENEN PSEN1	Nicastrin Presenelin enhancer 2 Presenelin 1	Cofactor subunit of γ-secretase, a glycoprotein transmembrane aspartyl protease cleaving over 30 type I integral membrane proteins, including Notch and Amyloid Precursor Protein Cofactor subunit of γ-secretase Catalytic subunit of γ-secretase	1 splice site, 1 truncating, 1 nonsense 1 truncating, 1 frameshift 1 truncating	Han Chinese	Familial
Liu et al., 2011[21(p201)]	NCSTN	Nicastrin	Cofactor subunit of γ-secretase	1 splice site, 1 truncating	Han Chinese	Familial
Chen et al., 2014[22]	NCSTN	Nicastrin	Cofactor subunit of γ-secretase	1 nonsense	African American	Familial
Faraji Zonooz et al. 2016[23]	NCSTN	Nicastrin	Cofactor subunit of γ-secretase	1 nonsense	Iranian	Familial
Takeichi et al., 2020[24]	NCSTN	Nicastrin	Cofactor subunit of γ-secretase	1 missense	Japanese	Familial
Genome-Wide Association Study						
Liu et al., 2019[27]	BCL2	BCL-2	Anti-apoptotic regulatory protein involved in skin homeostasis	5 single nucleotide polymorphisms associated with a positive response of HS to adalimumab	Not reported	Not reported
Target Candidate Gene Studies						
NCSTN Mutations						
Li et al., 2011[33]	NCSTN	Nicastrin	Cofactor subunit of γ-secretase	1 nonsense, 1 missense	Chinese	Familial
Pink et al., 2011[29]	NCSTN	Nicastrin	Cofactor subunit of γ-secretase	1 splice site	British	42% familial
Pink et al., 2012[58]	NCSTN	Nicastrin	Cofactor subunit of γ-secretase	1 missense, 2 splice site	Not reported	Sporadic
Haines et al., 2012[80]	NCSTN	Nicastrin	Cofactor subunit of γ-secretase	1 truncating	Singapore	Sporadic
Miskinyte et al., 2012[81]	NCSTN	Nicastrin	Cofactor subunit of γ-secretase	1 splice site, 2 truncating	French	Familial
Zhang et al., 2013[82]	NCSTN	Nicastrin	Cofactor subunit of γ-secretase	2 missense	Chinese	Familial
Nomura et al., 2013[83]	NCSTN	Nicastrin	Cofactor subunit of γ-secretase	1 splice site	Japanese	Familial

Study	Gene	Protein	Function	Finding/Mutation	Population	Familial/Sporadic
Jiao et al., 2013[84]	NCSTN	Nicastrin	Cofactor subunit of γ-secretase	1 missense	Han Chinese	Familial
Ma et al., 2013[85]	NCSTN	Nicastrin	Cofactor subunit of γ-secretase	1 truncating	Chinese	Familial
Nomura et al., 2014[60]	NCSTN	Nicastrin	Cofactor subunit of γ-secretase	1 truncating	Japanese	Familial
Yang et al., 2015[86]	NCSTN	Nicastrin	Cofactor subunit of γ-secretase	1 truncating	Chinese	Familial
Rathnamala et al., 2016[87]	NCSTN	Nicastrin	Cofactor subunit of γ-secretase	1 truncating	Indian	Familial
Zhang et al., 2016[34]	NCSTN	Nicastrin	Cofactor subunit of γ-secretase	1 missense	Chinese	Familial
Liu et al., 2016[88]	NCSTN	Nicastrin	Cofactor subunit of γ-secretase	1 truncating, 1 missense	Caucasian	Familial, Nonfamilial
Xiao et al., 2018[89]	NCSTN	Nicastrin	Cofactor subunit of γ-secretase	1 frameshift	Sporadic	Familial
Wu et al., 2018[32]	NCSTN	Nicastrin	Cofactor subunit of γ-secretase	1 truncating	Chinese	Familial
PSENEN						
Pink et al., 2011[29]	PSENEN	Presenelin enhancer 2	Cofactor subunit of γ-secretase	1 frameshift	British	Familial
Zhou et al., 2016[9](20)	PSENEN	Presenelin enhancer 2	Cofactor subunit of γ-secretase	1 missense, 1 splice site	Chinese	Familial
Kan et al., 2018[90]	PSENEN	Presenelin enhancer 2	Cofactor subunit of γ-secretase	1 frameshift	Japanese	Familial
Mutations in Other Genes						
Savva et al., 2013[35]	TNF	TNF-α	Pro-inflammatory cytokine elevated in HS lesional skin	SNP (−238G/A) in promoter region linked to HS susceptibility	Not reported	29% familial
Giatrakos et al., 2013[36]	IL12Rβ1	IL12Rβ1 receptor subunit	Part of IL-12 receptor complex; IL-12/IL-23 pathway involved in antigen presentation in HS	Haplotype (h2) associated with more severe disease vs. haplotype (h1) associated with an older age of onset	Caucasian	Sporadic
Giamarellos-Bourboulis et al., 2016[37]	DEFB (cluster of nine β—defensing genes)	β-defensin	Proinflammatory mediators; deposits of β-defensin-2 and -3 found in HS lesional skin	>6 copy number of DEFB (cluster of 9 beta-defensin genes) associated with a 6.72 OR for HS ($P < .0001$)	Greek (cohort 1), German (cohort 2)	20.9% and 37.1% familial in cohort one and two, respectively
Agut-Busquet et al., 2018[91]	MYD88	Myeloid differentiation primary response protein	Involved in innate and adaptive immune response and Toll-like receptor and IL-1 receptor signaling	SNP (GG genotype of rs6853) associated with an increased risk of severe HS	Caucasian	Not reported

HS, Hidradenitis suppurativa; SNP, single nucleotide polymorphisms.

TABLE 12.2 Mutations Identified in Syndromic Cases of Hidradenitis Suppurativa

Study	Gene	Protein	Function	Identified Mutation(s)	Ethnicity	Familial/Sporadic
HS + Nevus Comedonicus Syndrome (NCS)						
Higgins et al., 2017[45]	FGFR2	Fibroblast growth factor receptor 2	Expressed in keratinocytes, hair follicles, and sebaceous glands; substrate-receptor binding results in cell division and differentiation	1 missense	Unknown	Unknown
HS + Familial Mediterranean Fever						
Vural et al., 2019[50]	MEFV	Pyrin	Involved in regulating inflammasome activity	Frequency of pathogenic MEFV variants associated with risk of severe and complex HS	Not reported	Not reported
HS + Darier's Disease						
Ornelas et al., 2016[48]	ATP2A2	Sarcoplasmic reticulum calcium adenosine triphosphatase (SERCA) transport ATPase type 2 isoform pump	Important in maintaining calcium homeostasis; SERCA inhibition may affect Notch signaling	ATP2A2 mutation	Not reported	Not reported
HS + Dent Disease 2						
Marzuillo et al., 2018[47]	OCRL1	Inositol polyphosphate 5-phosphatase (OCRL1)	Forms a complex at maturing epidermal-dermal junction and regulates phosphoinositol-4,5-bisphosphate abundance (levels linked to inflammation)	OCRL1 mutation	Not reported	Not reported
HS + Pachyonychia Congenita						
Pedraz et al., 2008[51]	KRT6A	Keratin 6A	Provides strength to skin, nails, and hair	1 missense	Not reported	Not reported
HS + Down Syndrome						
Borbujo Martínez et al., 1992,[13] Mengesha et al., 1999,[11] Mebazaa et al., 2009,[12] Blok et al., 2016[92]	Chr 21	Primarily encodes Amyloid Precursor Protein	Integral membrane protein; competitive substrate for γ-secretase along with Notch	Trisomy 21	Not reported	Sporadic
HS + Keratitis-Ichthyosis-Deafness (KID)						
Montgomery et al., 2004,[15] Lazic et al., 2012[16]	GJB2 gene, G12R gene	Connexin-26 protein	Forms gap junctions key for tissue homeostasis, growth, and development	2 missense	Not reported	Sporadic
HS + Dowling-Degos Disease (DDD)						
Zhou et al., 2016[9]	PSENEN	Presenelin enhancer 2	Cofactor subunit of γ-secretase	1 missense, 1 splice site	Chinese	Familial
Ralser et al., 2017[10]	PSENEN	Presenelin enhancer 2	Cofactor subunit of γ-secretase	2 splice site, 2 nonsense	3 German, 2 Indian, 1 French patient	Not reported

Reference	Gene	Protein	Function	Mutation type	Ashkenazi Jewish	Familial
Pavlovsky et al., 2018[8]	PSEMEN	Presenelin enhancer 2	Cofactor subunit of γ-secretase	1 missense		Familial
González-Villanueva et al., 2018[7]	POFUT1	Protein O-Fucosyltransferase 1	Protein in endoplasmic reticulum; adds sugar moieties to Notch receptors	1 splice site	Not reported	Not reported
PASH (Pyoderma Gangrenosum, Acne, and Suppurativa Hidradenitis) and PAPASH Syndrome						
Braun-Falco et al., 2012,[39] Marzano et al., 2013,[42(p201)] Calderón-Castrat et al., 2016,[93] Saito et al., 2018[94]	PSTPIP1	Proline-serine-threonine phosphatase-interacting protein 1	Involved in regulating inflammasome activity	3 missense and 1 SNP with increased repetition of CCTG micro-satellite motif	Patient 1 Russian, Patient 2 German	Sporadic
Marzano et al., 2013[40]	NLRP3	Cryopyrin	Initiates and regulates the immune system's response to injury, invasion, or toxins	1 missense	Not reported	Not reported
	IL1RN	IL-1 receptor antagonist	Modulates the IL-1 mediated immune responses	1 missense		
	MEFV	Pyrin	Regulates inflammasome activity	2 missense		
	NOD2	Nucleotide-binding oligomerization domain-containing protein 2	Involved in autophagy; when triggered by a bacterial antigen, it activates NFκB that regulates the immune response	2 missense		
	PSMB8	Proteasome 20S Subunit Beta 8	Subunit of immunoproteosome important in detecting self v. non-self proteins in immune cells to guide immune response	1 missense		
Duchatelet et al., 2015[41]	NCSTN	Nicastrin	Cofactor subunit of γ-secretase	1 frameshift	Not reported	Not reported
Follicular Occlusion Triad						
Musumeci et al., 2019[43]	KR17	Keratin 17	Provides strength to skin, nails, and hair	1 missense	Not reported	Familial

HS, Hidradenitis suppurativa.

compared to healthy skin samples. However, no significant discrepancy in abundance of DNA methylation was detected between lesional HS, perilesional HS, and healthy skin samples, suggesting a role of DNA hydroxymethylation, but not methylation, in HS pathogenesis.[52]

The role of DNA hydroxymethylation in HS pathogenesis was further studied by Hessam et al. in 2018. The skin of HS patients (both lesional and nonlesional) and the skin of healthy controls underwent RT-PCR analysis for DNA hydroxymethylation regulators *TET1, TET2, TET3, IDH1, IDH2, IDH3A,* and *IDH3B.* The mRNA of these regulators was significantly under-expressed in lesional HS skin versus healthy skin, further supporting a role of DNA hydroxymethylation in HS pathogenesis.[53]

Hessam et al. also analyzed microRNA (miRNA) regulator expression profiles in HS inflammatory lesions in three independent studies. First, the authors assessed the expression of the miRNA regulatory machinery *Drosha, DGRC8 (Drosha* co-factor), *Dicer* and *Exportin-5* in lesional and non-lesional skin from HS patients, lesional skin from psoriasis patients, and skin from healthy controls using RT-qPCR. Results indicated downregulation of *Drosha* and *DGRC8* expression in non-lesional skin from HS patients. They hypothesized that, at early stages of HS inflammation, *Drosha* and *DGRC8* are active; however, *Dicer* and *Exportin-5* are observable only when clinical signs of inflammation become apparent.[54]

Second, the authors examined the expression of inflammation-related miRNAs (miRNA-155-5p, miRNA-223-5p, miRNA-31-5p, miRNA-21-5p, miRNA-125b-5p, and miRNA- 146) through RT-qPCR of HS lesional, HS perilesional, and healthy control skin. The expression of inflammation-related miRNAs was increased in HS lesional versus healthy control skin, suggesting a role of these miRNAs in modulating cutaneous inflammation in HS.[55]

Finally, Hessam et al. analyzed the expression profiles of RNA-induced silencing complex (RISC) components (specifically, transactivation-responsive RNA binding protein-1/2 [*TRBP1/2*], protein activator [*PACT*] of the interferon-induced protein kinase R, Argonaute RISC Catalytic Component-1 [*AGO1*] and Component- 2 [*AGO2*], metadherin, and staphylococcal nuclease and Tudor domain-containing-1 [*SND1*]) in inflammatory tissues of HS and psoriasis patients. They found that all RISC components demonstrated differential expression in skin biopsies of HS patients, psoriasis patients, and healthy controls, suggesting that they may play a role modulating cutaneous inflammation in HS as well.[56]

Discussion

Genetic and Epigenetic Architecture of Hidradenitis Suppurativa

This chapter highlights current genetic and epigenetic understandings of HS, but these domains are only part of HS's likely multifactorial pathogenesis, with other etiologies including microbiologic, endocrine, and environmental influences.[57] The degree to which genetics contributes to familial and sporadic HS is difficult to answer, and the general understanding in scientific literature has transformed over time. An early study by Fitzsimmons et al. noted vertical transmission of HS in five three-generational and six two-generational families, leading them to conclude that HS exhibits autosomal dominant inheritance, with incomplete penetrance as

only 34% versus 50% of first-degree relatives were affected.[5] Since then, several GWLA studies in HS families and target candidate gene studies sequencing γ-secretase genes, described above, have provided further evidence for monogenic forms of HS which a review Pink et al. found to include less than 7% of HS cases.[58] Familial clustering of HS, and studies showing altered expression of genes involved in epidermal proliferation and barrier integrity in HS lesional skin, however, support another subgroup of HS cases that have a polygenic predisposition.[59]

This review demonstrates the genetic heterogeneity of HS among familial and sporadic forms, as disease-related mutations have been found in a diverse number of loci. Since only 44 out of 67 identified genetic mutants linked to HS susceptibility have been localized to γ-secretase genes, it is clear that γ-secretase mutations do not account for all HS cases. In a study of 48 HS patients seen at a tertiary referral clinic, 19 of which had a positive family history of autosomal dominant inheritance, sequencing of γ-secretase genes *NCSTN, PSENEN,* and *PSEN1* identified only three *NCSTN* variants, with only two presumed to be pathogenic. This finding suggests that only a minority of cases are positive for γ-secretase mutations, and it is likely that many genes not yet identified are contributing to this disease.[58]

Additionally, γ-secretase mutations, when present, could be insufficient to cause HS. In a study by Nomura et al. researchers identified a nonsense *NCSTN* mutation in both the proband patient and his brother who had HS, as well as his 70-year-old sister who did not have HS. Evidence of an asymptomatic carrier of a likely pathogenic mutation suggests that a mutation in γ-secretase alone may not be enough to result in HS phenotype, potentially suggesting a polygenic inheritance pattern of HS in this family or highlighting the importance of environmental triggers in initiating the disease.[60]

In terms of HS's epigenetic architecture, research is preliminary. Despite the low number of individuals included in HS epigenetic studies and the lack of ethnic data in some of them, all have found evidence of novel epigenetic biomarkers correlating with skin inflammation in HS patients. However, the mechanisms by which these changes are driven are yet to be discovered.

γ-Secretase and Notch Signaling Structure and Function

With 30 mutations identified in *NCSTN,* 13 in *PSENEN,* and one in *PSEN1,* the major genetic predisposition to HS currently recognized is in genes encoding γ-secretase, a ubiquitous and heterogenous complex present in locations where HS occurs.[61] Notch, EGFR, and P13/AKT signaling pathways are all downstream of γ-secretase, and have been implicated in epidermal differentiation and homeostasis (Fig. 12.1).[15,35] Notch signaling, in particular, is involved in regulating the growth and differentiation of hair follicle and epithelial cells,[62,63] and the development and activities of immune cells, negatively influencing Toll-like receptor (TLR)-triggered innate immune responses.[64,65]

γ-Secretase and Notch Signaling in Skin Health and Hidradenitis Suppurativa Pathogenesis

Several human and animal studies have been done supporting a functional role of γ-secretase in maintaining skin homeostasis. In clinical trials for the γ-secretase inhibitors Niragacesta and Semagacestat, designed to treat desmoid tumor/aggressive fibromatosis and Alzheimer disease, respectively, subjects

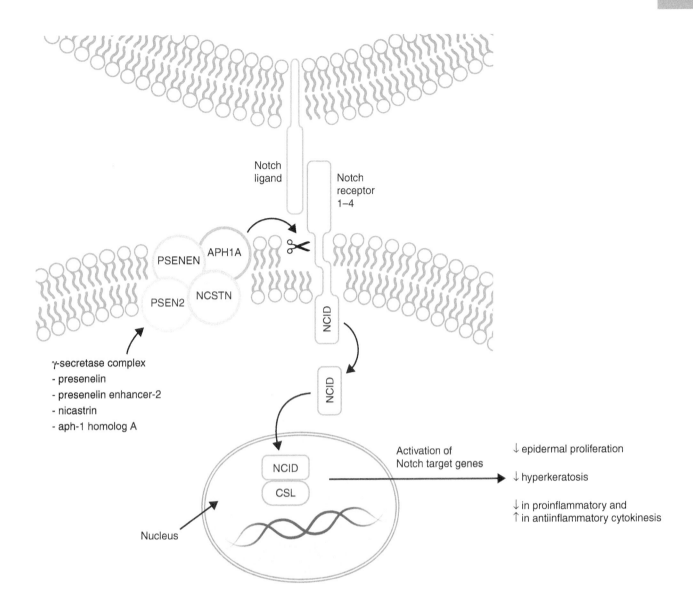

• **Fig. 12.1** Mutations in genes *NCSTN*, *PSENEN*, and *PSEN1*, which encode three out of the four gamma-secretase subunits, have been associated with hidradenitis suppurativa (HS) in a subset of patients. Gamma-secretase is an intramembranous complex involved in cleaving more than 30 type-1 transmembrane proteins including Notch. When cleaved, the intracellular cytoplasmic domain of Notch *(NCID)* enters the nucleus and interacts with CBF1, Suppressor of Hairless, Lag-1 (CSL), a DNA binding transcription factor, resulting in displacement of co-repressors and recruitment of co-activators to regulate the transcription of Notch target genes. Downstream effects include preventing epidermal hyperplasia, decreasing pro-inflammatory cytokines, and increasing anti-inflammatory cytokines. Mutations in genes *NCSTN*, *PSENEN*, and *PSEN1* have been shown to cause gamma-secretase insufficiency and impaired Notch signaling, leading to altered epidermal proliferation, hyperkeratosis, and inflammation of hair follicles, which are all characteristics of HS lesions.

reported a significant prevalence of skin side effects. In a phase II clinical trial for Niragacesta, 12 of 17 patients reported an adverse cutaneous reaction, with 6 out of 7 evaluated by dermatology demonstrating follicular and cystic lesions in intertriginous areas, with none of these patients having a personal or family history of HS.[66] In a phase II clinical trial for Semagacestat (*n* = 43), seven subjects reported a skin rash and three a change in hair color.[67] Taken together, these findings suggest a physiologic function of γ-secretase in hair follicles that, when deficient, results in development of HS-like lesions.

Knockdown and knockout experiments support an association between defective γ-secretase, Notch signaling, and HS-like manifestations. For example, a recent study by Yang et al. noted hyperkeratosis of hair follicles and inflammation, characteristic phenotypes of HS, in *NCSTN* conditional knockout mutant mice.[68] In another *NCSTN* knockdown study in human keratinocytes, Xiao et al. detected a correlation between deficient γ-secretase activity and altered keratinocyte proliferation and differentiation. They also noted similar modifications in Notch expression in mice *NCSTN*-silencing cells and human HS lesions. Significant elevations in phosphoinositide 3-kinase (PI3K) and

AKT were also detected, suggesting that *NCSTN* mutations could be impairing keratinocyte proliferation and differentiation via Notch and P13K/AKT pathways.[31]

This has been supported by other research demonstrating Notch to have tumor suppressor-like functions in skin, such as disrupted Notch signaling resulting in epidermal hyperplasia and basal cell carcinoma-like tumors in mice.[69] Another study by Xia et al. observed higher beta-catenin signaling in PSEN1 knockout mice that correlated with an increase in cell progression from G1 to S phase. This supports a role of γ-secretase and the beta-catenin pathway, which interacts with Notch signaling, in preventing epidermal hyperplasia, a pathologic feature of HS lesions.[70]

Notch signaling is also important in negatively regulating TLR-activated innate immunity, with immune imbalances in HS characterized by an overactivation of innate immunity and the IL-23/Th17 pathway.[71] In a study by Zhang et al., researchers observed an increase in anti-inflammatory cytokines, IL-10, and a decrease in proinflammatory cytokines, TNF-αα and IL-6, corresponding with an overexpression of Notch1 and Notch2, supporting an anti-inflammatory role of Notch signaling.[64] In HS lesional skin, IL-1b and TNF-αα have been detected at 31-fold and 5-fold greater abundance relative to healthy skin in non-HS subjects.[72] IL-1b amplifies TLR signaling, in turn affecting NFκB activity. NFκκB and TNF-α upregulate matrix metalloproteases, potentially resulting in destructive remodeling of skin as is seen in HS.[73]

POGLUT1 mutations, which have been identified in patients with both Dowling-Degos disease and HS, may confer disease susceptibility by affecting Notch signaling. *POGLUT1* (protein O-glucosyltransferase 1) adds glucose moieties to serine residues in Notch's transactivating intracellular domain. In a muscular dystrophy patient with a missense mutation in *POGLUT1*, muscle biopsy revealed a decrease in Notch signaling.[74] This link further supports a role of Notch signaling in HS pathogenesis and/or should direct future research to explore mutations in other genes encoding proteins involved in Notch signaling, beyond the γ-secretase complex.

Importantly, not all studies analyzing γ-secretase insufficiency support a primary Notch-driven HS pathogenesis. A *NCSTN* knockdown study in human keratinocytes by Cao et al. found enhanced expression of genes involved in type I interferon response, suggesting that an inflammatory reaction, independent of Notch signaling, is associated with *NCSTN* deficiency and may be important in HS pathogenesis.[75] Additionally, splice site mutations in *PSEN1* in zebrafish have been shown to have different effects on Notch signaling, with particular truncating mutations inhibiting or enhancing Notch signaling. They even found that a HS-associated truncating mutation reported by Wang et al.[20] actually resulted in an increase in Notch signaling, which could suggest the involvement of other pathways in linking γ-secretase insufficiency to HS disease.[76]

Hidradenitis Suppurativa Phenotype and γ-Secretase Mutations

A review by Pink et al. observed that most individuals reported to have γ-secretase mutations have HS that is more severe, widespread, and treatment-resistant, suggesting an association between *NCSTN*, *PSENEN*, and *PSEN1* mutations and disease severity.[77] Another study by Xu et al. characterized the clinical presentations of HS in six different families positive for *NCSTN* mutations (*n* = 53), noting that they corresponded with a follicular subtype of HS.[17,78] These studies suggest a possible correlation between

γ-secretase mutations and disease presentation, however further work is needed to better understand genotype and phenotype relationships in HS.

PSTPIP1 Mutations and Inflammasome Function in Hidradenitis Suppurativa

To date, six *PSTPIP1* mutations have been identified in HS patients, with five of them identified in PASH or PAPASH patients. PSTPIP1 binds pyrin, the protein that is mutated in FMF. PSTPIP1 and pyrin are co-expressed as part of an NLRP3 (NOD-, LRR-, and/or pyrin domain-containing protein 3) inflammasome in granulocytes and monocytes. *PSTPIP1* mutations in PAPA (pyogenic arthritis, pyogenic gangrenosum, acne) syndrome patients are thought to cause hyperphosphorylation of PSTPIP1, increasing its binding affinity to pyrin. As result, pyrin loses its ability to inhibit the NLRP3 inflammasome-driven and caspase-1 mediated proinflammatory signaling pathway involved in cleaving pro-IL-1B to active IL-1B. This promotes an IL-1B-dependent inflammatory reaction, dominated by granulocytes and monocytes,[39] with both of these cell types identified in increased abundance in HS lesions.[79] Thus, in a subset of cases, inflammasome dysfunction may be an important factor in HS pathogenesis.

Conclusion

The body of work in HS genetics and epigenetics literature supports a role of gene mutations, specifically those in γ-secretase and inflammation-related genes, and epigenetic changes, involving DNA hydroxymethylation and miRNA and RISC expression, in HS pathogenesis. Moving forward, it is critical to integrate findings of genomic and epigenomic studies with HS transcriptomic and proteomic studies to better understand the individual contributions to HS pathogenesis and recognize potential therapeutic targets.[30]

Areas of future exploration in HS genetic and epigenetic research include probing for susceptibility genes beyond γ-secretase, as studies suggest γ-secretase mutations are only seen in a minority of HS patients. Improved characterization of clinical and histological features of HS presentation is also important to improve genotype-phenotype correlations. Consensus regarding phenotypic categories of HS, such as those proposed by Canoui-Potrine et al. (axillary-mammary, follicular, and gluteal), will further assist with this.[78] In terms of future epigenetic investigations, the role of DNA hydroxymethylation and its regulating enzymes in HS (e.g., TET and IDH proteins) should be explored further to better understand the inflammatory profile of HS. While a significant reduction in global 5-hydroxymethylation is seen in HS patients, the mechanism by which it is altered is still unknown.[53] As associations between HS susceptibility, phenotype, and treatment response and genetic and epigenetic variants continue to be made, progress in identifying novel therapeutic targets and personalized approaches to HS treatment are likely to unfold.

References

1. Napolitano M, Megna M, Timoshchuk EA, et al. Hidradenitis suppurativa: from pathogenesis to diagnosis and treatment. *Clin Cosmet Investig Dermatol.* 2017;10:105–115. https://doi.org/10.2147/CCID.S111019.

2. Kimball AB, Sundaram M, Gauthier G, et al. The Comorbidity burden of hidradenitis suppurativa in the United States: a claims data analysis. *Dermatol Ther.* 2018;8(4):557–569. https://doi.org/10.1007/s13555-018-0264-z.

3. von Laffert M, Stadie V, Wohlrab J, Marsch WC. Hidradenitis suppurativa/acne inversa: bilocated epithelial hyperplasia with very different sequelae. *Br J Dermatol.* 2011;164(2):367–371. https://doi.org/10.1111/j.1365-2133.2010.10034.x.

4. Ingram JR, Abbott R, Ghazavi M, et al. The hidradenitis suppurativa priority setting partnership. *Br J Dermatol.* 2014;171(6):1422–1427. https://doi.org/10.1111/bjd.13163.

5. Fitzsimmons JS, Guilbert PR, Fitzsimmons EM. Evidence of genetic factors in hidradenitis suppurativa. *Br J Dermatol.* 1985;113(1):1–8. https://doi.org/10.1111/j.1365-2133.1985.tb02037.x.

6. Deckers IE, van der Zee HH, Boer J, Prens EP. Correlation of early-onset hidradenitis suppurativa with stronger genetic susceptibility and more widespread involvement. *J Am Acad Dermatol.* 2015;72(3):485–488. https://doi.org/10.1016/j.jaad.2014.11.017.

7. González-Villanueva I, Gutiérrez M, Hispán P, et al. Novel POFUT1 mutation associated with hidradenitis suppurativa-Dowling-Degos disease firm up a role for Notch signalling in the pathogenesis of this disorder. *Br J Dermatol.* 2018;178(4):984–986. https://doi.org/10.1111/bjd.16264.

8. Pavlovsky M, Sarig O, Eskin-Schwartz M, et al. A phenotype combining hidradenitis suppurativa with Dowling-Degos disease caused by a founder mutation in PSENEN. *Br J Dermatol.* 2018;178(2):502–508. https://doi.org/10.1111/bjd.16000.

9. Zhou C, Wen G-D, Soe LM, et al. Novel mutations in PSENEN gene in two chinese acne inversa families manifested as familial multiple comedones and Dowling-Degos Disease. *Chin Med J.* 2016;129(23):2834–2839. https://doi.org/10.4103/0366-6999.194648.

10. Ralser DJ, Basmanav FBÜ, Tafazzoli A, et al. Mutations in γ-secretase subunit-encoding PSENEN underlie Dowling-Degos disease associated with acne inversa. *J Clin Investig.* 2017;127(4):1485–1490. https://doi.org/10.1172/JCI90667.

11. Mengesha YM, Holcombe TC, Hansen RC. Prepubertal hidradenitis suppurativa: two case reports and review of the literature. *Pediat Dermatol.* 1999;16(4):292–296. https://doi.org/10.1046/j.1525-1470.1999.00077.x.

12. Mebazaa A, Ben Hadid R, Cheikh Rouhou R, et al. Hidradenitis suppurativa: A disease with male predominance in Tunisia. *Acta Dermatovenerologica Alpina, Pannonica, Et Adriatica.* 2009;18(4):165–172.

13. Borbujo Martínez J, Bastos Amigo J, Olmos Carrasco O, et al. Suppurative hidradenitis in Down's syndrome. Apropos of three cases. *Anales Espanoles De Pediatria.* 1992;36(1):59–61.

14. Blok J, Jonkman M, Horváth B. The possible association of hidradenitis suppurativa and Down syndrome: is increased amyloid precursor protein expression resulting in impaired Notch signalling the missing link? *Br J Dermatol.* 2014;170(6):1375–1377. https://doi.org/10.1111/bjd.12887.

15. Montgomery JR, White TW, Martin BL, et al. A novel connexin 26 gene mutation associated with features of the keratitis-ichthyosis-deafness syndrome and the follicular occlusion triad. *J Am Acad Dermatol.* 2004;51(3):377–382. https://doi.org/10.1016/j.jaad.2003.12.042.

16. Lazic T, Li Q, Frank M, et al. Extending the phenotypic spectrum of keratitis-ichthyosis-deafness syndrome: Report of a patient with GJB2 (G12R) Connexin 26 mutation and unusual clinical findings. *Pediat Dermatol.* 2012;29(3):349–357. https://doi.org/10.1111/j.1525-1470.2011.01425.x.

17. Xu H, Xiao X, Hui Y, et al. Phenotype of 53 Chinese individuals with nicastrin gene mutations in association with familial hidradenitis suppurativa (acne inversa). *Br J Dermatol.* 2016;174(4):927–929. https://doi.org/10.1111/bjd.14268.

18. Janse IC, Koldijk MJ, Spekhorst LM, et al. Identification of clinical and genetic parameters associated with hidradenitis suppurativa in inflammatory bowel disease. *Inflamm Bowel Dis.* 2016;22(1):106–113. https://doi.org/10.1097/MIB.0000000000000579.

19. Gao M, Wang PG, Cui Y, et al. Inversa acne (hidradenitis suppurativa): a case report and identification of the locus at chromosome 1p21.1-1q25.3. *J Investig Dermatol.* 2006;126(6):1302–1306. https://doi.org/10.1038/sj.jid.5700272.

20. Wang B, Yang W, Wen W, et al. Gamma-secretase gene mutations in familial acne inversa. *Science (New York, NY).* 2010;330(6007):1065. https://doi.org/10.1126/science.1196284.

21. Liu Y, Gao M, Lv Y, et al. Confirmation by exome sequencing of the pathogenic role of NCSTN mutations in acne inversa (hidradenitis suppurativa). *J Investig Dermatol.* 2011;131(7):1570–1572. https://doi.org/10.1038/jid.2011.62.

22. Chen S, Mattei P, You J, et al. γ-Secretase mutation in an African American family with hidradenitis suppurativa. *JAMA Dermatol.* 2015;151(6):668–670. https://doi.org/10.1001/jamadermatol.2014.5306.

23.. Zonooz FM, Sabbagh-Kermani F, Fattahi Z, et al. Whole genome linkage analysis followed by whole exome sequencing identifies nicastrin (NCSTN) as a causative gene in a multiplex family with γ-secretase spectrum of autoinflammatory skin phenotypes. *J Investig Dermatol.* 2016;136(6):1283–1286. https://doi.org/10.1016/j.jid.2016.02.801.

24. Takeichi T, Matsumoto T, Nomura T, et al. A novel NCSTN missense mutation in the signal peptide domain causes hidradenitis suppurativa, which has features characteristic of an autoinflammatory keratinization disease. *Br J Dermatol.* 2020;182(2):491–493. https://doi.org/10.1111/bjd.18445.

25. Pulst SM. Genetic linkage analysis. *Archiv Neurol.* 1999;56(6):667–672. https://doi.org/10.1001/archneur.56.6.667.

26. Abe Y, Tanaka N. Roles of the Hedgehog Signaling pathway in epidermal and hair follicle development, homeostasis, and cancer. *J Dev Biol.* 2017;5(4):12. https://doi.org/10.3390/jdb5040012.

27. Mohan L, Degner J, Georgantas RW, et al. A genetic variant in the BCL2 gene associates with adalimumab response in hidradenitis suppurativa clinical trials and regulates expression of BCL2. *J Investig Dermatol.* 2020;140(3):574–582. https://doi.org/10.1016/j.jid.2019.06.152 (web archive link).

28. Bergmans BA, De Strooper B. Gamma-secretases: from cell biology to therapeutic strategies. *Lancet Neurol.* 2010;9(2):215–226. https://doi.org/10.1016/S1474-4422(09)70332-1.

29. Pink AE, Simpson MA, Brice GW, et al. PSENEN and NCSTN mutations in familial hidradenitis suppurativa (Acne Inversa). *J Investig Dermatol.* 2011;131(7):1568–1570. https://doi.org/10.1038/jid.2011.42.

30. Tricarico PM, Boniotto M, Genovese G, et al. An Integrated Approach to Unravel Hidradenitis Suppurativa Etiopathogenesis. *Front Immunol.* 2019;10:892. https://doi.org/10.3389/fimmu.2019.00892.

31. Xiao X, He Y, Li C, et al. Nicastrin mutations in familial acne inversa impact keratinocyte proliferation and differentiation through the Notch and phosphoinositide 3-kinase/AKT signalling pathways. *Br J Dermatol.* 2016;174(3):522–532. https://doi.org/10.1111/bjd.14223.

32. Wu C, Yang J, Zhang S, et al. A novel NCSTN gene mutation in a Chinese family with acne inversa. *Mol Genet Genomics.* 2018;293(6):1469–1475. https://doi.org/10.1007/s00438-018-1475-9.

33. Li C-R, Jiang M-J, Shen D-B, et al. Two novel mutations of the nicastrin gene in Chinese patients with acne inversa. *Br J Dermatol.* 2011;165(2):415–418. https://doi.org/10.1111/j.1365-2133.2011.10372.x.

34. Zhang S, Meng J, Jiang M, Zhao J. Characterization of a novel mutation in the NCSTN Gene in a large Chinese family with acne inversa. *Acta Dermato-Venereologica.* 2016;96(3):408–409. https://doi.org/10.2340/00015555-2259.

35. Savva A, Kanni T, Damoraki G, et al. Impact of toll-like receptor-4 and tumour necrosis factor gene polymorphisms in patients with

hidradenitis suppurativa. *Br J Dermatol.* 2013;168(2):311–317. https://doi.org/10.1111/bjd.12105.

36. Giatrakos S, Huse K, Kanni T, et al. Haplotypes of IL-12Rβ1 impact on the clinical phenotype of hidradenitis suppurativa. *Cytokine.* 2013;62(2):297–301. https://doi.org/10.1016/j.cyto.2013.03.008.

37. Giamarellos-Bourboulis EJ, Platzer M, Karagiannidis I, et al. High copy numbers of β-defensin cluster on 8p23.1, confer genetic susceptibility, and modulate the physical course of hidradenitis suppurativa/acne inversa. *J Investig Dermatol.* 2016;136(8):1592–1598. https://doi.org/10.1016/j.jid.2016.04.021.

38. Shibuya Y, Morioka D, Nomura M, et al. Earwax of patients with hidradenitis suppurativa: a retrospective study. *Arch Plast Surg.* 2019;46(6):566–571. https://doi.org/10.5999/aps.2019.00290.

39. Braun-Falco M, Kovnerystyy O, Lohse P, Ruzicka T. Pyoderma gangrenosum, acne, and suppurative hidradenitis (PASH)—A new autoinflammatory syndrome distinct from PAPA syndrome. *J Am Acad Dermatol.* 2012;66(3):409–415. https://doi.org/10.1016/j.jaad.2010.12.025.

40. Marzano AV, Ceccherini I, Gattorno M, et al. Association of pyoderma gangrenosum, acne, and suppurative hidradenitis (PASH) shares genetic and cytokine profiles with other autoinflammatory diseases. *Medicine.* 2014;93(27), e187. https://doi.org/10.1097/MD.0000000000000187.

41. Duchatelet S, Miskinyte S, Join-Lambert O, et al. First nicastrin mutation in PASH (pyoderma gangrenosum, acne and suppurative hidradenitis) syndrome. *Br J Dermatol.* 2015;173(2):610–612. https://doi.org/10.1111/bjd.13668.

42. Marzano AV, Trevisan V, Gattorno M, et al. Pyogenic arthritis, pyoderma gangrenosum, acne, and hidradenitis suppurativa (PAPASH): A new autoinflammatory syndrome associated with a novel mutation of the PSTPIP1 gene. *JAMA Dermatol.* 2013;149(6):762–764. https://doi.org/10.1001/jamadermatol.2013.2907.

43. Musumeci ML, Fiorentini F, Bianchi L, et al. Follicular occlusion tetrad in a male patient with pachyonychia congenita: clinical and genetic analysis. *J Euro Acad Dermatol Venereol.* 2019;33(Suppl 6):36–39. https://doi.org/10.1111/jdv.15851.

44. Lleó A, Berezovska O, Ramdya P, et al. Notch1 competes with the amyloid precursor protein for gamma-secretase and down-regulates presenilin-1 gene expression. *The Journal of Biological Chemistry.* 2003;278(48):47370–47375. https://doi.org/10.1074/jbc.M308480200.

45. Higgins R, Pink A, Hunger R, et al. Generalized comedones, acne, and hidradenitis suppurativa in a patient with an FGFR2 missense mutation. *Front Med.* 2017;4:16. https://doi.org/10.3389/fmed.2017.00016.

46. Shi Y. *The role is phosphoinositol-4,5-bisphosphate in the cellular uptake of staphylococcus aureus.* Dissertation. University of Konstanz; 2016. Accessed September 17, 2021. https://d-nb.info/1114893846/34.

47. Marzuillo P, Piccolo V, Mascolo M, et al. Patients affected by dent disease 2 could be predisposed to hidradenitis suppurativa. *J Eur Acad Dermatol Venereol.* 2018;32(8):e309–e311. https://doi.org/10.1111/jdv.14860.

48. Ornelas J, Sivamani R, Awasthi S. A report of two patients with Darier disease and hidradenitis suppurativa. *Pediat Dermatol.* 2016;33(4):e265–e266. https://doi.org/10.1111/pde.12891.

49. Li M, Cheng R, Liang J, et al. Mutations in POFUT1, encoding protein O-fucosyltransferase 1, cause generalized Dowling-Degos disease. *Am J Hum Genet.* 2013;92(6):895–903. https://doi.org/10.1016/j.ajhg.2013.04.022.

50. Vural S, Gündoğdu M, Gökpınar İli E, et al. Association of pyrin mutations and autoinflammation with complex phenotype hidradenitis suppurativa: a case-control study. *Br J Dermatol.* 2019;180(6):1459–1467. https://doi.org/10.1111/bjd.17466.

51. Pedraz J, Peñas PF, Garcia-Diez A. Pachyonychia congenita and hidradenitis suppurativa: no response to infliximab therapy. *J Eur Acad Dermatol Venereol.* 2008;22(12):1500–1501. https://doi.org/10.1111/j.1468-3083.2008.02691.x.

52. Hessam S, Sand M, Lang K, et al. Altered global 5-hydroxymethylation status in hidradenitis suppurativa: support for an epigenetic background. *Dermatology.* 2017;233(2–3):129–135. https://doi.org/10.1159/000478043.

53. Hessam S, Gambichler T, Skrygan M, et al. Reduced ten-eleven translocation and isocitrate dehydrogenase expression in inflammatory hidradenitis suppurativa lesions. *Eur J Dermatol.* 2018;28(4):449–456. https://doi.org/10.1684/ejd.2018.3369.

54. Hessam S, Sand M, Skrygan M, et al. Inflammation induced changes in the expression levels of components of the microRNA maturation machinery Drosha, Dicer, Drosha co-factor DGRC8 and Exportin-5 in inflammatory lesions of hidradenitis suppurativa patients. *J Dermatol Sci.* 2016;82(3):166–174. https://doi.org/10.1016/j.jdermsci.2016.02.009.

55. Hessam S, Sand M, Skrygan M, et al. Expression of miRNA-155, miRNA-223, miRNA-31, miRNA-21, miRNA-125b, and miRNA-146a in the inflammatory pathway of hidradenitis suppurativa. *Inflammation.* 2017;40(2):464–472. https://doi.org/10.1007/s10753-016-0492-2.

56. Hessam S, Sand M, Skrygan M, Bechara FG. The microRNA effector RNA-induced silencing complex in hidradenitis suppurativa: a significant dysregulation within active inflammatory lesions. *Arch Dermatol Res.* 2017;309(7):557–565. https://doi.org/10.1007/s00403-017-1752-1.

57. Ingram JR. The genetics of hidradenitis suppurativa. *Dermatol Clin.* 2016;34(1):23–28. https://doi.org/10.1016/j.det.2015.07.002.

58. Pink AE, Simpson MA, Desai N, et al. Mutations in the γ-secretase genes NCSTN, PSENEN, and PSEN1 underlie rare forms of hidradenitis suppurativa (acne inversa). *J Invest Dermatol.* 2012;132(10):2459–2461. https://doi.org/10.1038/jid.2012.162.

59. Jfri AH, O'Brien EA, Litvinov IV, et al. Hidradenitis suppurativa: comprehensive review of predisposing genetic mutations and changes. *J Cutan Med Surg.* 2019;23(5):519–527. https://doi.org/10.1177/1203475419852049.

60. Nomura Y, Nomura T, Sakai K, et al. A novel splice site mutation in NCSTN underlies a Japanese family with hidradenitis suppurativa. *Br J Dermatol.* 2013;168(1):206–209. https://doi.org/10.1111/j.1365-2133.2012.11174.x.

61. Li T, Wen H, Brayton C, et al. Epidermal growth factor receptor and notch pathways participate in the tumor suppressor function of gamma-secretase. *J Bio Chem.* 2007;282(44):32264–32273. https://doi.org/10.1074/jbc.M703649200.

62. Rangarajan A, Talora C, Okuyama R, et al. Notch signaling is a direct determinant of keratinocyte growth arrest and entry into differentiation. *EMBO J.* 2001;20(13):3427–3436. https://doi.org/10.1093/emboj/20.13.3427.

63. Okuyama R, Tagami H, Aiba S. Notch signaling: its role in epidermal homeostasis and in the pathogenesis of skin diseases. *J Dermatol Sci.* 2008;49(3):187–194. https://doi.org/10.1016/j.jdermsci.2007.05.017.

64. Zhang Q, Wang C, Liu Z, et al. Notch signal suppresses toll-like receptor-triggered inflammatory responses in macrophages by inhibiting extracellular signal-regulated kinase 1/2-mediated nuclear factor κB activation. *J Bio Chem.* 2012;287(9):6208–6217. https://doi.org/10.1074/jbc.M111.310375.

65. Yuan JS, Kousis PC, Suliman S, et al. Functions of notch signaling in the immune system: consensus and controversies. *Ann Rev Immunol.* 2010;28(1):343–365. https://doi.org/10.1146/annurev.immunol.021908.132719.

66. O'Sullivan Coyne G, Woodring TS, Lee C-CR, et al. Hidradenitis suppurativa-like lesions associated with pharmacologic inhibition of gamma-secretase. *J Investig Dermatol.* 2018;138(4):979–981. https://doi.org/10.1016/j.jid.2017.09.051.

67. Fleisher AS, Raman R, Siemers ER, et al. Phase 2 safety trial targeting amyloid beta production with a gamma-secretase inhibitor in Alzheimer disease. *Arch Neurol.* 2008;65(8):1031–1038. https://doi.org/10.1001/archneur.65.8.1031.

68. Yang J, Wang L, Huang Y, et al. Keratin 5-Cre-driven deletion of Ncstn in an acne inversa-like mouse model leads to a markedly increased IL-36a and Sprr2 expression. *Fron Med.* 2020;14:305–317. https://doi.org/10.1007/s11684-019-0722-8.

69. Nicolas M, Wolfer A, Raj K, et al. Notch1 functions as a tumor suppressor in mouse skin. *Nat Genet.* 2003;33(3):416–421. https://doi.org/10.1038/ng1099.

70. Xia X, Qian S, Soriano S, et al. Loss of presenilin 1 is associated with enhanced β-catenin signaling and skin tumorigenesis. *Proc Natl Acad Sci U S A.* 2001;98(19):10863–10868. https://doi.org/10.1073/pnas.191284198.

71. Schlapbach C, Hänni T, Yawalkar N, Hunger RE. Expression of the IL-23/Th17 pathway in lesions of hidradenitis suppurativa. *J Am Acad Dermatol.* 2011;65(4):790–798. https://doi.org/10.1016/j.jaad.2010.07.010.

72. van der Zee HH, de Ruiter L, van den Broecke DG, et al. Elevated levels of tumour necrosis factor (TNF)-α, interleukin (IL)-1β and IL-10 in hidradenitis suppurativa skin: a rationale for targeting TNF-α and IL-1β. *Br J Dermatol.* 2011;164(6):1292–1298. https://doi.org/10.1111/j.1365-2133.2011.10254.x.

73. Mozeika E, Pilmane M, Nürnberg BM, Jemec GBE. Tumour necrosis factor-alpha and matrix metalloproteinase-2 are expressed strongly in hidradenitis suppurativa. *Acta Derm Venereol.* 2013;93(3):301–314. https://doi.org/10.2340/00015555-1492.

74. Servián-Morilla E, Takeuchi H, Lee TV, et al. A POGLUT1 mutation causes a muscular dystrophy with reduced Notch signaling and satellite cell loss. *EMBO Mol Med.* 2016;8(11):1289–1309. https://doi.org/10.15252/emmm.201505815.

75. Cao L, Morales-Heil DJ, Roberson EDO. Nicastrin haploinsufficiency alters expression of type I interferon-stimulated genes: The relationship to familial hidradenitis suppurativa. *Clin Exp Dermatol.* 2019;44(4):e118–e125. https://doi.org/10.1111/ced.13906.

76. Newman M, Wilson L, Verdile G, et al. Differential, dominant activation and inhibition of Notch signalling and APP cleavage by truncations of PSEN1 in human disease. *Hum Mol Genet.* 2014;23(3):602–617. https://doi.org/10.1093/hmg/ddt448.

77. Pink AE, Simpson MA, Desai N, et al. γ-Secretase mutations in hidradenitis suppurativa: new insights into disease pathogenesis. *J Investig Dermatol.* 2013;133(3):601–607. https://doi.org/10.1038/jid.2012.372.

78. Canoui-Poitrine F, Le Thuaut A, Revuz JE, et al. Identification of three hidradenitis suppurativa phenotypes: Latent class analysis of a cross-sectional study. *J Invest Dermatol.* 2013;133(6):1506–1511. https://doi.org/10.1038/jid.2012.472.

79. Vossen ARJV, van der Zee HH, Prens EP. Hidradenitis suppurativa: a systematic review integrating inflammatory pathways into a cohesive pathogenic model. *Front Immunol.* 2018;9. https://doi.org/10.3389/fimmu.2018.02965.

80. Haines RL, Common JE, Teo D, Tang MB, Lane EB. Sequencing of the γ-secretase complex in Singaporean patients with acne inversa reveals a novel mutation in nicastrin, but suggests other mechanisms must be present. *Br J Dermatol.* 2012;166:e33.

81. Miskinyte S, Nassif A, Merabtene F, et al. Nicastrin mutations in French families with hidradenitis suppurativa. *J Investig Dermatol.* 2012;132(6):1728–1730. https://doi.org/10.1038/jid.2012.23.

82. Zhang C, Wang L, Chen L, et al. Two novel mutations of the NCSTN gene in Chinese familial acne inverse. *J Eur Acad Dermatol Venereol.* 2013;27(12):1571–1574. https://doi.org/10.1111/j.1468-3083.2012.04627.x.

83. Nomura Y, Nomura T, Sakai K, et al. A novel splice site mutation in NCSTN underlies a Japanese family with hidradenitis suppurativa. *Br J Dermatol.* 2013;168(1):206–209. https://doi.org/10.1111/j.1365-2133.2012.11174.x.

84. Jiao T, Dong H, Jin L, et al. A novel nicastrin mutation in a large Chinese family with hidradenitis suppurativa. *Br J Dermatol.* 2013;168(5):1141–1143. https://doi.org/10.1111/bjd.12135.

85. Ma S, Yu Y, Yu G, Zhang F. Identification of one novel mutation of the NCSTN gene in one Chinese acne inversa family. *Dermatol Sin.* 2013;32:126–128. https://doi.org/10.1016/j.dsi.2013.06.003.

86. Yang J-Q, Wu X-J, Dou T-T, et al. Haploinsufficiency caused by a nonsense mutation in NCSTN underlying hidradenitis suppurativa in a Chinese family. *Clin Exp Dermatol.* 2015;40(8):916–919. https://doi.org/10.1111/ced.12724.

87. Ratnamala U, Jhala D, Jain NK, et al. Expanding the spectrum of γ-secretase gene mutation-associated phenotypes: two novel mutations segregating with familial hidradenitis suppurativa (acne inversa) and acne conglobata. *Exp Dermatol.* 2016;25(4):314–316. https://doi.org/10.1111/exd.12911.

88. Liu M, Davis JW, Idler KB, et al. Genetic analysis of NCSTN for potential association with hidradenitis suppurativa in familial and nonfamilial patients. *Br J Dermatol.* 2016;175(2):414–416. https://doi.org/10.1111/bjd.14482.

89. Xiao Y-J, Yang Y, Liang Y-H. hsa-miR-155 targeted NCSTN 3'UTR mutation promotes the pathogenesis and development of acne inversa. *Int J Clin Exp Pathol.* 2018;11(4). 1878–188.

90. Kan T, Takahagi S, Shindo H, et al. A unique clinical phenotype of a patient bearing a newly identified deletion mutation in the PSENEN gene along with the pathogenic serum desmoglein-1 antibody. *Clin Exp Dermatol.* 2018;43(3):329–332. https://doi.org/10.1111/ced.13326.

91. Papp K, Huang X, Gu Y, Fleischer A, Calimlim B. Abstracts. *Exp Dermatol.* 2018;27(S1):5–32. https://doi.org/10.1111/exd.13538.

92. Blok JL, Li K, Brodmerkel C, et al. Gene expression profiling of skin and blood in hidradenitis suppurativa. *Br J Dermatol.* 2016;174(6):1392–1394. https://doi.org/10.1111/bjd.14371.

93. Calderón-Castrat X, Bancalari-Díaz D, Román-Curto C, et al. PSTPIP1 gene mutation in a pyoderma gangrenosum, acne and suppurative hidradenitis (PASH) syndrome. *Br J Dermatol.* 2016;175(1):194–198. https://doi.org/10.1111/bjd.14383.

94. Saito N, Minami-Hori M, Nagahata H, et al. Novel PSTPIP1 gene mutation in pyoderma gangrenosum, acne and suppurative hidradenitis syndrome. *J Dermatol.* 2018;45(8):e213–e214. https://doi.org/10.1111/1346-8138.14259.

Clinician's Corner

13

Disease Evaluation and Outcome Measures

RYAN M. SVOBODA AND JOSLYN S. KIRBY

Introduction

Outcome measures play an important role in the field of dermatology, both in routine clinical practice and in clinical research trials. In clinical settings, robust outcome measures serve to classify disease severity, which can direct treatment choice. Outcome measures can also assess changes in disease severity over time.[1] Furthermore, these measures provide a common language between providers that can allow for effective communication of a patient's status, eliminating the subjectivity and ambiguity that arise from the use of clinical descriptors alone. In research settings, outcome measures allow for the systematic assessment of the efficacy of novel therapeutic interventions. Ideally, disease-specific outcome measures designed for use in clinical trials and applied uniformly between studies also make comparison of different treatment modalities between possible studies.[2]

Characteristics of Well-Designed Outcome Measures

Optimal outcome measures for clinical settings must allow for proper discrimination of disease severity. Measures that do not meet this specification may not detect small—but important—changes in disease.[3] Ideally, the outcome measure should demonstrate ease-of-use and have no significant learning curve. Outcome measures for clinical trials may be impractical for busy clinical settings. Outcome measures can be clinician-reported, which assess signs of disease activity, or can be patient-reported, which assess pain or quality of life. Both can support individualized care.[4] Composite measures also combine clinician-reported and patient-reported items into one scale.[5,6] Poorly designed outcome measures have negative consequences on both routine patient care and the results of clinical trials/drug discovery processes (Table 13.1).

The Hidradenitis Suppurativa Core Outcomes Set International Collaboration (HISTORIC): Addressing Current Challenges in Outcome Measure Development and Utilization

Hidradenitis suppurativa (HS) is a complex inflammatory disease which causes significant morbidity in affected patients.[7] Well-designed outcome measures are needed to support an efficient drug discovery and approval process. Currently, there is a wide variety of outcome measures for both clinical and trial use.[7] Many of these instruments are plagued by various shortcomings, including lack of precision, responsiveness to change, or patient-centeredness.[7,8] The use of various instruments across clinical trials has led to the systematic introduction of bias and makes comparison of results across studies difficult or impossible.[9]

In an effort to alleviate this problem, an international group of researchers, clinicians, and patient research partners are collaborating to develop an agreed-upon Core Outcome Set to be used in all clinical trials, examining possible treatment options for HS.[9] This ongoing multimodal effort—The Hidradenitis Suppurativa Core Outcomes Set International Collaboration (HISTORIC)—is working to develop a set of core outcome measures which pertains to all stakeholders, including patients, dermatologists, surgeons,

TABLE 13.1	Characteristics of a Well-Designed Outcome Measure		
Outcome Measure Characteristic	Description	Consequence(s) of Poorly Designed Measure	
Discrimination of disease severity	Ability to validly and reliably classify disease magnitude	• Enrollment of patients not well-suited for a clinical trial	
Responsiveness to change	Ability to detect meaningful small and large changes in disease severity over time	• Understatement of therapeutic effects in clinical trial settings • Inability to track improvement in clinical settings	
Reproducibility	Adequate interrater and intra rater reliability	• Imprecise, unreliable clinical trial results • Inability to reliably track clinical improvement over time	

TABLE 13.2	The Hurley Staging System for Hidradenitis Suppurativa
Stage I	≥1 abscesses
	No sinus tract or scar formation
Stage II	≥1 recurrent abscesses with associated sinus tract/scar formation
Stage III	Diffuse or near-diffuse involvement of affected region
	Multiple abscesses and interconnected sinus tracts
	Extensive scarring

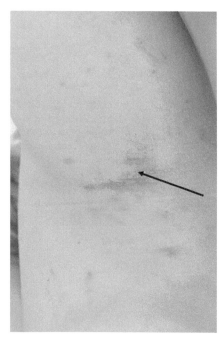

• **Fig. 13.1** Hurley stage I. Axilla with scattered inflammatory papules and pustules as well as a subcutaneous painful nodule *(arrow)*.

nurses, industry, and regulatory authorities. The core domains include (1) disease course; (2) physical signs; (3) HS-specific quality of life; (4) symptoms; (5) pain; and (6) Global assessments.[9] This ongoing international effort holds the promise of homogenizing outcome measures between trials to improve clinical trial design and ensure proper assessment of pertinent outcomes.

Current Outcome Measures for Hidradenitis Suppurativa

Clinician-Reported Outcome Measures

Hurley Staging System

First described in 1989, the Hurley Staging System (HSS) was originally developed to determine the best surgical approach for individual patients with HS based on the type of lesions in a given anatomic location.[10] However, despite not being the original intent of the scale, the HSS is now the most widespread outcome measure used for routine clinical assessment in HS.[7] Furthermore, the HSS is recommended by the United States and Canadian Hidradenitis Suppurativa Foundations for routine use in clinical settings due to its ease of application and the existence of therapeutic ladder recommendations based on the scale.[11]

The HSS categorizes patients into one of three groups based on their most severe area of involvement (Table 13.2).[12] Hurley Stage I disease represents the majority of patients with HS and is defined as the presence of one or more isolated abscesses in the absence of scar or sinus tract formation (Fig. 13.1). Hurley Stage II HS is characterized by the presence of recurrent abscesses with sinus tract formation or cicatrization (Fig. 13.2). Hurley Stage III disease is defined by diffuse or near-diffuse involvement across a body site with multiple abscesses and interconnected sinus tracts (Fig. 13.3).[13]

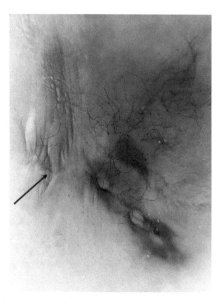

• **Fig. 13.2** Hurley stage II. Axilla with tunnel and scarring due to hidradenitis suppurativa and prior surgical excision *(arrow)*.

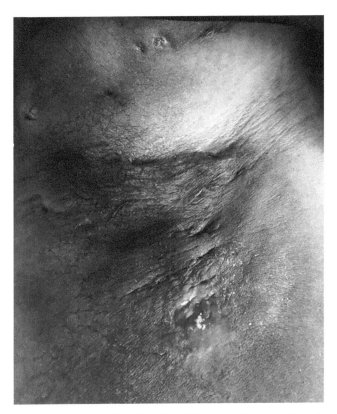

• **Fig. 13.3** Hurley stage III. Axilla with multiple tunnels throughout the axilla.

The advantages of the HSS include its ease of use and the minimal training required. It is quick to perform and can feasibly be integrated into busy clinical settings without significant difficulty.[11] Furthermore, the moderate-to-good interrater reliability of the HSS.[9,14] However, the HSS is a static measure initially designed to describe the severity of disease in individual regions in order to determine appropriateness of surgical therapy.[7] As such, it provides a measure of the most severely involved region, rather than an accurate assessment of the overall burden of disease. Additionally, with only three stages of disease, the HSS provides little granularity and demonstrates insufficient responsiveness to change, making it poorly suited for use as an outcome measure in research settings.

Modifications to the Hurley Staging System

A modification of the HSS was developed by the Dutch Hidradenitis Suppurativa Expert Group to further stratify HS into seven overall categories (Table 13.3). Unlike the traditional HSS, the refined HSS incorporates the degree of active inflammation as well as the magnitude of body surface involvement, based on the number of body regions involved.[15] The modifications introduced in this scale expands the stratification of patients traditionally defined as having Hurley Stage I or II disease. The changes may better classify patients who would benefit from systemic therapy and improve detection of small meaningful changes. The refined HSS remains a relatively simple, time-efficient measure that can easily be incorporated into daily clinical practice. However, a disadvantage of this revised scale is that it has fair interrater reliability, so raters may benefit from training or experience.[9]

Inflammatory Lesion Counts

Inflammatory lesion counts—which involve separately determining the number of inflammatory nodules, abscesses, and draining fistulae/sinus tracts in each patient—are a frequent method of assessing HS severity. Although inflammatory lesion counts form the basis of many other HS-specific outcome scales, they can also function in isolation and have been used in this manner in clinical trials.[16,17] In contrast to the HSS, which is a discrete measure ranging from 1 to 3, inflammatory lesion counts are open-ended with no upper limit. This allows for the detection of small changes in disease activity, as determined by either the resolution of existing lesions or the development of new lesions. However, the interrater reliability of lesion counts were found to be poorly to moderately reliable.[9] In addition, lesion counts are purely clinician-reported and do not take into account important patient-reported aspects of HS including pain; therefore, lesion counts (when used alone) may underestimate the severity of disease from the patient's perspective.[16] Reliability and error in the scales are important because there is a higher chance with lower reliability that a change in score could be due to measurement error rather than a real change in disease. Furthermore, clinician assessment of lesion counts at predetermined time points (such as routine office visits) will not capture changes in HS severity that occur between evaluations.[17] This section describes several of the lesion-count based outcome measures.

Sartorius Score (Hidradenitis Suppurativa Score)

The Sartorius score (also known as the Hidradenitis Suppurativa Score) was originally proposed as an alternative staging system for HS by Karin Sartorius in 2003 (Sartorius et al., 2003). The original purpose of the instrument was to serve as a uniform outcome measure that could be applied to cohort studies investigating

TABLE 13.3   The Modified Hurley Staging System

Sinus tracts?	No	≤2 regions AND <5 abscesses/nodules				Stage IA
		>2 regions OR ≥5 abscesses/nodules	Fixed lesions			Stage IB
			Migratory lesions			Stage IC
	Yes	Interconnected sinus tracts involving ≥1% BSA?	No	Inflammation?	No	Stage IIA
					Yes, ≤2 regions	Stage IIB
					Yes, >2 regions	Stage IIC
			Yes			Stage III

BSA, Body surface area.

surgical treatment of HS while providing a more dynamic and precise scale compared to the HSS.[18] The Sartorius score is an open-ended scoring system which takes into account four clinician-reported variables (Table 13.4). These include the number of anatomic regions involved, the number and types of lesions, the distance between lesions, and the absence or presence of normal intervening skin between lesions.[18] Each characteristic is attached to an assigned point value, which are summed to calculate an overall score that can track disease severity over time. Due to the dynamic and open-ended nature of the scale, it is more ideal for determining response to treatment than the traditional HSS.[18] For this reason, it has been used as an outcome measurement instrument in clinical trials.[19,20] Like the HSS, the Sartorius score is relatively easy to combine with patient-reported outcome measures like the Dermatology Life Quality Index (DLQI) and was designed with this purpose in mind.[5] Although the Sartorius scale provides a granular and dynamic measure of disease activity, it can be time consuming.[21] Therefore, additional training may be required and although it has been used successfully in research settings, implementation into ordinary clinical workflow is difficult.[22]

Modified Sartorius Score

The revised Sartorius score, like the original, considers the number and types of lesions present, the distance between lesions, and the absence or presence of normal skin between lesions.[22] However, the revised score involves a simplified assessment scale meant to make the instrument more practical to use by clinicians. For example, the number of lesion types in the revised score has been dichotomized into nodules and fistulae for simplicity (see Table 13.4). Furthermore, the number of points assigned to each variable has been altered to allow for more granular comparison of a patient's clinical status between time points. Although the modified Sartorius scale is still time consuming to perform compared to more traditional methods such as the HSS, after training, it can reliably be performed in about 5 minutes, depending on disease severity.[22]

Hidradenitis Suppurativa Clinical Response

The Hidradenitis Suppurativa Clinical Response (HiSCR) is a validated outcome measure which was specifically developed for the evaluation of anti-inflammatory treatments for HS.[23] The HiSCR was designed retrospectively using data from a Phase II trial.[23] Like Sartorius score, the HiSCR is based on inflammatory lesion counts; however, the HiSCR is a dichotomous outcome scale that divides patients into two groups: HiSCR achievers and non-achievers. HiSCR achievers are defined as those who demonstrate a (1) 50% or more reduction in the number of abscesses and inflammatory nodules, (2) lack of increase in the number of abscesses, and (3) lack of increase in the number of draining fistulae, compared to

TABLE 13.4 The Sartorius Score Versus the Modified Sartorius Score

	Original Sartorius Score		Modified Sartorius Score	
Anatomic regions considered	Points (3 per region involved)		Points (3 per region involved)	
	Axilla	Left	Axilla	Left
		Right		Right
	Groin	Left	Groin	Left
		Right		Right
	Gluteal	Left	Gluteal	Left
		Right		Right
	Inframammary	Left	Inframammary	Left
		Right		Right
	Other		Other	
Lesion type	Points (per lesion)		Points (per lesion)	
	Abscess/nodules	2	Nodules	1
	Fistulae	4	Fistulae	6
	Scars	1		
	Other	1		
Longest distance between two relevant lesions	Points		Points	
	<5 cm	2	<5 cm	1
	5–10 cm	4	5–10 cm	3
	>10 cm	8	>10 cm	9
Lesions clearly separated by normal skin?	Points		Points	
	Yes	0	Yes	0
	No	6	No	9

the baseline counts.[23] The HiSCR was validated against existing HS-specific outcome measures and is relatively simple to use.[23] HiSCR achievement has been shown to correlate both clinically meaningful changes in status as well as improvement in patient-reported outcomes (e.g., reduction in DLQI and visual analogue pain scales).[23] In a Phase II trial of adalimumab in the treatment of HS, the HiSCR demonstrated excellent responsiveness to change in clinical status.[24] However, because the HiSCR represents a dichotomous outcome, it has limited granularity compared to continuous outcome scales and therefore is not useful in further sub-stratifying patients with severe disease in clinical settings, although this was not its original intent.[23] Further, the interrater reliability for abscess and inflammatory nodule counts that serve as the basis of the HiSCR was demonstrated to be relatively low (interclass correlation coefficient 0.44) in a comparative study examining multiple outcome measures.[9]

International Hidradenitis Suppurativa Severity Scoring System

The International Hidradenitis Suppurativa Severity Scoring System (IHS4) is an expert consensus-based scale developed by members of the European Hidradenitis Suppurativa Foundation using the Delphi method.[25] After development of a preliminary scale, a multicenter, prospective validation study of 210 patients was performed in an effort to correlate the results of the IHS4 with other existing outcome measures and to determine strengths and weaknesses of the novel instrument.[25] Following this, a second Delphi voting procedure was undertaken in order to optimize the scale based on the findings from the validation study; from this, the finalized version of the IHS4 was developed. The clinician determines the number of inflammatory nodules, abscesses, and draining tunnels present. Each lesion has a differential weight (nodules x1, abscesses x2, and fistulae/sinuses x4); therefore, after multiplying the number of lesions by the weight, the sum of these is the total score (Table 13.5). The total score can be categorized as: mild ($\leq$3 points), moderate (4 to 10 points), or severe (>10 points)

disease.[25] One important feature of IHS4 is that the presence of a single draining tunnel (fistulae/sinus tract) automatically designates a patient as having at least moderate disease.

The IHS4 has several advantages. The use of a consensus-based Delphi technique and the prospective validation of the measure against pre-existing HS scoring systems provide strength to this method. The instrument was developed to be useful as both a severity staging system in clinical settings and an outcome measure instrument in research trials.[9] The lesion types utilized in the scale are well-defined with strict, objective definitions, thereby improving ease of use. Like the HSS, it categorizes patients as having mild, moderate, or severe disease. Despite its advantages, the IHS4 has demonstrated a lower interrater reliability.[9]

Hidradenitis Suppurativa Physician Global Assessment

The Hidradenitis Suppurativa Physician Global Assessment (HS-PGA) is a numerical scale that is similar in nature and design to PGA scores developed for other dermatologic diseases.[26] The HS-PGA is a six-point scale with scores from 0 (clear) to 5 (very severe). The specific scale values are determined by lesion counts of inflammatory nodules, abscesses, and draining fistulae (Table 13.6). The HS-PGA is advantageous in that clinicians are likely to be familiar with this type of scale, as PGA scales are favored by the FDA and exist for a multitude of dermatologic diseases.[26] However, there is potential for significant heterogeneity among patients with among the discrete values. In addition, due to the reliability issues with lesion counts, it is possible that changes in disease are not captured.[23]

Composite Outcome Measures

Some outcome measures combine items that are clinician-reported and patient-reported, which apply to the Hidradenitis Suppurativa Severity Index (HSSI) and Acne Inversa Severity Index (AISI). The HSSI is a numerical scale that was developed for use in an open label clinical trial of adalimumab and a randomized trial of

TABLE 13.5 The International Hidradenitis Suppurativa Severity Scoring System

Lesion Type	×	Weighting Factor	=	Subscores
Nodules (#)		1		
Abscesses (#)		2		
Draining tunnels (fistulae/ sinuses, #)		3		
				Overall IHS4 Score is the total sum of subscores

Overall HS Severity	IHS4 Score
Mild HS	$\leq$3
Moderate HS	4–10
Severe HS	$\geq$11

HS, Hidradenitis suppurativa, *IHS4,* International Hidradenitis Suppurativa Severity Scoring System.

TABLE 13.6 The Hidradenitis Suppurativa Physician Global Assessment

HS-PGA Score	Non-inflammatory Nodules	Inflammatory Nodules	Abscesses/ Draining Fistulae
0 (Clear)	0	0	0
1 (Minimal)	$\geq$1	0	0
2 (Mild)	Any number	1–4	0
	Any number	0	1
3 (Moderate)	Any number	$\geq$5	0
	Any number	$\geq$1	1
	Any number	<10	2–5
4 (Severe)	Any number	$\geq$10	2–5
5 (Very Severe)	Any number	Any number	>5

HS-PGA, Hidradenitis suppurativa physician global assessment.

infliximab in the treatment of HS.[27,28] The impetus for the development of this scale was to produce an outcome measure that would overcome the shortcomings of the HSS (insufficient responsiveness to change) and Sartorius score (time-consuming, difficult to interpret) while also addressing important patient-reported outcomes such as drainage and pain.[27] The HSSI contains multiple components which address different aspects of HS. These include traditional lesion counts, body surface area (BSA) involvement, drainage (as captured by number of dressing changes during working and leisure hours), and pain (via a visual analogue scale). An HSSI index is determined for each of the four individual variables; these are then summed to determine an overall score, which categorizes patients as having mild (0 to 7), moderate (8 to 12), and/or severe (≥13) disease (Table 13.7). The HSSI is relatively unique in that it combines objective data (lesion counts, BSA involvement) with patient-reported data (drainage, pain), thus incorporating both clinician-reported outcomes and patient-reported outcomes into a single score. However, while the HSSI does appear to be reproducible, it has not been used extensively in research or clinical practice.[21]

The AISI was proposed by Chiricozzi, et al. in 2015 as an analog to other severity indices used in both clinical trial and real-life practice settings to assess the severity of dermatologic diseases (e.g., Psoriasis Area Severity Index).[29] The AISI takes into account both type of lesions and the total number of anatomic regions affected by each lesion subtype. As opposed to other scales which consider lesion type (such as the HSS, the IHS4, the Sartorius score, and the HiSCR), the AISI includes a broader characterization scheme which takes into account abscess/inflammatory nodule, sinus tract, keloid/fibrotic adherence, and fibrosclerotic inflammatory plaque.[29] The AISI also includes a visual analog scale for patient-reported pain (Table 13.8). The AISI can be performed quickly (mean 46.4 seconds), making it potentially useful in clinical settings while also being dynamic enough to detect small changes in disease status necessary for research instruments.[29] Furthermore, it has demonstrated high correlation with the modified Sartorius score ($r = 0.973$) and Dermatology Life Quality Index ($r = 0.826$). Despite these advantages, the AISI incorporates lesion

types that are not standard in other HS-specific scales (e.g., fibrosclerotic inflammatory plaque) and therefore may require a significant learning curve. Perhaps for this reason, it has demonstrated lower interrater reliability in comparison to other instruments.[9]

New Directions—Body Surface Area Based Measures

The majority of early outcome measure instruments is developed for HS function on the basis of lesion counts, as previously discussed. However, the proposed Core Outcomes Set developed as part of the HISTORIC initiative includes BSA involvement as one of the physical signs to be assessed in HS clinical trials, despite the fact that this measure was, at the time, not part of existing HS severity indices, aside from the HSSI.[8] In order to rectify this, novel instruments based on this core domain have since been developed.

The Severity and Area Score for Hidradenitis (SASH) is a novel outcome measurement developed by Kirby, et al. in 2019. This instrument was constructed based on input from both dermatologic and gynecologic providers.[30] After development of the initial measure, cognitive debriefing interviews and focus groups of initial providers were conducted, and changes to the SASH were made based on the themes that emerged from this feedback to yield the finalized instrument (see Table 13.8). The SASH was evaluated in a multi-rater study which revealed interrater reliability on par with that of the modified Sartorius score and significantly higher than that of the HSS. The intra rater reliability of the SASH was excellent (intra-class correlation coefficient 0.98).[30]

The Hidradenitis Suppurativa Area and Severity Index (HASI) is another novel instrument that was developed to take BSA involvement into account. The HASI measures four signs of inflammation (erythema, thickness, drainage, and tenderness) each on a scale of 0 to 3 for each body region (see Table 13.8). The percentage of surface area involvement of each region is then used to determine an area score, which is multiplied by the sum of the four inflammation measure scores.[31] The scale is a composite measure with a clinician-reported items and patient-report needed for tenderness. There are plans to modify the new instrument and to investigate its reliability. Novel BSA-centric outcome measures such as the SASH and HASI demonstrate promise in improving the clinicians' ability to accurately and reliably assess disease severity and the effectiveness of therapy.[30]

Patient-Reported Outcome Measures

Patient-reported outcome measures provide important insight into the experience and impact of a conditions. In clinical settings, patient-reported outcomes have been shown to enhance patient-clinician communication and inform management decisions.[32,33] In the research setting, patient-reported measures are useful in evaluating outcomes important to patients.[34] Given the high morbidity related to HS, patient-reported outcomes can provide a crucial perspective on the impact of the condition.

Non-Hidradenitis Suppurativa-Specific Patient Reported Outcome Measures

Multiple patient-reported outcome measures exist which are not specific to HS. These include skin-specific health-related quality-of-life (HRQOL) scales, such as the DLQI, Skindex-29, and Skindex-16 instruments, designed to measure the burden of skin disease on quality of life.[35,36] Additionally, numerical rating and visual analog scales for pain exist and have been applied to assessment of patients with HS. Although these tools are useful in adding

---

TABLE 13.7 The Hidradenitis Suppurativa Severity Index

Individual Component Score	0	1	2	3	4
Body surface area (%)	0	1	2–3	4–5	>5
Number of erythematous, painful lesions	0	1–2	2–3	4–5	>5
Drainage (# of dressing changes during working hours)	0	-	1	>1	-
Pain (Visual Analog Scale)	0–1	1–2	2–4	5–7	8–10

Total HSSI Index = Sum of Individual Component Scores

Overall HS Severity	HSSI Score
Mild HS	0–7
Moderate HS	8–12
Severe HS	≥13

HS, Hidradenitis suppurativa; *HSSI*, Hidradenitis suppurativa severity index.

TABLE 13.8 Other Hidradenitis Suppurativa-Specific Outcome Measures

	Clinical Features Considered in Scale		
Composite Measure	Lesion Type	Anatomic Location	Patient-Reported
Acne Inversa Severity Index (AISI)	• Comedonic lesion *(1 point)* • Abscess/inflammatory nodule *(2 points)* • Sinus tract *(3 points)* • Keloid/fibrotic adherence *(4 points)* • Fibrosclerotic inflammatory plaque *(5 points)*	x # of body sites in which each lesion is located	Visual analog scale for patient-reported pain (0–10)
Body Surface Area Based Measures	Clinical Features Assessed	Body Sites Included	
Severity and Area Score for Hidradenitis (SASH)	• Inflammatory color change • Induration • Open Skin Surface	• Head and neck • Left axilla • Right axilla • Chest and abdomen • Pubis andr genitals	• Back • Buttocks/intergluteal cleft • Left thigh • Right thigh
Hidradenitis Suppurativa Area and Severity Index (HASI)	• Erythema • Thickness • Drainage • Tenderness	• Head • Left axilla • Right axilla • Anterior chest	• Back • Anterior bathing trunk • Posterior bathing trunk • Other
Hidradenitis Suppurativa-Specific Patient Reported Outcome Measures Hidradenitis Suppurativa Symptoms Assessment (HSSA)	Domain(s) Assessed • Signs • Symptoms	Concepts within Domain • Pain • Drainage • Redness • Tenderness	• Swollen • Hard skin • Hot skin • Bad smell • Itchy
Hidradenitis Suppurativa Impact Assessment (HSIA)	• Impacts	• Uncomfortableness of clothing • Arm movement • Exercise • Walking • Sitting • Wanting to be around others • Household activities • School/work presenteeism	• Self-conscious • Embarrassed • Sad • Worried • Bothered • Sexual activity • Satisfaction with treatment • Bothered by scars • School/work absenteeism
Hidradenitis Suppurativa Quality of Life (HiSQOL) Score	• Symptoms	• Pain • Itch	• Drainage • Odor
	• Psychosocial	• Down/depressed • Embarrassed • Anxious/nervous	• Concentration • Sexual desire
	• Activities/adaptations	• Walking • Exercising • Sleeping • Washing yourself	• Getting dressed • What you where • Ability to work/study • Sexual activity difficult

important information on disease severity and impact, these scales are not inherently specific to HS and therefore may overlook unique impacts of this disease.[37]

Hidradenitis Suppurativa-Specific Patient Reported Outcome Measures

In order to more accurately measure patient-reported outcomes specific to HS in clinical trials and efficacy studies, HS-specific patient-reported outcomes have been developed, as recommended by the HISTORIC consensus for an HS Core Outcomes Set.[8] The nine-item Hidradenitis Suppurativa Symptoms Assessment (HSSA) and the 17-item Hidradenitis Suppurativa Impact Assessment (HSIA) were developed simultaneously in order to better characterize the patient-level impacts of HS in a manner that could be measured in treatment studies (see Table 13.8).[38] The HSSA measures the burden of nine physical symptoms of HS (ranging from pain to pruritus) on patients, whereas the HSIA focuses on gauging the effects of the disease on daily activities.[38] Both scales have demonstrated the ability to generate content-valid, reliable results in research settings, although the results of studies with large sample sizes are lacking.

The Hidradenitis Suppurativa Quality of Life (HiSQOL) score is a more recently proposed HS-specific HRQOL instrument. This tool was developed by two groups who performed preliminary work to develop separate HS-specific HRQOL instruments; the Hidradenitis Suppurativa Quality of Life (HSQOL) measure and the preliminary HiSQOL.[39,40] Efforts of the two groups were combined in order to generate the finalized HiSQOL, which supersedes the two preliminary instruments. The HiSQOL's 17 items are separated into three subscales (symptoms, psychosocial, and activities-adaptations), which can be assessed independently or combined into an overall score (see Table 13.8).[41] Although the HiSQOL was originally developed to measure HS-specific quality-of-life in the clinical trial setting, future studies are planned in order to generate a reduced version for use in clinical settings.[41]

Conclusions and Future Directions

Outcome measures serve an important purpose in both clinical practice—as a means of gauging disease severity and monitoring response to therapy—and in research, in which they play a vital role in the drug approval process and in comparing the efficacy of different treatment modalities across trials. Poorly designed outcome measures can have a negative impact on direct patient care and can impede treatment innovation. Currently, multiple disparate outcome measures exist for HS and could be used in both routine clinical practice and for research. The HISTORIC group is working to achieve global consensus on a Core Outcomes Set for HS clinical trials that addresses all stakeholders and includes both objective clinician-reported measures of disease stage and severity as well as patient-reported measures of disease severity and impact. This Core Outcomes Set holds the promise of a more standardized assessment of potential treatments for HS. Ultimately, this may lead to a more efficient drug discovery and approval process, and a more transparent means of comparing different treatment options between trials.

References

1. Hatfield DR, Ogles BM. Why some clinicians use outcome measures and others do not. *Admin Policy Ment Health.* 2007;34:283–291.
2. Thorlacius L, Ingram JR, Garg A, et al. Protocol for the development of a core domain set for hidradenitis suppurativa trial outcomes. *BMJ Open.* 2017;7(2), e014733.
3. Dutmer AL, Reneman MF, Schiphorst Preuper HR, et al. The NIH minimal dataset for chronic low back pain: Responsiveness and minimal clinically important change. *Spine.* 2019;44(2):e1211–e1218.
4. Mason NR, Sox HC, Whitlock EP. A patient-centered approach to comparative effectiveness research focused on older adults: lessons from the patient-centered outcomes research institute. *J Am Geriatr Soc.* 2018;67:21–28.
5. Finlay AY, Khan GK. Dermatology Life Quality Index (DLQI)- -a simple practical measure for routine clinical use. *Clin Exp Dermatol.* 1994;9(3):210–216.
6. Chren MM, Lasek RJ, Sahay AP, Sands LP. Measurement properties of Skindex-16: a brief quality-of-life measure for patients with skin diseases. *J Cutan Med Surg.* 2001;5(2):105–110.
7. Revuz JE, Jemec GB. Diagnosing Hidradenitis Suppurativa. *Dermatol Clin.* 2016;34(1):1–5.
8. Thorlacius L, Ingram JR, Villumsen B, et al. A core domain set for hidradenitis suppurativa trial outcomes: an international Delphi process. *Br J Dermatol.* 2018;179(3):642–650.
9. Thorlacius L, Garg A, Riis PT, et al. Inter-rater agreement and reliability of outcome measurement instruments and staging systems used in hidradenitis suppurativa. *Br J Dermatol.* 2019;181(3):483–491.
10. Hurley HJ. Axillary hyperhidrosis, apocrine bromhidrosis, hidradenitis suppurativa, and familial benign pemphigus: surgical approach. In: Dermatologic Surgery, Roenigk RK, Roenigk HH (Eds), New York 1989. p.729.
11. Alikhan A, Sayed C, Alavi A, et al. North American clinical management guidelines for hidradenitis suppurativa: A publication from the United States and Canadian Hidradenitis Suppurativa Foundations: Part I: Diagnosis, evaluation, and the use of complementary and procedural management. *J Am Acad Dermatol.* 2019;81(1):76–90.
12. Canoui-Poitrine F, Revuz JE, Wolkenstein P, et al. Clinical characteristics of a series of 302 French patients with hidradenitis suppurativa, with an analysis of factors associated with disease severity. *J Am Acad Dermatol.* 2009;61(1):51–57.
13. DeFazio MV, Economides JM, King KS, et al. Outcomes after combined radical resection and targeted biologic therapy for the management of recalcitrant hidradenitis suppurativa. *Ann Plast Surg.* 2016;77(2):217–222.
14. Ovadja ZN, Schuit MM, van der Horst CMAM, Lapid O. Inter- and intrarater reliability of Hurley staging for hidradenitis suppurativa. *Br J Dermatol.* 2019;181(2):344–349.
15. Horvath B, Janse IC, Blok JL, et al. Hurley staging refined: A proposal by the Dutch hidradenitis suppurativa expert group. *Acta Derm Venereol.* 2017;97(3):412–413.
16. Jemec GB, Wendelboe P. Topical clindamycin versus systemic tetracycline in the treatment of hidradenitis suppurativa. *J Am Acad Dermatol.* 1998;39(6):971–974.
17. Ingram JR, Hadjieconomou S, Piguet V. Development of core outcome sets in hidradenitis suppurativa: systematic review of outcome measure instruments to inform the process. *Br J Dermatol.* 2016;175(2):263–272.
18. Sartorius K, Lapins J, Emtestam L, Jemec GB. Suggestions for uniform outcome variables when reporting treatment effects in hidradenitis suppurativa. *Br J Dermatol.* 2003;149(1):211–213.
19. Maarouf M, Clark AK, Lee DE, Shi VY. Targeted treatments for hidradenitis suppurativa: a review of the current literature and ongoing clinical trials. *J Dermatolog Treat.* 2018;29(5):441–449.
20. Giamarellos-Bourboulis EJ, Pelekanou E, Antonopoulou A, Petropoulou H, et al. An open-label phase II study of the safety and efficacy of etanercept for the therapy of hidradenitis suppurativa. *Br J Dermatol.* 2008;158(3):567–572.
21. Włodarek K, Stefaniak A, Matusiak Ł, Szepietowski JC. Could residents adequately assess the severity of hidradenitis suppurativa? Inter-rater and intrarater reliability assessment of major scoring systems. *Dermatol.* 2020;236(1):8–14.
22. Sartorius K, Emtestam L, Jemec GB, Lapins J. Objective scoring of hidradenitis suppurativa reflecting the role of tobacco smoking and obesity. *Br J Dermatol.* 2009;161(4):831–839.
23. Kimball AB, Jemec GB, Yang M, et al. Assessing the validity, responsiveness and meaningfulness of the Hidradenitis Suppurativa Clinical Response (HiSCR) as the clinical endpoint for hidradenitis suppurativa treatment. *Br J Dermatol.* 2014;171(6):1434–1442.
24. Kimball AB, Ganguli A, Fleischer A. Reliability of the hidradenitis suppurativa clinical response in the assessment of patients with hidradenitis suppurativa. *J Eur Acad Dermatol Venereol.* 2018;32(12):2254–2256.
25. Zouboulis CC, Tzellos T, Kyrgidis A, et al. Development and validation of the International Hidradenitis Suppurativa Severity Score System (IHS4), a novel dynamic scoring system to assess HS severity. *Br J Dermatol.* 2017;177(5):1401–1409.

26. Robinson A, Kardos M, Kimball AB. Physician global assessment (PGA) and psoriasis area and severity index (PASI): why do both? A systematic analysis of randomized controlled trials of biologic agents for moderate to severe plaque psoriasis. *J Am Acad Dermatol.* 2012;66(3):369–375.

27. Amano M, Grant A, Kerdel FA. A prospective open-label clinical trial of adalimumab for the treatment of hidradenitis suppurativa. *Int J Dermatol.* 2010;49(8):950–955.

28. Grant A, Gonzalez T, Montgomery MO, et al. Infliximab therapy for patients with moderate to severe hidradenitis suppurativa: a randomized, double-blind, placebo-controlled crossover trial. *J Am Acad Dermatol.* 2010;62(2):205–217.

29. Chiricozzi A, Faleri S, Franceschini C, et al. AISI: A new disease severity assessment tool for hidradenitis suppurativa. *Wounds.* 2015;27(10):258–264.

30. Kirby JS, Butt M, King T. Severity and area score for hidradenitis (SASH): a novel outcome measurement for hidradenitis suppurativa. *Br J Dermatol.* 2020;940–948.

31. Goldfarb N, Ingram JR, Jemec GBE, et al. Hidradenitis suppurativa area and severity index (HASI): a pilot study to develop a novel instrument to measure the physical signs of hidradenitis suppurativa. *Br J Dermatol.* 2020;182(1):240–242.

32. Snyder CF, Aaronson NK, Choucair AK, et al. Implementing patient-reported outcomes assessment in clinical practice: a review of the options and considerations. *Qual Life Res.* 2012;21(8):1305–1314.

33. Greenhalgh J, Meadows K. The effectiveness of the use of patient-based measures of health in routine practice in improving the process and outcomes of patient care: a literature review. *J Eval Clin Pract.* 1999;5(4):401–406.

34. Frank L, Basch E, Selby JV, Institute P-COR. The PCORI perspective on patient-centered outcomes research. *JAMA.* 2014;312(15):1513–1514.

35. Rogers A, LK DeLong, Chen SC. Clinical meaning in skin-specific quality of life instruments: a comparison of the Dermatology life quality index and skindex banding systems. *Dermatol Clin.* 2012;30(2):333–342.

36. Chren MM. The Skindex instruments to measure the effects of skin disease on quality of life. *Dermatol Clin.* 2012;30(2):231–236.

37. Kouris A, Platsidaki E, Christodoulou C, et al. Quality of life and psychosocial implications in patients with hidradenitis suppurativa. *Dermatol.* 2016;232(6):687–691.

38. Kimball AB, Sundaram M, Banderas B, et al. Development and initial psychometric evaluation of patient-reported outcome questionnaires to evaluate the symptoms and impact of hidradenitis suppurativa. *J Dermatolog Treat.* 2018;29(2):152–164.

39. Sisic M, Kirby JS, Boyal S, et al. Development of a quality-of-life measure for hidradenitis suppurativa. *J Cutan Med Surg.* 2017;21(2):152–155.

40. Thorlacius L, Esmann S, Miller I, et al. Development of HiSQOL: A hidradenitis suppurativa-specific quality of life instrument. *Skin Appendage Disord.* 2019;5(4):221–229.

41. Kirby JS, Thorlacius L, Villumsen B, et al. The hidradenitis suppurativa quality of life (HiSQOL) score: development and validation of a measure for clinical trials. *Br J Dermatol.* 2020;183:340–348.

14

Overview and Comparison of Hidradenitis Suppurativa Management Guidelines

ALEKSI J. HENDRICKS, JENNIFER L. HSIAO, AND VIVIAN Y. SHI

Introduction

Long considered an orphan disease until recent years, hidradenitis suppurativa (HS) is rapidly gaining attention in the healthcare field with a growing spotlight on investigating HS pathogenesis, epidemiology, and treatment options. To better navigate the expanding therapeutic options available, a number of HS management guidelines have been published by international expert organizations from North America, South America, and Europe between 2015 and July 2020 (Fig. 14.1). These groups include the British Association of Dermatologists,[1] U.S. and Canadian HS Foundations,[2,3] HS ALLIANCE,[4] Canadian Dermatology Association,[5,6] European HS Foundation,[7] European Academy of Dermatology and Venereology,[8] Swiss Consensus Group,[9] and Brazilian Society of Dermatology.[10] These guidelines encompass therapeutic modalities ranging from lifestyle modifications and topical therapies to systemic medications and procedural interventions. While significant overlap exists between the therapeutic ladders proposed by each set of guidelines, there are also abundant variations in recommendations across organizations. International recommendations and practice guidelines have been collated and compared in recent summaries,[11,12] allowing for review and discussion of practices with the best evidence and efficacy in HS treatment.

The management of HS often requires a comprehensive approach comprised of lifestyle modifications, mental healthcare, and depending on disease severity, topical antimicrobials, systemic antibiotics, hormonal and immune modulators, light-based therapies, and procedural interventions.[13] In this chapter, which is modified from our recent publication,[11] we compare the similarities and differences among the nine published guidelines and highlight knowledge and practice gaps that remain to be addressed. Specific management modalities are discussed in detail in Section 3: Clinician's Corner, Chapters 13 to 28.

General Guideline Comparison

International guidelines emphasize a multidisciplinary approach to HS management, including primary care providers, dermatologists, surgeons, pain management, and mental health specialists. All nine guidelines propose lifestyle modifications (such as weight loss and smoking cessation) and topical antimicrobials as first-line medical therapy, followed by systemic antibiotics, then systemic immunomodulators (such as adalimumab) for severe widespread disease. All guidelines include procedural modalities, such as intralesional corticosteroids recommended for isolated inflammatory lesions and light-based procedures (including laser hair reduction) as second- or third-line therapeutic considerations. Guideline recommendations vary in the order of use for systemic retinoids and

International Hidradenitis Suppurativa Management Guideline Publications
2015 – 2020

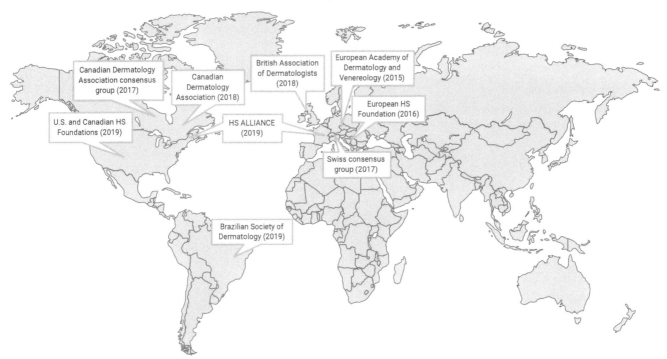

• **Fig. 14.1** International Hidradenitis Suppurativa Management Guideline Publications. Guidelines to manage hidradenitis suppurativa (HS) have been published by international expert organizations from North America, South America, and Europe between 2015 and July 2020. These groups include the British Association of Dermatologists,[1] U.S. and Canadian HS Foundations,[2,3] HS ALLIANCE,[4] Canadian Dermatology Association,[5,6] European HS Foundation,[7] European Academy of Dermatology and Venereology,[8] Swiss Consensus Group,[9] and Brazilian Society of Dermatology.[10] (Illustration created with BioRender.com.)

hormonal agents. The North American guideline presents a broader discussion on classification criteria, biomarker and genetic testing, comorbidities screening, and procedural interventions than European and Brazilian groups. Additionally, while other guidelines utilize a therapeutic ladder approach, the North American and HS ALLIANCE guidelines display treatment modalities according to level of evidence. The North American guidelines also incorporate a more in-depth discussion of complementary and alternative medicine treatment modalities.

Detailed Comparison by HS Treatment Modality

Non-Pharmacological Approaches

Several lifestyle modifications are recommended as components of a comprehensive HS treatment plan. Universally supported lifestyle approaches include smoking cessation and weight reduction.[1,2,4-10] While existing data is inconsistent in characterizing the relationship between tobacco use and HS severity, the prevalence of HS is higher among individuals who smoke compared to those who do not, and tobacco cessation should be encouraged for general health benefits. Similarly, there is limited evidence to support an association between higher body mass index and more severe HS, but proposed contributing factors include proinflammatory cytokines from adipose tissue and increased friction and inflammation in intertriginous areas. Tobacco cessation and weight

loss counseling should be incorporated in routine HS management where relevant. Additionally, mental health is recognized in all guidelines as a critical factor in treatment of HS due to the psychological impact of chronic pain, skin disfigurement, and variable efficacy of treatment.[1,2,4-10] All expert guidelines support screening for depression and anxiety in routine clinical visits with referral to psychiatric care as appropriate, further emphasizing the importance of a multidisciplinary healthcare team in managing HS.

Pain Management

The pain burden of HS remains a challenging aspect of disease management. Most guidelines recommend assessing pain severity using validated patient-reported outcome tools such as a pain visual analogue scale or numeric rating scale.[1,2,4-8] Guidance regarding selection of analgesic agents is limited, but those guidelines that do address specific agents recommend topical analgesics and nonsteroidal antiinflammatories as first-line treatment, with opioids reserved only for severe pain refractory to first-line agents and to be used under the supervision of pain management specialists.[2,6,8]

Topical Analgesics

The North American and Canadian consensus guidelines cite topical lidocaine as a first-line option for HS pain management,[2,6] with diclofenac gel suggested as an alternative in the Canadian consensus guidelines.[6]

Non-Steroidal Antiinflammatory Drugs (NSAIDs)

North American, Canadian consensus, and European S1 guidelines discuss nonsteroidal antiinflammatory drug (NSAIDs) as first-line systemic pain management in HS.[2,6,8] NSAID use should be reviewed regularly during clinical visits with special dosing consideration or use of alternate agents in patients with impaired hepatic or renal function.

Neuropathic Pain Agents

Gabapentin and pregabalin are mentioned in the North American and Canadian consensus guidelines as therapeutic options for neuropathic pain associated with HS.[2,6]

Tramadol

The opioid-like analgesic tramadol is cited in the North American guidelines as an agent for HS-associated pain that does not respond to topical analgesics or NSAIDs, although specific dosing is not discussed.[2]

Opioids

Opioid use in selected patients (those with severe pain unresponsive to first-line agents) is discussed in the North American, Canadian consensus, and European S1 guidelines.[2,6,8] These three guidelines underscore the importance of judicious opioid prescribing and recommend involvement of pain specialists in managing HS patients who are candidates for opioid use. However, the Canadian consensus and European S1 guidelines highlight the lack of evidence for opioid use in treating HS.[6,8]

Topical Modalities

The nine guidelines recommend topical therapies for use in mild HS, localized disease, or as an adjunct to systemic therapies. Recommendations for these modalities are summarized in Table 14.1.

Topical Keratolytics

Keratolytics aim to reduce follicular plugging thought to exacerbate the cycle of follicular occlusion and inflammation in HS. Resorcinol 15% cream is a keratolytic with antiseptic properties mentioned in six of the nine guidelines,[3,5-8,10] and recommended as second-line therapy in the European HS Foundation and Canadian Dermatology Association guidelines.[5,7] While more readily available in Europe, resorcinol cream requires compounding by a specialty pharmacy in the United States.

Topical Antiseptics

Topical antiseptics are used to inhibit bacterial colonization and resulting cutaneous inflammation. Recommendations for various antiseptic agents are included in the North American, Swiss, and Brazilian guidelines,[3,9,10] although the North American guideline cites a lack of evidence to support specific formulations.[3] Recommended topical antiseptics include chlorhexidine, benzoyl peroxide, zinc pyrithione, triclosan, and ammonium bituminosulfonate (ichthammol). Availability of these agents varies by region, as triclosan was removed from the U.S. market in 2018 due to lack of efficacy and safety data. Ichthammol is available over the counter as a cream or ointment formulation in the United States but is more frequently recommended and used for dermatologic purposes in Europe.[14]

Topical Antibiotics

Clindamycin is a topical antibiotic available as a 1% lotion or solution that decreases cutaneous inflammation and inhibits biofilm formation.[15] There is consensus across all guidelines in recommending topical clindamycin as a first-line therapy in mild HS with predominantly superficial pustules and no deep abscesses.[1,3-10] Recommended application as proposed by the European S1, European HS Foundation, and HS ALLIANCE guidelines is twice daily for up to 3 months,[4,7,8] with caution against long-term use due to risk of bacterial resistance.

Systemic Therapies

Guideline recommendations regarding systemic therapeutic agents in HS are summarized in Table 14.2.

Systemic Antibiotics

Systemic antibiotics are widely used in HS management for their antiinflammatory and antibacterial effects; they are more practical than topical antibiotics for treatment of widespread disease. Several antibiotic regimens are cited by the nine guidelines, with uniform recommendation of oral tetracyclines (doxycycline or minocycline) as first-line agents in mild-to-moderate HS (although tetracyclines are not recommended in children due to potential teeth discoloration).[1,3,4,10] Clindamycin and rifampicin in combination are cited as second-line therapy in all guidelines,[1,3-10] but recommendations for third-line options are less consistent, including metronidazole, moxifloxacin and rifampin triple therapy,[3,4,8] dapsone,[1,3,5,7,9,10] and intravenous ertapenem as rescue therapy or bridge to surgery.[3,4]

Systemic Retinoids

Retinoids are vitamin A analogs that regulate keratinocyte turnover and are used in HS to combat keratin plugging and resulting inflammation in pilosebaceous units. Acitretin is recommended across all guidelines as second- or third-line therapy following failure of topical and oral antibiotics,[1,3-10] with suggested dosing regimens ranging from 0.2 to 0.88 mg/kg daily. Isotretinoin use is controversial, with Canadian consensus and European S1 guidelines citing lack of demonstrated efficacy,[6,8] while British and North American guidelines recommend its use as a second- or third-line agent in patients with concomitant moderate to severe acne,[1,3] and Canadian Dermatology Association and European HS Foundation guidelines suggest use only as a third-line agent.[5,7] Brazilian guidelines specifically recommend preferential use of isotretinoin over acitretin in women of childbearing age.[10] While appropriate in men and post-menopausal women without additional precautions, use of systemic retinoids in women of childbearing potential requires concomitant use of reliable contraception due to the teratogenic effects of retinoids.

Biologics and Immunomodulators

Guidelines recommend consideration of biologics in moderate-to-severe HS refractory to systemic antibiotics. Targets of these immunomodulatory agents include tumor necrosis factor-alpha (TNF-α) (adalimumab, infliximab), interleukin (IL)-1 (anakinra, canakinumab), IL-12/23 (ustekinumab), and IL-17 (secukinumab), which have been shown to be elevated in the skin and serum of HS patients.[16-19]

TABLE 14.1 Topical and Intralesional Therapy for HS—International Guideline Recommendations

Modality	British Association of Dermatologists[1]	North American (US and Canadian HS Foundations)[3]	HS ALLIANCE[4]	Canadian Dermatology Association[5]	Canadian Consensus Group[6]	European HS Foundation[7]	European S1[8]	Swiss Consensus Group[9]	Brazilian Society of Dermatology[10]
				RECOMMENDATIONS PER GUIDELINE					
Topical Therapies (Further discussed in Chapter 15)									
Resorcinol 15% cream	–	Recommended (may induce contact dermatitis)	–	2nd line	Resolve/prevent follicular blockage in mild HS	2nd line	For recurrent lesions in Hurley stage I/II HS[a] BID application during flares	–	Can be useful to shorten mean duration of painful nodule or abscess
Antiseptics	–	Chlorhexidine, benzoyl peroxide zinc pyrithione supported by expert opinion	–	–	–	–	–	Triclosan, ammonium bituminosulfate for all Hurley stages[a]	Advise on adequate local hygiene; no need for soaps with high concentrations of chlorhexidine
Clindamycin 1% solution	Consider in patients with HS	May reduce pustules; carries risk of bacterial resistance	Recommended BID × ≤ 3 months in Hurley I/II[a] with localized lesions, especially without deep inflammatory lesions	1st line tx for mild HS; 1% lotion applied BID × 12 weeks	Use as topical antiinflammatory agent and to prevent secondary infection[b]	Recommended BID ×3 months as 1st line tx in Hurley stage II,[a] especially without deep inflammatory lesions[b]	BID × 3 months in localized Hurley stage I or mild stage II,[a] can be prolonged if clinically indicated[b]	Recommended in Hurley I/II[a] HS to avoid bacterial superinfection and reduce inflammation	Recommended for Hurley stage I[a] or in cases of superficial lesions during exacerbation

–Not specifically mentioned

[a]Hurley staging

Hurley stage I—single or multiple abscesses without scarring

Hurley stage II—limited scarring and/or sinus tracts

Hurley stage III—extensive scarring and/or sinus tracts

[b]Recommendation based on randomized controlled trial(s) in HS

BID, Twice daily; *HS,* hidradenitis suppurativa; *tx,* treatment,

From Hendricks AJ, Hsiao JL, Lowes MA, Shi VY. A comparison of international management guidelines for hidradenitis suppurativa. *Dermatol.* 2021;237(1):81–96. doi:10.1159/000503605.

TABLE 14.2 Systemic Therapy for HS—International Guideline Recommendations

Systemic Antibiotics (Further discussed in Chapter 16)

Modality	British Association of Dermatologists[1]	North American (US and Canadian HS Foundations)[3]	HS Alliance[4]	Canadian Dermatology Association[5]	Canadian Consensus Group[6]	European HS Foundation[7]	European S1[8]	Swiss Consensus Group[9]	Brazilian Society of Dermatology[10]
				RECOMMENDATIONS PER GUIDELINE					
Tetracyclines	Doxycycline or lymecycline for ≥12 weeks. Consider tx breaks to assess efficacy and decrease risk of antimicrobial resistance	In mild to moderate HS × 12 weeks or as long-term maintenance[a]	Recommended in Hurley I/II[b] × ≤12 weeks[a]	500 mg BID × 4 months for mild HS (1st line)[a]	500 mg BID[a]	500 mg BID as 1st line tx in moderate HS or widespread Hurley I/II[b] for up to 4 months[a]	500 mg BID × 4 months; can be prolonged if clinically indicated[a]	Doxycycline 50–200 mg daily × 3–6 months in Hurley I/II[b] HS	500 mg BID × 10–12 weeks, 1–2 courses
Clindamycin + rifampicin	Clindamycin 300 mg BID and rifampicin 300 mg BID × 10–12 weeks for patients unresponsive to oral tetracyclines[a]	2nd line for mild-moderate HS, 1st line or adjunct for severe HS[a]	Clindamycin and rifampicin 300 mg each BID × 10 weeks[a]	Clindamycin 300 mg BID + rifampicin 600 mg daily × 10 weeks in moderate HS or mild-moderate HS unresponsive to tetracyclines (1st line)[a]	Clindamycin 300 mg BID + rifampicin 600 mg once daily or 300 mg BID × 10 weeks[a]	Clindamycin 300 mg BID + rifampicin 600 mg once daily or 300 mg BID × 10 weeks as 1st line tx for moderate PGA[a]	Clindamycin 300 mg BID + rifampicin 600 mg once daily or 300 mg BID × 10 weeks[a]	Clindamycin and rifampicin each 300 mg BID × 3 months	Clindamycin 300 mg BID + rifampicin 600 mg daily × 10 weeks
Rifampin/Moxifloxacin/Metronidazole/	—	2nd /3rd line in moderate to severe HS	Rifampicin 10 mg/kg once daily + moxifloxacin 400 mg once daily + metronidazole 500 mg TID (×6 weeks only) may have efficacy in Hurley I/II[a] patients	—	—	—	Effective in tx-resistant Hurley stage II/III[b] HS at 12 weeks	—	—
Dapsone	Consider in HS unresponsive to antibiotic therapies	May be effective for minority of Hurley I/II[a] patients as long-term maintenance	Evidence from single study	3rd line	Efficacy in HS reported in case reports	3rd line	Reserve for patients with mild to moderate HS when standard 1st and 2nd line agents fail	50–150 mg daily in refractory Hurley II/III[b] disease	May be considered after failure of 1st or 2nd line antibiotics
Ertapenem	—	For severe disease as one-time rescue, bridge to surgery or maintenance tx	IV ertapenem 1 g/d In selected patients with severe HS ×6 weeks	—	—	—	—	—	—

Supplements (Further discussed in Chapter 28)

Drug									
Zinc	Insufficient evidence	–	Combination tx of oral zinc gluconate 30 mg TID + topical triclosan 2% in Hurley I/II[b]	Zinc gluconate as 2nd line tx	Zinc sulfate recommended as adjuvant therapy	Zinc gluconate as 2nd line tx	Zinc gluconate initiated at 90 mg/day as maintenance tx in Hurley I/II[b]	Zinc gluconate 30 mg TID as adjunct to antibiotics in Hurley I/II[b] HS	30 mg TID as maintenance tx in Hurley stage I/II[b] HS. Long-term use limited by zinc-induced impairment of iron and copper absorption

Retinoids (Further discussed in Chapter 17)

Drug									
Acitretin	0.3–0.5 mg/kg daily in men and non-fertile women unresponsive to antibiotics	Consider as 2nd/3rd line tx; contraindicated in women of reproductive potential	3rd line tx for mild-moderate HS	2nd line	0.25–0.88 mg/kg daily can be initiated in early HS stages, may be used in chronic stages with sinus tracts and scarring	2nd line	Can be initiated in early HS stages, may be used in chronic stages with sinus tracts and scarring. Dosing ranges from 0.25–0.88 mg/kg daily × 3–12 months	0.2–0.5 mg/kg daily in Hurley II/III[b] HS refractory to antibiotics	Preferred over isotretinoin due to higher response rates, but not appropriate in women of childbearing age
Isotretinoin	Do not offer unless concomitant moderate to severe acneiform lesions of face or trunk	Consider only as 2nd/3rd line tx or in patients with severe concomitant acne	–	3rd line	Not proven effective in HS even with concomitant acne	3rd line	Not recommended for use in tx of HS	–	Use of isotretinoin over acitretin justified in women of childbearing age

Biologics (Further discussed in Chapter 18)

Drug									
Adalimumab (anti-TNF-α)	40 mg SC weekly for patients ≥12 yo with moderate-severe HS unresponsive to conventional systemic tx[a]	Recommended at 40 mg SC weekly to improve HS severity and QoL in moderate-severe HS[a]	First choice biologic in moderate to severe HS after failure of conventional tx[a]	160 mg SC week 0, 80 mg week 2, then 40 mg weekly for moderate to severe HS unresponsive to antibiotics (1st line)[a]	40 mg SC weekly for patients with moderate to severe HS[a]	40 mg SC weekly for moderate-severe HS[a]	160 mg SC week 0, 80 mg week 2, then 40 mg weekly for moderate-severe HS[a]. Consider other tx modalities if HiSCR not achieved by 16 weeks	160 mg SC weekly for Hurley II/III[b] HS refractory to antibiotics	160 mg SC week 0, 80 mg week 2, then 40 mg weekly[a]. Once inflammation is controlled, consider excision of residual active areas or scarring

(Continued)

TABLE 14.2

Systemic Therapy for HS—International Guideline Recommendations—cont'd

Modality	British Association of Dermatologists[1]	North American (US and Canadian HS Foundations)[3]	HS Alliance[4]	Canadian Dermatology Association[5]	Canadian Consensus Group[6]	European HS Foundation[7]	European S1[8]	Swiss Consensus Group[9]	Brazilian Society of Dermatology[10]
					RECOMMENDATIONS PER GUIDELINE				
Infliximab (anti-TNF-α)	Consider at 5 mg/kg q8 weeks in moderate-severe HS unresponsive to adalimumab	Recommended for moderate to severe HS. Dose ranging studies needed to determine optimal dosage	Consider as 2nd line biologic for moderate to severe HS	2nd line[a]	No significant difference vs. placebo in HiSCR[a]	5 mg/kg IV at weeks 0, 2, 6 and q2 months thereafter x 12 weeks as 2nd line in moderate to severe HS unresponsive to adalimumab	5 mg/kg IV at weeks 0, 2, 6, then q2 months[a]	–	5 mg/kg IV at weeks 0, 2, 6, then q2 months[a]
Anakinra (anti-IL-1)	Insufficient evidence	100 mg daily may be effective; dose ranging studies needed to determine optimal dosage	Consider as 3rd line biologic for moderate to severe HS	–	Significant improvement in disease severity score and HiSCR[a]	–	–	–	Not available in Brazil
Canakinumab (anti-IL-1β)	–	–	–	–	–	–	–	–	Used successfully in sparse care reports
Ustekinumab (anti-IL-12/23)	Insufficient evidence	45–90 mg q12 weeks may be effective; dose ranging studies needed to determine optimal dosage	Potentially effective tx for moderate-severe HS	–	–	–	Three 45 mg SC injections at 0, 4, and 16 weeks with cumulative 33% response rate in 3-patient case series	–	45–90 mg SC q12 weeks; higher dose may be needed for HS tx
Secukinumab (anti-IL-17A)	–	–	–	–	–	–	–	–	Success in a case of severe tx-refractory HS
Etanercept (anti-TNF-α)	Do not offer[a]	Limited evidence does not support use in HS management[a]	Not effective[a]	–	No significant difference vs. placebo[a]	–	No significant difference vs. placebo[a]	–	Variable data on efficacy in HS; unable to draw conclusions about its potential utility

Immunosuppressive agents (Further discussed in Chapter 17)

Systemic corticosteroids	–	Short-term steroid pulse can be considered for acute flares or bridge to other tx Long-term: taper to lowest possible dose in severe HS	2nd line	–	2nd line	Recommend dose of 0.5–0.7 mg/kg oral prednisolone for short-term use in acute flares, taper over following weeks	Prednisolone 0.5–0.7 mg/kg daily in refractory disease	Short course may be indicated for tx of flares
Cyclosporine		Low-dose prednisolone 10 mg/day (or equivalent) may be effective adjunct tx in recalcitrant HS Use with caution long-term	2nd line	Efficacy in HS reported in case reports	3rd line	Reserved for cases unresponsive to standard 1st, 2nd, or 3rd line tx Reported dosing in HS varies from 2–6 mg/kg for 6 weeks to 7 months	2–6 mg/kg daily in refractory disease	Data not robust; consider only as 3rd line option for long-term control of inflammation

Hormonal agents (Further discussed in Chapter 17)

Metformin	Consider in HS patients with concomitant DM, PCOS, or pregnancy	Consider metformin 500 mg BID-TID in appropriate female patients as monotherapy for mild-moderate or as adjunctive tx in severe HS[a]	–	May be beneficial in patients with HS and PCOS	–	–	500–1500 mg daily in refractory disease	May consider in women of childbearing age who have failed systemic antibiotics
Cyproterone acetate + ethinyl estradiol	Insufficient evidence	Consider in appropriate female patients as monotherapy for mild to moderate or as adjunctive tx in severe HS[a]	–	~1/2 of patients exhibited clearance No significant difference in PaGA between cyproterone acetate + ethinyl estradiol vs. ethinyl estradiol + norgestrel at 6 months[a]	3rd line	100 mg cyproterone acetate daily for female patients with menstrual abnormalities, signs of hyperandrogenism, or high levels of DHEA, androstenedione, or SHBP	–	May consider in women of childbearing age who have failed systemic antibiotics

(Continued)

					RECOMMENDATIONS PER GUIDELINE					
Modality	British Association of Dermatologists[1]	North American (US and Canadian HS Foundations)[3]	HS Alliance[4]	Canadian Dermatology Association[5]	Canadian Consensus Group[6]	European HS Foundation[7]	European S1[8]	Swiss Consensus Group[9]	Brazilian Society of Dermatology[10]
Finasteride	Insufficient evidence	Consider 1.25–5 mg/d in appropriate female patients as monotherapy for mild to moderate or as adjunctive tx in severe HS	—	—	—	—	—	—	1–5 mg/d in children <12 yo with HS refractory to topical/oral antibiotics
Spironolactone	Insufficient evidence	Consider spironolactone 100–150 mg daily as monotherapy in women with mild-moderate HS or as adjunctive tx in severe HS	—	—	—	—	—	—	Consider in female HS patients who have failed systemic antibiotics

—Not specifically mentioned

[a]Recommendation based on randomized controlled trial(s) in HS

[b]Hurley staging

Hurley stage I—single or multiple abscesses without scarring

Hurley stage II—limited scarring and/or sinus tracts

Hurley stage III—extensive scarring and/or sinus tracts

abx, Antibiotics; *BID*, twice daily; *DHEA*, dehydroepiandrosterone; *DLQI*, Dermatology Life Quality Index; *DM*, diabetes mellitus; *HS*, hidradenitis suppurativa; *IV*, intravenous; *PGA*, Physician's Global Assessment; *PaGA*, Participant's Global Assessment; *PCOS*, polycystic ovary syndrome; *QoL*, quality of life; *SC*, subcutaneously; *SHBP*, sex hormone-binding protein; *TID*, three times daily; tx, treatment

Modified from Hendricks *et al.* 2019[11].

Adalimumab

Adalimumab is a fully human monoclonal IgG1 antibody that targets both soluble and receptor-bound TNF-α, one of the main pathogenic cytokines in HS. Adalimumab is one of the few HS treatments that has been evaluated in large randomized double-blind placebo-controlled trials.[20-22] In the United States, adalimumab was FDA-approved in 2015 for treatment of moderate-to-severe HS and is currently available for both adult and adolescent (age 12 and older) HS management.

All guidelines recommend adalimumab as the first-line biologic;[1,3-10] however, variations exist on the indication to start adalimumab. While all guidelines state that adalimumab should be considered in moderate to severe cases of HS (also commonly defined as Hurley stage II/III HS), the British and HS ALLIANCE guidelines add that patients should first have been unresponsive to conventional systemic treatments; the European HS Foundation and Swiss guidelines state that patients should have been refractive to antibiotics. The remaining guidelines make little to no mention of specific prior therapy failure before considering adalimumab.

Infliximab

Infliximab is a chimeric monoclonal antibody against TNF-α that is recommended by seven out of nine guidelines as the second-line biologic to adalimumab for moderate to severe HS refractory,[1,3-5,7,8,10] but it has not received regulatory approval for HS. Intravenous infliximab at 5 mg/kg administered at weeks 0, 2, and 6 has been evaluated in a small randomized controlled trial (RCT).[23]

Anakinra, Canakinumab, Secukinumab, and Ustekinumab

Several other biologics are cited in various guidelines as potential third-line therapeutic agents following failure of adalimumab and infliximab. These include the IL-1 receptor antagonist anakinra,[3,4,6] IL-1β monoclonal antibody canakinumab,[10] IL-12/IL-23 modulator ustekinumab,[3,4,8,10] and IL-17A monoclonal antibody secukinumab.[10] These agents have demonstrated some success in small RCTs, pilot studies, and case series, but have not been evaluated in large-scale RCTs approved or published at this time. Consideration of their use as third-line agents is variably recommended in international guidelines, but HS-specific dosing and efficacy have not yet been established.

Etanercept

Etanercept is a fusion recombinant protein TNF receptor that interferes with TNF-α signaling.[24] Five out of nine guidelines recommend not using etanercept in HS,[1,3,4,6,8] citing a double-blind RCT that demonstrated no significant difference in HS severity between etanercept 50 mg subcutaneous injection versus placebo twice weekly after 3 months.[24] Brazilian guidelines are not for or against etanercept use, but assert that conclusions about its efficacy in HS cannot be drawn due to conflicting study results and insufficient data.[10]

Traditional Immunosuppressive Agents

Systemic corticosteroids and cyclosporine are included in the majority of international guidelines as third-line treatments for refractory HS. Per the North American, HS ALLIANCE, Canadian Dermatology Association, European HS Foundation, European S1, Swiss, and Brazilian guidelines, corticosteroid use should be restricted to short courses for acute flares or as bridge therapy to another systemic agent.[3-5,7-10] If considered for longer term use, corticosteroids should be tapered to the lowest effective dose. Cyclosporine is cited in seven out of nine guidelines as an

alternative immunosuppressive agent to be considered for treatment-refractory HS,[3,5-10] with a proposed dosing of 2 to 6 mg/kg daily (as suggested in the Swiss guideline.)[9]

Hormonal Modulators

Fluctuating hormone levels are thought to play a role in the pathogenesis of HS, as many female patients report disease flares associated with menses and improvement in symptoms during pregnancy.[25,26] Hormonal modulators are recommended by several guidelines for female HS patients with coexisting diabetes, polycystic ovary syndrome (PCOS), or hyperandrogenism.

Metformin

The hypoglycemic agent metformin has been found to be effective in the treatment of HS, which often coexists with and may be exacerbated by the proinflammatory states of insulin resistance and metabolic syndrome.[27] British, North American, Canadian Dermatology Association, Swiss, and Brazilian guidelines discuss use of metformin in HS patients with diabetes, PCOS or during pregnancy,[1,3,6,9,10] at a recommended dosing of 500 mg two to three times daily.[3,9]

Antiandrogens

As hyperandrogenism promotes excess sebum production and follicular occlusion,[28] antiandrogen agents are thought to be beneficial in certain subsets of HS patients. Cyproterone acetate is an antiandrogen studied in combination with ethinyl estradiol that demonstrated efficacy in reducing HS lesions,[29] and is included in the North American, Canadian consensus, European HS Foundation, European S1, and Brazilian guidelines.[3,6-8,10] Although available in other countries, cyproterone acetate is not approved for use in the United States. Finasteride is a 5α-reductase inhibitor that blocks peripheral testosterone conversion and is discussed in the North American and Brazilian guidelines at doses of 1 to 5 mg daily as a third-line treatment option for use in female or pediatric HS patients.[3,10]

Spironolactone

The aldosterone receptor antagonist spironolactone has antiandrogenic properties and is recommended by two guidelines for use in female HS patients.[3,10] North American guidelines suggest spironolactone as monotherapy for women with mild to moderate HS or as adjunctive treatment in severe HS,[3] and Brazilian guidelines recommend spironolactone for use in women who have failed systemic antibiotics.[10]

Procedural Modalities

Procedural interventions for HS range from intralesional corticosteroid injections to light-based therapy, lasers, and surgical excision. International guideline recommendations on these modalities are varied but include relatively uniform support for carbon dioxide ablative laser treatment, deroofing, and wide local excision. Procedural recommendations are summarized in Table 14.3.

Intralesional Corticosteroids

Intralesional corticosteroid injections can reduce acute lesion pain and inflammation, and are cited universally across guidelines for use in acute, isolated HS lesions either as monotherapy or concomitantly with systemic treatment.[1,3-10] Triamcinolone 5 to 10 mg/mL has demonstrated efficacy in reducing size, redness, edema, suppuration, and pain associated with HS lesions.[3,6,30]

TABLE 14.3 Laser, Phototherapy and Surgical Approaches for HS—International Guideline Recommendations

Modality		RECOMMENDATIONS PER GUIDELINE							
	British Association of Dermatologists[1]	North American (US and Canadian HS Foundations)[2]	HS ALLIANCE[4]	Canadian Dermatology Association[5]	Canadian consensus group[6]	European HS Foundation[7]	European S1[8]	Swiss consensus group[9]	Brazilian Society of Dermatology[10]
Intralesional corticosteroid injections	Consider for individual lesions in the acute phase	Injection of inflamed lesions or short-term control of flares	May be helpful for acute inflammatory nodules in combination with other tx at all Hurley stages	2nd line	TAC 5–10 mg/mL for rapid reduction of inflammation in acute flares or as rescue therapy adjunctive to systemic tx	2nd line	TAC 5–10 mg/mL for rapid reduction of inflammation in acute flares and for recalcitrant nodules and sinus tracts	Injection of inflamed nodules in Hurley I/II[a] HS	TAC 5–10 mg/mL for tx of acute inflammation and abscesses, refractory nodules, tunnels
Light-based therapy (Further discussed in Chapter 25)									
Photodynamic therapy	Insufficient evidence	Variable success based on small, uncontrolled studies	—	—	Cited	—	Variable success reported with PDT. Additional studies needed to establish role of PDT in HS tx	—	—
Intense pulsed light	Insufficient evidence	Supported by case reports	—	—	Cited	Significant improvement maintained at 12 months	Additional studies needed to establish role of IPL in HS tx	—	Option for laser hair removal as adjuvant tx to reduce flares and appearance of new lesions. Can provide favorable results even in Hurley II/III[a] disease
Lasers (Further discussed in Chapter 25)									
Nd:YAG laser	Insufficient evidence	Recommended in Hurley II/III[a] disease[b]. Recommended in Hurley stage I HS based on expert consensus	—	—	Cited	Significant improvement in HS-LASI at 3 months at sites treated with Nd:YAG monthly + topical antimicrobials vs. topical antimicrobials alone[b]	Significant improvement at sites treated with Nd:YAG monthly + topical antimicrobials vs. topical antimicrobials alone[b]. Additional studies needed to establish Nd:YAG as standard HS tx	—	Option for laser hair removal or treatment of superficial lesions

TABLE 14.3 Laser, Phototherapy and Surgical Approaches for HS—International Guideline Recommendations—cont'd

Modality	British Association of Dermatologists	North American (US and Canadian HS Foundations)	HS ALLIANCE	Canadian Dermatology Association	Canadian consensus group	European HS Foundation	European S1	Swiss consensus group	Brazilian Society of Dermatology
					RECOMMENDATIONS PER GUIDELINE				
CO$_2$ ablative laser	–	Appropriate for extensive chronic lesions in Hurley II/III[a] HS	Effective alternative to electrosurgical or cold steel techniques	Consider for Hurley stage II/III[a] disease	Cited	Recurrence rate in treated areas ranging from 1.1%–29%	Can be used for excision and marsupialization of skin areas with less bleeding and better visualization than in standard excisions	Consider in widespread or severe HS	Consider for targeted vaporization and excision of lesions separated by healthy tissue
Procedural and surgical interventions (Further discussed in Chapters 22–24, 26)									
Incision and drainage	–	Recommended only for acute abscesses to relieve pain	May be performed in acute situations for tense/painful abscesses; recurrence nearly inevitable	–	May be performed in patients with mild HS	–	–	–	Performed on acute lesions for symptomatic relief
Deroofing or limited excision	–	Recommended for recurrent nodules and tunnels	May be used for solitary lesions, recurrent lesions at fixed locations, or fistula formation in limited areas	Consider for Hurley stage II/III[a] disease	Can be attempted in early/mild disease	17% lesion recurrence rate after deroofing	Effective and fast surgical technique that can be performed in-office	Recommended only in localized, well-circumscribed Hurley I/II[a] HS	For localized disease
Wide local excision	To minimize recurrence when conventional systemic tx have failed	Appropriate for extensive chronic lesions. Post-surgical healing by secondary intention, primary closure, delayed primary closure, flaps, grafts, and/or skin substitutes	Perform in Hurley stage III[a] HS to prevent further recurrence	Consider for Hurley stage II/III[a] disease	Only potentially curative tx for severe HS	Accepted therapeutic modality	Treatment of choice for HS with healing by secondary intention, primary closure, grafts, or flaps according to size/location of defect	Consider in widespread or severe HS. Recommend healing by secondary intention ± partial closure ± negative pressure-assisted healing	In chronic cases of moderate-severe HS. Recommend healing by secondary intention > primary closure > grafts > flaps

–Not specifically mentioned

[a]Hurley staging

[b]Recommendation based on randomized controlled trial(s) in HS

Hurley stage I—single or multiple abscesses without scarring

Hurley stage II—limited scarring and/or sinus tracts

Hurley stage III—extensive scarring and/or sinus tracts

CO$_2$, Carbon dioxide; f/u, follow-up; HS, hidradenitis suppurativa; HS-LASI, HS Lesion, Area and Severity Index; IPL, intense pulsed light; Nd:YAG, neodymium-doped yttrium aluminum garnet; PDT, photodynamic therapy; TAC, triamcinolone acetonide; tx, treatment; WLE, wide local excision.

Modified from Hendricks et al.[11]

Adverse effects of repeated corticosteroid injections may include skin atrophy and telangiectasias, the use of which is contraindicated in the setting of suspected bacterial infection.[8,10]

Light-Based Therapy

Photodynamic Therapy

In photodynamic therapy (PDT), a photosensitizing agent and light source are used to generate free radicals in the skin that result in localized cell death, which may promote remodeling of chronic structural changes (such as fistulas and recurrent nodules) or disruption of bacterial biofilms.[31] Reports of PDT in HS have yielded conflicting results,[32-36] and its use is mentioned in only the North American, Canadian consensus, and European S1 guidelines as a potential treatment option.[2,6,8] No recommendations specify a sensitizing agent or red versus blue light PDT.

Intense Pulsed Light

Intense pulsed light (IPL) as a hair reduction modality in HS is discussed in five out of nine guidelines, including the North American, Canadian consensus, European HS Foundation, European S1, and Brazilian publications.[2,6-8,10] A single split-body RCT evaluated IPL in Hurley stage II/III patients twice weekly and demonstrated significant improvement of HS in treated versus untreated sites.[37]

Lasers

Neodymium-Doped Yttrium Aluminum Garnet

Neodymium-doped yttrium aluminum garnet (Nd:YAG) laser treatment targets the dark pigment of hair follicles to reduce hair growth, aiming to break the cycle of follicular occlusion and inflammation in HS.[38-40] Nd:YAG laser therapy is recommended for Hurley stage II/III disease by the majority of international groups, including the North American, Canadian Dermatology Association, European HS Foundation, European S1, and Brazilian guidelines.[2,6-8,10] The North American guidelines also propose Nd:YAG as a therapeutic option in Hurley stage I HS on the basis of expert consensus.[2] In an RCT, Nd:YAG in combination with topical antimicrobials has demonstrated improvement compared to topical antimicrobials alone.[39]

Carbon Dioxide Ablative Laser

Carbon dioxide (CO_2) ablative laser treatment vaporizes layers of affected skin to expose and excise the base of HS lesions and connecting sinus tracts.[41] CO_2 ablative laser therapy is recommended by eight of nine guidelines for chronic lesions in moderate to severe HS,[2,4-10] citing less bleeding and sparing of healthy tissue as advantages over traditional excision.[8,10]

Surgical Procedures

Incision and Drainage

Incision and drainage (I&D) involves incising and draining purulent contents from pustules and abscesses. It is recommended in the North American, HS ALLIANCE, Canadian consensus, and Brazilian guidelines for pain relief associated with acute, isolated, and inflammatory HS lesions.[2,4,6,10]

Deroofing

Deroofing refers to removal of the skin overlying an abscess or sinus tract to allow for drainage and healing by secondary intention.[42] Deroofing is discussed by the majority of guidelines as an intervention for recurrent nodules and sinus tracts, either in localized areas of mild disease or in more extensive Hurley stage II/III HS.[2,4-10]

Wide Local Excision

Wide local excision (WLE) involves surgical removal of an entire affected anatomical region with a wide margin of clear skin, rather than the limited excision of isolated HS lesion(s) while leaving intervening skin intact.[41] WLE is recommended consistently across all guidelines for treatment-refractory advanced localized disease.[1,2,4-10] Recommendations for post-surgical healing options vary and may include healing by secondary intention, primary closure, grafts, or flaps based on the size and location of the surgical defect.[2,8-10]

Conclusion

Existing HS guidelines uniformly support lifestyle modifications, with emphasis on weight loss and smoking cessation. The use of topical and oral antibiotics is generally recommended as first-line therapy for mild to moderate disease, with immunomodulators added for more severe disease. Hormonal therapies and systemic retinoids are typically mentioned as adjunctive therapy, but guidelines vary on when these modalities should be implemented. Procedural interventions such as intralesional corticosteroids provide rapid relief of individual lesions during the acute stage, while wide local excision offers more permanent improvement over an entire anatomical region; however, patients need to be appropriate surgical candidates. With the exception of adalimumab, most recommended therapies have not been evaluated in large randomized controlled trials.

Despite similarities across guidelines, a truly international consensus on optimal HS management has still not been achieved. Current guidelines lack recommendations on which specialist should be the principal provider for HS and how the principal providers can educate and collaborate with healthcare professionals in different specialties to treat HS using a multidisciplinary approach (e.g., emergency medicine, infectious disease, general surgery, plastic surgery, wound care, urology, obstetrics and gynecology, and mental health specialists). However, this may also be a reflection of the different resources and variations in scopes of practice for specialties in different countries. Additionally, complementary and alternative medicine-based modalities are not routinely mentioned in guideline recommendations despite widespread use among HS patients.[43] Future guidelines should also aim to include recommendations on appropriate early screening and management for HS in the pediatric population so that we can shift the paradigm for HS management from disease control to disease prevention.[44]

Practical considerations in HS management include insurance coverage and patient out-of-pocket costs, as the majority of recommended therapies are not specifically approved for use in HS. It is also noteworthy that current guidelines are written by experts from developed regions (Europe, North America, Brazil), and many treatment modalities may not be available to providers and patients in less-developed countries. There is an urgent need to encourage communication with more international groups to involve providers and researchers from developing countries who face unique challenges in managing HS using limited resources. As novel treatment options and evidence supporting their use continue to emerge, guidelines will need to be regularly updated to reflect the rapidly advancing therapeutic landscape.

References

1. Ingram JR, Collier F, Brown D, et al. British association of dermatologists guidelines for the management of hidradenitis suppurativa (acne inversa) 2018. *Br J Dermatol*. 2019;180(5):1009–1017. https://doi.org/10.1111/bjd.17537.
2. Alikhan A, Sayed C, Alavi A, et al. North American clinical management guidelines for hidradenitis suppurativa: a publication from the United States and Canadian hidradenitis suppurativa foundations. Part I: Diagnosis, evaluation, and the use of complementary and procedural management. *J Am Acad Dermatol*. 2019;81(1):76–90. https://doi.org/10.1016/j.jaad.2019.02.067.
3. Alikhan A, Sayed C, Alavi A, et al. North American clinical management guidelines for hidradenitis suppurativa: a publication from the United States and Canadian Hidradenitis suppurativa foundations. Part ii: topical, intralesional, and systemic medical management. *J Am Acad Dermatol*. 2019;81:76–90. https://doi.org/10.1016/j.jaad.2019.02.068.
4. Zouboulis CC, Bechara FG, Dickinson-Blok JL, et al. Hidradenitis suppurativa/acne inversa: a practical framework for treatment optimization - systematic review and recommendations from the HS ALLIANCE working group. *J Eur Acad Dermatol Venereol*. 2019;33(1):19–31. https://doi.org/10.1111/jdv.15233.
5. Gulliver W, Landells IDR, Morgan D, Pirzada S. Hidradenitis suppurativa: a novel model of care and an integrative strategy to adopt an orphan disease. *J Cutan Med Surg*. 2018;22(1):71–77.
6. Alavi A, Lynde C, Alhusayen R, et al. Approach to the management of patients with hidradenitis suppurativa: a consensus document. *J Cutan Med Surg*. 2017;21(6):513–524.
7. Gulliver W, Zouboulis CC, Prens E, et al. Evidence-based approach to the treatment of hidradenitis suppurativa/acne inversa, based on the European guidelines for hidradenitis suppurativa. *Rev Endocr Metab Disord*. 2016;17(3):343–351.
8. Zouboulis CC, Desai N, Emtestam L, et al. European S1 guideline for the treatment of hidradenitis suppurativa/acne inversa. *J Eur Acad Dermatol Venereol*. 2015;29(4):619–644. https://doi.org/10.1111/jdv.12966.
9. Hunge RE, Laffitte E, Lauchli S, et al. Swiss Practice Recommendations for the management of hidradenitis suppurativa/acne inversa. *Dermatol*. 2017;233(2–3):113–119. https://doi.org/10.1159/000477459.
10. Magalhaes RF, Rivitti-Machado MC, Duarte GV, et al. Consensus on the treatment of hidradenitis suppurativa - Brazilian Society of Dermatology. *An Bras Dermatol*. 2019;94(2 Suppl 1):7–19. https://doi.org/10.1590/abd1806-4841.20198607.
11. Hendricks AJ, Hsiao JL, Lowes MA, Shi VY. A comparison of international management guidelines for hidradenitis suppurativa. *Dermatol*. 2021;237(1):81–96. https://doi.org/10.1159/000503605.
12. Orenstein LAV, Nguyen TV, Damiani G, et al. Medical and surgical management of hidradenitis suppurativa: a review of international treatment guidelines and implementation in general dermatology practice. *Dermatol*. 2020;1–20. https://doi.org/10.1159/000507323.
13. Collier EK, Hsiao JL, Shi VY, Naik HB. Comprehensive approach to managing hidradenitis suppurativa patients. *Int J Dermatol*. 2020;59(6):744–747. https://doi.org/10.1111/ijd.14870.
14. Boyd AS. Ichthammol revisited. *Int J Dermatol*. 2010;49(7):757–760. https://doi.org/10.1111/j.1365-4632.2010.04551.x.
15. Ring HC, Bay L, Nilsson M, et al. Bacterial biofilm in chronic lesions of hidradenitis suppurativa. *Br J Dermatol*. 2017;176(4):993–1000. https://doi.org/10.1111/bjd.15007.
16. van der Zee HH, de Ruiter L, van den Broecke DG, et al. Elevated levels of tumour necrosis factor (TNF)-alpha, interleukin (IL)-1beta and IL-10 in hidradenitis suppurativa skin: a rationale for targeting TNF-alpha and IL-1beta. *Br J Dermatol*. 2011;164(6):1292–1298.
17. Witte-Handel E, Wolk K, Tsaousi A, et al. The IL-1 pathway is hyperactive in hidradenitis suppurativa and contributes to skin infiltration and destruction. *J Invest Dermatol*. 2019;139(6):1294–1305.
18. Thomi R, Cazzaniga S, Seyed Jafari SM, et al. Association of hidradenitis suppurativa With T helper 1/T helper 17 phenotypes: a semantic map analysis. *JAMA Dermatol*. 2018;154(5):592–595.
19. Matusiak L, Szczech J, Bienick A, et al. Increased interleukin (IL)-17 serum levels in patients with hidradenitis suppurativa: Implications for treatment with anti-IL-17 agents. *J Am Acad Dermatol*. 2017;76(4):670–675.
20. Kimball AB, Kerdel F, Adams D, et al. Adalimumab for the treatment of moderate to severe Hidradenitis suppurativa: a parallel randomized trial. *Ann Intern Med*. 2012;157(12):846–855.
21. Kimball AB, Okun MM, Williams DA, et al. Two Phase 3 Trials of Adalimumab for Hidradenitis Suppurativa. *N Engl J Med*. 2016;375(5):422–434.
22. Miller I, Lynggaard CD, Lophaven S, Zachariae C, et al. A double-blind placebo-controlled randomized trial of adalimumab in the treatment of hidradenitis suppurativa. *Br J Dermatol*. 2011;165(2):391–398.
23. Grant A, Gonzalez T, Montgomery MO, et al. Infliximab therapy for patients with moderate to severe hidradenitis suppurativa: a randomized, double-blind, placebo-controlled crossover trial. *J Am Acad Dermatol*, 62(2):205–217.
24. Adams DR, Yankura JA, Fogelberg AC, Anderson BE. Treatment of hidradenitis suppurativa with etanercept injection. *Arch Dermatol*. 2010;146(5):501–504.
25. Vossen AR, van Straalen KR, Prens EP, van der Zee HH. Menses and pregnancy affect symptoms in hidradenitis suppurativa: A cross-sectional study. *J Am Acad Dermatol*. 2017;76(1):155–156.
26. Riis PT, Ring HC, Themstrup L, Jemec GB. The role of androgens and estrogens in hidradenitis suppurativa - a systematic review. *Acta Dermatovenerol Croat*. 2016;24(4):239–249.
27. Jennings L, Hambly R, Hughes R, et al. Metformin use in hidradenitis suppurativa. *J Dermatolog Treat*. 2020;31(3):261–263. https://doi.org/10.1080/09546634.2019.1592100.
28. Clayton RW, Gobel K, Niessen CM, et al. Homeostasis of the sebaceous gland and mechanisms of acne pathogenesis. *Br J Dermatol*. 2019;181:677–690.
29. Mortimer PS, Dawber RP, Gales MA, Moore RA. A double-blind controlled cross-over trial of cyproterone acetate in females with hidradenitis suppurativa. *Br J Dermatol*. 1986;115(3):263–268. Accessed from https://onlinelibrary.wiley.com/doi/abs/10.1111/j.1365-2133.1986.tb05740.x?sid=nlm%3Apubmed.
30. Riis PT, Boer J, Prens EP, et al. Intralesional triamcinolone for flares of hidradenitis suppurativa (HS): A case series. *J Am Acad Dermatol*. 2016;75(6):1151–1155.
31. Suárez Valladares MJ, Eiris Salvado N, Rodríguez Prieto MA. Treatment of hidradenitis suppurativa with intralesional photodynamic therapy with 5-aminolevulinic acid and 630 nm laser beam. *J Dermatol Sci*. 2017;85(3):241–246. https://doi.org/10.1016/j.jdermsci.2016.12.014.
32. Gold M, Bridges TM, Bradshaw VL, Boring M. ALA-PDT and blue light therapy for hidradenitis suppurativa. *J Drugs Dermatol*. 2004;3(1 Suppl):S32–S35.
33. Saraceno R, Teoli M, Casciello C, Chimenti S. Methyl aminolaevulinate photodynamic therapy for the treatment of hidradenitis suppurativa and pilonidal cysts. *Photodermatol Photoimmunol Photomed*. 2009;25(3):164–165. https://doi.org/10.1111/j.1600-0781.2009.00428.x.
34. Schweiger ES, Riddle CC, Aires DJ. Treatment of hidradenitis suppurativa by photodynamic therapy with aminolevulinic acid: preliminary results. *J Drugs Dermatol*. 2011;10(4):381–386.
35. Strauss RM, Pollock B, Stables GI, et al. Photodynamic therapy using aminolaevulinic acid does not lead to clinical improvement in hidradenitis suppurativa. *Br J Dermatol*. 2005;152(4):803–804. https://doi.org/10.1111/j.1365-2133.2005.06475.x.
36. Rose RF, Stables GI. Topical photodynamic therapy in the treatment of hidradenitis suppurativa. *Photodiagnosis Photodyn Ther*. 2008;5(3):171–175. https://doi.org/10.1016/j.pdpdt.2008.07.002.

37. Highton L, Chan WY, Khwaja N, Laitung JK. Treatment of hidradenitis suppurativa with intense pulsed light: a prospective study. *Plast Reconstr Surg.* 2011;128(2):459–465. https://doi.org/10.1097/PRS.0b013e31821e6fb5.

38. Naouri M, Maruani A, Lagrange S, et al. Treatment of hidradenitis suppurativa using long-pulsed hair removal Nd:Yag laser. A multicentric prospective randomized intra-individual comparative trial. *J Am Acad Dermatol.* 2021;84:203–205.

39. Mahmoud BH, Tierney E, Hexsel CL, et al. Prospective controlled clinical and histopathologic study of hidradenitis suppurativa treated with the long-pulsed neodymium:yttrium-aluminium-garnet laser. *J Am Acad Dermatol.* 2010;62(4):637–645. https://doi.org/10.1016/j.jaad.2009.07.048.

40. Tierney E, Mahmoud BH, Hexsel C, et al. Randomized control trial for the treatment of hidradenitis suppurativa with a neodymium-doped yttrium aluminium garnet laser. *Dermatol Surg.* 2009;35(8): 1188–1198. https://doi.org/10.1111/j.1524-4725.2009.01214.x.

41. Danby FW, Hazen PG, Boer J. New and traditional surgical approaches to hidradenitis suppurativa. *J Am Acad Dermatol.* 2015;73(5 Suppl 1):S62–S65. https://doi.org/10.1016/j.jaad.2015.07.043.

42. van der Zee HH, Prens EP, Boer J. Deroofing: a tissue-saving surgical technique for the treatment of mild to moderate hidradenitis suppurativa lesions. *J Am Acad Dermatol.* 2010;63(3):475–480. https://doi.org/10.1016/j.jaad.2009.12.018.

43. Price KN, Thompson AM, Rizvi O, et al. Complementary and alternative medicine use in patients with hidradenitis suppurativa. *JAMA Dermatol.* 2020;156:345–348. https://doi.org/10.1001/jamadermatol.2019.4595.

44. Paek SY, Hamzavi I, Danby FW, Qureshi AA. Disease modification for hidradenitis suppurativa: A new paradigm. *J Am Acad Dermatol.* 2017;76(4):772–773. https://doi.org/10.1016/j.jaad.2016.12.015.

15

Topical Therapeutics

CONNOR R. BUECHLER AND STEVEN D. DAVELUY

Introduction

Topical therapy is a mainstay of dermatological treatment and holds many advantages, including ease of use, relative lack of systemic side effects, and patient-directed application. In hidradenitis suppurativa (HS), topical therapeutics are often used for early-stage lesions or as a complement to systemic or surgical treatments. The four categories of disease-modifying topical therapy for HS are antibiotics, antiseptics, keratolytics, and bathing additives (each of which will be discussed in this chapter), while symptom-control therapies such as topical analgesia and antipruritics are reviewed in Chapter 19. Some complementary and alternative therapies are also thought to be helpful when applied topically, and these will be briefly reviewed as well.

Unfortunately, the level of evidence supporting the use of most topical therapies in HS is low (Table 15.1). This chapter will provide an overview of dosing schedules, drug mechanisms of action (Fig. 15.1), and contraindications of topical therapeutics for HS to better inform these decisions.

Antibiotics

The occlusion of the folliculopilosebaceous unit that heralds the onset of HS is followed by bacterial growth, inducing inflammation that leads to abscesses, sinus tracts, and destruction of adnexal structures. Given that bacteria are thought to contribute to the development and perpetuation of these lesions, it is no surprise that antibiotic therapy can be a useful approach to treatment. Topical antibiotics are postulated to work by two complementary methods in the treatment of HS: the reduction of bacterial burden and the prevention of inflammation.[1] Their antibacterial effects decrease bacterial colonization, which then tempers the local inflammation associated with the body's response to the resident bacteria. A number of topical antibiotics also have antiinflammatory effects independent of their antibacterial properties, and many are also delivered in vehicles that themselves may soothe inflamed skin via emollient, cooling, hydrating, or barrier-forming properties.[2] In this section, various topical antibiotics that have been used in the treatment of HS will be discussed.

Clindamycin

Clindamycin is a broad-spectrum antibiotic of the lincosamide class that interferes with the synthesis of bacterial proteins by binding to the 50S ribosomal subunit, providing a bacteriostatic effect with concentration-dependent bactericidal activity against staphylococci, streptococci, and some anaerobes.[3] It also boasts independent immunomodulatory effects. Though the mechanism of these additional properties is poorly understood, studies have postulated that clindamycin may inhibit complement-derived chemotaxis of polymorphonuclear leukocytes,[4–6] potentiate the uptake of microorganisms by phagocytic cells of the innate immune system,[7] and inhibit biofilm formation,[8] thus assisting in the clearance of bacteria without drawing in additional inflammatory milieu. Given its localized effect, topical clindamycin is most effective for limited disease in the absence of deep abscesses and sinus tracts. Treatment has been shown to reduce pustules but has limited effect on abscesses and nodules.[9,10] However, it can be used as an adjunct in more severe stages of HS along with the addition of systemic medications and surgical intervention.

Clindamycin is the only topical antibiotic treatment for HS to have been validated in randomized controlled trials.[9,10] In these trials, topical clindamycin treatment was responsible for a significant reduction in the number of abscesses, inflammatory nodules, and pustules compared to the placebo, with effects equivalent to systemic tetracycline. Interestingly, the efficacy of clindamycin in

TABLE 15.1 Topical Therapeutics for Hidradenitis Suppurativa

			TOPICAL ANTIBIOTICS			
Therapy Name	Mechanism of Action	Dosing	Contraindications	Adverse Effects	Level of Evidence[a]	Notes on Use
Clindamycin	Inhibit bacterial ribosome, inhibit PMN chemotaxis, inhibit biofilm formation, potentiate phagocytosis of bacteria	BID Limit monotherapy to 3 months	Hypersensitivity to clindamycin or lincomycin derivatives, history of regional enteritis or ulcerative colitis, history of antibiotic-associated colitis	Pruritis, xeroderma, erythema, burning, exfoliation, oily skin, bacterial resistance	B	Strongly consider in all mild HS patients and as adjunct therapy in moderate to severe cases. Safe for pregnant patients.
Fusidic Acid	Bind to elongation factor-G on bacterial ribosome inhibiting translation, suppress cytokine signaling	TID	Hypersensitivity to therapeutic vehicle or FA itself	Mild irritant or allergic contact dermatitis, bacterial resistance	B	Consider for Hurley stage 1 and early lesions. Avoid prolonged monotherapy as bacterial resistance is common.
Dapsone	Halt bacterial folate metabolism, reduce oxidative damage to tissue	BID	Hypersensitivity to therapeutic vehicle or dapsone itself	Methemoglobinemia, mild irritant or allergic contact dermatitis, bacterial resistance	D	Consider for Hurley I and early lesions or as adjunct therapy in later stages for patients who cannot use topical clindamycin.
Gentamicin	Inhibit bacterial ribosome	TID following surgery	Hypersensitivity to therapeutic vehicle or gentamicin itself	Mild irritant or allergic contact dermatitis, bacterial resistance	E	Use after de-roofing or local excision procedures. Consider for a secondarily infected HS lesion that grows gram negative species.
Topical Keratolytics						
Resorcinol	Cytotoxic, modulate cytokine/chemokine release	BID with increasing concentration to therapeutic level (typically 15%–20%)	Concomitant use of intense pulsed light therapy, hypersensitivity to therapeutic vehicle or resorcinol itself	Desquamation, depigmentation, mild irritation, or allergic contact dermatitis	B	Use for acute lesions and to maintain quiescence. Check baseline pregnancy test. Not for use in women actively trying to get pregnant.
Azelaic Acid	Modulate keratinocyte proliferation	BID	Hypersensitivity to therapeutic vehicle or azelaic acid itself	Photosensitivity, desquamation, depigmentation, mild irritant or allergic contact dermatitis	E	Consider in children given low risk profile.
Bathing Additives and Complementary Therapies						
Bleach baths	Creation of superoxide radicals, modulate NF-κB signaling	2–3 times weekly	None	Caustic effects, bleaching of hair and fabrics	E	Consider in combination with other topical therapies for mild disease.
Magnesium Sulfate	Unknown	PRN	None known	Unknown	E	Not enough evidence to make a definitive conclusion.
CBD oil	Decrease pain perception, inhibit keratinocyte proliferation while regulating cellular differentiation and	PRN	None known	Unknown	E	Not enough evidence to make a definitive conclusion.

TABLE 15.1	Topical Therapeutics for Hidradenitis Suppurativa—cont'd						
			TOPICAL ANTIBIOTICS				
Therapy Name	Mechanism of Action	Dosing	Contraindications	Adverse Effects	Level of Evidence	Notes on Use	
	promoting apoptosis of both keratinocytes and sebocytes						
Turmeric	Disrupt bacterial membranes, inhibit bacterial replication, disrupt microbial biofilms	PRN	None known	Unknown	E	Not enough evidence to make a definitive conclusion.	

BID, Two times per day; *CBD*, cannabidiol; *NF-kB*, nuclear factor kappa B; *PMN*, polymorphonuclear leukocyte; *PRN*, as needed; *TID*, three times per day.

[a]Lebwohl's Levels of Evidence:

Grade A: Double-blind study. At least one prospective randomized, double-blind, controlled trial without major design flaws (in the author's view).

Grade B: Clinical trial ≥ 20 subjects. Prospective clinical trials with 20 or more subjects; trials lacking adequate controls or another key facet of design that would normally be considered desirable (in the author's opinion).

Grade C: Clinical trial < 20 subjects. Small trials with fewer than 20 subjects with significant design limitations, very large numbers of case reports (at least 20 cases in the literature), or retrospective analyses of data.

Grade D: Series ≥ 5 subjects. Series of patients reported to respond (at least five cases in the literature).

Grade E: Anecdotal case reports. Individual case reports amounting to published experience of fewer than five cases.

one trial was independent of the presence of bacteria at the onset of treatment, as measured by culture of aseptic aspirate from inflamed HS lesions,[10,11] indicating that the antiinflammatory properties of the drug may have played a major role.

Though HS treatment guidelines recommend various formulations of topical clindamycin such as solution,[12–14] gel,[15] or lotion,[16,17] the original studies demonstrating efficacy were performed using clindamycin 1% solution.[9,10] Availability, price, and patient preference are all considerations when choosing the most appropriate vehicle. Most consensus clinical guidelines[13,16–18] recommend twice-daily application of topical clindamycin to areas affected by HS. However, use as monotherapy should not exceed 3 months, as studies have shown the emergence of resistant *Staphylococcus aureus* in the lesions of patients treated for prolonged periods.[10] The addition of benzoyl peroxide (BPO) can mitigate the development of bacterial resistance and allow prolonged use.[19]

Contraindications to the use of topical clindamycin either alone or in combination with other therapies are rare and limited to those with a history of hypersensitivity to preparations containing clindamycin or lincomycin derivatives, a history of regional enteritis or ulcerative colitis, or a history of antibiotic-associated colitis.[20] Cutaneous adverse effects experienced by some patients include pruritis, xeroderma, erythema, burning, exfoliation, or oily skin.

Fusidic Acid

Fusidic acid (FA) inhibits the activity of the bacterial ribosome. FA binds to elongation factor G on the ribosome, preventing translocation of the bacterial ribosome.[21,22] FA is most active against gram-positive bacteria, particularly *Staphylococcus* species (which are one of the most commonly found bacteria in HS wound cultures),[23,24] and likely responsible for a significant amount of subsequent inflammation. Although biochemically comparable to many steroids, FA does not possess any steroid activity. There is excellent penetration of FA into deeper layers of the skin due to

its lipophilic steroid-like structure and independent antiinflammatory activity due to suppression of cytokine signaling.[25]

Evidence for FA utility in HS patients is limited to case reports and a single prospective cohort study.[26] In this study involving 627 patients with Hurley stage 1 axillary HS, FA 2% ointment was applied thrice daily after washing with antibacterial soap.[26] All patients had complete healing within 4 weeks of treatment. These data have, to our knowledge, not yet been replicated elsewhere.

FA for treatment of HS is typically formulated as a 2% sodium fusidate ointment or cream. Other formulations of FA are available and used for dermatologic conditions, such as combination formulations of FA with 1% hydrocortisone or 0.1% betamethasone, which can be used to treat eczema complicated by staphylococcal infection.[22] While each of these formulations is available to those suffering from HS, further study of the relative efficacy of combined versus FA-only topicals is needed before a particular formulation can be recommended. There are significant concerns about the development of resistant bacteria with FA monotherapy, given that a single point mutation is enough to confer significant resistance[21,22,27] and contribute to outbreaks of multi-drug-resistant bacteria. Prolonged monotherapy with FA is therefore generally avoided. Adverse events during treatment are uncommon and generally limited to reactions to components of the vehicle, which can lead to mild allergies or irritant contact dermatitis. Contraindications are limited to hypersensitivity to components of the topical therapeutic vehicle or FA itself.

Dapsone

Dapsone is an antibiotic with significant independent antiinflammatory activity commonly used for the treatment of a variety of dermatological conditions. The antibiotic activity of dapsone is mediated through the inhibition of dihydropteroate synthesis, halting folate metabolism and resulting in the stasis of bacterial growth. Its antiinflammatory activity is accomplished through inhibition of

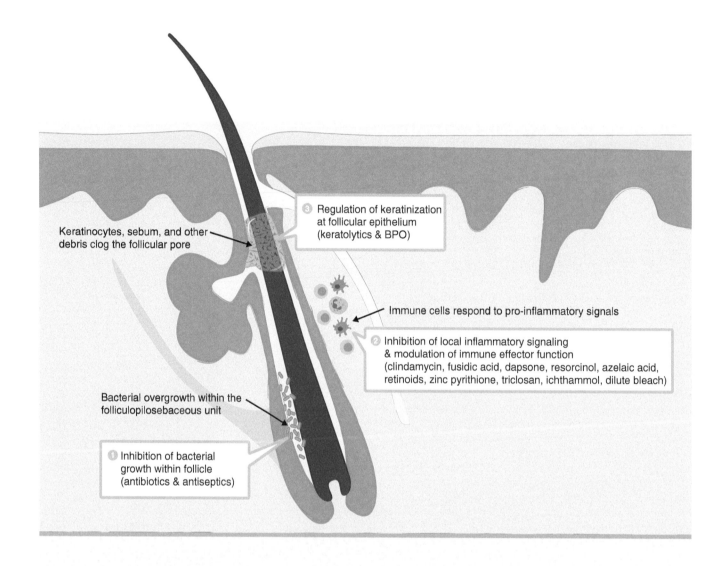

Keratinocytes, sebum, and other debris clog the follicular pore

❸ Regulation of keratinization at follicular epithelium (keratolytics & BPO)

Immune cells respond to pro-inflammatory signals

❷ Inhibition of local inflammatory signaling & modulation of immune effector function (clindamycin, fusidic acid, dapsone, resorcinol, azelaic acid, retinoids, zinc pyrithione, triclosan, ichthammol, dilute bleach)

Bacterial overgrowth within the folliculopilosebaceous unit

❶ Inhibition of bacterial growth within follicle (antibiotics & antiseptics)

• **Fig. 15.1** Mechanisms of Action of Topical Medications Used to Treat Hidradenitis Suppurativa. Key therapies are listed alongside their mechanism. Topical complementary and alternative therapies are not shown. *BPO*, benzoyl peroxide.

myeloperoxidase, an enzyme vital for oxidative destruction of microbes by neutrophils that often causes simultaneous damage to local tissues.[28] Dapsone has also been postulated to inhibit neutrophil chemotaxis,[29] a function that may serve to lessen inflammation in HS abscesses and sinus tracts. Limited evidence based on expert opinion suggests topical dapsone may be useful in early disease.[30]

Commercially available topical dapsone for use in dermatological conditions is currently limited to gel form, with 5% and 7.5% formulations available. Initial dosing begins at twice-daily application, which is the recommended frequency for treatment of acne vulgaris.[31] While concerns of antibiotic resistance would theoretically also apply to the use of topical dapsone, the literature currently suggests that monotherapy over periods up to 12 weeks does not lead to bacterial resistance.[32] However, further study must be undertaken over longer periods to establish the safety of long-term dapsone monotherapy for conditions such as HS, which often requires more than 12 weeks of therapy.

While dapsone is structurally similar to sulfonamide drugs, allergy to sulfonamides is not a contraindication to its use. Although various dermatological side-effects of oral dapsone have been described, including severe reactions (such as toxic epidermal necrolysis), these effects have not been seen with topical dapsone.[33] Unlike with the use of systemic dapsone, a glucose-6-phosphate dehydrogenase (G6PD) level does not need to be checked before commencing treatment with topical dapsone[34] as there is no evidence of clinically relevant hemolysis or anemia after topical administration.[33] Dapsone may also induce methemoglobinemia in the presence of other pharmaceuticals with similar propensities (such as local anesthetics), and this is true of both oral and topical dapsone.[33]

Gentamicin

Gentamicin is an aminoglycoside antibiotic that inhibits the production of bacterial proteins by binding to ribosomal subunits, preventing the translation of messenger ribonucleic acid. Its broad spectrum of action makes it an attractive candidate for use in treating infected wounds. Thus far, study of topical gentamicin in HS has been limited to postoperative application as a strategy to reduce the rate of post-operative infection.[35] While short-term complications, including dehiscence and infection, were mitigated by topical gentamicin use, the rate of recurrence of HS lesions was unaffected in the long term.

Gentamicin is available commercially as gentamicin sulfate 0.1% cream and ointment. Given the paucity of data and the lack of published success in treating HS lesions, guidelines tend to recommend that topical gentamicin be used only if other topical antibiotics are not available or cannot be used.[15] Generally, topical gentamicin can be applied 3 to 4 times daily for treatment of superficial skin and soft tissue infections.

Contraindications are limited to hypersensitivity to product components, and adverse effects include skin irritation and the potential emergence of superinfection with atypical, resistant organisms.[36–38] Given the varied bacterial milieu within HS wounds and the importance of bacterial control for mitigation of HS symptoms, such emergence should not be taken lightly.

Antiseptics

As opposed to the more narrowly targeted effects of antibiotic compounds, antiseptic washes are not absorbed into the body and have a broad spectrum of antimicrobial activity that relies on a variety of mechanisms to slow or stop microbial growth, resulting in reduced selective pressure and rare development of resistance.[39] Antiseptic washes provide an additional method of minimizing bacterial colonization and reducing concomitant inflammation for HS patients, and are even more frequently utilized in some practices than topical antibiotics (though they are often used in tandem.)[12] Given that lesions of HS are often polymicrobial on culture, antiseptic washes are theorized to be of similar utility to antibiotics without the risk of bacterial resistance or insufficient breadth of coverage that can accompany antibiotic use. However, such intervention comes with risk of both allergic and irritant contact dermatitis. There are few studies evaluating their effectiveness in preventing and treating HS flares. Patient adherence to using antiseptic washes has been reported to be low, with only 70% of patients using the recommended wash at all, and only 30% of those patients using it daily. Reported barriers to use included difficulty finding and affording the recommended wash with little perceived benefit.[40] In this section, antiseptic washes commonly prescribed as treatment for early-stage HS will be discussed.

Chlorhexidine

Chlorhexidine is a cationic biguanide surfactant compound that destabilizes bacterial cell walls and membranes with residual activity lasting several hours after initial application.[41] Commonly used as a disinfectant scrub prior to surgery or a mouthwash for gingivitis, it is also used topically by those with HS for this broad-spectrum antibacterial effect. Current evidence for utility of topical chlorhexidine is limited only to expert opinion.

Unfortunately, chlorhexidine has difficulty overcoming the biofilms that characterize many HS lesions,[42–44] and is thus thought to be less able to affect the inflammation caused by secondary bacterial colonization. Patients should be counseled that chlorhexidine's activity can be diminished through the concomitant use of incompatible products that include anionic surfactants

commonly found in laundry detergents, handwashes, bodywashes, and household cleaners.[45] Use of chlorhexidine on open wounds weeping purulent discharge, serum, or blood is also ineffective, as presence of excess phospholipids similarly blunts its antimicrobial activity.[45] Chlorhexidine is available over the counter, and side effects include irritation and, more rarely, allergic contact dermatitis.[46]

Benzoyl Peroxide

Use of benzoyl peroxide (BPO) as a topical treatment for HS is based on its use for the same theoretical reason—decreased bacterial colonization—in other dermatological conditions such as acne vulgaris. The compound destroys bacteria by creating free radicals that disrupt bacterial proteins via oxidation[47] and also exhibits a mild sebostatic and keratolytic effect[48] postulated to be beneficial in treatment of HS. In one randomized trial, BPO was used along with topical clindamycin in both arms of therapy as the standard of care; laser therapy was added in the treatment arm.[49] Both arms of this study showed improvement in HS from baseline.

BPO washes are available over the counter in formulations between 2.5% and 10%. Patients may continue their regular bathing schedule while simply replacing other soaps or cleansers with a BPO-containing wash. Given its keratolytic effects, BPO-based washes can lead to irritation and desquamation in addition to rare allergic hypersensitivity reactions. Patients should also be counseled to rinse thoroughly before initiating contact with hair or fabrics, as the reactive oxygen species created by BPO have been known to have a bleaching effect.

Zinc Pyrithione

Although best known as a topical antifungal agent for treatment of seborrheic dermatitis, zinc pyrithione has antiinflammatory and antiproliferative properties that also make it a theoretically effective choice as a topical antiseptic for HS. As a positively charged ion coordination complex, it derives its antimicrobial properties through cell membrane depolarization and inhibition of substrate transport and ATP synthesis.[50,51] Its antiinflammatory and antiproliferative effects are due to modulation of dendritic cell activity and an accompanying reduction of inflammatory signaling.[52] Expert opinion suggests zinc pyrithione may be non-inferior to chlorhexidine wash for HS[53]; however, there are currently no studies examining its therapeutic efficacy. Studies have indicated that the antimicrobial effects of zinc pyrithione outlast those of chlorhexidine,[54] making it a theoretically better choice for those who desire long-lasting antiseptic effect from a single wash. There are no absolute contraindications for zinc pyrithione use; patients should be cautioned to watch for allergic or irritant contact dermatitis.

Zinc pyrithione is available for patients as a 0.25% spray and a wash up to 2% concentration. These formulations are easily applied to the hair-bearing areas typically affected by HS. In addition, these products are usually less expensive than other medicated washes such as chlorhexidine and are available without a prescription.

Triclosan

Triclosan is a halogenated bisphenol compound that acts via disruption of the bacterial cell wall and fatty acid synthesis.[55,56] It is also active against biofilms,[57] an important consideration in the treatment of HS, and has demonstrated notable antiinflammatory effects in ex vivo studies via the suppression of both acute and chronic mediators of inflammation.[58] While it is recommended by several expert-developed guidelines,[59] well-controlled studies are lacking at this time to support specific usage directions.

Of note, there is significant controversy regarding the safety and effectiveness of triclosan as an antiseptic. Due to concern regarding its role in bacterial resistance,[60] potential endocrine toxicity,[61,62] evidence of accumulation of triclosan in wastewater,[63] and questionable efficacy as compared to other antimicrobial options,[64] the United States Food and Drug Administration banned its inclusion in antiseptic washes in 2016.[65] However, the product continues to be available outside of the United States, and many non-US dermatologists continue to recommend its use in the treatment of HS.[14,59]

Ammonium Bituminosulfate (Ichthammol)

Ammonium bituminosulfate, also known as ichthammol, is a topical medication that has been used to treat a variety of cutaneous conditions. It is thought to have both antiinflammatory and antimicrobial properties[66] through the inhibition of inflammatory cell-to-cell signaling, modulation of superoxide production, and mild inhibition of bacterial growth.[67–69] It is recommended by multiple expert guidelines for treatment of HS[59]; however, no studies have been done to date that prove efficacy in prevention or treatment of HS-related inflammation or lesions.

Ichthammol is available over the counter in multiple forms but is most commonly used for HS as a 20% ointment. Though this compound is available worldwide, ichthammol is more commonly recommended by European clinicians than their US counterparts.[59] There are no absolute contraindications to the use of ichthammol, and adverse effects are limited to skin irritation,[70] though the sulfur-like odor of topical preparations may prove bothersome to many patients. Patients should be advised of the potential for staining of fabrics, skin, and hair with certain preparations.

Keratolytics

As HS is theorized to begin with follicular occlusion due to hyperkeratosis, preventing this initial event is another promising therapeutic target in the treatment of HS lesions. Keratolytics, which lead to separation and desquamation of the cornified epithelium, help to unblock occluded follicles and prevent future occlusion. In this section, the mechanism of action, level of supportive evidence, dosing schedule, contraindications, adverse effects, and available formulations will be discussed for keratolytics used in the treatment of HS.

Resorcinol

Resorcinol is a benzenediol chemical with keratolytic properties mediated through cytotoxicity and cytokine modulation,[71] as well as antipruritic and antimycotic properties.[72] It has been shown to decrease both pain and duration of HS abscesses with adequate treatment,[73] with over 80% clinical resolution of lesions in a 1-month-long trial.[74] However, there have to date been no controlled trials of resorcinol treatment, with current data limited to case-reports and open-label studies. It is also important to note that studies have been limited to lesions that do not have scarring or fistulas, as pilot data[23] showed that such lesions were not amenable to resorcinol treatment.

Dosing of resorcinol is carefully titrated to reach a therapeutic concentration where adverse effects are still tolerable. Generally, a 10% cream is applied twice daily for the first week, with concentration then increased by 5% each week until lesions and pain begin to resolve, at which point the concentration is kept constant.[23] The final prescription is usually for at least a 15% cream as keratolysis is minimal below this concentration, though creams up to 30% concentration have also been used for other dermatologic indications.[75] Maintenance therapy involves prophylactic application twice weekly. Resorcinol is not available in the United States except via specialty compounding pharmacies, which can significantly increase the price and be an inconvenience for both patient and physician.

There is risk of contact dermatitis with use of resorcinol, as well as brownish hyperpigmentation of the skin.[72,74] Resorcinol is not recommended for concurrent use with intense pulsed light (IPL) for HS due to the combined irritative effect.[76] Resorcinol will also cause desquamation in most patients, and moisturizers may be used to mitigate this side effect. Of note, resorcinol also has potential to interfere with thyroid hormone synthesis at elevated concentrations in the bloodstream, and thus should be avoided in open wounds of pregnant patients in the absence of sufficient safety data.[77,78]

Azelaic Acid

Azelaic acid is commonly used in the treatment of acne and has been postulated to have a theoretical benefit for patients with HS. Its major mechanism of action is the modulation of keratinocyte proliferation,[79] though it has been shown to dampen inflammatory cytokine signaling[80] and exhibit antifungal and bacteriostatic properties.[81] No formal studies are available to demonstrate its benefit in HS, so it is generally not used for this indication. There is limited expert opinion that discusses use of azelaic acid cream in pediatric HS.[82]

Formulations of azelaic acid consist of gels, creams, and foams with up to 20% concentration. For acne and acne rosacea, dosing schedule is up to twice daily; however, optimal dosing schedule has not been independently investigated in HS. Patients should be cautioned about the drying effect of azelaic acid preparations, as well as the potential for photosensitivity, irritant or allergic contact dermatitis, and changes of skin color in darker-skinned individuals. There are no absolute contraindications to the use of azelaic acid.

Retinoids

Retinoids, such as tretinoin and adapalene, are structurally related to vitamin A and promote keratinocyte maturation via transcription factor modulation.[83] They also have antiinflammatory properties via alterations to multiple pathways in the inflammatory response, from reactive oxygen species release to cytokine signaling.[84,85] While these properties would carry a theoretical benefit for the treatment of HS, this has not been true in clinical practice, and current expert opinion is that topical retinoids are not recommended in the treatment of HS.[86]

Bathing Additives

While bathing additives can provide an antimicrobial strategy similar to the antiseptic washes previously discussed, emerging evidence suggests that some bathing additives are associated with antiinflammatory, reparative, or antioxidative properties,[87] which could provide additional benefit in the treatment of HS. Current expert opinion on bathing additives in HS is limited to that of bleach (sodium hypochlorite) baths. Though magnesium sulfate (Epsom salt) baths and other soaks are popular among patients, there is a lack of scientific support or clinical evidence from similar dermatological conditions for such therapies. In this section, both bleach baths and Epsom salt baths will be discussed, with Epsom salt baths serving as the bridge to the concluding section of this chapter, "complementary and alternative therapies."

Bleach Baths

Bleach (sodium hypochlorite) is best known as an antimicrobial household cleaner, for which it relies on the creation of superoxide radicals to destroy bacteria, spores, viruses, and fungi. Previous studies have found that dilute (0.005%) bleach baths create a bacteriostatic effect in as little as 5 minutes,[56] and the superoxide radicals exhibit a concentration-dependent ability to penetrate and dissipate biofilms created by bacteria.[88] However, it is important to note that recent evidence suggests dilute bleach baths have no direct antimicrobial ability,[89] thus any benefits may not be due to the previously presumed antiseptic properties. Bleach also exhibits antiinflammatory properties[90] that have made it an important part of dermatological therapy in recent years, particularly as treatment for acute flares of atopic dermatitis.[91] This antiinflammatory effect is postulated to be due to the modulation of nuclear factor kappa B transcription factor, signaling and resulting in decrease of inflammatory cytokine levels.[92] While there have, as yet, been no studies of the efficacy of bleach baths for HS, their use is recommended by several treatment guidelines developed by expert committees.[78,93,94]

Bleach baths are typically kept to 0.005% bleach (0.5 cup of household bleach per standard 40 gallon [150 L] bathtub) for optimal benefit while avoiding caustic damage to the skin. More concentrated preparations have been known to cause urticaria and irritant contact dermatitis. There are no clinical studies demonstrating the effect of varying frequency of bleach baths for treatment of HS, but 2 to 3 times weekly at 0.005% concentration is thought to produce benefit.[93] Patients should be cautioned regarding the caustic effects of concentrated bleach on the skin, as well as the potential for bleaching of hair and fabrics. Although pigmentation changes may occur with more concentrated preparations, skin pigmentation should not occur at the recommended 0.005% concentration.

Magnesium Sulfate Baths

Magnesium sulfate baths, colloquially known as "Epsom salt soaks," have long been a favorite of those seeking non-pharmacological treatment for dermatological or musculoskeletal complaints, with claims of healing illnesses, reducing bodily aches and pains, and tempering inflammation. Unfortunately, no study has been able to prove an antimicrobial, analgesic, or antiinflammatory benefit to these soaks. However, patients have anecdotally reported both in the clinic and in online forums that they find these baths soothing and perceive benefits in their daily function. While reports of toxicity secondary to hypermagnesemia from Epsom salt enemas have been published,[95–97] there are no reports of adverse effects from these baths. Given the lack of evidence of harm, patients can be advised to continue such regimens if desired, though counseling regarding proven disease-modifying interventions should also be offered.

Complementary Therapies

Many patients with chronic diseases that prove recalcitrant to conventional medication regimens explore complementary and alternative medicines (CAM), and those who suffer from HS are certainly no exception. These therapies often appear on online message boards and support groups, and it is common for HS patients to not inform their healthcare provider about their use of CAM.[98] Topical CAM that have been purported as helpful (but that lack studies in HS) include turmeric, cannabidiol (CBD) oil, menthol, aloe vera, tea tree oil, apple cider vinegar, iodine, zinc paste, and others.[98,99] CAM therapies are discussed extensively in Chapter 28; however, the most widely used topical CAM therapies will be covered in this chapter (including magnesium sulfate baths, CBD oil, and turmeric).

Cannabidiol Oil

CBD oil is thought to assist in wound healing and pain relief. In addition to its ability to decrease pain perception, in vitro studies have also shown CBD to inhibit keratinocyte proliferation while regulating cellular differentiation and promoting apoptosis of both keratinocytes and sebocytes.[100–103] Current evidence beyond patient anecdotes is lacking for its long-term safety and effectiveness in treating HS.

Turmeric

In vitro, turmeric has been shown to disrupt bacterial membranes,[104] inhibit bacterial replication,[105] and disrupt microbial biofilms.[106] It may possess antiinflammatory and antiproliferative potential via modulation of NF-κB signaling and phosphorylase kinase activity.[107,108] While it can be taken as a systemic medication, it has a long history of use as a topical therapeutic. However, studies of topical turmeric in HS are needed to determine efficacy.

Summary

Topical therapies are an important part of the clinician's treatment arsenal for HS. While their use has the potential to provide more complete relief in the case of mild or Hurley stage 1 disease, utilization as an adjunct in later stage disease can still provide benefit. Most lack large-scale or well-controlled studies, and as such the decision of the optimal topical regimen must be an open dialogue between the clinician and patient based on expert opinion, clinical experience, and the trajectory of the individual patient's disease. Owing to their relative ease of use and very low risk of side effects, most experts recommend all patients with HS use a daily antiseptic wash (most commonly BPO, chlorhexidine, or zinc pyrithione) and a topical antibiotic (most commonly clindamycin solution or lotion).

References

1. Nazary M, van der Zee HH, Prens EP, et al. Pathogenesis and pharmacotherapy of Hidradenitis suppurativa. *Eur J Pharmacol.* 2011;672(1–3):1–8.
2. Kurian A, Barankin B. Delivery vehicle advances in dermatology. *Skin Therapy Letter.* 2011;7(2):4–5.
3. Nastro LJ, Finegold SM. Bactericidal activity of five antimicrobial agents against *Bacteroides fragilis. J Infect Dis.* 1972;126(1):104–107.
4. Pasquale TR, Tan JS. Nonantimicrobial effects of antibacterial agents. *Clin Infect Dis.* 2005;40(1):127–135.

5. Stevens DL, Maier KA, Mitten JE. Effect of antibiotics on toxin production and viability of *Clostridium perfringens*. *Antimicrob Agents Chemother*. 1987;31(2):213–218.

6. Ras GJ, Anderson R, Taylor GW, et al. Clindamycin, erythromycin, and roxithromycin inhibit the proinflammatory interactions of *Pseudomonas aeruginosa* pigments with human neutrophils in vitro. *Antimicrob Agents Chemother*. 1992;36(6):1236–1240.

7. Gemmell CG, Peterson PK, Schmeling D, et al. Potentiation of opsonization and phagocytosis of *Streptococcus pyogenes* following growth in the presence of clindamycin. *J Clin Invest*. 1981;67(5):1249–1256.

8. Ardon CB, Prens EP, Fuursted K, et al. Biofilm production and antibiotic susceptibility of Staphylococcus epidermidis strains from Hidradenitis Suppurativa lesions. *J Eur Acad Dermatol Venereol*. 2019;33(1):170–177.

9. Clemmensen OJ. Topical treatment of hidradenitis suppurativa with clindamycin. *Int J Dermatol*. 1983;22(5):325–328.

10. Jemec GB, Wendelboe P. Topical clindamycin versus systemic tetracycline in the treatment of hidradenitis suppurativa. *J Am Acad Dermatol*. 1998;39(6):971–974.

11. Jemec GB, Faber M, Gutschik E, Wendelboe P. The bacteriology of hidradenitis suppurativa. *Dermatology*. 1996;193(3):203–206.

12. Ingram JR, McPhee M. Management of hidradenitis suppurativa: a U.K. survey of current practice. *Br J Dermatol*. 2015;173(4):1070–1072.

13. Alikhan A, Sayed C, Alavi A, et al. North American clinical management guidelines for hidradenitis suppurativa: A publication from the United States and Canadian Hidradenitis Suppurativa Foundations: Part II: topical, intralesional, and systemic medical management. *J Am Acad Dermatol*. 2019;81(1):91–101.

14. Hunger RE, Laffitte E, Lauchli S, et al. Swiss practice recommendations for the management of Hidradenitis Suppurativa/acne inversa. *Dermatol*. 2017;233(2–3):113–119.

15. Magalhaes RF, Rivitti-Machado MC, Duarte GV, et al. Consensus on the treatment of hidradenitis suppurativa–Brazilian Society of Dermatology. *An Bras Dermatol*. 2019;94(2 Suppl 1):7–19.

16. Gulliver W, Zouboulis CC, Prens E, et al. Evidence-based approach to the treatment of hidradenitis suppurativa/acne inversa, based on the European guidelines for hidradenitis suppurativa. *Rev Endocr Metab Disord*. 2016;17(3):343–351.

17. Zouboulis CC, Bechara FG, Dickinson-Blok JL, et al. Hidradenitis suppurativa/acne inversa: a practical framework for treatment optimization–systematic review and recommendations from the HS ALLIANCE working group. *J Eur Acad Dermatol Venereol*. 2019;33(1):19–31.

18. Zouboulis CC, Desai N, Emtestam L, et al. European S1 guideline for the treatment of hidradenitis suppurativa/acne inversa. *J Eur Acad Dermatol Venereol*. 2015;29(4):619–644.

19. Harkaway KS, McGinley KJ, Foglia AN, et al. Antibiotic resistance patterns in coagulase-negative staphylococci after treatment with topical erythromycin, benzoyl peroxide, and combination therapy. *Br J Dermatol*. 1992;126(6):586–590.

20. Food US, Administration Drug. *Clindamycin phosphate gel package insert*; 2001. https://www.accessdata.fda.gov/drugsatfda_docs/label/2001/50782lbl.pdf. Accessed 30 January 2020.

21. Besier S, Ludwig A, Brade V, Wichelhaus TA. Molecular analysis of fusidic acid resistance in *Staphylococcus aureus*. *Mol Microbiol*. 2003;47(2):463–469.

22. Schofer H, Simonsen L. Fusidic acid in dermatology: an updated review. *Eur J Dermatol*. 2010;20(1):6–15.

23. Sartorius K, Boer J, Jemec GB. Topical treatment. In: Jemec GBE, Revuz J, Leyden JJ, editors. *Hidradenitis Suppurativa*. Berlin, Heidelberg: Springer; 2006:150–160.

24. Ring HC, Riis Mikkelsen P, Miller IM, et al. The bacteriology of hidradenitis suppurativa: a systematic review. *Exp Dermatol*. 2015;24(10):727–731.

25. Christiansen K. Fusidic acid non-antibacterial activity. *Int J Antimicrob Agents*. 1999;12(Suppl 2):S73–S78.

26. Shirah BH, Shirah HA. Effective modified conservative tissue preserving protocol to treat stage I axillary hidradenitis suppurativa: a prospective cohort study of 627 patients with five years follow-up. *J Dermatolog Treat*. 2017;28(5):458–463.

27. Shah M, Mohanraj M. High levels of fusidic acid-resistant *Staphylococcus aureus* in dermatology patients. *Br J Dermatol*. 2003;148(5):1018–1020.

28. Kosseifi SG, Guha B, Nassour DN, et al. The Dapsone hypersensitivity syndrome revisited: a potentially fatal multisystem disorder with prominent hepatopulmonary manifestations. *J Occup Med Toxicol*. 2006;1:9.

29. Abramovits W. Dapsone in dermatology. In: Yamauchi PS, editor. *Biologic and Systemic Agents in Dermatology*. Springer: Cham; 2018:517–524.

30. Scheinfeld N. Hidradenitis suppurativa: A practical review of possible medical treatments based on over 350 hidradenitis patients. *Dermatol Online J*. 2003;19(4):1.

31. Wozel G, Blasum C. Dapsone in dermatology and beyond. *Arch Dermatol Res*. 2014;306(2):103–124.

32. Kircik LH. Use of dapsone 5% gel as maintenance treatment of acne vulgaris following completion of oral doxycycline and dapsone 5% gel combination treatment. *J Drugs Dermatol*. 2016;15(2):191–195.

33. Food US, Administration Drug. *Aczone gel package insert*; 2018. https://www.accessdata.fda.gov/drugsatfda_docs/label/2018/021794s016lbl.pdf. Accessed 30 January 2020.

34. Zaenglein AL, Pathy AL, Schlosser BJ, et al. Guidelines of care for the management of acne vulgaris. *J Am Acad Dermatol*. 2016;74(5):945–973. e933.

35. Buimer MG, Ankersmit MF, Wobbes T, Klinkenbijl JH. Surgical treatment of hidradenitis suppurativa with gentamicin sulfate: a prospective randomized study. *Dermatol Surg*. 2008;34(2):224–227.

36. Gentamicin Cream - FDA prescribing information, side effects and uses. https://www.drugs.com/pro/gentamicin-cream.html. Accessed January 30, 2020.

37. Lo MW, Mak SK, Wong YY, et al. Atypical mycobacterial exit-site infection and peritonitis in peritoneal dialysis patients on prophylactic exit-site gentamicin cream. *Perit Dial Int*. 2013;33(3):267–272. https://doi.org/10.3747/pdi.2011.00184.

38. Wyatt TD, Ferguson WP, Wilson TS, McCormick E. Gentamicin resistant *Staphylococcus aureus* associated with the use of topical gentamicin. *J Antimicrob Chemother*. 1977;3(3):213–217.

39. Leaper DJ, Schultz G, Carville K, et al. Extending the TIME concept: what have we learned in the past 10 years? *Int Wound J*. 2012;9:1–19.

40. Leiphart P, Kitts S, Sciacca Kirby J. Adherence to over-the-counter antimicrobial washes in hidradenitis suppurativa patients. *Dermatol*. 2019;235(5):440–441.

41. Kuyyakanond T, Quesnel LB. The mechanism of action of chlorhexidine. *FEMS Microbiol Lett*. 1992;100(1–3):211–215.

42. Bonez PC, Dos Santos Alves CF, Dalmolin TV, et al. Chlorhexidine activity against bacterial biofilms. *Am J Infect Control*. 2013;41(12):e119–e122.

43. Ring HC, Bay L, Nilsson M, et al. Bacterial biofilm in chronic lesions of hidradenitis suppurativa. *Br J Dermatol*. 2017;176(4):993–1000.

44. Kathju S, Lasko LA, Stoodley P. Considering hidradenitis suppurativa as a bacterial biofilm disease. *FEMS Immunol Med Microbiol*. 2012;65(2):385–389.

45. Russell AD, Day MJ. Antibacterial activity of chlorhexidine. *J Hosp Infect*. 1993;25(4):229–238. https://doi.org/10.1016/0195-6701(93)90109-d.

46. Toholka R, Nixon R. Allergic contact dermatitis to chlorhexidine. *Australas J Dermatol*. 2013;54(4):303–306. https://doi.org/10.1111/ajd.12087.

47. Nacht S, Yeung D, Beasley JN, et al. Benzoyl peroxide: percutaneous penetration and metabolic disposition. *J Am Acad Dermatol*. 1981;4(1):31–37.

48. Kircik LH. The role of benzoyl peroxide in the new treatment paradigm for acne. *J Drugs Dermatol.* 2013;12(6):s73–s76.

49. Mahmoud BH, Tierney E, Hexsel CL, et al. Prospective controlled clinical and histopathologic study of hidradenitis suppurativa treated with the long-pulsed neodymium:yttrium-aluminium-garnet laser. *J Am Acad Dermatol.* 2010;62(4):637–645.

50. Dinning AJ, Al-Adham IS, Austin P, et al. Pyrithione biocide interactions with bacterial phospholipid head groups. *J Appl Microbiol.* 1998;85(1):132–140.

51. Chandler CJ, Segel IH. Mechanism of the antimicrobial action of pyrithione: effects on membrane transport, ATP levels, and protein synthesis. *Antimicrob Agents Chemother.* 1978;14(1):60–68.

52. Kitamura H, Morikawa H, Kamon H, et al. Toll-like receptor-mediated regulation of zinc homeostasis influences dendritic cell function. *Nat Immunol.* 2006;7(9):971–977.

53. Danesh MJ, Kimball AB. Pyrithione zinc as a general management strategy for hidradenitis suppurativa. *J Am Acad Dermatol.* 2015;73 (5), e175.

54. Guthery E, Seal LA, Anderson EL. Zinc pyrithione in alcohol-based products for skin antisepsis: persistence of antimicrobial effects. *Am J Infect Control.* 2015;33(1):15–22.

55. Levy CW, Roujeinikova A, Sedelnikova S, et al. Molecular basis of triclosan activity. *Nature.* 1999;398(6726):383–384.

56. McDonnell G, Russell AD. Antiseptics and disinfectants: activity, action, and resistance. *Clin Microbiol Rev.* 1999;12(1):147–179.

57. Lubarsky HV, Gerbersdorf SU, Hubas C, et al. Impairment of the bacterial biofilm stability by triclosan. *PLoS One.* 2012;7(4), e31183. https://doi.org/10.1371/journal.pone.0031183.

58. Barros SP, Wirojchanasak S, Barrow DA, et al. Triclosan inhibition of acute and chronic inflammatory gene pathways. *J Clin Periodontol.* 2010;37(5):412–418.

59. Hendricks AJ, Hsiao JL, Lowes MA, Shi VY. A comparison of international management guidelines for hidradenitis suppurativa. *Dermatology.* 2019;1–16.

60. Yazdankhah SP, Scheie AA, Hoiby EA, et al. Triclosan and antimicrobial resistance in bacteria: an overview. *Microb Drug Resist.* 2006;12(2):83–90.

61. Koeppe ES, Ferguson KK, Colacino JA, Meeker JD. Relationship between urinary triclosan and paraben concentrations and serum thyroid measures in NHANES 2007-2008. *Sci Total Environ.* 2013;445–446:299–305.

62. Dann AB, Hontela A. Triclosan: environmental exposure, toxicity and mechanisms of action. *J Appl Toxicol.* 2011;31(4):285–311.

63. Dhillon GS, Kaur S, Pulicharla R, et al. Triclosan: current status, occurrence, environmental risks and bioaccumulation potential. *Int J Environ Res Public Health.* 2015;12(5):5657–5684.

64. Giuliano CA, Rybak MJ. Efficacy of triclosan as an antimicrobial hand soap and its potential impact on antimicrobial resistance: a focused review. *Pharmacotherapy.* 2015;35(3):328–336. https://doi.org/10.1002/phar.1553.

65. McNamara PJ, Levy SB. Triclosan: an Instructive Tale. *Antimicrob Agents Chemother.* 2016;60(12):7015–7016. https://doi.org/10.1128/AAC.02105-16.

66. Warnecke J, Wendt A. Anti-inflammatory action of pale sulfonated shale oil (ICHTHYOL pale) in UVB erythema test. *Inflamm Res.* 1998;47(2):75–78. https://doi.org/10.1007/s000110050282.

67. Boyd AS. Ichthammol revisited. *Int J Dermatol.* 2010;49(7):757–760. https://doi.org/10.1111/j.1365-4632.2010.04551.x.

68. Rabe KF, Perkins RS, Dent G, et al. Inhibitory effects of sulfonated shale oil fractions on the oxidative burst and Ca++ mobilization in stimulated macrophages. *Arzneimittelforschung.* 1994;44(2):166–170. https://www.ncbi.nlm.nih.gov/pubmed/7908522.

69. Nilssen E, Wormald PJ, Oliver S. Glycerol and ichthammol: medicinal solution or mythical potion? *J Laryngol Otol.* 1996;110(4):319–321.

70. Lawrence CM, Smith AG. Ichthammol sensitivity. *Contact Dermatitis.* 1981;7(6):335.

71. Newby CS, Barr RM, Greaves MW, Mallet AI. Cytokine release and cytotoxicity in human keratinocytes and fibroblasts induced by phenols and sodium dodecyl sulfate. *J Invest Dermatol.* 2000;115 (2):292–298.

72. Atkins D, Frodel J. Skin rejuvenation in facial surgery. *Facial Plast Surg.* 2006;22(2):129–139. https://doi.org/10.1055/s-2006-947719.

73. Boer J, Jemec GB. Resorcinol peels as a possible self-treatment of painful nodules in hidradenitis suppurativa. *Clin Exp Dermatol.* 2010;35(1):36–40. https://doi.org/10.1111/j.1365-2230.2009.03377.x.

74. Pascual JC, Encabo B, Ruiz de Apodaca RF, et al. Topical 15% resorcinol for hidradenitis suppurativa: An uncontrolled prospective trial with clinical and ultrasonographic follow-up. *J Am Acad Dermatol.* 2017;77(6):1175–1178.

75. Polano MK. *Topical Therapeutics.* Edinburgh: Churchill Livingstone; 1984.

76. Theut Riis P, Saunte DM, Sigsgaard V, et al. Intense pulsed light treatment for patients with hidradenitis suppurativa: beware treatment with resorcinol. *J Dermatolog Treat.* 2018;29(4):385–387.

77. Lynch BS, Delzell ES, Bechtel DH. Toxicology review and risk assessment of resorcinol: thyroid effects. *Regul Toxicol Pharmacol.* 2002;36(2):198–210.

78. Perng P, Zampella JG, Okoye GA. Management of hidradenitis suppurativa in pregnancy. *J Am Acad Dermatol.* 2017;76 (5):979–989.

79. Detmar M, Mayer-da-Silva A, Stadler R, Orfanos CE. Effects of azelaic acid on proliferation and ultrastructure of mouse keratinocytes in vitro. *J Invest Dermatol.* 1989;93(1):70–74.

80. Mastrofrancesco A, Ottaviani M, Aspite N, et al. Azelaic acid modulates the inflammatory response in normal human keratinocytes through PPARgamma activation. *Exp Dermatol.* 2010;19(9):813–820.

81. Sieber MA, Hegel JK. Azelaic acid: Properties and mode of action. *Skin Pharmacol Physiol.* 2014;27(Suppl 1):9–17. https://doi.org/10.1159/000354888.

82. Scheinfeld N. Hidradenitis Suppurativa in prepubescent and pubescent children. *Clin Dermatol.* 2015;33(3):316–319. https://doi.org/10.1016/j.clindermatol.2014.12.007.

83. Fisher GJ, Voorhees JJ. Molecular mechanisms of retinoid actions in skin. *FASEB J.* 1996;10(9):1002–1013. https://doi.org/10.1096/fasebj.10.9.8801161.

84. Wolf Jr JE. Potential anti-inflammatory effects of topical retinoids and retinoid analogues. *Adv Ther.* 2002;19(3):109–118. https://doi.org/10.1007/BF02850266.

85. Schmidt N, Gans EH. Tretinoin: a review of its anti-inflammatory properties in the treatment of acne. *J Clin Aesthet Dermatol.* 2011;4(11):22–29. https://www.ncbi.nlm.nih.gov/pubmed/22125655.

86. Wollina U, Brzezinski P, Koch A. Retinoids in Hidradenitis suppurativa/acne inversa. In: Karadag AS, Aksoy B, Parish LC, editors. *Retinoids in Dermatology.* Boca Raton: CRC Press; 2019.

87. Maarouf M, Hendricks AJ, Shi VY. Bathing additives for atopic dermatitis - a systematic review. *Dermatitis.* 2019;30(3):191–197. https://doi.org/10.1097/DER.0000000000000459.

88. Eriksson S, van der Plas MJA, Morgelin M, Sonesson A. Antibacterial and antibiofilm effects of sodium hypochlorite against *Staphylococcus aureus* isolates derived from patients with atopic dermatitis. *Br J Dermatol.* 2017;177(2):513–521. https://doi.org/10.1111/bjd.15410.

89. Sawada Y, Tong Y, Barangi M, et al. Dilute bleach baths used for treatment of atopic dermatitis are not antimicrobial in vitro. *J Allergy Clin Immunol.* 2019;143(5):1946–1948. https://doi.org/10.1016/j.jaci.2019.01.009.

90. Fukuyama T, Martel BC, Linder KE, et al. Hypochlorous acid is antipruritic and anti-inflammatory in a mouse model of atopic dermatitis. *Clin Exp Allergy.* 2018;48(1):78–88. https://doi.org/10.1111/cea.13045.

91. Maarouf M, Shi VY. Bleach for atopic dermatitis. *Dermatitis.* 2018;29(3):120–126. https://doi.org/10.1097/DER.0000000000000358.

92. Leung TH, Zhang LF, Wang J, et al. Topical hypochlorite ameliorates NF-kappaB-mediated skin diseases in mice. *J Clin Invest.* 2013;123(12):5361–5370. https://doi.org/10.1172/JCI70895.

93. Woodruff CM, Charlie AM, Leslie KS. Hidradenitis suppurativa: A guide for the practicing physician. *Mayo Clin Proc.* 2015;90 (12):1679–1693. https://doi.org/10.1016/j.mayocp.2015.08.020.

94. Isak V, Feldman S, Pichardo R. Hidradenitis suppurativa: A comparison of guidelines. *J Dermatol Dermatolo Surg.* 2018;22(2): 48–59. https://doi.org/10.4103/jdds.jdds_19_18.

95. Leap J, Baltaji S, Singh A. Fatal epsom salt overdose. *Am J Respir Crit Care Med.* 2019;199:A4826.

96. Shoaib Khan M, Zahid S, Ishaq M. Fatal hypermagnesemia: an acute ingestion of Epsom Salt in a patient with normal renal function. *Caspian J Intern Med.* 2018;9(4):413–415. https://doi.org/10.22088/cjim.9.4.413.

97. Bokhari SR, Siriki R, Teran FJ, Batuman V. Fatal Hypermagnesemia due to laxative use. *Am J Med Sci.* 2018;355(4):390–395. https://doi.org/10.1016/j.amjms.2017.08.013.

98. Price KN, Thompson AM, Rizvi O, et al. Complementary and Alternative Medicine Use in Patients With Hidradenitis Suppurativa. *JAMA Dermatol.* 2020;156(3):345–348. https://doi.org/10.1001/jamadermatol.2019.4595 (web archive link).

99. Kearney N, Byrne N, Kirby B, Hughes R. Complementary and alternative medicine use in hidradenitis suppurativa. *Br J Dermatol.* 2020;182(2):484–485. https://doi.org/10.1111/bjd.18426.

100. Wilkinson JD, Williamson EM. Cannabinoids inhibit human keratinocyte proliferation through a non-CB1/CB2 mechanism and have a potential therapeutic value in the treatment of psoriasis. *J Dermatol Sci.* 2007;45(2):87–92. https://doi.org/10.1016/j.jdermsci.2006.10.009.

101. Maccarrone M, Di Rienzo M, Battista N, et al. The endocannabinoid system in human keratinocytes. Evidence that anandamide inhibits epidermal differentiation through CB1 receptor-dependent inhibition of protein kinase C, activation protein-1, and transglutaminase. *J Biol Chem.* 278(36):33896–33903. https://doi.org/10.1074/jbc.M303994200.

102. Toth BI, Dobrosi N, Dajnoki A, et al. Endocannabinoids modulate human epidermal keratinocyte proliferation and survival via the sequential engagement of cannabinoid receptor-1 and transient receptor potential vanilloid-1. *J Invest Dermatol.* 2011;131(5): 1095–1104. https://doi.org/10.1038/jid.2010.421.

103. Olah A, Toth BI, Borbiro I, et al. Cannabidiol exerts sebostatic and antiinflammatory effects on human sebocytes. *J Clin Invest.* 2014;124(9):3713–3724. https://doi.org/10.1172/JCI64628.

104. Tyagi P, Singh M, Kumari H, et al. Bactericidal activity of curcumin I is associated with damaging of bacterial membrane. *PLoS One.* 2015;10(3), e0121313. https://doi.org/10.1371/journal.pone.0121313.

105. Rai D, Singh JK, Roy N, Panda D. Curcumin inhibits FtsZ assembly: an attractive mechanism for its antibacterial activity. *Biochem J.* 2008;410(1):147–155. https://doi.org/10.1042/BJ20070891.

106. Vaughn AR, Haas KN, Burney W. Potential role of curcumin against biofilm-producing organisms on the skin: a review. *Phytother Res.* 2017;31(12):1807–1816. https://doi.org/10.1002/ptr.5912.

107. Allegra A, Innao V, Russo S, et al. Anticancer activity of curcumin and its analogues: preclinical and clinical studies. *Cancer Invest.* 2017;35 (1):1–22. https://doi.org/10.1080/07357907.2016.1247166.

108. Reddy S, Aggarwal BB. Curcumin is a non-competitive and selective inhibitor of phosphorylase kinase. *FEBS Lett.* 1994;341(1):19–22. https://doi.org/10.1016/0014-5793(94)80232-7.

16

Systemic Antibiotics in Hidradenitis Suppurativa

AUDE NASSIF, MAYUR RAMESH, ILTEFAT HAMZAVI, AND OLIVIER JOIN-LAMBERT, SR.

CHAPTER OUTLINE

Introduction

Antibiotics alone, or in combination with other therapeutic strategies, have been empirically used in hidradenitis suppurativa (HS) with variable success, resulting only in temporary symptom relief in the disease process. Although very few randomized controlled studies have been performed to confirm their efficacy, antibiotics are currently recommended worldwide as first-line therapy by several guidelines issued from scientific dermatological societies.

Rationale for the Use of Antibiotics in Hidradenitis Suppurativa

Role of Bacterial Dysbiosis in the Pathophysiology of Hidradenitis Suppurativa

The pathogenesis of HS has not been fully elucidated, but is associated with genetic, immunological, hormonal, environmental, and microbiological factors. The recently unraveled microbiology of HS suggests abnormal host-microbiome cross-talks, bacterial pathogenicity, and dysbiotic variations according to the clinical severity of the disease (Fig. 16.1). The persistence of bacteria within highly inflammatory lesions probably results from both an immune skin defect in HS and bacterial pathogenic properties.

Considering the results of pathological studies,[1] the initial pathologic process results from hair follicle (HF) plugging, which, in case of rupture, leads to the release of keratin debris and bacteria within the dermis. Extensive bacteriological studies of HS lesions have shown that mild HS lesions (Hurley stage I nodules and abscesses) are associated with low virulent skin colonizers such as *Cutibacterium* (formerly *Propionibacterium*) *avidum*, and coagulase negative staphylococci, including the virulent *Staphylococcus lugdunensis* and *Corynebacterium* spp.[2,3] Anaerobes are associated with 50% of Hurley stage I lesions. Some patients develop more severe and chronic lesions with scarring (Hurley stage II and III). The microbiology of these lesions, as assessed before antibiotic

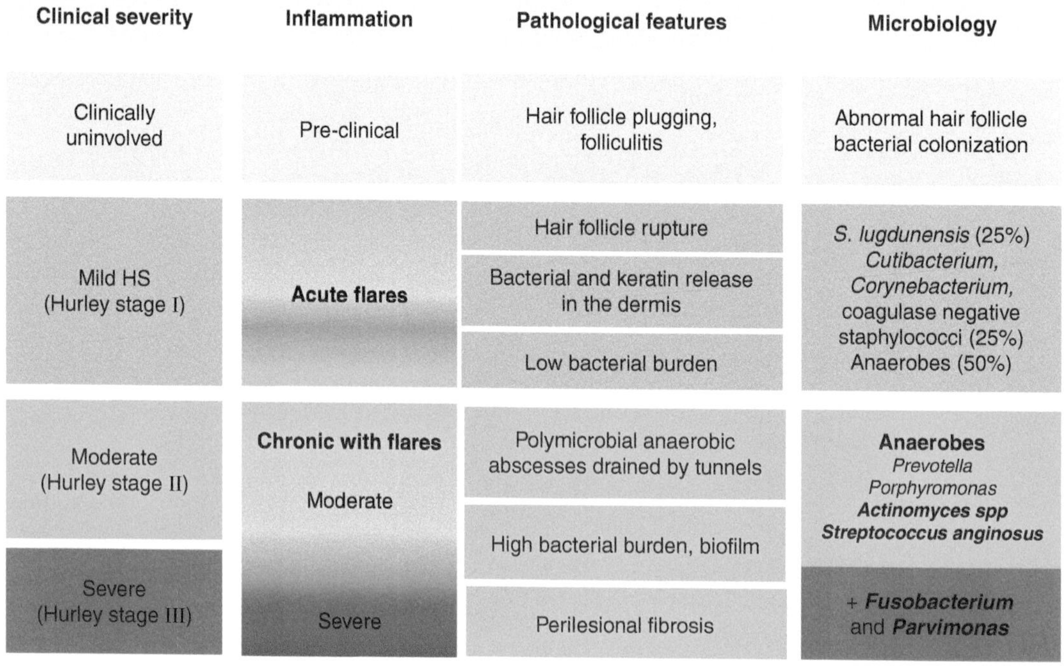

Clinical severity	Inflammation	Pathological features	Microbiology
Clinically uninvolved	Pre-clinical	Hair follicle plugging, folliculitis	Abnormal hair follicle bacterial colonization
Mild HS (Hurley stage I)	Acute flares	Hair follicle rupture	*S. lugdunensis* (25%) *Cutibacterium*, *Corynebacterium*, coagulase negative staphylococci (25%) Anaerobes (50%)
		Bacterial and keratin release in the dermis	
		Low bacterial burden	
Moderate (Hurley stage II)	Chronic with flares	Polymicrobial anaerobic abscesses drained by tunnels	**Anaerobes** *Prevotella Porphyromonas* **Actinomyces spp Streptococcus anginosus**
	Moderate	High bacterial burden, biofilm	
Severe (Hurley stage III)	Severe	Perilesional fibrosis	+ **Fusobacterium** and **Parvimonas**

• **Fig. 16.1** Clinico-Pathological Staging of Hidradenitis Suppurativa With Corresponding Microbiology.

treatments, is constituted of anaerobes, with a predominance of *Prevotella* and *Porphyromonas*, two gram-negative anaerobic rods. *Parvimonas* and *Fusobacterium* are associated with Hurley stage III lesions.[4]

Chronic HS lesions are associated with bacterial biofilms,[5] which are made of dormant bacteria surrounded by a gelatinous substance. Biofilms are associated with chronic infections in humans, reflecting the inability of the immune system to clear these bacteria. Indeed, biofilms are notably difficult to treat using antibiotics, which are poorly active on dormant bacteria and may not diffuse properly into biofilms. Biofilm presence may explain constant relapses after antibiotic treatments, usually occurring in previous scars.

The role of fungibiomes has not been specifically studied in HS using new generation sequencing technology. In our experience, *Candida* spp. can be grown on culture media used for prolonged bacterial cultures of HS suppurative lesions, but always in patients having received prolonged and potent antibiotic course, with clinical signs of candidiasis and rarely in patients naïve from any antibiotic treatment. Moreover, systemic treatment of candidiasis does not improve HS. Therefore, a role for fungal microbiome in HS pathogenesis seems unlikely.

Arguments for a Rational Use of Antibiotics in Hidradenitis Suppurativa

HS is a chronic dermatological disease with a significant negative impact on quality of life due to unmet needs. Continuous or repeated intermittent antibiotic courses are regularly employed in 70% of HS patients by general practitioners as well as specialists,[6] with few validated alternative and satisfactory treatment options.
- Systemic nonsteroidal antiinflammatory drugs (NSAIDs) and corticosteroids are typically used as supportive care to decrease symptoms such as pain, but no controlled studies have proved their efficacy and harmlessness.
- Antitumor necrosis factor (TNF)-alpha agents are only approved for moderate and severe HS, but not for mild cases.

Moreover, anti-TNF-alpha agents such as adalimumab provide significant improvement (reaching HiSCR) in only 50% of the patients[7] and, although rarely, they can cause worrisome/significant side effects.
- Surgery, although a cornerstone treatment of HS, cannot always be performed due to the multiplicity, size, and/or localization of lesions, as well as lack of access to surgical experts specialized in HS procedures. Recurrences in the surgical margins can occur in up to 50% of cases.

Although antibiotics may be useful in the management of HS, their long-term risks include *Clostridioides difficile* infections and the emergence of resistance.

Antibiotics in Hidradenitis Suppurativa: Literature Review

A search through PUBMED, performed from 1950 to 2020, using the MeSH terms "hidradenitis suppurativa," "acne inversa," and "antibiotic" resulted in 311 references. We excluded reviews and articles that were not in English. Parameters analyzed in our report included design, primary outcome, number of patients, initial severity, disease severity assessment, treatments, adverse events, follow-up, and limitations.

Single Oral Antibiotics

Tetracyclines
- A randomized trial compared the efficacy of oral tetracycline 500 mg bid versus topical clindamycin (1%) in 46 Hurley stage I and II patients,[8] 34 patients being evaluable. Primary outcome was improvement in a composite score consisting of subjective and objective data at month 3. Compared to baseline, there was a 30% to 40% improvement as assessed by the number of nodules or abscesses in both groups with no statistical difference. Considering the low number of patients, the high

number of patients lost to follow-up, and the absence of placebo control group, the results of this study (which was performed in the late 1990s) are difficult to interpret.

- In a recent retrospective multi-center descriptive study performed in adolescents, Riis et al. reported the efficacy of tetracycline in 16/32 patients with a median age of 16 and an interquartile range of 3,[9] but no details were specified on the disease severity, associated treatments, or outcome measures.

- A retrospective study compared the outcomes of 10 patients who were treated with doxycycline 200 mg/d (7 Hurley stage I, 2 Hurley stage II, and 1 Hurley stage III) and of 35 patients treated with the rifampin-clindamycin combination (7 Hurley stage I, 19 Hurley stage II, and 9 Hurley stage III).[10] Hidradenitis suppurativa clinical response (HiSCR) was achieved at month 3 in 60% of patients treated with doxycycline and in 46% of patients treated with the rifampin-clindamycin combination.

- Armyra et al. reported a series of 20 HS patients treated with minocycline 100 mg/d combined with colchicine 1 mg/d for 6 months, followed by 6 months of colchicine alone.[11] Hurley staging and PGA (Physician Global Assessment) score were used. The series consisted of 1 Hurley stage I, 15 Hurley stage II, and 4 Hurley stage III patients. Primary objective of clinical improvement was obtained in all subjects. No patients achieved complete remission. The part played by colchicine alone and minocycline alone in the management of HS cannot be ascertained from this study.

Trimethoprim-Sulfamethoxazole

Trimethoprim-sulfamethoxazole (TMP-SMX) is commonly used in the long term to prevent *Pneumocystis jiroveci* pneumonia in HIV and immunosuppressed patients (80/400 mg/d or 160/800 mg/d) and has a good safety profile.[12] In one retrospective and one uncontrolled prospective study totaling 56 patients conducted by the same researchers, TMP-SMX was given as maintenance treatment to prevent flares (80/400 mg/d under 80 kg, 160/800 mg/d above 80 kg) after clinical remission of all lesions.[13,14] Notably, no new sites affected with HS were observed during the 6-month follow-up in the retrospective study and during the 9-month follow-up in the prospective study. A limited number of relapses occurred only in scars, suggesting bacterial persistence of biofilms, and these were easily controlled by pristinamycin +/– metronidazole prescribed for 3 weeks. These findings suggest that a low maintenance treatment with an appropriate antibiotic such as TMP-SMX may limit relapses and prevent HS progression in new areas.

Dapsone

Dapsone is known for its antimicrobial properties in leprosy and is additionally used as an antiinflammatory agent in several dermatological diseases. Most reports of dapsone use in HS involve a combination of dapsone with different drugs (anti-androgens, anti-TNF agents, cyclosporine, metformin, liraglutide, and finasteride). With these combination treatments, clinical improvement of HS has been reported using various non-validated criteria.[15-17] A G6PD deficiency should be ruled out before starting dapsone and regular monitoring for anemia and methemoglobinemia is recommended during this treatment.

Combination of Oral Antibiotics

Clindamycin-Rifampin

- Mendonça et al. first reported the efficacy of the clindamycin-rifampin (CR) combination (600 mg/d each) in a retrospective study of 14 HS patients without any information on clinical severity.[18] Remission (not defined) was achieved in 8 patients

"between 1 and 4 years" after a single course of 10 weeks and in 2 other patients after adding minocycline 100 mg/d; 4 patients stopped the combination because of diarrhea.

- Gener et al. reported a retrospective series of 116 patients treated with the CR combination (600 mg daily for each antibiotic).[19] Out of 116, only 70 patients were evaluable (51 Hurley stage I, 57 Hurley stage II, and 8 Hurley stage III). Median Sartorius score dropped from 28 to 19, with only 8 patients in complete remission (modified Sartorius 0). Adverse effects were predominantly diarrhea; follow-up data were not available.

- Van der Zee et al. reported a retrospective series of 34 HS patients (4 Hurley stage I, 20 Hurley stage II, and 10 Hurley stage III) treated with different dosing and duration of the CR combination.[20] Assessment relied on global evaluation of inflammation by physician, remission being defined as at least 75% of improvement from baseline. A total of 16/34 patients obtained "remission," 12 patients only had a partial response, and 6 had no improvement, or worsening. Nine patients stopped treatment due to diarrhea. Relapses without maintenance antibiotics occurred within 5 months.

- Bettoli et al. reported a prospective series of 23 moderate to severe patients[21] with 20 evaluable patients. No remission was observed, but an improvement was noted in 17/20 subjects, with a median Sartorius score decreasing from 132 to 71.

- Dessinioti et al. reported a prospective series of 26 patients (4 Hurley stage I, 16 Hurley stage II, and 6 Hurley stage III) treated with the CR combination (600 mg each daily) for 12 weeks starting with 5 day-intravenous (IV) administration of clindamycin 900 mg/d.[22] Response was defined as an improvement of >50% in nodules and abscesses count. Clinical improvement was noted in 19/26 patients. During the subsequent one year follow-up in 17 patients, 10 had relapses within a 4-month median without maintenance treatment.

- Marasca et al. reported a retrospective series in moderate to severe HS patients with no reported Hurley staging,[23] comparing 30 subjects on CR combination (rifampin being given alone for the first week at 600 mg daily, then adding clindamycin 600 mg daily) with 30 patients on adalimumab for 10 weeks. Clinical outcomes were an improvement in modified Sartorius, HiSCR and HIDRAdisk scores at week 10, in comparison to baseline. Only 10/30 patients achieved HiSCR in the antibiotic combination group, with a decrease in modified Sartorius from 69 to 58. Further follow-up was not reported.

Rifampin is never used alone because of a high risk of emergence of resistant mutants during treatment. The CR combination should theoretically prevent this phenomenon. However, rifampin is a strong inductor of P450 cytochrome, which can result in an increased metabolism of clindamycin. In 10 patients using the oral combination, a dramatic decrease of clindamycin plasma level was observed at day 10 (up to 82% of the peak concentration, undetectable trough levels).[24] Increasing dosage of clindamycin did not help to improve its level. These interactions and clinical findings were subsequently confirmed in another study.[25] Therefore, it is likely that the CR combination is in fact a monotherapy of rifampin after 10 days of use. Even though rifampin may work in mild HS, because of a low bacterial load and the highly bactericidal activity of rifampin, it should ideally be avoided as a single agent in the management of HS.[26]

The above findings led to reconsideration of the long-term utility of the CR combination in HS. Caposiena Caro et al.

prospectively compared the efficacy of the CR combination to clindamycin alone in 2 groups of 30 HS (11 Hurley stage I, 30 Hurley stage II, and 19 Hurley stage III) patients.[27] HiSCR at week 8 was achieved in 57% and 63% of patients, respectively. During the 1-year follow-up, 8 and 10 patients of the two groups respectively remained in remission without a maintenance treatment.

In a recent retrospective multicenter Spanish study on 509 HS patients treated with the CR combination, 26.5% stopped the CR combination before week 10, mostly due to gastro-intestinal intolerance.[28] *C. difficile* infections are rarely reported in HS patients with this combination and prevalence was identical to a large non-HS control group in a recent study.[29]

Clindamycin-Ofloxacin

This alternative was proposed to spare rifampin use in HS. Delaunay et al. reported a retrospective series of 65 HS patients (21 Hurley stage I, 21 Hurley stage II, and 23 Hurley stage III) treated at two different centers using a weight-based regimen of ofloxacin 200 to 400 mg/d and clindamycin 600 to 1800 mg/d for 3 months.[30] Clinical response was assessed after 3 months as complete, partial (reduction without disappearance), or none (stability or worsening). Twenty-two (34%) patients achieved clinical remission and 38 (58%) reported partial improvement.

Rifampin, Moxifloxacin and Metronidazole

Join-Lambert et al. reported a retrospective series of 28 HS patients (6 Hurley stage I, 10 Hurley stage II, and 12 Hurley stage III) treated with the combination of rifampin (10 mg/kg/d), moxifloxacin (400 mg/d), and metronidazole (500 mg tid) for 6 weeks, followed by 1 to 3 months with only rifampin and moxifloxacin.[14] Remission, defined by absence of any inflammation in scars, was observed in 6/6 Hurley stage I and 8/10 Hurley stage II subjects within 2 to 4 months. Of note, severe patients received a 2-week induction of IV ceftriaxone and oral metronidazole, and after clinical remission, patients were given TMP-SMX for maintenance treatment. Adverse events included gastro-intestinal side-effects, candidiasis, reversible tendonitis, and increase of liver enzymes. During the follow-up under TMP-SMX maintenance, seven patients had no relapse within 6 months and seven experienced relapses occurring only in previously involved areas (scars containing biofilms). The same team reported a prospective study of 28 severe Hurley stage I HS patients using this treatment strategy.[13] The median-modified Sartorius score dropped from 14 to 0 at week 12, with 75% being in remission. The median number of flares dropped from 21/year to 1/year during the 12-month follow-up with TMP-SMX maintenance treatment.

Intravenous Beta-Lactam Antibiotics

The efficacy of once-daily intravenous (IV) broad-spectrum beta-lactams has been reported in both a 3 to 6 week induction or when used as a rescue treatment strategy in moderate and severe HS.

Ceftriaxone in Combination with Oral Metronidazole

In the retrospective study of Join-Lambert et al. (see above) on the moxifloxacin-rifampin-metronidazole combination for moderate (Hurley stage II) and severe (Hurley stage III) HS, patients received a 2-week induction course of IV ceftriaxone 1g daily associated with metronidazole (500 mg 3 times daily orally).[14] The efficacy of the induction treatment was not specifically reported in this study, the primary endpoint being the percentage of clinical remissions at week 12. However, all patients were clinically improved

with this partial induction regimen at the 6-week visit as assessed by the size and number of active lesions (authors' personal data).

In a prospective study, Delage et al.[31] reported a small series of 17 Hurley II HS patients treated with a 3-week IV induction of ceftriaxone 1g daily associated with metronidazole (500 mg 3 times daily orally), followed by 3 weeks of the combination of rifampin (10 mg/kg/d), moxifloxacin, (400 mg/d), and metronidazole (500 mg tid) for 3 weeks, then by 6 weeks of only rifampin and moxifloxacin, then cotrimoxazole for maintenance. The primary endpoint was remission at week 12, which was obtained in 11 patients (65%) and subsequently in 3 other patients during the 1-year follow-up. Many mild side effects were reported.

Ertapenem

Join-Lambert et al. reported a retrospective series of 30 severe (17 refractory Hurley stage II and 13 Hurley stage III) HS patients treated with an IV ertapenem induction (1g daily) through a PICC-line for 6 weeks, followed by the combination of oral rifampin, moxifloxacin, and metronidazole.[32] Median-modified Sartorius improved from 49 to 19 and median pain level dropped from 6/10 to 0 at week 6. At the 6-month follow-up, 59% (16) of the patients who underwent oral consolidation after ertapenem course were in remission. In patients who stopped treatment after ertapenem, Sartorius score stopped improving or returned to baseline.

Braunberger et al. reported a retrospective series of 36 severe and refractory HS patients treated with ertapenem (28 evaluable) along with anti-TNF-alpha agents biotherapy in 4 patients and systemic corticosteroids in 5 patients.[33] Seventy-one percent were very satisfied or satisfied, with a quality of life notably improved in 86%. Although based on subjective criteria, such a level of satisfaction from patients with any treatment within 6 weeks has rarely been reported so far in HS.

Chahine et al. reported a case of severe and refractory HS with a high suspicion of septicemia, which was dramatically improved with ertapenem.[34]

Based on unpublished and personal communications (Hamzavi et al. and Nassif et al.), IV ertapenem as a bridge to surgery for 2 to 3 weeks prior has been successfully used to control severe/refractory Hurley stage III HS. Also, in some patients, IV ertapenem has been used to control symptoms until patients are able to use biologic therapy such as anti-TNF-alpha agents.

Antibiotic Resistance in Hidradenitis Suppurativa

Mechanisms of Acquired Resistance in Bacteria

Mutation of the antimicrobial target gene is the most rapid mechanism of acquired resistance. Risk of resistance among different antibiotic families is variable and compounded by the bacterial bioburden within HS lesions. Rifampin, when used alone, is particularly prone to select resistant mutants.

High-level resistance against clindamycin and tetracycline are usually mediated by chromosomal insertion of mobile genetic elements carrying resistance genes such as *erm* and *tet* genes, respectively. Transfer of mobile genetic elements is favored by low antibiotic concentrations and prolonged treatments.

Depending on the bacterial species, beta-lactam resistance usually occurs by target mutation, resistance gene acquisition (beta-lactamases, target variants), or impermeability due to porin loss or efflux. Compared to fluoroquinolones and rifampin, the risk of mutant selection is much lower using betalactam antibiotics. However, it can occur with repeated antibiotic treatments.

Impact of Low Antibiotic Dosages on the Emergence of Antimicrobial Resistance

In dermatology, antibiotics are often given as "immunomodulating" treatments for prolonged periods and in low dosages to reduce adverse events. However, bacterial resistance emerges quickly with low antibiotic concentrations.[35]

Antimicrobial Resistance in Hidradenitis Suppurativa

Bacteria associated with HS are intrinsically susceptible to a wide range of antibiotics (Table 16.1). We have little data on antimicrobial resistance in HS. However, recent reports indicate an increase in antibiotic resistance, particularly to clindamycin and, to a lesser extent, rifampin.[36-39] In addition, clindamycin resistance in anaerobes has emerged in the community (10% to 30% depending on the species).[40,41] This may account for antibiotic failures in HS.

Biofilms as a Cause of Resistance to Antibiotics

Bacterial biofilms are associated with indwelling devices, endocarditis, and chronic infections. The immune system has little ability to eradicate biofilms. Also, they are difficult to treat using antibiotics, independently of any antimicrobial resistance, since antibiotics and many drugs cannot penetrate into the biofilms. Chronic HS lesions are associated with bacterial biofilms.[5] This could account for why relapses always occur in scars and for the lower efficacy of antibiotics in severe HS. The role of biofilms in HS is still unclear but argues in favor of surgery when possible, when medical treatments are not satisfactory.

Antibiotics in Hidradenitis Suppurativa Guidelines

In an effort to standardize HS treatments, recommendations from various dermatology societies have been released during the past years.[42-47]

- Tetracyclines are recommended as first-line therapy. Short courses of treatment of flares (7 to 21 days) using oral antibiotics are recommended by the French guidelines in Hurley stage I and II patients.
- The combination of CR is recommended by many societies as second-line therapy in Hurley stage I patients and as first-line in Hurley II and III HS.
- The rifampin-moxifloxacin-metronidazole combination is recommended as a first-line consideration in Hurley stage I and II patients by the HS Alliance and as second line in Hurley II and III patients by the European S1 and North American guidelines.
- IV ceftriaxone and oral metronidazole are recommended for severe HS by the French guidelines. IV ertapenem is recommended as a rescue therapy by the North American guidelines.
- Efficacy is generally assessed after a 10- to 12-week course of antibiotics.

TABLE 16.1 Usual Susceptibility Rate of Bacteria Associated with Hidradenitis Suppurativa

ANTIBIOTICS		AEROBES				ANAEROBES		
Family	Name	CoNS	SLU	Cor	Str	Cocci	G+ rods	G- rods
Betalactam antibiotics	Amoxicillin	V	V	S	S	S	S	S
	Amoxicillin + clavulanic acid	V	S	S	S	S	S	S
	(IV) Piperacillin + tazobactam	V	S	S	S	S	S	S
	(IV) Ceftriaxone	V	S	S	S	S	S	V
	(IV) Ertapenem	V	S	S	S	S	S	S
Macrolides	Clindamycin	V	V	V	V	V	V	V
	Pristinamycin[a]	S	S	S	S	S	S	S
Tetracyclines	Doxycycline	V	S	S	S	S	S	S
	Minocycline	S	S	S	S	S	S	S
Fluoroquinolones	Ofloxacin	V	S	V	S	V	V	V
	Levofloxacin[b]	V	S	V	S	V	V	V
	Moxifloxacin[b]	V	S	S	S	S	V	S
Other	Trimethoprim-sulfamethoxazole	Nr	Nr	Nr	Nr	Nr	Nr	Nr
	Rifampin	S	S	S	S	S	S	S
	Metronidazole	R	R	R	R	S	V	S
	Linezolid	S	S	S	S	S	S	V

CoNS, Coagulase negative staphylococci (community resistance rate); Cor: Corynebacterium spp.; G- rods: anaerobic gram-negative rods (Prevotella, Porphyromonas, Fusobacterium, Bacteroides); G+ rods: anaerobic gram-positive rods (Cutibacterium, Actinomyces); IV, intravenous; Nr, not relevant (low dosage); R, resistant; S, susceptible; SLU, Staphylococcus lugdunensis; Str, Streptococcus anginosus group, S. agalactiae, S. dysgalactiae; V: variable (intrinsic or acquired resistance).

[a]Not available worldwide.

[b]Moxifloxacin shows an extended spectrum on anaerobes compared to older fluoroquinolones. Levofloxacin shows an improved coverage of anaerobes compared to ofloxacin.

TABLE 16.2	Recommended Use of Antibiotic by Dermatology Societies Guidelines in HS				
	Hurley	1st line	2nd line	3rd line	Maintenance
Swiss guidelines[42]	Stage 1	tetracycline	rifampin-clindamycin		tetracycline
	Stage 2	tetracycline	rifampin-clindamycin	dapsone or metformin	tetracycline
	Stage 3	rifampin-clindamycin	dapsone + metformin		tetracycline
British guidelines[43]	Stage 1, 2, and 3	tetracycline	dapsone or metformin (diabetes, PCOS, or pregnancy)	none	
North American guidelines[44]	Stage 1	tetracycline	rifampin-clindamycin		dapsone
	Stage 2	tetracycline	rifampin-clindamycin or rifampin-moxifloxacin-metronidazole	rifampin-moxifloxacin-metronidazole	dapsone
	Stage 3	rifampin-clindamycin	rifampin-moxifloxacin-metronidazole	rifampin-moxifloxacin-metronidazole ertapenem as rescue therapy	
Brazilian guidelines [45]	Stage 1, 2, and 3	tetracycline or TMP-SMX	rifampin-clindamycin or ofloxacin-clindamycin	dapsone or metformin	
European Alliance guidelines [46]	Continuous Stage 1	tetracycline or rifampin-moxifloxacin-metronidazole	rifampin-moxifloxacin-metronidazole		tetracycline
	Stage 2	rifampin-clindamycin	rifampin-moxifloxacin-metronidazole	dapsone	tetracycline
	Stage 3	rifampin-clindamycin		ertapenem followed by rifampin-moxifloxacin-metronidazole	tetracycline
French guidelines [47]	Intermittent Stage 1	intermittent stage 1: AMC or PST on demand continuous stage 1: doxy or TMP-SMX, AMC, or PST on demand	doxy or TMP-SMX, + AMC, or PST on demand	none	tetracycline
	Stage 2	doxy or TMP-SMX, AMC, or PST on demand	ceftriaxone + metronidazole or levofloxacin + metronidazole	none	doxy or TMP-SMX
	Stage 3	ceftriaxone + metronidazole or levofloxacin + metronidazole		none	doxy or TMP-SMX

Other treatment options are not presented here. *AMC*, Amoxicillin-clavulanate; doxy: doxycycline; *HS*, hidradenitis suppurativa; *PST*, pristinamycin; *PCOS*, polycystic ovary syndrome; *TMP-SMX*, trimethoprim-sulfamethoxazole.

The heterogeneity of these guidelines summarized in Table 16.2 probably reflects variable experts' opinions due to the poor level of evidence from the literature on antibiotics in HS.

Approach to Antibiotic Treatments in Hidradenitis Suppurativa

Pre-Antibiotic Evaluation and Follow-Up of Patients

Indication of Antibiotics in Hidradenitis Suppurativa

The basic principle of antibiotic treatments in HS is that all clinical signs of the disease, from nodules and abscesses to chronic suppurative lesions, are partly due to abnormal proliferation of bacteria within lesions and can be melted into mere scars with targeted antibiotics.

Considering the global problem of antimicrobial resistance, antibiotics must be given and managed as antiinfectious and not as immunomodulating treatments, except for tetracycline antibiotics. Antibiotics should only be given to patients with acute lesions (nodules), acute flares, and chronic suppurative lesions.

Assessment of *Hidradenitis Suppurativa* Clinical Severity

The clinical severity of HS should be carefully evaluated before starting a treatment in order to define the optimal strategy and assess its efficacy during follow-up: number and size of lesions, Hurley stage and other clinical scores, activity (number of flares, duration), pain, and impact on quality of life.

Management of Coexisting Clinical Conditions

Treating coexisting conditions helps improve HS and spares antibiotics use. Patients with diabetes mellitus (DM) are prone to infections[48] and DM is associated with HS in up to 30% of cases.[49] Being overweight is associated with DM and HS. The proliferation of anaerobes in skinfolds may have an adverse impact on HS clinical course.[50]

HS patients frequently use NSAIDs as painkillers for HS or other unrelated conditions (e.g., headaches, painful periods, joint pain). NSAIDs can promote skin bacterial infections and a recent report suggests that NSAID may induce, aggravate, or prolong HS flares, with improvement after stopping these treatments.[51] In the authors' opinion, stopping systemic NSAIDs and corticosteroids when feasible may decrease HS activity and spare concurrent antibiotic treatments.

Clinical History and Testing Needed Before Initiation of Antibiotics

Before initiating antibiotics, allergies or previous intolerances should be ascertained. Comorbidities and medical treatments should be listed to assist in searching for potential drug-drug interactions (e.g., rifampin has significant interactions with contraceptive pills, anti-epileptics, and immune suppressive drugs used in transplantation). Antibiotics should be used with caution in preexisting conditions: peripheral neuropathy (contraindication for metronidazole), tendonitis (contraindication for fluoroquinolones), chronic hepatitis (contraindication for rifampin), cardiac abnormal rhythm and/or conduction abnormalities (contraindication for fluoroquinolones).

Based on the adverse effect profile, certain blood tests are recommended before initiation of antibiotics as well. A complete blood count, blood liver function testing, chest radiograph, and tuberculin test are suggested before initiation of rifampin. Women of child-bearing age should be warned about need for alternate methods of contraception due to reduced levels of contraceptive drugs. Prior to starting a long course of moxifloxacin, an EKG should be performed (due to risk of prolonged QTc interval). G6PD deficiency should be ruled out before starting dapsone.

Considering that prolonged cultures (at least one week) are required to grow anaerobes and that the variety of bacterial species associated with HS lesions cannot be identified in a routine laboratory, it is not recommended to sample HS lesions for bacteriological studies before starting a first treatment.

However, one should consider a sampling of HS lesions in severe patients who received numerous and/or repeated antibiotic courses with refractory severe disease or in severe or moderate patients with antibiotic-resistant lesions. In these cases, the aim of microbiological sampling will be to adapt the treatment to atypical bacteria not usually associated with untreated HS, such as *Pseudomonas aeruginosa* and *Enterococcus* spp., which are naturally resistant and can be selected by ertapenem (authors' unpublished data).

Bacteriologists should be informed of the clinical context and describe the results of bacterial cultures, including predominant aerobic bacteria and the presence or absence of anaerobes.

Only suppurative lesions should be sampled. Sampling can be performed by careful topical swabbing of pus from suppurative lesions after topical antiseptic disinfection of the skin surface and pressure over the lesion. Fresh pus should be immediately poured in a transport medium in order to avoid anaerobes death in the air oxygen.

Patients Follow-Up

Clinical efficacy and tolerance of antibiotics should be assessed periodically during the first 6 to 12 weeks and then as needed, once remission has been obtained. Monitoring for adverse effects such as mucosal candidiasis is essential.

The Antibiotic Toolbox in Hidradenitis Suppurativa

Doxycycline as First-Line Therapy

In current international guidelines, antibiotics of the tetracycline family are considered as first-line therapy in patients with continuous or frequently relapsing HS to spare the use of broad-spectrum antibiotics. In severe patients, the efficacy of tetracycline family is mild and temporary, and should not postpone more effective treatments. With a similar antimicrobial spectrum, doxycycline (100 to 200 mg/d) is a better therapeutic option because, contrary to tetracycline drug, its absorption is not markedly affected by food.

Oral Treatment of Flares

There is currently no standardized definition of flare. Therefore, we propose to define an HS flare as inflammation with erythema, edema, and increase in local temperature and pain compared to baseline and involving a surface >3 cm in an HS site lasting more than 5 days.

The treatment of HS flares is typically using standard oral antimicrobial treatments of skin and soft tissue infections. However, short treatments for 5 to 7 days carry the risk of immediate relapses in HS.

Amoxicillin-clavulanic acid (1000/250 mg orally, 3 times daily) or pristinamycin (1 g orally, 3 times daily) alone or combined with metronidazole (250 to 500 mg orally, 3 times daily) can be used for 7 to 21 days, depending on the initial clinical severity. Pristinamycin, a streptogramin group antibiotic, is a combination of two components that exhibit synergistic antibacterial activity and are active against various gram-positive cocci and anaerobes.[52] This antibiotic is not available worldwide.

Antibiotic Treatments for Management of Moderate and Severe Hidradenitis Suppurativa

Induction IV beta-lactam agents are generally used to treat severe infections before switching to an oral regimen. In moderate and severe HS, they are used before consolidation treatments to decrease bacterial burden prior to oral antibiotic combinations to prevent the emergence of resistant mutants.[14,32] They are usually well-tolerated, ensuring a better adherence to treatment.

IV/IM ceftriaxone (1-2g daily) in association with oral metronidazole is suggested to be used as first line for moderate HS. Ertapenem use (1g/d for ertapenem daily) is restricted to hospital prescription and must be reserved for severe HS or patients not responding to ceftriaxone and metronidazole or presenting with a contraindication against metronidazole.

Oral antibiotics as consolidation therapy: the CR combination is considered the cornerstone of antibiotic treatments for chronic HS. However, it results in a rifampin quasi-monotherapy after 10 days of treatment with a dramatic decrease in clindamycin serum concentrations.

Reported alternatives are clindamycin alone, the clindamycin-ofloxacin combination or levofloxacin (optimized antimicrobial spectrum in HS compared to ofloxacin),[53,54] and the rifampin-moxifloxacin-metronidazole combination, the latter ensuring an optimal coverage of aerobic and anaerobic HS bacteria.[55] The combinations of clindamycin-metronidazole, levofloxacin-metronidazole, and spiramycin-metronidazole are also likely effective in HS.

Of note, metronidazole has potent activity against most anaerobic bacteria, but it must be used in association with other antibiotics in HS to cover aerobic species present in lesions including *Streptococcus* and *Staphylococcus*. Other anaerobic bacteria such as *Actinomyces* and *Cutibacterium* (formerly *Propionibacterium*) are naturally resistant to metronidazole. Importantly, prolonged metronidazole therapy beyond 6 weeks is not recommended because of a risk of peripheral neuropathy. It may be resumed after at least a 4 to 6 week washout period if needed.[14]

Oral Maintenance Regimens

Maintenance regimens are given for at least several months after the initial induction and consolidation antibiotic regimens in order to obtain long-term control of disease activity. Antibiotics used for prolonged maintenance treatment must be well tolerated and must be different from those used to treat flares and chronic HS because antimicrobial resistance may emerge against these drugs.

Doxycycline (100 to 200 mg/d) or a low dosage of TMP-SMX (80/400 mg/d) can be used.

Severity-Guided Antibiotic Management of Hidradenitis Suppurativa

The antibiotic treatment options in HS according to Hurley stage are summarized in Table 16.3 and key information in Box 16.1. Hurley Stage II and III patients should be treated in centers with a multidisciplinary team including dermatologists, infectious diseases specialists, surgeons, and other specialists (endocrinology, rheumatology, gastro-enterology). To optimize the management of these patients, each center should build an algorithm based on updated knowledge of the available scientific literature. An example of a treatment algorithm based on literature data is presented in Fig. 16.2. A multidisciplinary approach to HS management is further discussed in Chapter 32.

Mild Hidradenitis Suppurativa (Hurley Stage I)

In HS, and particularly in Hurley stage I patients, treating or removing flare favoring factors such as overweight/obesity, diabetes, and potentially systemic NSAIDs, and systemic steroids can result in improvement of HS and should be the first treatment consideration. The clinical severity of the disease should be reassessed after at least 3 months of starting a treatment regimen.

In Hurley stage I, clinical remission of flares (i.e., nodules and abscesses) can be obtained in most patients using appropriate antibiotic treatments. Flares should be treated as soon as possible to limit bacterial overgrowth within lesions and secondary pain and inflammation. Patients often feel prodromes of flares, but do not receive immediate treatment because they often wait to see a dermatologist. Patients should have an antibiotic prescription for self-management of flares.

Hurley stage I flares should be treated for 1 to 3 weeks according to baseline severity and clinical evolution (see Fig 16.2). Treatments that are too short put patients at risk for rapid relapses. Surgical drainage may be necessary to alleviate pain, but relapses can still occur if antibiotics are not used. In an attempt to spare more potent antibiotics, amoxicillin/clavulanic acid or pristinamycin and metronidazole can be used in patients with limited activity of the disease. In severe Hurley Stage I patients (above 5 nodules and ≥4 flares a year), the oral combination of rifampin, moxifloxacin, and metronidazole can be used.[13]

A maintenance treatment should be given to prevent flares only when they are frequent (French guidelines: ≥4 flares/year), such as doxycycline or cotrimoxazole daily.

In case of repeated and frequent flares in the same site (≥1 flare within 6 months), suggesting biofilm persistence, surgery should

be performed after a new flare treatment. If surgery is not feasible, starting a Hurley stage II intravenous induction treatment before surgery should be considered.

Moderate and Severe Hidradenitis Suppurativa (Hurley Stage II and III)

In moderate and severe HS, maintenance treatments can be proposed as a first attempt to control the disease (usually unsatisfactory) or while in wait for more potent antibiotic courses and/or biologics. The use of oral treatments in mild HS flares as first-line therapy can improve patients, but only temporarily and incompletely.

Using IV beta-lactams as induction treatment calms lesions and decreases the bacterial load, thus optimizing the success rate of subsequent oral combination of antibiotics. Combining antibiotics with good diffusion properties such as rifampin, fluoroquinolones, and tetracycline antibiotics allows for enhancement of the antimicrobial spectrum, and the ability to obtain synergistic bactericidal activity and to overcome resistance to one of the drugs.

Moderate Hidradenitis Suppurativa

In Hurley stage II patients, clinical remission of lesions can be obtained with an IV or IM ceftriaxone and oral metronidazole combination for 3 weeks followed by an oral consolidation treatment for 2 months. Relapses in scars occurring within 6 months after remission should be an indication for a localized or semi-wide surgery after a new IV treatment.

Severe Hidradenitis Suppurativa

Antibiotics significantly improve Hurley stage III patients, but relapses usually occur after switching to oral treatments, after stopping metronidazole, or after switching to maintenance treatment, again demonstrating the necessity for surgery or other long-term treatment plan after 1 or 2 early and/or close relapses.

In Hurley stage III patients, either IV ceftriaxone and oral metronidazole (3 weeks) or preferably ertapenem (6 weeks), which allows a more prolonged optimal coverage of anaerobes (allowing 6 more weeks of oral combination treatment including metronidazole), may be used as induction treatment to decrease bacterial load before switching to an optimized oral combination of antibiotics such as rifampin-moxifloxacin-metronidazole for 3 to 6 weeks, then rifampin and moxifloxacin alone for 6 weeks (metronidazole must not be given for more than 6 weeks, but can be used again after a 6-week washout period).[32] Ertapenem alone or associated with oral linezolid is also an option in these patients as a second IV line therapy to lead them to surgery. Importantly, repeated use of ertapenem or ceftriaxone may select bacteria intrinsically resistant to these antibiotics (*Pseudomonas aeruginosa* and *Enterococcus* spp.) (A. Nassif and O. Join-Lambert, personal communication).

In patients previously treated with many courses of different antibiotics without clear efficacy, or in cases of a resistant area after IV induction, a swab should be performed for bacterial cultures to adapt the treatment.

Management of "Relapsing" and of "Antibiotic Resistant" Lesions

Lesions relapsing after effective treatments are not always synonymous with antimicrobial resistance and may be due to reactivation of bacterial biofilms present in the scar. Depending on the clinical severity, a first line 1-to 3-week oral antibiotic course for flare treatment should be attempted before a more aggressive management strategy.

TABLE 16.3 Therapeutic Options of Hidradenitis Suppurativa Using Antibiotics

Treatment Type	HURLEY STAGE/LINE OF TREATMENT				Recommended Dosing Regimen	Duration	Notes
	HI (i)	HI (c)	HII	HIII			
First-Line Therapy							
Doxycycline	NR-G	1	1[a]	1[a]	100–200mg/d	3 months–1 year	Doxycycline is a better therapeutic option compared to tetracycline because, contrary to tetracycline, the absorption of doxycycline is not markedly affected by food. Stopped temporarily in case of flare treatment.
Flare Treatment							
Amoxicillin + clavulanic acid	1	1	a	a	1000mg/250mg tid	1–3 weeks	Hurley 2 and 3: for limited flares. If active disease, consider chronic HS treatment. Metronidazole can be added to increase activity on anaerobes. Metronidazole must not be given over 6 weeks to prevent peripheral neuropathy.
Pristinamycin[c]	1	1	a	a	1g tid		
Pristinamycin[c] + metronidazole	1	1	a	a	1g tid + 250–500mg tid		
Chronic HS intravenous induction treatments							
Ceftriaxone + oral metronidazole	NR-G	3	1	1	1–2g daily + 250–500mg tid	3–6 weeks	Followed by chronic HS oral consolidation treatments. Metronidazole must not be given over 6 weeks to prevent peripheral neuropathy.
Ertapenem	NR-G	NR-G	3	1, 2 or 3[b]	1g daily	6 weeks	
Chronic HS oral consolidation treatments (recommended use after IV induction treatment)							
Rifampin + clindamycin LD	NR-G	NR-G	1 NR-A	1 NR-A	600mg + 600mg daily	12 weeks	Not recommended by the French guidelines (pharmacokinetic interaction, clindamycin at dose of zero in blood).
Clindamycin alone	NR-G	2	1 NR-A	1 NR-A	600mg tid	12 weeks	Normal clindamycin dosage may improve efficacy. Safety not assessed. Association with metronidazole may prevent *Clostridium difficile* infections. Levofloxacin is more active than ofloxacin on streptococci and anaerobes. Metronidazole must not be given over 6 weeks to prevent peripheral neuropathy.
Clindamycin + metronidazole		2	1 ND	1 ND	600mg tid + 500mg tid		
Clindamycin + ofloxacin		2	1	1	600mg TID + 400mg daily		
Clindamycin + levofloxacin		2	1	1	600mg TID + 500–1000mg daily		
Levofloxacin + metronidazole		2	1	1 ND	500–1000mg daily + 500mg TID		
Rifampin + moxifloxacin + metronidazole followed by rifampin + moxifloxacin	NR-G	2	1	1	10mg/kg/d + 400mg/d + 250–500mg tid for 6 weeks followed by 10mg/kg/d + 400mg/d for 6 weeks	12 weeks	Follow liver enzymes, platelet count. EKG recommended before treatment (QTc). Moxifloxacin has extended spectrum on anaerobes compared to older fluoroquinolones. Metronidazole must not be given over 6 weeks to prevent peripheral neuropathy. Rifampin should be taken on an empty stomach to optimize absorption.
Maintenance Treatment							
Doxycycline	NR-G	1	1	1	100–200 mg/d	≥6 months	Doxycycline is a better therapeutic option compared to tetracycline because, contrary to tetracycline, the absorption of doxycycline is not markedly affected by food. Trimethoprim/sulfamethoxazole can rarely be associated with severe cutaneous reactions. Maintenance treatments should be stopped temporarily in case of flare treatment.
Trimethoprim/sulfamethoxazole LD	NR-G	1	1	1	80mg/400mg/d, double dose if weight >80kg		

HI: Hurley stage I, (i): intermittent (<4 flares/year), (c): continuous (≥4 flares /year); HII: Hurley stage II, HIII: Hurley stage III. Numbers 1, 2, and 3 refer to first, second, and third line (rescue / preoperative) therapy. *HS*, Hidradenitis suppurativa; *LD*, low dosage; *ND*, no data in the literature; *NR-A*, not recommended by authors: risk of failure due to preexisting resistance or emergence of resistance; *NR-G*, not recommended by guideline; *tid*: *ter in die*, three times a day.

[a]These treatments may improve Hurley stage II and III patients temporarily.

[b]After failure of biotherapy and/or standard antimicrobial treatments as rescue therapy or preoperatively.

[c]Not available worldwide.

a. HS is a chronic condition and, except for acute flares, there is no emergency for prescribing antibiotics.

b. Antibiotics should be considered as part of a global treatment strategy, including other treatment options (surgery and biotherapy) depending on the clinical severity of the disease. Severe patients should be treated in specialized multidisciplinary centers.

c. Stopping/treating flare triggers should be tried first, as it can significantly improve patients and may avoid antibiotic treatments.

d. Using low dosages of antibiotics is not recommended except for maintenance treatments. Clinically inefficacious treatments should not be continued.

e. In Hurley stage II and II patients, IV betalactams should be used as

induction for 3–6 weeks before starting oral consolidation antibiotic treatments to optimize their efficacy. Rifampin should never be used alone and should be taken on an empty stomach (1 h before or 2 h after a meal) to optimize absorption.

f. Maintenance treatments should be given to patients with chronic or active hidradenitis suppurativa after clinical remission to prevent relapses or new HS active areas and to spare concurrent treatments. Doxycycline is a better therapeutic option than tetracycline because its absorption is not markedly affected by food.

g. Surgery should be planned if possible after 2 or more close relapses in the same scar to limit the repeated use of antibiotics.

Clinically refractory lesions, while on antibiotics adapted to severity, may be due to selection of antimicrobial resistant bacteria. For resistant Hurley stage I lesions, a Hurley stage II IV ceftriaxone and oral metronidazole induction treatment for 3 weeks can be proposed and will usually obtain remission so that the patient can be switched to maintenance treatment and/or treated by surgery in case of repeated relapses in the same scar. If Hurley stages II and III prove resistant to the strategies recommended above, a swab for microbiologic cultures should be performed under treatment to identify resistant bacteria and alter management accordingly.

After more than 1 relapse within a 6-month period after remission has been observed, escalation of antibiotics is not recommended, except as a prelude to a planned surgery or initiation of biologic therapy.

Antibiotics Before Surgery

Antibiotics (oral in Hurley stage I, IV in Hurley stages II and III) are frequently given for 1-3 weeks before surgery and one week thereafter to prevent relapses in the margins (I. Hamzavi, A. Nassif, and O. Join-Lambert, personal communications). This strategy usually helps to suppress inflammation with consequent faster healing of the surgical site.

In the authors' opinion, NSAIDs should not be used as pain killers postoperatively as they may promote bacterial infections.

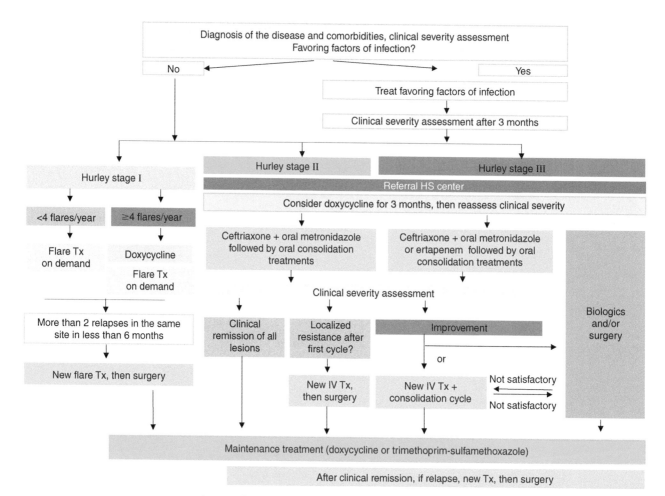

• **Fig. 16.2** Example of Treatment Algorithm: Antibiotic Treatment.

Antibiotics Combined with Other Hidradenitis Suppurativa Treatments

Antibiotics and Biotherapies

Considering HS as a host-microbiome disease, combining biotherapies and optimized antibiotic treatments appears to be logical to treat the inflammatory trigger and the dysregulated immune response. In routine practice, antibiotics are often given before starting a biotherapy or can be given as rescue therapy.[34] A combination of IV antibiotics and biotherapies may be beneficial for moderate to severe HS patients. Prospective Randomized Controlled Trials (RCTs) comparing one arm with only a biotherapy, one arm with only IV antibiotics, and one arm combining both treatments, should be initiated in order to demonstrate treatment synergy, allowing shorter antibiotic treatments to obtain remission and therefore less risk of side effects.

Antibiotics and Systemic Retinoids

A combination of antibiotics and systemic retinoids may be an option in Hurley stage I patients with the follicular phenotype, cautiously avoiding a concomitant tetracycline because of the risk of intra-cranial hyper-pressure.

Antibiotics and NSAIDs or Systemic Corticosteroids

The authors do not recommend associating these treatments with antibiotics for HS, since they probably alter their efficacy, with a usual delay of 3 weeks, as very often observed in routine practice (personal communication, A. Nassif).

Antibiotics and Immunosuppressive Treatments

Data on immunosuppressive drugs such as cyclosporine or methotrexate in HS are scarce in HS (not reviewed here). Most studies had a retrospective design, included few patients, often with severe recalcitrant HS or comorbidities justifying their use. Moreover, some of them may induce HS.[56] Associating antibiotics with immunosuppressive treatments in severe patients may be used as compassionate treatment in specialized centers in an attempt to improve their outcome.

Conclusion

HS is an enigmatic inflammatory disease, which is associated with specific dysbiotic features. Targeted antibiotics and a mild antibiotic maintenance treatment after remission can both be helpful to control the disease, but RCTs are needed to assess their efficacy and optimal use in HS. The repeated use of potent antibiotics may result in antimicrobial resistance. Therefore, antibiotics should not be used in HS without combining with a long-term treatment plan in place such as surgery or non-antibiotic systemic therapies.

References

1. van der Zee HH, de Ruiter L, Boer J, et al. Alterations in leucocyte subsets and histomorphology in normal-appearing perilesional skin and early and chronic hidradenitis suppurativa lesions. *Br J Dermatol.* 2012;166(1):98–106.
2. Ring HC, Thorsen J, Saunte DM, et al. The Follicular skin microbiome in patients with hidradenitis suppurativa and healthy controls. *JAMA Dermatol.* 2017;153(9):897–905.
3. Guet-Revillet H, Coignard-Biehler H, Jais JP, et al. Bacterial pathogens associated with hidradenitis suppurativa, france. *Emerg Infect Dis.* 2014;20(12):1990–1998.
4. Guet-Revillet H, Jais JP, Ungeheuer MN, et al. The Microbiological landscape of anaerobic Infections in hidradenitis suppurativa: a prospective metagenomic study. *Clin Infect Dis.* 2017;65(2):282–291.
5. Ring HC, Bay L, Nilsson M, et al. Bacterial biofilm in chronic lesions of hidradenitis suppurativa. *Br J Dermatol.* 2017;176(4):993–1000.
6. Kohorst JJ, Kimball AB, Davis MD. Systemic associations of hidradenitis suppurativa. *J Am Acad Dermatol.* 2015;73(5 Suppl 1):S27–S35.
7. Kimball AB, Okun MM, Williams DA, et al. Two phase 3 trials of adalimumab for hidradenitis suppurativa. *N Engl J Med.* 2016;375(5):422–434.
8. Jemec GB, Wendelboe P. Topical clindamycin versus systemic tetracycline in the treatment of hidradenitis suppurativa. *J Am Acad Dermatol.* 1998;39(6):971–974.
9. Riis PT, Saunte DM, Sigsgaard V, et al. Clinical characteristics of pediatric hidradenitis suppurativa: a cross-sectional multicenter study of 140 patients. *Arch Dermatol Res.* 2020;312(10):715–724.
10. Vural S, Gundogdu M, Akay BN, et al. Hidradenitis suppurativa: Clinical characteristics and determinants of treatment efficacy. *Dermatol Ther.* 2019;32(5), e13003.
11. Armyra K, Kouris A, Markantoni V, et al. Hidradenitis suppurativa treated with tetracycline in combination with colchicine: a prospective series of 20 patients. *Int J Dermatol.* 2017;56(3):346–350.
12. Di Cocco P, Orlando G, Bonanni L, et al. A systematic review of two different trimetoprim-sulfamethoxazole regimens used to prevent Pneumocystis jirovecii and no prophylaxis at all in transplant recipients: appraising the evidence. *Transplantation Proceedings.* 2009;41(4):1201–1203.
13. Delage M, Jais JP, Lam T, et al. Rifampin-moxifloxacin-metronidazole combination therapy for severe Hurley Stage 1 Hidradenitis Suppurativa: prospective short-term trial and one-year follow-up in 28 consecutive patients. *J Am Acad Dermatol.* 2020;S0190-9622(20):30049-9. Advance online publication. https://doi.org/10.1016/j.jaad.2020.01.007
14. Join-Lambert O, Coignard H, Jais JP, et al. Efficacy of rifampin-moxifloxacin-metronidazole combination therapy in hidradenitis suppurativa. *Dermatol.* 2011;222(1):49–58.
15. Kaur MR, Lewis HM. Hidradenitis suppurativa treated with dapsone: A case series of five patients. *J Dermatol Treat.* 2006;17(4):211–213.
16. Yazdanyar S, Boer J, Ingvarsson G, et al. Dapsone therapy for hidradenitis suppurativa: a series of 24 patients. *Dermatol.* 2011;222(4):342–346.
17. Staub J, Pfannschmidt N, Strohal R, et al. Successful treatment of PASH syndrome with infliximab, cyclosporine and dapsone. *J Eur Acad Dermatol Venereol.* 2015;29(11):2243–2247.
18. Mendonca CO, Griffiths CE. Clindamycin and rifampicin combination therapy for hidradenitis suppurativa. *Br J Dermatol.* 2006;154(5):977–978.
19. Gener G, Canoui-Poitrine F, Revuz JE, et al. Combination therapy with clindamycin and rifampin for hidradenitis suppurativa: a series of 116 consecutive patients. *Dermatol.* 2009;219(2):148–154.
20. van der Zee HH, Boer J, Prens EP, Jemec GB. The effect of combined treatment with oral clindamycin and oral rifampicin in patients with hidradenitis suppurativa. *Dermatol.* 2009;219(2):143–147.
21. Bettoli V, Zauli S, Borghi A, et al. Oral clindamycin and rifampicin in the treatment of hidradenitis suppurativa-acne inversa: a prospective study on 23 patients. *J Eur Acad Dermatol Venereol.* 2014;28(1): 125–126.
22. Dessinioti C, Zisimou C, Tzanetakou V, et al. Oral clindamycin and rifampicin combination therapy for hidradenitis suppurativa: a prospective study and 1-year follow-up. *Clin Exp Dermatol.* 2016;41(8):852–857.
23. Marasca C, Annunziata MC, Villani A, et al. Adalimumab versus rifampicin plus clindamycin for the treatment of moderate to severe hidradenitis suppurativa: a retrospective study. *J Drugs Dermatol.* 2019;18(5):437–438.
24. Join-Lambert O, Ribadeau-Dumas F, Jullien V, et al. Dramatic reduction of clindamycin plasma concentration in hidradenitis

suppurativa patients treated with the rifampin-clindamycin combination. *Eur J Dermatol.* 2014;24(1):94–95.

25. Bernard A, Kermarrec G, Parize P, et al. Dramatic reduction of clindamycin serum concentration in staphylococcal osteoarticular infection patients treated with the oral clindamycin-rifampicin combination. *J Infect.* 2015;71(2):200–206.

26. Albrecht J, Barbaric J, Nast A. Rifampicin alone may be enough: is it time to abandon the classic oral clindamycin-rifampicin combination for hidradenitis suppurativa? *Br J Dermatol.* 2019;180(4):949–950.

27. Caposiena Caro RD, Cannizzaro MV, Botti E, et al. Clindamycin versus clindamycin plus rifampicin in hidradenitis suppurativa treatment: Clinical and ultrasound observations. *J Am Acad Dermatol.* 2019;80(5):1314–1321.

28. Schneller-Pavelescu L, Vergara-de Caso E, Martorell A, et al. Interruption of oral clindamycin plus rifampicin therapy in patients with hidradenitis suppurativa: An observational study to assess prevalence and causes. *J Am Acad Dermatol.* 2019;80(5):1455–1457.

29. Lyons AB, Kaddurah H, Peacock A, et al. Hidradenitis suppurativa and risk for development of *Clostridium difficile* colitis. *Int J Dermatol.* 2020;59(6):e218–e219.

30. Delaunay J, Villani AP, Guillem P, et al. Oral ofloxacin and clindamycin as an alternative to the classic rifampicin-clindamycin in hidradenitis suppurativa: retrospective analysis of 65 patients. *Br J Dermatol.* 2018;178(1). e15–e6.

31. Delage M, Join-Lambert O, Guet-Revillet H, et al. *Observational study of 17 Hurley Stage 2 HS patients treated by targetted antibiotherapy: efficacy, tolerance and 1 year follow-up.* EHSF session, communication. Vienna: EADV; 2016.

32. Join-Lambert O, Coignard-Biehler H, Jais JP, et al. Efficacy of ertapenem in severe hidradenitis suppurativa: a pilot study in a cohort of 30 consecutive patients. *J Antimicrob Chemother.* 2016;71(2): 513–520.

33. Braunberger TL, Nartker NT, Nicholson CL, et al. Ertapenem - a potent treatment for clinical and quality of life improvement in patients with hidradenitis suppurativa. *Int J Dermatol.* 2018;57(9):1088–1093.

34. Chahine AA, Nahhas AF, Braunberger TL, et al. Ertapenem rescue therapy in hidradenitis suppurativa. *JAAD Case Rep.* 2018; 4(5):482–483.

35. Greenfield BK, Shaked S, Marrs CF, et al. Modeling the emergence of antibiotic resistance in the environment: an analytical solution for the minimum selection concentration. *Antimicrob Agents Chemother.* 2018;62(3).

36. Bettoli V, Manfredini M, Massoli L, et al. Rates of antibiotic resistance/sensitivity in bacterial cultures of hidradenitis suppurativa patients. *J Eur Acad Dermatol Venereol.* 2019;33(5):930–936.

37. Fischer AH, Haskin A, Okoye GA. Patterns of antimicrobial resistance in lesions of hidradenitis suppurativa. *J Am Acad Dermatol.* 2017;76(2):309–313. e2.

38. Hem S, Delage M, Nassif A, et al. Antimicrobial resistance of anaerobic actinomyces: a retrospective monocentric study focusing on Hidradenitis suppurativa. *Exp Dermatol.* 2017;(special issue: 6th conference of the EHSF 2017, European Hidradenitis suppurativa foundation e.V., 8–10 February, Copenhagen, Denmark). O04–3.

39. Malandain D, Join-Lambert O, Auzou M, Cattoir V. Antimicrobial susceptibility and molecular mechanisms of acquired resistance in Actinotignum (Actinobaculum) schaalii isolated in patients with hidradenitis suppurativa. In: *26th European Conference on Clinical Microbiology and Infectious Diseases, Amsterdam, The Netherlands*; 2016.

40. Boyanova L, Mitev A, Gergova G, et al. High prevalence and resistance rates to antibiotics in anaerobic bacteria in specimens from patients with chronic balanitis. *Anaerobe.* 2012;18(4):414–416.

41. Dubreuil L, Odou MF. Anaerobic bacteria and antibiotics: What kind of unexpected resistance could I find in my laboratory tomorrow? *Anaerobe.* 2010;16(6):555–559.

42. Hunger RE, Laffitte E, Lauchli S, et al. Swiss Practice Recommendations for the Management of Hidradenitis Suppurativa/Acne Inversa. *Dermatology.* 2017;233(2-3):113–119.

43. Ingram JR, Collier F, Brown D, et al. British Association of Dermatologists guidelines for the management of hidradenitis suppurativa (acne inversa) 2018. *Br J Dermatol.* 2019;180(5):1009–1017.

44. Alikhan A, Sayed C, Alavi A, et al. North American clinical management guidelines for hidradenitis suppurativa: A publication from the United States and Canadian Hidradenitis Suppurativa Foundations: Part II: Topical, intralesional, and systemic medical management. *J Am Acad Dermatol.* 2019;81(1):91–101.

45. Magalhaes RF, Rivitti-Machado MC, Duarte GV, et al. Consensus on the treatment of hidradenitis suppurativa - Brazilian Society of Dermatology. *An Bras Dermatol.* 2019;94(2 Suppl 1):7–19.

46. Zouboulis CC, Bechara FG, Dickinson-Blok JL, et al. Hidradenitis suppurativa/acne inversa: a practical framework for treatment optimization - systematic review and recommendations from the HS ALLIANCE working group. *J Eur Acad Dermatol Venereol.* 2019; 33(1):19–31.

47. Société Française de Dermatologie. *Prise en charge de l'hidradénite suppurée*; 2019. accessed May, 2020.

48. Pearson-Stuttard J, Blundell S, Harris T, et al. Diabetes and infection: assessing the association with glycaemic control in population-based studies. *Lancet Diabetes Endocrinol.* 2016;4(2):148–158.

49. Bui TL, Silva-Hirschberg C, Torres J, Armstrong AW. Hidradenitis suppurativa and diabetes mellitus: A systematic review and meta-analysis. *J Am Acad Dermatol.* 2018;78(2):395–402.

50. Riverain-Gilet E, Guet-Revillet H, Jais J-P, et al. The surface microbiome of clinically unaffected skinfolds in hidradenitis suppurativa: a cross-sectional culture based and 16S ribosomal RNA gene amplicon sequencing study in 60 patients. *J Invest Dermatol.* 2020; [accepted for publication].

51. Bécherel P, Thomas M, Moreno J, et al. NSAIDs and pain management in HS: important risk of flares (a series of 62 cases). In: *9th Conference of the EHSF 2020, European Hidradenitis Suppurativa Foundation eV, 5-7 February, Athens, Greece*; 2020:C152.

52. Cooper EC, Curtis N, Cranswick N, Gwee A. Pristinamycin: old drug, new tricks? *J Antimicrob Chemother.* 2014;69(9):2319–2325.

53. Nightingale CH, Grant EM, Quintiliani R. Pharmacodynamics and pharmacokinetics of levofloxacin. *Chemotherapy.* 2000;46(Suppl 1): 6–14.

54. Stein GE, Goldstein EJ. Review of the in vitro activity and potential clinical efficacy of levofloxacin in the treatment of anaerobic infections. *Anaerobe.* 2003;9(2):75–81.

55. Behra-Miellet J, Dubreuil L, Jumas-Bilak E. Antianaerobic activity of moxifloxacin compared with that of ofloxacin, ciprofloxacin, clindamycin, metronidazole and beta-lactams. *Int J Antimicrob Agents.* 2002;20(5):366–374.

56. Mahé E, Morelon E, Lechaton S, et al. Cutaneous adverse events in renal transplant recipients receiving sirolimus-based therapy. *Transplantation.* 2005;79(4):476–482.

17

Non-Antibiotic and Non-Biologic Systemic Therapeutics

SURYA A. VEERABAGU AND TARANNUM JALEEL

Introduction

The pathogenesis of hidradenitis suppurativa (HS) remains to be fully elucidated. Genetic susceptibility along with hormonal fluctuations and immune dysregulation are all thought to contribute to HS development.[1] HS tends to occur in patients with comorbid conditions associated with hyperandrogenism, insulin resistance, and inflammation including acne vulgaris, hirsutism, diabetes, and polycystic ovary syndrome (PCOS). Utilizing multimodal treatment regimens including hormonal therapies (anti-androgens, anti-diabetics), systemic immunomodulators (oral retinoids), and immunosuppressants may alleviate HS symptoms and aid in recovery. This chapter discusses non-antibiotic and non-biologic systemic therapies for HS. Table 17.1 summarizes the mechanism of action, other indications, dosing regimen, contraindications, and adverse effects for the medications discussed in this chapter. Table 17.2 outlines the levels of evidence and recommendations regarding the use of these therapies according to the 2019 North American guidelines.

Hyperandrogenism and Hidradenitis Suppurativa

Small questionnaire-based studies conducted in the U.K. found that approximately 50% of women with HS report acute flares which are temporally related to menstruation.[45,46] In one cross-sectional study in the Netherlands, patients reported frequent changes in disease activity during pregnancy. Furthermore, improvement in HS symptoms during pregnancy was associated with a history of premenstrual disease flares.[45] These findings suggest that disease activity in women with HS may be strongly correlated with hormonal fluctuations.

The skin has the unique ability to synthesize androgens de novo from cholesterol in the epidermis and sebaceous glands.[47–49] However, the main source of androgens are the testes, ovaries, and adrenal glands. The circulating androgens, dehydroepiandrosterone (DHEA) and androstenedione, are converted into testosterone in sebocytes, sweat glands, and dermal papilla cells. In the skin, the enzyme 5α-reductase metabolizes testosterone into a more potent androgen, dihydrotestosterone (DHT). In comparison to testosterone, DHT binds to androgen receptors with 10 times higher affinity and with greater stability.[50–52] Androgen metabolism is depicted in Fig. 17.1.

In the skin, androgen receptors are primarily located in the dermal papillae, sebaceous epithelium, eccrine sweat epithelium, and, to a lesser degree, in basal epidermal cells and reticular dermal fibroblasts. They are also present in pilosebaceous duct keratinocytes and, to a lesser degree, in interfollicular keratinocytes, and could play a role in acne and HS via promotion of follicular hyperkeratinization.[53,54] According to the acne model, hyperproliferation of the infrainfundibular keratinocytes is one of the initial and most crucial events in the development of microcomedones, and is also characteristic of HS.[55] Infrainfundibular hyperkeratosis, hyperplasia of the follicular epithelium, and perifolliculitis lead to localized inflammation and precede follicular rupture in HS.[56,57] In one study, anti-androgens were shown to decrease follicular debris at the hair follicle, raising the possibility that androgens could play a role in hyperkeratinization. Additionally, increased 5α-reductase activity in infrainfundibular keratinocytes—as opposed to interfollicular epidermal cells—suggests that DHT could affect follicular keratinization; however, this remains to be fully explored.[58]

Androgens may also modulate the inflammatory milieu important in HS pathogenesis. It is postulated that Tumor Necrosis

TABLE 17.1 Mechanism of Action, Other Uses, Dosage, Relative and Absolute Contraindications, and Side Effects of Systemic Non-Antibiotic and Non-Biologic Therapeutics

Medication	Mechanism of Action	Other HS-related Indications	Dosing Regimen	Absolute Contraindications	Relative Contraindications	Adverse Effects
Combined Oral Contraceptives[2-5]	• Inhibit ovulation via inhibiting FSH and LH. • Increase SHBG.	• Acne vulgaris	Estrogen content <50 mcg/day PO. Avoid progestogen-only regimens.	• Pregnancy • Liver tumor • Active or history of breast or endometrial cancer • Ischemic/valvular heart disease • History of thromboembolic disorders • Smokers over age 35 • Migraines with aura • Valvular heart disease	• Uncontrolled HTN • Uncontrolled DM	• Bleeding • Nausea • Headaches • Abdominal cramping • Breast tenderness • Vaginal discharge • Decreased libido
Spironolactone[5-7]	• Aldosterone antagonist, K+ sparing diuretic. • Androgen antagonist. • Androgen biosynthesis inhibitor.	• Acne vulgaris • PCOS	25–50 mg/day titrate as needed to a dose of 50–200 mg/day, PO	• Addison disease • Serum Cr >4 mg/dL • Serum K+ >5 mmol/L • Concurrent use of potassium sparing diuretics • Pregnancy	• Uncontrolled DM • Respiratory or metabolic acidosis • Hepatic disease with biliary cirrhosis or ascites • Menstrual irregularity	• Arrythmia • Hyperkalemia • Hepatotoxicity • Renal failure • Gynecomastia
Finasteride[8-11]	• Inhibitor of type II 5α-reductase that decreases DHT.	• PCOS	2.5–10 mg/day PO	• Pregnancy	• Breast-feeding • Hepatic disease	• Impotence • Orthostatic hypotension • Decreased libido • Sexual dysfunction • Rhinitis • Prostate cancer • Depression and self-harm behavior • Infertility (rare reports post-marketing)
Metformin[12-15]	• Inhibit hepatic gluconeogenesis and the action of glucagon by inhibiting mGPD. • Increases glycolysis and peripheral glucose uptake. • Increases insulin sensitivity. • Promotes weight loss.	• Type 2 DM • PCOS	1500–2000 mg PO	• Renal or hepatic insufficiency • Acute hypoxia and acute cardiac disease • Acidemia (lactic acidosis/ metabolic acidosis)	• Iodinated contrast • Acute MI • Alcoholism • Pernicious anemia • Uncontrolled adrenal insufficiency, pituitary insufficiency, or hypothyroidism	• GI disturbance • Lactic acidosis • B12 deficiency
Liraglutide[16]	• GLP-1 analog. • Decreases glucagon release and gastric emptying. • Increases glucose-dependent insulin release and satiety.	• Type 2 DM • Weight reduction and maintenance in obese and overweight individuals	0.6–1.8 mg injection/day	• Certain types of thyroid cancer • Diabetic Ketoacidosis, Type 1 DM • Pregnancy • History of suicide attempts or active suicidal ideation	• Renal insufficiency • Gastroparesis • Cholelithiasis • Gallbladder disease • Hepatic disease • Breast-feeding • Pancreatitis	• Palpitations • Nausea • Vomiting • Cholecystitis • Pancreatitis • Renal failure • Suicidal ideation • Heart block

Drug	Mechanism	Indications	Dosing	Contraindications	Side effects
Oral Retinoids: Acitretin/ Isotretinoin[17-19]	• Activates nuclear receptors to produce anti-keratinizing, anti-inflammatory, and anti-proliferative effects in the skin.	• Acne vulgaris • Severe psoriasis	0.5–0.6 mg/kg/day PO	• Breast-feeding • Pregnancy • Acitretin should be avoided in women of childbearing age.	• Xerosis • Alopecia • Teratogenic • Pseudotumor cerebri • Tinnitus • Epistaxis • Hepatotoxicity • Hypertriglyceridemia • Dysglycemias • Visual disturbance • Hepatic insufficiency
Colchicine[20-25]	• Anti-inflammatory, disrupts microtubule polymerization. • Prevents activation, degranulation, and migration of neutrophils.	• Behçet	0.5 mg PO BID	• Both hepatic and renal insufficiency • Pregnancy • Myopathy	• Nausea • Diarrhea • Neutropenia • Infertility (rare) • Renal insufficiency • Hepatic insufficiency • Biliary obstruction • Bone marrow suppression
Methotrexate[26-29]	• Dihydrofolate reductase inhibitor that prevents conversion of folic acid into tetrahydrofolate, inhibiting DNA synthesis in the S-phase of the cell cycle. • Causes adenosine accumulation, inhibiting neutrophil chemotaxis.	• Psoriasis	Start: 15 mg/week with laboratory monitoring Dose adjustments: increase by 5 mg/week at week 8 if no response	• Severe renal insufficiency • Pregnancy • Breastfeeding • Blood disorders: blood marrow hypoplasia, leukopenia, thrombocytopenia, anemia • Alcoholism • Active tuberculosis	• Myelosuppression • Pulmonary toxicity • GI disorders • Hepatotoxicity • Lymphoma • Renal or hepatic insufficiency • Ascites • HIV/AIDS • GI disease • Radiation therapy
Dapsone[30-36]	• Inhibits bacterial dihydropteroate synthetase and synthesis of dihydrofolic acid. • Anti-inflammatory.	• Pyoderma gangrenosum • Dissecting cellulitis of the scalp • Acne vulgaris	Start at 25 mg daily and titrate to 100 mg PO BID	• G6PD deficiency • Agranulocytosis • Aplastic anemia	• Agranulocytosis • Methemoglobinemia • Cardiopulmonary disease • Renal or hepatic insufficiency • Allergy to sulfonamide antibiotics • Neuropathy
Prednisone[37-41]	• Inhibits synthesis of leukotrienes. • Diminishes production of proinflammatory cytokines. • Inhibits cytotoxic T-cell activation.	• Ankylosing spondylitis	10 mg/day PO	• Uncontrolled DM	• Hyperglycemia • Sleep disturbances • Psychomotor agitation • Avascular necrosis • Visual impairment • Warfarin use • DM • Infections • Peptic ulcers • Congestive heart failure • Recent MI • Glaucoma • Seizure disorder
Cyclosporine[42-44]	• Calcineurin inhibitor. • Inhibits T-lymphocytes.	• Refractory psoriasis	1–6 mg/kg/day	• Active infection	• Nephrotoxicity • HTN • Hyperlipidemia • Neurotoxicity • Gingival hyperplasia • Hirsutism • Renal insufficiency • Uncontrolled HTN • Asthma • Blood disorders: aplastic anemia

BID, Twice per day; Cr, creatinine; DHT, dihydrotestosterone; DM, diabetes mellitus; FSH, follicle stimulating hormone; G6PD, glucose 6 phosphate dehydrogenase; GI, gastrointestinal; GLP-1, glucagon like peptide-1; HTN, hypertension; K+, potassium; LH, luteinizing hormone; mGPD, mitochondrial glycerophosphate dehydrogenase; MI, myocardial infarction; PCOS, polycystic ovary syndrome; PO, per os (oral administration); SHBG, sex hormone binding globulin.

TABLE 17.2 Evidence Levels: Non-Antibiotic and Non-Biologic Systemic Therapeutics for Hidradenitis Suppurativa

Therapy Name	Evidence Level	Recommended Use
OCPs	A	Consider in female patients with no contraindications.
Spironolactone	C	Consider in female patients with no contraindications.
Finasteride	D	Not enough evidence to make a definitive conclusion.
Metformin	C	Strongly consider in patients with obesity, insulin resistance and/or PCOS.
Liraglutide	E	Not enough evidence to make a definitive conclusion.
Isotretinoin	C	Not enough evidence to make a definitive conclusion. Consider in patients with severe concomitant acne.
Acitretin	B	Consider in patients with recalcitrant HS with failure to respond to first-line therapy.
Colchicine	B	Consider in patients with refractory mild-moderate disease who can tolerate colchicine and minocycline combination therapy.
Methotrexate	C	Not enough evidence to make a definitive conclusion.
Dapsone	B	May be effective for select patients without contraindications.
Prednisone	C	Can be used as rescue therapy or bridge-therapy to other long-term treatment option.
Cyclosporine	E	Consider in patients with recalcitrant moderate to severe HS who have failed or are not candidates for standard therapy.

Evidence Levels:
A: At least one prospective, randomized, double-blind, controlled trial without major design flaws (in the authors' view).
B: Prospective clinical trials with 20 or more subjects; trials lacking adequate controls or another key facet of design that would normally be considered desirable.
C: Small trials with fewer than 20 subjects with specific design limitations, very large numbers of case reports (at least 20 cases in the literature), or retrospective analysis of data.
D: Series of greater than or equal to five patients reported to respond.
E: Anecdotal case reports individual case reports amounting to published experience of fever than five cases
HS, Hidradenitis suppurativa; *OCPs*, oral contraceptive pills; *PCOS*, polycystic ovary syndrome.

Factor alpha (TNF-α expression, interleukin (IL)-1β, and IL-17 are prominent inflammatory actors in HS.[59,60] Multiple independent studies have indicated increased IL-17 expression in HS lesions compared with control skin.[60–63] IL-17 is produced by T-helper-17 (Th17) cells, innate lymphoid cells, T cells, mast cells, and neutrophils.[64–66] IL-1β, IL-6, TGF-β, and IL-2, produced by innate immune cells, can further upregulate IL-17 production. Testosterone and DHT modulate TGF-β, IL-6, and TNF-α production,

indicating that there is a potential for these androgens to exacerbate HS lesions via the Th17 inflammatory pathway.[67,68] In a rat model, androgens were shown to exacerbate inflammatory responses resulting in delayed skin healing. Androgens specifically promote inflammation by enhancing local TNF-α expression of TLR stimulated macrophages, thereby inducing the release of proinflammatory cytokines. Androgen receptor signaling also upregulates TNF-α expression via other avenues, including increasing the inflammatory monocyte population via upregulation of CCR2, thereby enhancing monocyte chemotaxis.[69] Gilliver et al. conducted a study in which a 5α-reductase inhibitor administered to a rat model resulted in significantly decreased inflammatory markers such as TNF-α and IL-6 in the skin and markedly accelerated wound healing.[67]

Studies have demonstrated improvement in HS disease activity with the use of both antiandrogens (e.g., finasteride, flutamide, spironolactone) and oral contraceptive pills (OCPs).[70–75] While the exact mechanism remains unclear, clinical evidence suggests that blocking the androgenic pathway is effective in management and will be discussed below in further detail.

Oral Contraceptives

Combined OCPs contain both progesterone and estrogen and act primarily by preventing ovulation through the inhibition of follicular stimulating hormone (FSH) and luteinizing hormone (LH).[76] Oral estrogens produce an anti-androgenic effect by increasing the concentration of circulating sex hormone binding globulin (SHBG). SHBG binds more avidly to androgens than estrogens, rendering androgens less bioavailable to interact with the androgen receptor as demonstrated in Fig. 17.2.[77–79]

Several studies have evaluated the use of OCPs in HS. One study evaluated ethinyl estradiol/cyproterone (CPA) versus ethinyl estradiol/norgestrel in women with HS. There was no clinically significant difference as evaluated by visual analogue scales (VAS) and disease activity scores in response to the two treatments among the 18 patients who completed the trial, but there was significant improvement overall in comparison to baseline HS status. Seven (39%) patients' HS lesions completely cleared while five (28%) patients improved, four (22%) remain unchanged, and two (11%) patients' conditions deteriorated.[73] In another case series evaluating a combination treatment of ethinyl estradiol and CPA, all 4 individuals exhibited improvement after 3 to 7 months of treatment.[72] In both studies, free androgen index, defined as the ratio of total testosterone divided by SHBG, was decreased in response to treatment, which may explain patients' HS improvement.[72,73]

While these two studies show some promise for OCPs, more randomized-controlled studies must be conducted to better understand the potential benefits of OCPs. Small sample sizes, variable outcome measures and methods, and reporting bias limit the evidence available to make fully informed recommendations for OCPs at this time. The 2019 North American HS management guidelines suggest OCP usage as monotherapy for mild to moderate HS or in combination with other agents for more severe disease for appropriate female patients, such as those with HS flares around menses or those with PCOS. When selecting an OCP, progestogen-only regimens should be avoided as anecdotal concerns suggest that they may worsen HS.[80] The 2015 European guidelines suggest antiandrogen therapy such as CPA in female patients with menstrual abnormalities, signs of hyperandrogenism, or upper-normal or high serum levels of DHEA, androstenedione, and/or SHBG.[81] A comparison of HS management guidelines

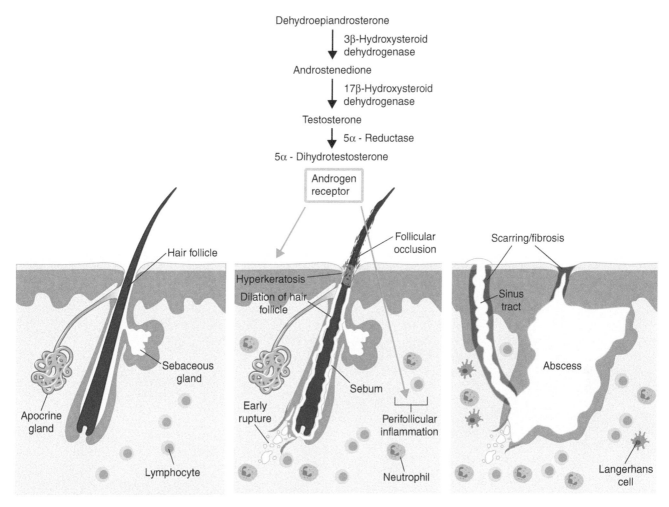

• **Fig. 17.1** Androgen Metabolism in the Skin. The skin contains all the necessary substrates and enzymes to synthesize androgens. Additionally, the skin can synthesize androgens de novo from cholesterol. These androgens contribute to follicular hyperkeratosis and inflammation.

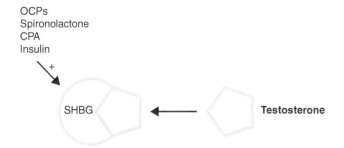

• **Fig. 17.2** Sex Hormone Binding Globulin Mechanism. Sex hormone binding globulin (SHBG) binds androgens rendering them unable to bind to the androgen receptor. Oral contraceptives, spironolactone, cyproterone acetate, and insulin all increase SHBG, decreasing bioavailable testosterone. *OCPs*, Oral contraceptive pills.

published by different international expert organizations can be found in Chapter 14.

Spironolactone

Spironolactone is another antiandrogen used in HS treatment. It is an aldosterone antagonist and competitively inhibits active sodium transport.[82] While originally used for its potassium-sparing diuretic effects, spironolactone is commonly used off-label for skin conditions such as acne vulgaris due to its anti-androgenic properties.[83]

The anti-androgenic properties of spironolactone are most likely attributable to the structural similarities between the mineralocorticoid and androgen receptors. Although the exact mechanism of its anti-androgenic effects are unknown, spironolactone inhibits the activity of 5α-reductase in vitro, decreasing the conversion of testosterone to DHT.[84] It also increases the level of SHBG, depleting bioavailable testosterone.[47,85] An active metabolite of spironolactone also inhibits 17α-hydroxylase and desmolase, two enzymes necessary for adrenal and gonadal androgen synthesis.[82,86,87] Spironolactone's therapeutic effects in skin could be due to inhibition of 17α-hydroxylase within the cytoplasm of sebocytes and keratinocytes, although this has not been directly demonstrated.[47] Spironolactone also modulates the deposition of extracellular matrix in human skin. Spironolactone's capacity as a potential scar and keloid treatment is under investigation; preliminary results have revealed decreased collagen expression in spironolactone-treated skin.[88]

A single center retrospective study of 67 female HS patients treated with spironolactone from 2000 to 2017 exhibited promising results. The study showed statistically significant improvement in the Numeric Rating Scale (NRS)-pain score (-1.5, $P = .01$), lesion count (-1.3, $P = .02$), and the Hidradenitis Suppurativa-Physicians Global Assessment (HS-PGA) score (-0.6, $P < .001$). The average daily spironolactone dose was 75 mg (range: 25 to 200 mg) and the average duration of treatment was 7.1 months (range: 0 to 28 months). There was no difference in change in NRS-pain score, lesion counts, or HS-PGA score between subjects who received less than 75 mg versus those who received greater than 100 mg daily. A sub-analysis of groups stratified by race, Body Mass Index (BMI), comorbidities, and concomitant HS treatments did not show any significant differences in treatment response.[89]

Two smaller retrospective studies evaluated a total of 46 patients on spironolactone with 7 patients on concurrent OCPs and 17 patients on concurrent metformin. Overall, 26/46 (57%) exhibited clinical improvement.[74,90] Another retrospective study reviewed 31 HS patients on different combination therapies. All six patients with mild and moderate disease on combinations containing spironolactone (combined with either isotretinoin or adalimumab) exhibited clinical improvement.[91] Finally, another retrospective review with 64 patients found that patient response rate to antiandrogen therapy (including Diane-35 (ethinyl estradiol 35 μg and CPA 2 mg), CPA, spironolactone, and OCPs), was significantly superior to oral antibiotics (55% vs. 26%, respectively).[92]

Spironolactone is a potent therapeutic agent to consider for patients suffering from HS. There is an ongoing investigation regarding the optimal dosage of spironolactone in the treatment of HS.[93] Similar to OCPs, spironolactone should be considered as monotherapy for appropriate female patients (such as those with HS flares around menses or those with PCOS) with moderate HS or in combination with other agents for more severe disease.[80,94]

Finasteride

There are two types of 5α-reductase enzymes; type I 5α-reductase is found in both hair follicles and apocrine glands, whereas type II 5α-reductase is found only in hair follicles.[9,47,95] Finasteride inhibits type II 5α-reductase while dutasteride inhibits both type I and type II.[47] While the exact mechanism of finasteride's effects in HS is unknown, it is hypothesized that finasteride modulates HS disease activity by reducing the concentration of hair follicle DHT levels.[71]

Khandalavala et al. conducted a systematic review in 2016 which summarized 5 publications detailing 13 individual cases of HS treated with finasteride. Notably, the cases included four male and nine female patients. Dosages ranged from 2.5 to 10 mg daily. It was effective for both men and women, especially those with metabolic or hormonal alterations present such as PCOS, metabolic syndrome, obesity, and precocious puberty. Of the 13 cases, 3 (23%) patients had complete responses and 10 (77%) patients experienced partial responses. Due to recurrence of symptoms upon cessation of finasteride therapy, some patients used finasteride continuously or as needed for up to 6 years. Khandalavala et al. suggested that finasteride could be used as a monotherapy or additional therapy for advanced HS as it could increase time between flares.[8] In one case series of five pre-pubescent patients, including one male patient, finasteride treatment decreased the frequency and intensity of flares for all patients.[96]

Similar to other hormonal modulators finasteride should be considered as monotherapy for appropriate female patients (such as those with HS flares around menses or those with PCOS) with moderate HS or in combination with other agents for more severe disease.[80] There is not enough conclusive evidence at this time to

make a distinction between finasteride's efficacy in men compared to women. Therefore, finasteride could be considered for males who have other stigmata of hyperandrogenism such as androgenetic alopecia.

Insulin Resistance and Obesity

HS tends to occur in patients with comorbid medical conditions associated with insulin resistance such as diabetes and PCOS.[97] A case control study in Spain demonstrated that patients with HS were found to have elevated levels of insulin resistance, even when controlling for age, gender, and BMI.[98] Elevated insulin levels affect the levels of circulating insulin growth factor-1 (IGF-1) and insulin growth factor binding protein (IGFBP-3), which regulate keratinocyte proliferation and apoptosis, respectively. Typically these two factors are in balance, however, in insulin resistant states, IGF-1 increases and IGFBP-3 decreases, causing increased keratinocyte proliferation and decreased keratinocyte apoptosis, amplifying the likelihood of follicular hyperkeratinization.[99–105] Increased IGF-1 also increases levels of androgens, growth hormone, and glucocorticoids through various pathways. Elevated androgens in turn increase IGF-1, and promote insulin resistance in peripheral tissues further propagating this cycle.[104] This pathway is depicted in Fig. 17.3 below.

Burghen et al. compared serum insulin and androgen levels in obese women with PCOS and control obese women. A positive correlation was found between elevated insulin levels and increased androgen levels in both groups of women.[106] Insulin can both increase circulating androgens and decrease serum SHBG resulting in increased free serum testosterone levels. Increased insulin influences pituitary release of gonadotrophins, increasing ovarian androgen production.[107] Notably, abnormally high insulin states decrease insulin responses in the liver and muscles but increase insulin-dependent ovarian androgen production.[108] It is unclear whether the reverse is possible—that hyperandrogenism can cause hyperinsulinemia. Few studies have demonstrated that androgen reduction or blockade resulted in improved insulin sensitivity.[109]

Studies have found a correlation between the severity of HS and increased BMI.[110,111] The rate of long-term self-reported remission, defined as no inflammatory boils in the last 6 months, is lower in obese patients.[112] Obesity may be strongly associated with HS and other autoimmune disorders because adipose tissue produces pro-inflammatory mediators, including IL-6, TNF-α, inducible nitric oxide synthase, and TGF-β1.[113,114] In addition, obesity causes mechanical stress, increased moisture, and increased friction in skin folds, which can promote follicular hyperkeratinization and occlusion, key instigating factors of HS pathogenesis.[115–117]

Anti-Diabetic Medications

Given the interconnections between obesity, hyperinsulinemia, and HS, medications such as metformin and liraglutide have been explored for therapeutic potential.

Metformin

Metformin is the first-line oral therapeutic agent for type 2 diabetes and prediabetes. Although the Food and Drug Administration has yet to approve it for PCOS, metformin is one of the most commonly prescribed medications for this indication.[13] Metformin decreases insulin levels in the body resulting in decreased androgen levels in PCOS patients. Given the known association between HS

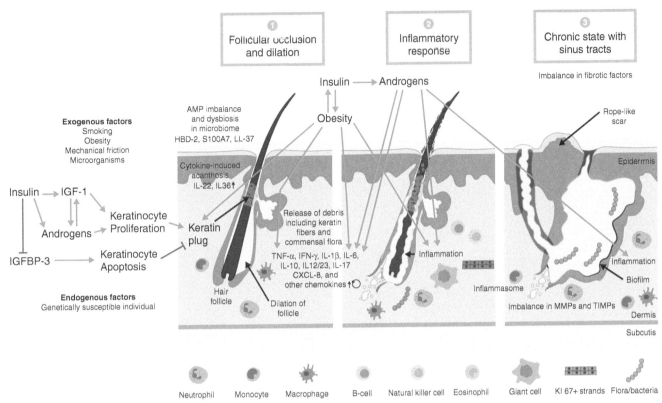

• **Fig. 17.3** Elevated insulin levels increase the levels of circulating insulin growth factor-1 *(IGF-1)* and decrease insulin growth factor binding protein *(IGFBP-3)*, which regulate keratinocyte proliferation and apoptosis, respectively. This promotes follicle plugging. Additionally, increased IGF-1 increases androgens. Increased insulin and insulin resistance may increase risk of obesity, which can affect hidradenitis suppurativa *(HS)* as excessive fat can secrete inflammatory markers like interleukin (IL)-6, TNF-α, inducible nitric oxide synthase, and TGF-β1. (Burghen GA, Givens JR, Kitabchi AE. Correlation of hyperandrogenism with hyperinsulinism in polycystic ovarian disease. *J Clin Endocrinol Metab.* 1980;50[1]:113–116. https://doi.org/10.1210/jcem-50-1-113 [web archive link]; Kahn BB, Flier JS. Obesity and insulin resistance. *J Clin Invest.* 2000;106[4]:473–481.)

and PCOS, HS patients exhibiting symptoms of androgen excess are recommended to be screened for PCOS.[97] Unlike other diabetes medications, metformin does not usually cause hypoglycemia as it functions to increase end-organ insulin sensitivity and does not increase insulin release. Metformin specifically inhibits mitochondrial glycerophosphate dehydrogenase (mGPD) which in turn prevents hepatic gluconeogenesis and decreases glucagon release. Metformin also increases insulin sensitivity by promoting peripheral glucose uptake and utilization while decreasing gastrointestinal glucose absorption.[14]

In addition to attenuating HS patients' insulin resistance, metformin promotes weight loss in diabetic and nondiabetic patients alike. While the mechanism behind the weight reduction remains controversial, some studies indicate that metformin decreases total caloric intake by decreasing production of appetite-inducing peptides such as neuropeptide-Y and agouti-related protein (AgRP) in the hypothalamus.[118,119] Metformin decreases gastrointestinal absorption of glucose, further curbing caloric intake. Metformin also improves leptin sensitivity as evidenced by decreased circulating leptin and increased leptin receptor expression in rat models.[118,120] Leptin is known to decrease appetite, and leptin resistance can cause obesity.[121]

Small studies, including case reports, have identified metformin as a possible therapeutic agent in HS.[122,123] In a retrospective study of 53 HS patients, 36 (68%) had subjective clinical response;

response to metformin was independent of concomitant insulin resistance.[124] Verdolini et al. reported 25 patients, majority of whom were female and overweight, treated with metformin 1000 to 1500 mg/day for 6 months. Of the 25 patients, 18 (72%) had a significant average reduction of Sartorius score of 12.7 and 16 (64%) patients also had a significant improvement in DLQI score of 7.6. Diabetic patients who had HS and had been previously treated with metformin were excluded from the study. Patients did not experience any side effects of hypoglycemia, and glucose remained within the normal range on blood tests.[125]

Metformin may be considered as monotherapy or adjunct therapy for patients with concomitant diabetes mellitus and females with PCOS and/or pregnancy.[80,126]

Liraglutide

Liraglutide is a glucagon-like-peptide (GLP-1) receptor agonist and is typically added to metformin for treatment in diabetic patients if weight loss is desired. GLP-1 stimulates glucose-dependent insulin secretion, inhibits glucagon secretion, slows gastric emptying, and decreases appetite.[16] When studied in patients with both diabetes and psoriasis, liraglutide improved disease activity as demonstrated by Psoriasis Area and Severity Index (PASI) and DLQI scores.[127] However, this result has not been reproduced by placebo-controlled trials in glucose tolerant patients.[128] In patients with both diabetes and psoriasis, proinflammatory markers in psoriatic lesions, including IL-17, TNF-α, and nuclear factor-κB, have been found to be decreased after liraglutide treatment.[127]

There are few studies describing liraglutide's efficacy in HS. One case report detailed a 31-year-old female smoker with Hurley stage II disease who had significant improvement on liraglutide after previously failing rifampicin-clindamycin, metformin, spironolactone, adalimumab, etanercept, and dapsone. She had a 6.5-kg weight loss after 8 weeks of liraglutide therapy.[129] Another report detailed a 19-year-old woman with an 8-year history of advanced HS who was successfully treated with a combined regimen of metformin, liraglutide, dapsone, and finasteride.[123] Further studies are needed to evaluate therapeutic efficacy of liraglutide but it could be considered as adjunct therapy in patients who are obese and/or have findings of insulin resistance.[80]

Immune System Regulation

It is suggested that in a genetically predisposed individual, follicular occlusion and rupture leads to a cycle of chronic inflammation, as evidenced by the upregulation of innate and adaptive immune cells in the lesional and perilesional skin of HS patients.[59,60] A systematic review presented multiple studies reporting elevated levels of cytokines in the skin of HS patients including, but not limited to, Interferon gamma IFN-γ, TNF-α, TNF-β, IL-1β, IL-8, IL-17A, and IL-32, IL-36/IL-36α/IL-36/IL-36γ.[130–133] Elevated levels of inflammatory mediators in the serum of HS patients have been reported as well including, but not limited to, IL-1β, IL-6, IL-8, IL-10, and IL-17.[134,135]

Treatment of HS patients with medications that can modulate follicular keratinization or immune response such as oral retinoids, colchicine, methotrexate, cyclosporine, and dapsone have been reported with varying therapeutic efficacy.

Oral Retinoids

Oral retinoids are anti-keratinizing, anti-inflammatory, and anti-proliferative.[18] They inhibit IL-6-driven induction of Th17 cells via regulation of TGF-β dependent immune responses, thereby decreasing inflammation.[136] In addition, retinoids can impede neutrophil superoxide anion production and lysosomal enzyme release while not having a significant effect on chemotaxis.[133,137] One study reported a high prevalence of hyper-homocystinemia in patients with HS in comparison to healthy controls, with a significant correlation between plasma levels of homocysteine and disease severity using Sartorius score.[138] Isotretinoin has demonstrated homocysteine reduction in acne patients with corresponding symptomatic relief,[139] and could also correspond to alleviating HS symptoms in a similar process.

Data for the use of isotretinoin has been mixed. Studies with isotretinoin dosages ranging from 0.5 to 1.2 mg/kg/day (range 4 to 10 months) reported improvement of symptoms in 15.9% to 68% of patients. While not all studies reported Hurley stages and disease severity, 99 out of 273 (36.3%) patients improved, with better responses in patients with mild HS.[80,140–147] Another study reported a significant association between previous history of a pilonidal cyst and response to isotretinoin in HS.[140]

Of note, some cases in the literature suggest that isotretinoin could worsen HS. In one cohort of 8 patients with severe acne treated with isotretinoin, 4 (50%) patients developed a flare of HS at week 10 of treatment and the rest developed it at different time points (4 to 12 weeks). Half of the patients had no prior history of HS.[148] Another retrospective study reported that 5/6 patients on isotretinoin had worsening of their HS, and 1/6 had no change.[149] One study from 2011 compared biopsies of HS lesions and showed a reduction or absence of sebaceous glands in comparison with normal skin in patients with HS.[150] Isotretinoin decreases the size and action of sebaceous glands, which results in efficacy in the treatment of acne; however, it is a potential explanation for its limited therapeutic ability in HS as sebaceous glands have been shown to be reduced in fully evolved HS lesions.[148,151] Given the variable data in the literature at this time, isotretinoin may be considered in patients with severe concomitant acne.[80]

Acitretin is often considered to be superior to isotretinoin in treatment of HS; however, comparative data is lacking. Three retrospective studies with a total of 31 patients report clinical improvement in 75% to 100% of patients on acitretin monotherapy or as combination therapy.[146,152,153] Matusiak et al. conducted a prospective study in which all nine patients on an average daily dose of 0.56 mg/kg acitretin monotherapy for 9 months achieved significant improvement or complete remission. However, it should be noted that the study began with 17 patients and 8 (47%) patients dropped out due to reasons such as lack of clinical effectiveness, visual disturbance, alopecia, and retinoid-induced dermatitis.[154] There have also been reported cases of HS flare with acitretin.[155]

More studies are needed to determine the therapeutic efficacy of oral retinoids for HS and to determine whether there are specific clinical phenotypes that are more likely to be responsive as well as the optimal setting for their use, including as monotherapy versus combination therapy.

Systemic Immunomodulators

Colchicine

Colchicine is an immunomodulator that prevents the release of inflammatory glycoproteins from phagocytes, decreases phagocytosis, and disrupts production, intracellular transport, and secretion of cytokines/leukotrienes, especially IL-1β in lymphocytes.[23] Through this mechanism, it decreases neutrophil chemotaxis and neutrophil adhesion molecules. Within neutrophils, colchicine binds tubulin, dampening neutrophil motility.[23] Furthermore, colchicine disrupts mitotic spindle formation in leukocytes, preventing replication past metaphase.[24]

In one prospective pilot study, 20 patients with a wide range of disease activity were treated with combination therapy with colchicine 0.5 mg twice daily and minocycline 100 mg daily for 6 months, followed by a maintenance regimen of colchicine 0.5 mg twice daily for 3 months. Treatment was associated with a marked improvement in PGA, Hurley stage, and DLQI scores starting at 3 months and improving substantially over the next 6 months. Additionally, patients reported decreased drainage and pain.[156] Colchicine monotherapy has not been supported by the literature. A prospective single-arm study reported a lack of clinical response among eight patients who were treated with colchicine monotherapy at a dose of 0.5 mg twice daily for 4 months.[157] Larger prospective studies are needed to evaluate colchicine's therapeutic benefit. Proper dosage and monotherapy versus adjunct therapy also need to be assessed.

Methotrexate

Methotrexate, another systemic immunomodulator, is an antimetabolite analog of folic acid that inactivates dihydrofolate reductase, an enzyme necessary for nucleotide synthesis. Methotrexate reduces inflammation by inhibiting T-lymphocyte proliferation, and may also downregulate neutrophil chemotaxis.[27] In studies of psoriatic and rheumatoid arthritis patients, methotrexate was shown to decrease the major proinflammatory markers IL-17 and nuclear factor-κB.[158–160] While these effects have not yet been demonstrated in HS, they have been used as justification for the initial evaluation of methotrexate in HS patients. In another retrospective study analyzing patients with HS (3/3) or concomitant HS and pyoderma gangrenosum (3/3) on infliximab with human anti-chimeric antibodies, 6/8 were placed on methotrexate, which allowed patients to remain on infliximab for at least 7 more months with clinical improvement.[161]

Savage et al. conducted a retrospective study of 15 HS patients; 7 were treated with methotrexate alone and 8 treated with methotrexate in combination with biologic agents (adalimumab, infliximab, or ustekinumab). Patients were on an average cumulative dose of 520.1 mg and duration of treatment of 11.7 months, and all failed to demonstrate reductions in HS-PGA, nodule count, and abscess count.[162] Two case reports described clinical improvement after treatment with methotrexate in combination with adalimumab/infliximab in patients with concomitant SAPHO (synovitis, acne, pustulosis, hyperostosis, and osteitis) syndrome and HS.[163,164] In one case series, three patients with recalcitrant HS were treated with methotrexate monotherapy at doses ranging from 12.5 to 15.0 mg weekly for 6 to 24 months without benefit.[165] Larger prospective studies are needed before any conclusion can be made regarding the utility of methotrexate in the management of HS. Overall, the available limited evidence at this time does not support the use of methotrexate in the treatment of HS.[80,126]

Dapsone

Dapsone is both an antimicrobial and antiinflammatory agent. Its antibacterial properties derive from its inhibition of dihydropteroate synthetase, an enzyme necessary for bacterial replication. Dapsone suppresses the myeloperoxidase-peroxide halide-mediated cytotoxic system, a component of the neutrophil respiratory burst that normally induces chemotactic migration of neutrophils.[33] Dapsone also inhibits β-2 integrin-mediated adherence of neutrophils.[34] Lastly, it protects cells from neutrophil-mediated injury by inhibiting production of toxic oxygen-derived radicals.[166,167]

Yazdanyar et al. described the treatment of 24 patients with dapsone 50 to 200 mg daily and reported clinically significant improvement as measured by global physician assessment in 6 (25%) of the patients and slight improvement in 3 patients (12.5%).[168] Kaur and Lewis reported clinical improvement in a case series of five patients with refractory HS who were treated with dapsone 50 to 150 mg daily. Patients were treated initially for 8 weeks; however, discontinuation or dose-reduction of dapsone led to immediate relapse of HS symptoms. Median duration to follow up was 24 months and up to that point all patients had exhibited continued improvement while remaining on dapsone.[169] Another study in Germany described five patients with HS who experienced complete resolution of their symptoms at 2 to 4 weeks after initiation of dapsone therapy.[170] Another study described 16/25 (64%) patients with recalcitrant HS on 50 to 150 mg dapsone daily experiencing clinical improvement.[171] Lastly, two additional case reports of patients with severe refractory HS treated with dapsone in combination with other immunosuppressants described significant improvement.[172,173] While these initial reports are promising, prospective randomized-controlled trials are needed.

Overall, dapsone may be effective for a minority of patients with Hurley stage 1 to 2 as long-term maintenance.[80,81,94]

Immunosuppressants as Bridge Therapy

Prednisone

Prednisone is a well-known glucocorticoid that is a broad immunosuppressant. It blocks the synthesis of leukotrienes, diminishes the production of proinflammatory cytokines such as IL-1, and inhibits cytotoxic T-cell activation. Steroids and other immunosuppressive agents, such as methotrexate, have also been used to suppress antibody formation against biologic agents.[174]

In one retrospective study, low-dose systemic corticosteroids were used in combination with other medical therapies such as rifampin, clindamycin, acitretin, dapsone, doxycycline, isotretinoin, and adalimumab in 13 patients with recalcitrant HS. The patients received prednisone 10 mg per day and assessments were done at 2- and 4-week intervals. After 4 to 12 weeks of therapy, five (38%) patients' HS completely resolved and six (46%) patients had partial responses. Three (23%) patients continued on low-dose prednisone for more than 6 months. Patients experienced side effects such as hyperglycemia, sleep disturbance, and mild psychomotor agitation.[37] Prednisone can be considered as rescue therapy for flares or as a bridge therapy to a more long-term treatment.[80]

Cyclosporine

Cyclosporine has limited data in the literature as a treatment for HS. As a calcineurin inhibitor, it blocks lymphocytes in the G0 or G1 phase of the cell cycle and preferentially inhibits T-lymphocytes and T-helper cells. Cyclosporine inhibits lymphokine production and release.[42] More specifically, the IL-12/IL-23 proinflammatory pathway, found to be elevated in HS and a multitude of other autoimmune diseases, promotes differentiation of Th17 toward producing pro-inflammatory cytokines such as TNF-β, granulocyte-macrophage colony-stimulating factor (GM-CSF), IL-17A, and IL-22.[175,176] Cyclosporine has been shown to inhibit pro-inflammatory Th17 polarization, differentiation, and activation. In addition, corticosteroid-resistant human Th17 cells are attenuated by cyclosporine as demonstrated in patients with steroid-refractory uveitis and steroid-resistant asthma.[177–181]

Case reports with a total of five patients on cyclosporine at doses ranging from 2 to 6 mg/kg/day described notable clinical improvement in all patients.[182–185] Of note, in one patient who developed HS after renal transplantation, remission of HS occurred after switching immunosuppressant therapy from cyclosporine to oral tacrolimus.[186] More studies are needed to evaluate cyclosporine's effects in HS. At this time, cyclosporine may be considered in patients with recalcitrant HS who have failed standard treatment regimens.[80,81,187]

Conclusions

There are numerous potential targets for HS therapy. Given the absence of high-level evidence to support many of the therapies that are currently in clinical use, treatments should be individualized based on a patient's comorbidities and disease severity. Although the pathogenesis of HS remains to be fully elucidated, this chapter details the possible mechanisms by which hyperandrogenism, insulin resistance, and dysregulated inflammation contribute to disease activity. Current treatment approaches target the pathways thought to be important in the development and

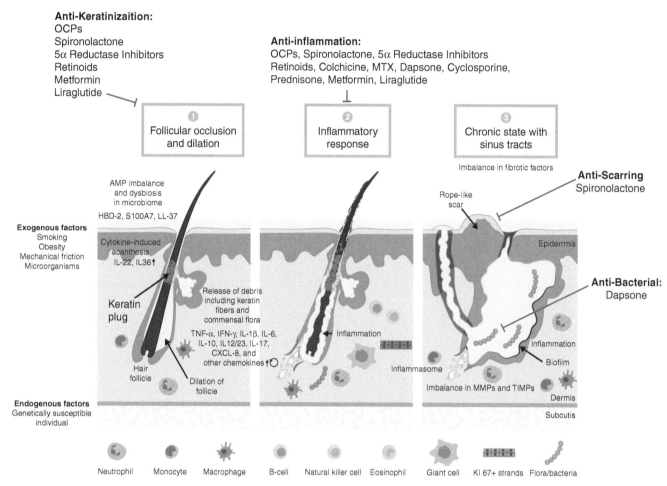

Anti-Keratinizaition:
OCPs
Spironolactone
5α Reductase Inhibitors
Retinoids
Metformin
Liraglutide

Anti-inflammation:
OCPs, Spironolactone, 5α Reductase Inhibitors
Retinoids, Colchicine, MTX, Dapsone, Cyclosporine,
Prednisone, Metformin, Liraglutide

① Follicular occlusion and dilation

② Inflammatory response

③ Chronic state with sinus tracts

Imbalance in fibrotic factors

Anti-Scarring
Spironolactone

Anti-Bacterial:
Dapsone

AMP imbalance
and dysbiosis
in microbiome
HBD-2, S100A7, LL-37

Exogenous factors
Smoking
Obesity
Mechanical friction
Microorganisms

Cytokine-induced
acanthosis
IL-22, IL36↑

Keratin
plug

Release of debris
including keratin
fibers and
commensal flora

Rope-like
scar

Epiderrmis

TNF-α, IFN-γ, IL-1β, IL-6,
IL-10, IL12/23, IL-17,
CXCL-8, and
other chemokines↑○

Inflammation

Inflammation

Biofilm

Hair
follicle

Dilation of
follicle

Inflammasome

Inflammation

Endogenous factors
Genetically susceptible
individual

Imbalance in MMPs and TIMPs

Dermis

Subcutis

Neutrophil Monocyte Macrophage B-cell Natural killer cell Eosinophil Giant cell KI 67+ strands Flora/bacteria

• **Fig. 17.4** Non-Antibiotic and Non-Biologic Systemic Therapeutics. Direct antikeratinizing medications include oral contraceptives *(OCPs)*, spironolactone, retinoids, 5-α reductase inhibitors, and those with indirect effects via the insulin pathway include metformin and liraglutide. Retinoids, colchicine, *MTX*, dapsone, cyclosporine, and prednisone all directly decrease inflammation. Metformin and liraglutide decrease inflammation due to indirect actions via aiding weight loss, which can potentially result in a decrease of adipocytokines. Dapsone has both antibacterial and antiinflammatory effects.

propagation of HS symptomatology (Fig. 17.4). Most therapies have yet to be evaluated with high-quality clinical trials. While data is primarily limited to case reports, retrospective case series, and small prospective trials, promising results have nonetheless been reported for several of the therapies discussed in this chapter.

References

1. Vekic DA, Frew J, Cains GD. Hidradenitis suppurativa, a review of pathogenesis, associations and management. Part 1. *Australas J Dermatol.* 2018;59(4):267–277. https://doi.org/10.1111/ajd.12770.
2. Brown EJ, Deshmukh P, Antell K. Contraception Update: Oral Contraception. *FP Essent.* 2017;462:11–19.
3. Cooper DB, Mahdy H. *Oral Contraceptive Pills.* In: *StatPearls.* StatPearls Publishing; 2019. http://www.ncbi.nlm.nih.gov/books/NBK430882/. Accessed 5 January 2020.
4. Committee on Gynecologic Practice. ACOG Committee Opinion Number 540: Risk of venous thromboembolism among users of drospirenone-containing oral contraceptive pills. *Obstet Gynecol.* 2012;120(5):1239–1242. https://doi.org/10.1097/aog.0b013e318277c93b.
5. Zaenglein AL, Pathy AL, Schlosser BJ, et al. Guidelines of care for the management of acne vulgaris. *J Am Acad Dermatol.* 2016;74(5):945–973.e33. https://doi.org/10.1016/j.jaad.2015.12.037.
6. Aldactone (spironolactone) dose, indications, adverse effects, interactions... from PDR.net. Accessed April 21, 2020. https://www.pdr.net/drug-summary/Aldactone-spironolactone-978.2934.
7. Barrionuevo P, Nabhan M, Altayar O, et al. Treatment Options for Hirsutism: A Systematic Review and Network Meta-Analysis. *J Clin Endocrinol Metab.* 2018;103(4):1258–1264. https://doi.org/10.1210/jc.2017-02052.
8. Khandalavala BN, Do MV. Finasteride in Hidradenitis Suppurativa. *J Clin Aesthet Dermatol.* 2016;9(6):44–50.
9. Propecia (finasteride) dose, indications, adverse effects, interactions... from PDR.net. Accessed April 21, 2020. https://www.pdr.net/drug-summary/Propecia-finasteride-378.609.
10. Welk B, McArthur E, Ordon M, et al. Association of Suicidality and Depression With 5α-Reductase Inhibitors. *JAMA Intern Med.* 2017;177(5):683–691. https://doi.org/10.1001/jamainternmed.2017.0089.
11. Farrell AM, Randall VA, Vafaee T, Dawber RP. Finasteride as a therapy for hidradenitis suppurativa. *Br J Dermatol.* 1999;141(6):1138–1139. https://doi.org/10.1046/j.1365-2133.1999.03224.x.

12. Metformin for treatment of the polycystic ovary syndrome—UpTo-Date. Accessed January 10, 2020. https://www.uptodate.com/contents/metformin-for-treatment-of-the-polycystic-ovary-syndrome?search=metformin&source=search_result&selectedTitle=4~148&usage_type=default&display_rank=3#H5.

13. Sam S, Ehrmann DA. Metformin therapy for the reproductive and metabolic consequences of polycystic ovary syndrome. *Diabetologia.* 2017;60(9):1656–1661. https://doi.org/10.1007/s00125-017-4306-3.

14. Rena G, Hardie DG, Pearson ER. The mechanisms of action of metformin. *Diabetologia.* 2017;60(9):1577–1585. https://doi.org/10.1007/s00125-017-4342-z.

15. Fortamet (metformin hydrochloride) dose, indications, adverse effects, interactions... from PDR.net. Accessed July 6, 2020. https://www.pdr.net/drug-summary/Fortamet-metformin-hydrochloride-1924.

16. Victoza (liraglutide) dose, indications, adverse effects, interactions... from PDR.net. Accessed April 21, 2020. https://www.pdr.net/drug-summary/Victoza-liraglutide-459.5943.

17. Ortiz NEG, Nijhawan RI, Weinberg JM. Acitretin. *Dermatol Ther.* 2013;26(5):390–399. https://doi.org/10.1111/dth.12086.

18. Zouboulis CC, Korge B, Akamatsu H, et al. Effects of 13-cis-retinoic acid, all-trans-retinoic acid, and acitretin on the proliferation, lipid synthesis and keratin expression of cultured human sebocytes in vitro. *J Invest Dermatol.* 1991;96(5):792–797. https://doi.org/10.1111/1523-1747.ep12471782.

19. Zito PM, Mazzoni T. *Acitretin.* In: *StatPearls.* StatPearls Publishing; 2019. http://www.ncbi.nlm.nih.gov/books/NBK519571/. Accessed 3 January 2020.

20. Dalbeth N, Lauterio TJ, Wolfe HR. Mechanism of action of colchicine in the treatment of gout. *Clin Ther.* 2014;36(10):1465–1479. https://doi.org/10.1016/j.clinthera.2014.07.017.

21. Colcrys (colchicine) dose, indications, adverse effects, interactions... from PDR.net. Accessed April 21, 2020. https://www.pdr.net/drug-summary/Colcrys-colchicine-592.

22. Cocco G, Chu DCC, Pandolfi S. Colchicine in clinical medicine. A guide for internists. *Eur J Intern Med.* 2010;21(6):503–508. https://doi.org/10.1016/j.ejim.2010.09.010.

23. Stack JR, Ryan J, McCarthy GM. Colchicine: New Insights to an Old Drug. *Am J Ther.* 2015;22(5):e151–e157. Published online 2015 https://doi.org/10.1097/01.mjt.0000433937.07244.e1.

24. Hastie SB. Interactions of colchicine with tubulin. *Pharmacol Ther.* 1991;51(3):377–401. https://doi.org/10.1016/0163-7258(91)90067-v.

25. Sahin MT, Oztürkcan S, Türel-Ermertcan A, et al. Behçet's disease associated with hidradenitis suppurativa. *J Eur Acad Dermatol Venereol.* 2007;21(3):428–429. https://doi.org/10.1111/j.1468-3083.2006.01922.x.

26. METHOTREXATE (methotrexate) Indications and Clinical Use | Pfizer Medical Information—Canada. Accessed April 22, 2020. https://www.pfizermedicalinformation.ca/en-ca/methotrexate/indications-and-clinical-use#.

27. Cronstein BN, Eberle MA, Gruber HE, Levin RI. Methotrexate inhibits neutrophil function by stimulating adenosine release from connective tissue cells. *PNAS.* 1991;88(6):2441–2445. https://doi.org/10.1073/pnas.88.6.2441.

28. Kalb RE, Strober B, Weinstein G, Lebwohl M. Methotrexate and psoriasis: 2009 National Psoriasis Foundation Consensus Conference. *J Am Acad Dermatol.* 2009;60(5):824–837. https://doi.org/10.1016/j.jaad.2008.11.906.

29. Menting SP, Dekker PM, Limpens J, et al. Methotrexate Dosing Regimen for Plaque-type Psoriasis: A Systematic Review of the Use of Test-dose, Start-dose, Dosing Scheme, Dose Adjustments, Maximum Dose and Folic Acid Supplementation. *Acta Derm Venereol.* 2016;96(1):23–28. https://doi.org/10.2340/00015555-2081.

30. Lang PG. Sulfones and sulfonamides in dermatology today. *J Am Acad Dermatol.* 1979;1(6):479–492. https://doi.org/10.1016/S0190-9622(79)80088-2.

31. Liang SE, Hoffmann R, Peterson E, Soter NA. Use of Dapsone in the Treatment of Chronic Idiopathic and Autoimmune Urticaria. *JAMA Dermatol.* 2019;155(1):90–95. https://doi.org/10.1001/jamadermatol.2018.3715.

32. Kurien G, Jamil RT, Preuss CV. *Dapsone.* In: *StatPearls.* StatPearls Publishing; 2019. http://www.ncbi.nlm.nih.gov/books/NBK470552/. Accessed 8 January 2020.

33. Harvath L, Yancey KB, Katz SI. Selective inhibition of human neutrophil chemotaxis to N-formyl-methionyl-leucyl-phenylalanine by sulfones. *J Immunol.* 1986;137(4):1305–1311.

34. Webster GF, Alexander JC, McArthur WP, Leyden JJ. Inhibition of chemiluminescence in human neutrophils by dapsone. *Br J Dermatol.* 1984;110(6):657–663. https://doi.org/10.1111/j.1365-2133.1984.tb04701.x.

35. Dapsone (dapsone) dose, indications, adverse effects, interactions... from PDR.net. Accessed August 9, 2020. https://www.pdr.net/drug-summary/Dapsone-dapsone-261.

36. Ghaoui N, Hanna E, Abbas O, et al. Update on the use of dapsone in dermatology. *Int J Dermatol.* 2020;59(7):787–795. https://doi.org/10.1111/ijd.14761.

37. Wong D, Walsh S. Low-dose systemic corticosteroid treatment for recalcitrant hidradenitis suppurativa. *J Am Acad Dermatol.* 2016;75(5):1059–1062. https://doi.org/10.1016/j.jaad.2016.06.001.

38. Prednisone- ClinicalKey. Accessed May 1, 2020. https://www-clinicalkey-com.libproxy.tulane.edu/#!/content/6-s2.0-505?scrollTo=%23MonitoringParameters.

39. Frey BM, Frey FJ. Clinical pharmacokinetics of prednisone and prednisolone. *Clin Pharmacokinet.* 1990;19(2):126–146. https://doi.org/10.2165/00003088-199019020-00003.

40. Walton RG, Farber EM. Systemic use of corticosteroids in dermatology. *Calif Med.* 1961;94(4):209–210.

41. Prednisone Tablets (prednisone) dose, indications, adverse effects, interactions... from PDR.net. Accessed July 6, 2020. https://www.pdr.net/drug-summary/Prednisone-Tablets-prednisone-3516.6194.

42. Cyclosporine. *LiverTox: Clinical and Research Information on Drug-Induced Liver Injury.* National Institute of Diabetes and Digestive and Kidney Diseases; 2012. http://www.ncbi.nlm.nih.gov/books/NBK548753/. Accessed 8 January 2020.

43. Fahr A. Cyclosporin clinical pharmacokinetics. *Clin Pharmacokinet.* 1993;24(6):472–495. https://doi.org/10.2165/00003088-199324060-00004.

44. Cyclosporine- ClinicalKey. Accessed May 1, 2020. https://www-clinicalkey-com.libproxy.tulane.edu/#!/content/6-s2.0-158?scrollTo=%23MonitoringParameters.

45. Vossen ARJV, van Straalen KR, Prens EP, van der Zee HH. Menses and pregnancy affect symptoms in hidradenitis suppurativa: a cross-sectional study. *J Am Acad Dermatol.* 2017;76(1):155–156. https://doi.org/10.1016/j.jaad.2016.07.024.

46. Barth JH, Layton AM, Cunliffe WJ. Endocrine factors in pre- and postmenopausal women with hidradenitis suppurativa. *Br J Dermatol.* 1996;134:1057–1059.

47. Chen W, Thiboutot D, Zouboulis CC. Cutaneous androgen metabolism: basic research and clinical perspectives. *J Invest Dermatol.* 2002;119(5):992–1007. https://doi.org/10.1046/j.1523-1747.2002.00613.x.

48. Smythe CDW, Greenall M, Kealey T. The Activity of HMG-CoA Reductase and Acetyl-CoA Carboxylase in Human Apocrine Sweat Glands, Sebaceous Glands, and Hair Follicles Is Regulated by Phosphorylation and by Exogenous Cholesterol. *J Invest Dermatol.* 1998;111(1):139–148. https://doi.org/10.1046/j.1523-1747.1998.00246.x.

49. Menon GK, Feingold KR, Moser AH, et al. De novo sterologenesis in the skin. II. Regulation by cutaneous barrier requirements. *J Lipid Res.* 1985;26(4):418–427.

50. Lai JJ, Chang P, Lai KP, et al. The role of androgen and androgen receptor in the skin-related disorders. *Arch Dermatol Res.* 2012;304(7):499–510. https://doi.org/10.1007/s00403-012-1265-x.

51. Chen W, Zouboulis CC, Fritsch M, et al. Evidence of heterogeneity and quantitative differences of the type 1 5alpha-reductase expression in cultured human skin cells—evidence of its presence in melanocytes. *J Invest Dermatol.* 1998;110(1):84–89. https://doi.org/10.1046/j.1523-1747.1998.00080.x.

52. Anderson KM, Liao S. Selective retention of dihydrotestosterone by prostatic nuclei. *Nature.* 1968;219(5151):277–279. https://doi.org/10.1038/219277a0.

53. Deplewski D, Rosenfield RL. Role of hormones in pilosebaceous unit development. *Endocr Rev.* 2000;21(4):363–392. https://doi.org/10.1210/edrv.21.4.0404.

54. Choudhry R, Hodgins MB, Van der Kwast TH, et al. Localization of androgen receptors in human skin by immunohistochemistry: implications for the hormonal regulation of hair growth, sebaceous glands and sweat glands. *J Endocrinol.* 1992;133(3):467–475. https://doi.org/10.1677/joe.0.1330467.

55. Anina Lambrechts I, Nuno de Canha M, Lall N. Chapter 4—Exploiting medicinal plants as possible treatments for acne vulgaris. In: Lall N, ed. *Medicinal Plants for Holistic Health and Well-Being.* London, United Kingdom: Academic Press; 2018:117–143. https://doi.org/10.1016/B978-0-12-812475-8.00004-4.

56. von Laffert M, Stadie V, Wohlrab J, Marsch WC. Hidradenitis suppurativa/acne inversa: bilocated epithelial hyperplasia with very different sequelae. *Br J Dermatol.* 2011;164(2):367–371. https://doi.org/10.1111/j.1365-2133.2010.10034.x.

57. von Laffert M, Helmbold P, Wohlrab J, et al. Hidradenitis suppurativa (acne inversa): early inflammatory events at terminal follicles and at interfollicular epidermis*. *Exp Dermatol.* 2010;19(6):533–537. https://doi.org/10.1111/j.1600-0625.2009.00915.x.

58. Thiboutot DM, Knaggs H, Gilliland K, Hagari S. Activity of type 1 5α–reductase is greater in the follicular infrainfundibulum compared with the epidermis. *Br J Dermatol.* 1997;136(2):166–171. https://doi.org/10.1046/j.1365-2133.1997.d01-1162.x.

59. Kelly G, Sweeney CM, Tobin AM, Kirby B. Hidradenitis suppurativa: the role of immune dysregulation. *Int J Dermatol.* 2014;53(10):1186–1196. https://doi.org/10.1111/ijd.12550.

60. Kelly G, Hughes R, McGarry T, et al. Dysregulated cytokine expression in lesional and nonlesional skin in hidradenitis suppurativa. *Br J Dermatol.* 2015;173(6):1431–1439. https://doi.org/10.1111/bjd.14075.

61. Schlapbach C, Hänni T, Yawalkar N, Hunger RE. Expression of the IL-23/Th17 pathway in lesions of hidradenitis suppurativa. *J Am Acad Dermatol.* 2011;65(4):790–798. https://doi.org/10.1016/j.jaad.2010.07.010.

62. Wolk K, Warszawska K, Hoeflich C, et al. Deficiency of IL-22 contributes to a chronic inflammatory disease: pathogenetic mechanisms in acne inversa. *J Immunol.* 2011;186(2):1228–1239. https://doi.org/10.4049/jimmunol.0903907.

63. van der Zee HH, Laman JD, de Ruiter L, et al. Adalimumab (antitumour necrosis factor-α) treatment of hidradenitis suppurativa ameliorates skin inflammation: an in situ and ex vivo study. *Br J Dermatol.* 2012;166(2):298–305. https://doi.org/10.1111/j.1365-2133.2011.10698.x.

64. O'Brien RL, Born WK. Dermal γδ T cells—What have we learned? *Cell Immunol.* 2015;296(1):62–69. https://doi.org/10.1016/j.cellimm.2015.01.011.

65. Amatya N, Garg AV, Gaffen SL. IL-17 Signaling: The Yin and the Yang. *Trends Immunol.* 2017;38(5):310–322. https://doi.org/10.1016/j.it.2017.01.006.

66. Cua DJ, Tato CM. Innate IL-17-producing cells: the sentinels of the immune system. *Nat Rev Immunol.* 2010;10(7):479–489. https://doi.org/10.1038/nri2800.

67. Gilliver SC, Ashworth JJ, Mills SJ, et al. Androgens modulate the inflammatory response during acute wound healing. *J Cell Sci.* 2006;119(4):722–732. https://doi.org/10.1242/jcs.02786.

68. Arredouani MS. New insights into androgenic immune regulation. *Oncoimmunology.* 2014;3(9):e954968. https://doi.org/10.4161/21624011.2014.954968.

69. Lai JJ, Lai KP, Chuang KH, et al. Monocyte/macrophage androgen receptor suppresses cutaneous wound healing in mice by enhancing local TNF-alpha expression. –*J Clin Invest.* Accessed March 3, 2020. https://www.ncbi.nlm.nih.gov/pubmed/19907077.

70. Randhawa HK, Hamilton J, Pope E. Finasteride for the treatment of hidradenitis suppurativa in children and adolescents. *JAMA Dermatol.* 2013;149(6):732–735. https://doi.org/10.1001/jamadermatol.2013.2874.

71. Khandalavala BN, Do MV. Finasteride in Hidradenitis Suppurativa: A "Male" Therapy for a Predominantly "Female" Disease. *J Clin Aesthet Dermatol.* 2016;9(6):44–50.

72. Sawers RS, Randall VA, Ebling FJ. Control of hidradenitis suppurativa in women using combined antiandrogen (cyproterone acetate) and oestrogen therapy. *Br J Dermatol.* 1986;115(3):269–274. https://doi.org/10.1111/j.1365-2133.1986.tb05741.x.

73. Mortimer PS, Dawber RP, Gales MA, Moore RA. A double-blind controlled cross-over trial of cyproterone acetate in females with hidradenitis suppurativa. *Br J Dermatol.* 1986;115(3):263–268. https://doi.org/10.1111/j.1365-2133.1986.tb05740.x.

74. Lee A, Fischer G. A case series of 20 women with hidradenitis suppurativa treated with spironolactone. *Australas J Dermatol.* 2015;56(3):192–196. https://doi.org/10.1111/ajd.12362.

75. Li C, Xu H, Zhang X, et al. Hidradenitis suppurativa is treated with low-dose flutamide. *J Dermatol.* 2019;46(2):e52–e54. https://doi.org/10.1111/1346-8138.14541.

76. Rivera R, Yacobson I, Grimes D. The mechanism of action of hormonal contraceptives and intrauterine contraceptive devices. *Am J Obstet Gynecol.* 1999;181(5):1263–1269. https://doi.org/10.1016/S0002-9378(99)70120-1.

77. Trivedi MK, Shinkai K, Murase JE. A review of hormone-based therapies to treat adult acne vulgaris in women. *Int J Womens Dermatol.* 2017;3(1):44–52. https://doi.org/10.1016/j.ijwd.2017.02.018.

78. Haider A, Shaw JC. Treatment of Acne Vulgaris. *JAMA.* 2004;292(6):726–735. https://doi.org/10.1001/jama.292.6.726.

79. Redmond GP, Olson WH, Lippman JS, et al. Norgestimate and ethinyl estradiol in the treatment of acne vulgaris: a randomized, placebo-controlled trial. *Obstet Gynecol.* 1997;89(4):615–622. https://doi.org/10.1016/S0029-7844(97)00059-8.

80. Alikhan A, Sayed C, Alavi A, et al. North American clinical management guidelines for hidradenitis suppurativa: a publication from the United States and Canadian Hidradenitis Suppurativa Foundations: Part II: Topical, intralesional, and systemic medical management. *J Am Acad Dermatol.* 2019;81(1):76–90. https://doi.org/10.1016/j.jaad.2019.02.067.

81. Zouboulis CC, Desai N, Emtestam L, et al. European S1 guideline for the treatment of hidradenitis suppurativa/acne inversa. *J Eur Acad Dermatol Venereol.* 2015;29(4):619–644. https://doi.org/10.1111/jdv.12966.

82. Corvol P, Michaud A, Menard J, et al. Antiandrogenic effect of spirolactones: mechanism of action. *Endocrinology.* 1975;97(1):52–58. https://doi.org/10.1210/endo-97-1-52.

83. Spironolactone: Drug information—UpToDate. Accessed January 10, 2020. https://www.uptodate.com/contents/spironolactone-drug-information?search=spironolactone&source=panel_search_result&selectedTitle=1~148&usage_type=panel&kp_tab=drug_general&display_rank=1#references.

84. Serafini PC, Catalino J, Lobo RA. The effect of spironolactone on genital skin 5 alpha-reductase activity. *J Steroid Biochem.* 1985;23(2):191–194. https://doi.org/10.1016/0022-4731(85)90236-5.

85. Kim GK, Del Rosso JQ. Oral Spironolactone in Post-teenage Female Patients with Acne Vulgaris. *J Clin Aesthet Dermatol.* 2012;5(3):37–50.

86. Stripp B, Taylor AA, Bartter FC, et al. Effect of spironolactone on sex hormones in man. *J Clin Endocrinol Metab.* 1975;41(5):777–781. https://doi.org/10.1210/jcem-41-4-777.

87. Menard RH, Guenthner TM, Kon H, Gillette JR. Studies on the destruction of adrenal and testicular cytochrome P-450 by

spironolactone. Requirement for the 7alpha-thio group and evidence for the loss of the heme and apoproteins of cytochrome P-450. *J Biol Chem.* 1979;254(5):1726–1733.

88. Mitts TF, Bunda S, Wang Y, Hinek A. Aldosterone and mineralocorticoid receptor antagonists modulate elastin and collagen deposition in human skin. *J Invest Dermatol.* 2010;130(10):2396–2406. https://doi.org/10.1038/jid.2010.155.

89. Golbari NM, Porter ML, Kimball AB. Antiandrogen therapy with spironolactone for the treatment of hidradenitis suppurativa. *J Am Acad Dermatol.* 2019;80(1):114–119. https://doi.org/10.1016/j.jaad.2018.06.063.

90. Quinlan C, Kirby B, Hughes R. Spironolactone therapy for hidradenitis suppurativa. *Clin Exp Dermatol.* 2020 Jun;45(4):464–465. https://doi.org/10.1111/ced.14119. Epub 2019 Nov 17. PMID: 31602704.

91. McPhie ML, Bridgman AC, Kirchhof MG. Combination Therapies for Hidradenitis Suppurativa: A Retrospective Chart Review of 31 Patients. *J Cutan Med Surg.* 2019;23(3):270–276. https://doi.org/10.1177/1203475418823529.

92. Kraft JN, Searles GE. Hidradenitis suppurativa in 64 female patients: retrospective study comparing oral antibiotics and antiandrogen therapy. *J Cutan Med Surg.* 2007;11(4):125–131. https://doi.org/10.2310/7750.2007.00019.

93. Spironolactone for Hidradenitis Suppurativa—Full Text View—ClinicalTrials.gov. Accessed April 23, 2020. https://clinicaltrials.gov/ct2/show/NCT04100083.

94. Orenstein LAV, Nguyen TV, Damiani G, et al. Medical and Surgical Management of Hidradenitis Suppurativa: A Review of International Treatment Guidelines and Implementation in General Dermatology Practice. *Dermatology (Basel).* 2020;1–20. https://doi.org/10.1159/000507323. Published online May 14.

95. Makrantonaki E, Ganceviciene R, Zouboulis C. An update on the role of the sebaceous gland in the pathogenesis of acne. *Dermatoendocrinol.* 2011;3(1):41–49. https://doi.org/10.4161/derm.3.1.13900.

96. Mota F, Machado S, Selores M. Hidradenitis Suppurativa in Children Treated with Finasteride—A Case Series. *Pediatr Dermatol.* 2017;34(5):578–583. https://doi.org/10.1111/pde.13216.

97. Garg A, Neuren E, Strunk A. Hidradenitis Suppurativa Is Associated with Polycystic Ovary Syndrome: A Population-Based Analysis in the United States. *J Invest Dermatol.* 2018;138(6):1288–1292. https://doi.org/10.1016/j.jid.2018.01.009.

98. Vilanova I, Hernández JL, Mata C, et al. Insulin resistance in hidradenitis suppurativa: a case-control study. *J Eur Acad Dermatol Venereol.* 2018;32(5):820–824. https://doi.org/10.1111/jdv.14894.

99. Wolf R, Matz H, Orion E. Acne and diet. *Clin Dermatol.* 2004;22(5):387–393. https://doi.org/10.1016/j.clindermatol.2004.03.007.

100. Kucharska A, Szmurło A, Sińska B. Significance of diet in treated and untreated acne vulgaris. *Postepy Dermatol Alergol.* 2016;33(2):81–86. https://doi.org/10.5114/ada.2016.59146.

101. Barbieri RL, Hornstein MD. Hyperinsulinemia and ovarian hyperandrogenism. Cause and effect. *Endocrinol Metab Clin North Am.* 1988;17(4):685–703.

102. Barbieri RL, Smith S, Ryan KJ. The role of hyperinsulinemia in the pathogenesis of ovarian hyperandrogenism. *Fertil Steril.* 1988;50(2):197–212. https://doi.org/10.1016/s0015-0282(16)60060-2.

103. Escobar-Morreale HF, Serrano-Gotarredona J, García-Robles R, et al. Abnormalities in the serum insulin-like growth factor-1 axis in women with hyperandrogenism. *Fertil Steril.* 1998;70(6):1090–1100. https://doi.org/10.1016/s0015-0282(98)00388-4.

104. Livingstone C, Collison M. Sex steroids and insulin resistance. *Clin Sci.* 2002;102(2):151–166. https://doi.org/10.1042/cs1020151.

105. De Mellow JS, Handelsman DJ, Baxter RC. Short-term exposure to insulin-like growth factors stimulates testosterone production by testicular interstitial cells. *Acta Endocrinol.* 1987;115(4):483–489. https://doi.org/10.1530/acta.0.1150483.

106. Burghen GA, Givens JR, Kitabchi AE. Correlation of hyperandrogenism with hyperinsulinism in polycystic ovarian disease. *J Clin Endocrinol Metab.* 1980;50(1):113–116. https://doi.org/10.1210/jcem-50-1-113.

107. Nestler JE. Insulin regulation of human ovarian androgens. *Hum Reprod.* 1997;12(suppl 1):53–62. https://doi.org/10.1093/humrep/12.suppl_1.53.

108. Poretsky L. On the paradox of insulin-induced hyperandrogenism in insulin-resistant states. *Endocr Rev.* 1991;12(1):3–13. https://doi.org/10.1210/edrv-12-1-3.

109. Corbould A. Effects of androgens on insulin action in women: is androgen excess a component of female metabolic syndrome? *Diabetes Metab Res Rev.* 2008;24(7):520–532. https://doi.org/10.1002/dmrr.872.

110. Canoui-Poitrine F, Revuz JE, Wolkenstein P, et al. Clinical characteristics of a series of 302 French patients with hidradenitis suppurativa, with an analysis of factors associated with disease severity. *J Am Acad Dermatol.* 2009;61(1):51–57. https://doi.org/10.1016/j.jaad.2009.02.013.

111. Sartorius K, Emtestam L, Jemec GBE, Lapins J. Objective scoring of hidradenitis suppurativa reflecting the role of tobacco smoking and obesity. *Br J Dermatol.* 2009;161(4):831–839. https://doi.org/10.1111/j.1365-2133.2009.09198.x.

112. Kromann CB, Deckers IE, Esmann S, et al. Risk factors, clinical course and long-term prognosis in hidradenitis suppurativa: a cross-sectional study. *Br J Dermatol.* 2014;171(4):819–824. https://doi.org/10.1111/bjd.13090.

113. Gisondi P, Galvan A, Idolazzi L, Girolomoni G. Management of moderate to severe psoriasis in patients with metabolic comorbidities. *Front Med (Lausanne).* 2015;2:1. https://doi.org/10.3389/fmed.2015.00001.

114. Greenberg AS, Obin MS. Obesity and the role of adipose tissue in inflammation and metabolism. *Am J Clin Nutr.* 2006;83(2):461S–465S. https://doi.org/10.1093/ajcn/83.2.461S.

115. Yazdanyar S, Jemec GBE. Hidradenitis suppurativa: a review of cause and treatment. *Curr Opin Infect Dis.* 2011;24(2):118–123. https://doi.org/10.1097/QCO.0b013e3283428d07.

116. Sabat R, Chanwangpong A, Schneider-Burrus S, et al. Increased prevalence of metabolic syndrome in patients with acne inversa. *PLoS ONE.* 2012;7(2). https://doi.org/10.1371/journal.pone.0031810, e31810.

117. Kelly G, Prens EP. Inflammatory Mechanisms in Hidradenitis Suppurativa. *Dermatol Clin.* 2016;34(1):51–58. https://doi.org/10.1016/j.det.2015.08.004.

118. Malin SK, Kashyap SR. Effects of metformin on weight loss: potential mechanisms. *Curr Opin Endocrinol Diabetes Obes.* 2014;21(5):323–329. https://doi.org/10.1097/MED.0000000000000095.

119. Stevanovic D, Janjetovic K, Misirkic M, et al. Intracerebroventricular administration of metformin inhibits ghrelin-induced Hypothalamic AMP-kinase signalling and food intake. *Neuroendocrinology.* 2012;96(1):24–31. https://doi.org/10.1159/000333963.

120. Aubert G, Mansuy V, Voirol MJ, et al. The anorexigenic effects of metformin involve increases in hypothalamic leptin receptor expression. *Metab Clin Exp.* 2011;60(3):327–334. https://doi.org/10.1016/j.metabol.2010.02.007.

121. Gruzdeva O, Borodkina D, Uchasova E, et al. Leptin resistance: underlying mechanisms and diagnosis. *Diabetes Metab Syndr Obes.* 2019;12:191–198. https://doi.org/10.2147/DMSO.S182406.

122. Arun B, Loffeld A. Long-standing hidradenitis suppurativa treated effectively with metformin. *Clin Exp Dermatol.* 2009;34(8):920–921. https://doi.org/10.1111/j.1365-2230.2008.03121.x.

123. Khandalavala BN. A Disease-Modifying Approach for Advanced Hidradenitis Suppurativa (Regimen with Metformin, Liraglutide, Dapsone, and Finasteride): A Case Report. *Case Rep Dermatol.* 2017;9(2):70–78. https://doi.org/10.1159/000473873.

124. Jennings L, Hambly R, Hughes R, et al. Metformin use in hidradenitis suppurativa. *J Dermatolog Treat.* 2020;31(3):261–263. https://doi.org/10.1080/09546634.2019.1592100.

125. Verdolini R, Clayton N, Smith A, et al. Metformin for the treatment of hidradenitis suppurativa: a little help along the way. *J Eur Acad*

Dermatol Venereol. 2013;27(9):1101–1108. https://doi.org/10.1111/j.1468-3083.2012.04668.x.

126. Ingram JR, Collier F, Brown D, et al. British Association of Dermatologists guidelines for the management of hidradenitis suppurativa (acne inversa) 2018. *Br J Dermatol.* 2019;180(5):1009–1017. https://doi.org/10.1111/bjd.17537.

127. Buysschaert M, Baeck M, Preumont V, et al. Improvement of psoriasis during glucagon-like peptide-1 analogue therapy in type 2 diabetes is associated with decreasing dermal γδ T-cell number: a prospective case-series study. *Br J Dermatol.* 2014;171(1):155–161. https://doi.org/10.1111/bjd.12886.

128. Faurschou A, Gyldenløve M, Rohde U, et al. Lack of effect of the glucagon-like peptide-1 receptor agonist liraglutide on psoriasis in glucose-tolerant patients—a randomized placebo-controlled trial. *J Eur Acad Dermatol Venereol.* 2015;29(3):555–559. https://doi.org/10.1111/jdv.12629.

129. Jennings L, Nestor L, Molloy O, et al. The treatment of hidradenitis suppurativa with the glucagon-like peptide-1 agonist liraglutide. *Br J Dermatol.* 2017;177(3):858–859. https://doi.org/10.1111/bjd.15233.

130. Moran B, Sweeney CM, Hughes R, et al. Hidradenitis Suppurativa Is Characterized by Dysregulation of the Th17:Treg Cell Axis, Which Is Corrected by Anti-TNF Therapy. *J Invest Dermatol.* 2017;137(11):2389–2395. https://doi.org/10.1016/j.jid.2017.05.033.

131. Thomi R, Schlapbach C, Yawalkar N, et al. Elevated levels of the antimicrobial peptide LL-37 in hidradenitis suppurativa are associated with a Th1/Th17 immune response. *Exp Dermatol.* 2018;27(2):172–177. https://doi.org/10.1111/exd.13482.

132. Jiménez-Gallo D, de la Varga-Martínez R, Ossorio-García L, et al. The Clinical Significance of Increased Serum Proinflammatory Cytokines, C-Reactive Protein, and Erythrocyte Sedimentation Rate in Patients with Hidradenitis Suppurativa. *Mediators Inflamm.* 2017;2017:2450401. https://doi.org/10.1155/2017/2450401.

133. Lima AL, Karl I, Giner T, et al. Keratinocytes and neutrophils are important sources of proinflammatory molecules in hidradenitis suppurativa. *Br J Dermatol.* 2016;174(3):514–521. https://doi.org/10.1111/bjd.14214.

134. Nazary M, van der Zee HH, Prens EP, et al. Pathogenesis and pharmacotherapy of Hidradenitis suppurativa. *Eur J Pharmacol.* 2011;672(1–3):1–8. https://doi.org/10.1016/j.ejphar.2011.08.047.

135. Frew JW, Hawkes JE, Krueger JG. A systematic review and critical evaluation of inflammatory cytokine associations in hidradenitis suppurativa. *F1000Res.* 2018;7. https://doi.org/10.12688/f1000research.17267.1.

136. Mucida D, Park Y, Kim G, et al. Reciprocal TH17 and regulatory T cell differentiation mediated by retinoic acid. *Science.* 2007;317(5835):256–260. https://doi.org/10.1126/science.1145697.

137. Camisa C, Eisenstat B, Ragaz A, Weissmann G. The effects of retinoids on neutrophil functions in vitro. *J Am Acad Dermatol.* 1982;6(4 Pt 2 Suppl):620–629. https://doi.org/10.1016/s0190-9622(82)70051-9.

138. Marasca C, Donnarumma M, Annunziata MC, Fabbrocini G. Homocysteine plasma levels in patients affected by hidradenitis suppurativa: an Italian experience. *Clin Exp Dermatol.* 2019;44(3):e28–e29. https://doi.org/10.1111/ced.13798.

139. Marasca C, Donnarumma M, Annunziata MC, Fabbrocini G. Comment on "The effects of isotretinoin therapy on serum homocysteine, folate and vitamin B12 levels in patients with acne": may retinoids be useful to treat hyperhomocysteinemia found in patients affected by hidradenitis suppurativa? *J Eur Acad Dermatol Venereol.* 2020;34(3):e120–e121. https://doi.org/10.1111/jdv.16039.

140. Patel N, McKenzie SA, Harview CL, et al. Isotretinoin in the treatment of hidradenitis suppurativa: a retrospective study. *J Dermatolog Treat Published online September.* 2019;26:1–3. https://doi.org/10.1080/09546634.2019.1670779.

141. Dicken CH, Powell ST, Spear KL. Evaluation of isotretinoin treatment of hidradenitis suppurativa. *J Am Acad Dermatol.* 1984;11(3):500–502. https://doi.org/10.1016/s0190-9622(84)70199-x.

142. Norris JFB, Cunliffe WJ. Failure of treatment of familial widespread hidradenitis suppurativa with isotretinoin. *Clin Exp Dermatol.* 1986;11(6):579–583. https://doi.org/10.1111/j.1365-2230.1986.tb00512.x.

143. Soria A, Canoui-Poitrine F, Wolkenstein P, et al. Absence of efficacy of oral isotretinoin in hidradenitis suppurativa: a retrospective study based on patients' outcome assessment. *Dermatology (Basel).* 2009;218(2):134–135. https://doi.org/10.1159/000182261.

144. Boer J, van Gemert MJP. Long-term results of isotretinoin in the treatment of 68 patients with hidradenitis suppurativa. *J Am Acad Dermatol.* 1999;40(1):73–76. https://doi.org/10.1016/S0190-9622(99)70530-X.

145. Poli F, Wolkenstein P, Revuz J. Back and face involvement in hidradenitis suppurativa. *Dermatology (Basel).* 2010;221(2):137–141. https://doi.org/10.1159/000315508.

146. Vural S, Gündoğdu M, Akay BN, et al. Hidradenitis suppurativa: clinical characteristics and determinants of treatment efficacy. *Dermatol Ther.* 2019;32(5). https://doi.org/10.1111/dth.13003, e13003.

147. Brown CF, Gallup DG, Brown VM. Hidradenitis suppurativa of the anogenital region: response to isotretinoin. *Am J Obstet Gynecol.* 1988;158(1):12–15. https://doi.org/10.1016/0002-9378(88)90766-1.

148. Gallagher CG, Kirthi SK, Cotter CC, et al. Could isotretinoin flare hidradenitis suppurativa? A case series. *Clin Exp Dermatol.* 2019;44(7):777–780. https://doi.org/10.1111/ced.13944.

149. Jørgensen AR, Thomsen SF, Ring HC. Isotretinoin and hidradenitis suppurativa. *Clin Exp Dermatol.* 2019;44(4):e155–e156. https://doi.org/10.1111/ced.13953.

150. Kamp S, Fiehn AM, Stenderup K, et al. Hidradenitis suppurativa: a disease of the absent sebaceous gland? Sebaceous gland number and volume are significantly reduced in uninvolved hair follicles from patients with hidradenitis suppurativa. *Br J Dermatol.* 2011;164(5):1017–1022. https://doi.org/10.1111/j.1365-2133.2011.10224.x.

151. Poli F, Revuz J. Acne flare on isotretinoin: A pointer to diagnosis of hidradenitis suppurativa. *Ann Dermatol Venereol.* 2019;146(1):4–8. https://doi.org/10.1016/j.annder.2018.07.020.

152. Tan MG, Shear NH, Walsh S, Alhusayen R. Acitretin: Monotherapy or Combined Therapy for Hidradenitis Suppurativa? *J Cutan Med Surg.* 2017;21(1):48–53. https://doi.org/10.1177/1203475416659858.

153. Boer J, Nazary M. Long-term results of acitretin therapy for hidradenitis suppurativa. Is acne inversa also a misnomer? *Br J Dermatol.* 2011;164(1):170–175. https://doi.org/10.1111/j.1365-2133.2010.10071.x.

154. Matusiak Ł, Bieniek A, Szepietowski JC. Acitretin treatment for hidradenitis suppurativa: a prospective series of 17 patients. *Br J Dermatol.* 2014;171(1):170–174. https://doi.org/10.1111/bjd.12884.

155. Caro RDC, Bianchi L. Can retinoids flare hidradenitis suppurativa? A further case series. *Clin Exp Dermatol.* 2019;44(4):e153–e154. https://doi.org/10.1111/ced.13956.

156. Armyra K, Kouris A, Markantoni V, et al. Hidradenitis suppurativa treated with tetracycline in combination with colchicine: a prospective series of 20 patients. *Int J Dermatol.* 2017;56(3):346–350. https://doi.org/10.1111/ijd.13428.

157. van der Zee HH, Prens EP. The anti-inflammatory drug colchicine lacks efficacy in hidradenitis suppurativa. *Dermatology (Basel).* 2011;223(2):169–173. https://doi.org/10.1159/000332846.

158. Methotrexate pharmacogenetics in the treatment of rheumatoid arthritis | Pharmacogenomics. Accessed April 23, 2020. https://www-futuremedicine-com.libproxy.tulane.edu/doi/abs/10.2217/pgs-2019-0121.

159. Methotrexate restores the function of peripheral blood regulatory T cells in psoriasis vulgaris via the CD73/AMPK/mTOR pathway—Yan—2018—British Journal of Dermatology—Wiley Online Library. Accessed April 23, 2020. https://onlinelibrary-wiley-com.libproxy.tulane.edu/doi/full/10.1111/bjd.16560.

160. Bedoui Y, Guillot X, Sélambarom J, et al. Methotrexate an Old Drug with New Tricks. *Int J Mol Sci.* 2019;20(20). https://doi.org/10.3390/ijms20205023.

161. Wang LL, Micheletti RG. Low-dose methotrexate as rescue therapy in patients with hidradenitis suppurativa and pyoderma

gangrenosum developing human antichimeric antibodies to infliximab: a retrospective chart review. *J Am Acad Dermatol.* 2020;82 (2):507–510. https://doi.org/10.1016/j.jaad.2019.09.012.

162. Savage KT, Brant EG, Santillan MR, et al. Methotrexate shows benefit in a subset of patients with severe hidradenitis suppurativa. *Int J Women's Dermatol.* 2020. https://doi.org/10.1016/j.ijwd.2020.02.007. Published online February 25.

163. De Souza A, Solomon GE, Strober BE. SAPHO syndrome associated with hidradenitis suppurativa successfully treated with infliximab and methotrexate. *Bull NYU Hosp Jt Dis.* 2011;69(2): 185–187.

164. Vekic DA, Woods J, Lin P, Cains GD. SAPHO syndrome associated with hidradenitis suppurativa and pyoderma gangrenosum successfully treated with adalimumab and methotrexate: a case report and review of the literature. *Int J Dermatol.* 2018;57(1):10–18. https://doi.org/10.1111/ijd.13740.

165. Jemec GBE. Methotrexate is of limited value in the treatment of hidradenitis suppurativa. *Clin Exp Dermatol.* 2002;27(6):528–529. https://doi.org/10.1046/j.1365-2230.2002.11125.x.

166. Martin WJ, Kachel DL. Reduction of neutrophil-mediated injury to pulmonary endothelial cells by dapsone. *Am Rev Respir Dis.* 1985;131 (4):544–547. https://doi.org/10.1164/arrd.1985.131.4.544.

167. Kanoh S, Tanabe T, Rubin BK. Dapsone inhibits IL-8 secretion from human bronchial epithelial cells stimulated with lipopolysaccharide and resolves airway inflammation in the ferret. *Chest.* 2011;140(4):980–990. https://doi.org/10.1378/chest.10-2908.

168. Yazdanyar S, Boer J, Ingvarsson G, et al. Dapsone therapy for hidradenitis suppurativa: a series of 24 patients. *Dermatology.* 2011;222 (4):342–346. https://doi.org/10.1159/000329023.

169. Kaur MR, Lewis HM. Hidradenitis suppurativa treated with dapsone: a case series of five patients. *J Dermatolog Treat.* 2006;17 (4):211–213. https://doi.org/10.1080/09546630600830588.

170. Hofer T, Itin PH. Acne inversaEine Dapson-sensitive Dermatose. *Hautarzt.* 2001;52(1):989–992. https://doi.org/10.1007/s001050170015.

171. Murray G, Hollywood A, Kirby B, Hughes R. Dapsone therapy for hidradenitis suppurativa. *Br J Dermatol.* 2020. https://doi.org/10.1111/bjd.19136. Published online April 15.

172. Staub J, Pfannschmidt N, Strohal R, et al. Successful treatment of PASH syndrome with infliximab, cyclosporine and dapsone. *J Eur Acad Dermatol Venereol.* 2015;29(11):2243–2247. https://doi.org/10.1111/jdv.12765.

173. Kozub P, Simaljakova M. Hidradenitis suppurativa treated with combination of infliximab and dapsone. *Bratisl Lek Listy.* 2012;113(5):319–323. https://doi.org/10.4149/bll_2012_074.

174. Krishna M, Nadler SG. Immunogenicity to Biotherapeutics—The Role of Anti-drug Immune Complexes. *Front Immunol.* 2016;7. https://doi.org/10.3389/fimmu.2016.00021.

175. Burkett PR, GM zu Horste GM, Kuchroo VK. Pouring fuel on the fire: Th17 cells, the environment, and autoimmunity. *J Clin Invest.* 2015;125(6):2211–2219. https://doi.org/10.1172/JCI78085.

176. Weaver CT, Elson CO, Fouser LA, Kolls JK. The Th17 pathway and inflammatory diseases of the intestines, lungs, and skin. *Annu Rev Pathol Mech Dis.* 2013;8(1):477–512. https://doi.org/10.1146/annurev-pathol-011110-130318.

177. Gartlan KH, Varelias A, Koyama M, et al. Th17 plasticity and transition toward a pathogenic cytokine signature are regulated by cyclosporine after allogeneic SCT. *Blood Adv.* 2017;1(6):341–351. https://doi.org/10.1182/bloodadvances.2016002980.

178. Schewitz-Bowers LP, Lait PJP, Copland DA, et al. Glucocorticoid-resistant Th17 cells are selectively attenuated by cyclosporine A. *Proc Natl Acad Sci U S A.* 2015;112(13):4080–4085. https://doi.org/10.1073/pnas.1418316112.

179. Wang K, Shi L, Yu Z, et al. Cyclosporine A Suppresses the Activation of the Th17 Cells in Patients with Primary Sjögren's Syndrome. *Iran J Allergy Asthma Immunol.* 2015;14(2):198–207.

180. Copland DA, Schewitz-Bowers LP, Dick AD, Lee RW. Th17 Cells Are Refractory To Dexamethasone But Sensitive To Cyclosporine A. *Invest Ophthalmol Vis Sci.* 2012;53(14):4167.

181. McKinley L, Alcorn JF, Peterson A, et al. TH17 cells mediate steroid-resistant airway inflammation and airway hyperresponsiveness in mice. *J Immunol.* 2008;181(6):4089–4097. https://doi.org/10.4049/jimmunol.181.6.4089.

182. Bianchi L, Hansel K, Stingeni L. Recalcitrant severe hidradenitis suppurativa successfully treated with cyclosporine A. *J Am Acad Dermatol.* 2012;67(6):e278–e279. https://doi.org/10.1016/j.jaad.2012.06.011.

183. Buckley DA, Rogers S. Cyclosporin-responsive hidradenitis suppurativa. *J R Soc Med.* 1995;88(5):289P–290P.

184. Rose RF, Goodfield MJD, Clark SM. Treatment of recalcitrant hidradenitis suppurativa with oral ciclosporin. *Clin Exp Dermatol.* 2006;31 (1):154–155. https://doi.org/10.1111/j.1365-2230.2005.01983.x.

185. Gupta AK, Ellis CN, Nickoloff BJ, et al. Oral cyclosporine in the treatment of inflammatory and noninflammatory dermatoses: a clinical and immunopathologic analysis. *Arch Dermatol.* 1990;126(3):339–350. https://doi.org/10.1001/archderm.1990.01670270071012.

186. Ducroux E, Ocampo MA, Kanitakis J, et al. Hidradenitis suppurativa after renal transplantation: complete remission after switching from oral cyclosporine to oral tacrolimus. *J Am Acad Dermatol.* 2014;71 (5):e210–e211. https://doi.org/10.1016/j.jaad.2014.06.031.

187. Hunger RE, Laffitte E, Läuchli, et al. Swiss Practice Recommendations for the Management of Hidradenitis Suppurativa/Acne Inversa | Kopernio. Accessed June 7, 2020. https://kopernio.com/viewer?doi=10.1159%2F000477459&token=WzlzMDIzNDUsIjEwLjExNTkvMDAwNDc3NDU5Il0.kXKH7EpaTs431QQW3Z8sgTecdu4.

18

Targeted Therapeutics: Biologics, Small Molecules

ALEXANDRA P. CHARROW AND ROBERT G. MICHELETTI

CHAPTER OUTLINE

Introduction

Hidradenitis suppurativa (HS) is a chronic inflammatory disorder with a complex, multifactorial, and incompletely elucidated pathophysiology. Among relevant host factors are a number of important inflammatory pathways, including increased production of oxygen free radicals, enhanced expression of toll-like receptors and release of pro-inflammatory cytokines, increased tumor necrosis factor (TNF)-α expression, activation of the interleukin-23 (IL-23)/T helper-17 (TH-17) pathway, overproduction of interleukin-1 (IL-1), and others (Fig. 18.1). Historically, antibiotic and surgical treatments were the mainstay of HS therapy, but in the last decade a growing number of biologic therapies which modulate these inflammatory pathways have become available and have been investigated for treatment of moderate-to-severe HS. The appropriate candidate for biologic therapy has moderate or severe HS (correlating with Hurley stage II or III) and has either failed appropriate non-biologic therapy (e.g., 3 months or longer of doxycycline) or has inflammatory HS, which would benefit from the use of a biologic as initial therapy.[1] This chapter will review in detail the evidence for these targeted therapeutics, including adverse effects, monitoring recommendations, treatment pearls, and considerations for successful treatment of HS in the setting of relevant patient comorbidities (Table 18.1).

Tumor Necrosis Factor Inhibition

Adalimumab (TNF-α Inhibitor)

Adalimumab is the first FDA-approved medication for the treatment of HS and is thus the first-line agent for treatment of moderate or severe HS which has failed to respond to non-biologic therapies. Efficacy was established with publication of the Pioneer I and II trials in 2016. Pioneer I and II demonstrated a modest but significant improvement in disease for roughly half of patients.[3,4] The two trials included anti-TNF treatment-naive patients with Hurley Stage II or III disease and at least 3 inflammatory nodules. Treatment included a loading dose followed by maintenance dosing at 40 mg weekly. HS Clinical Response, termed the HiSCR, was defined as a 50% reduction in inflammatory nodule count. HiSCR was achieved in 41.8% of patients in the adalimumab arm of Pioneer I and 58.9% of patients in the adalimumab arm of Pioneer II, compared to 26% and 27.6% of patients in the placebo arms, respectively. Health-related quality-of-life measures also improved significantly among patients in the treatment arm, including better pain numeric rating scale scores and improvements in Dermatology Life Quality Index (DLQI) measures.[3,4] Based on this and subsequent data, adalimumab has become the mainstay of therapy for patients with moderate-to-severe HS following antibiotic failure.

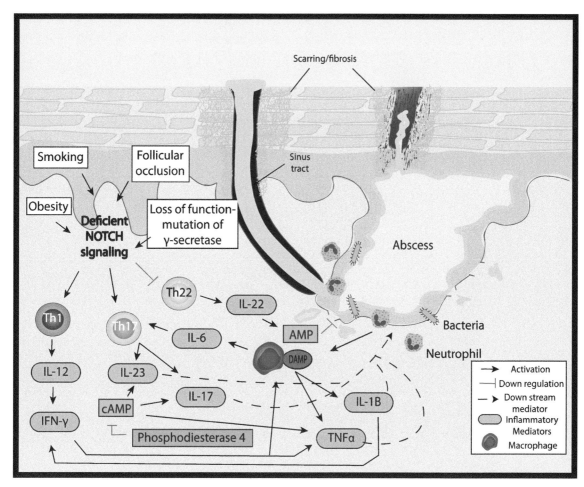

• **Fig. 18.1** Illustration of Proposed Mechanism of Hidradenitis Suppurativa and Targets of Inquiry. *IL*, Interleukin; *Th*, T helper; *TNF-α*, tumor necrosis factor-α. *AMP*, Adenosine Monophosphate; *cAMP*, cyclic Adenosine Monophosphate; *DAMP*, Deoxyadenosine monophosphate; *IFN*, Interfeuron (From Maarouf M, Clark AK, Lee DE, Shi VY. Targeted treatments for hidradenitis suppurative: a review of the current literature and ongoing clinical trials. *J Dermatol Treat*. 2018 Aug;29(5):441–449. https://doi.org/10.1080/09546634.2017.1395806)

Pioneer I and II demonstrated efficacy in HS through the use of higher dosages than were previously standard for other inflammatory conditions; psoriasis, rheumatoid arthritis, inflammatory bowel disease (IBD), and psoriatic arthritis all utilize every-other-week maintenance dosing of adalimumab. However, in studies comparing weekly with every-other-week dosing of adalimumab for HS, patients receiving every-other-week dosing (or decreasing to every-other-week dosing after initial response to weekly dosing) experienced reduced efficacy.[5] Standard treatment based on these and other trials has established the need for a loading dose of 160 mg at week 0, followed by 80 mg at week 2, and then continued use of 40 mg weekly thereafter beginning at day 28.[1]

While adalimumab has clear efficacy for the treatment of HS, outcomes from the PIONEER trials were also notable for the number of non-responders. Roughly half of PIONEER I and PIONEER II patients did not achieve HiSCR (50% disease response) with the use of weekly adalimumab.[1] Patients experiencing a partial response to therapy at week 12 frequently achieve HiSCR by week 36 with continued therapy, but those who do not show at least a partial response by week 12 are unlikely to

benefit from continued treatment and should be considered for alternative therapies.[5] Among responders, continued weekly dosing of adalimumab is considered the most effective strategy, yet those who achieve HiSCR generally continue to have flares and waxing and waning disease activity.[5]

Infliximab (TNF-α Inhibitor)

Patients with inadequate response to therapy with adalimumab frequently benefit from a switch to infliximab. While infliximab has not been studied in a randomized controlled trial for HS comparable in size to those for adalimumab, it nevertheless offers an evidence-based alternative for treatment of moderate or severe HS, as outlined in the European and American treatment guidelines and a Cochrane Review.[6,7] Infliximab is an anti-TNF-α therapy administered intravenously in a weight-based fashion. Loading doses at weeks 0, 2, and 6 are followed by maintenance dosing every 4 to 8 weeks thereafter. Randomized controlled trials of Infliximab have demonstrated significant disease improvement over placebo; however, sample sizes are small.[8,9]

TABLE 18.1 Biologics Used for Treatment of Hidradenitis Suppurativa

Biologics and Small Molecules	Mechanism of Action	Comorbidity Use (FDA-approved for use in below conditions)	Contraindication	Efficacy Data and Level of Evidence[63]	Major Adverse Events	Additional Notes
Adalimumab	Fully humanized IgG1 monoclonal antibody against TNF-α	FDA approved for use in: Rheumatoid arthritis (RA), psoriatic arthritis (PsA), ankylosing spondylitis (AS), Crohn's disease and ulcerative colitis (IBD), psoriasis (PsO), hidradenitis suppurativa (HS) uveitis[64]	Demyelinating conditions such as multiple sclerosis (MS); congestive heart failure (CHF); Lupus (SLE)[64]	A, I[65]	• Injection site reactions • Increased risk of rare serious infections and TB reactivation • Lupus-like syndrome • Worsening of MS and CHF[66]	• The only FDA-approved medication for HS • Injectable medication, available as pen or syringe • Loaded as 160 mg at day 0, 80 mg at day 14, 40 mg weekly at day 28 • Citrate-free formulations may be less painful to inject
Infliximab	IgG1 monoclonal antibody against TNF-α	IBD, RA, AS, PsO, PsA[64]	MS; Relative contraindication: CHF and SLE[2]	B, II[65]	• Infusion reactions • Increased risk of rare serious infections and TB reactivation • Lupus-like syndrome • Worsening of MS and CHF[67]	• Intravenous infusion dosed at 5–10 mg/kg every 4–8 weeks • Anti-Infliximab antibody production is common and necessitates use of MTX 5–10 mg or Azathioprine 50 mg[68]
Anakinra	IgG1 monoclonal antibody IL-1-α and 1β inhibitor	RA, Cryopyrin-Associated Periodic Syndromes (CAPS)[69]	Known hypersensitivity to *E. coli*-derived proteins, Anakinra[7]	B, II[65]	• Site injection reactions • Infections at doses higher than 100 mg daily[70]	• Dosed as a daily injection at 100 mg
Canakinumab	IgG1 monoclonal antibody to IL-1β inhibitor	CAPS, Muckle-Wells (MW), Familial Cold Autoinflammatory Syndrome (FCAS)[71]	Known hypersensitivity to Canakinumab[9]	C, III[72]	• Increase risk of infection • Arthritis • Leukopenia[73]	• Dosed as a 150 mg injection every q8wk
Ustekinumab/ IL12/23 inhibitors	IgG1 monoclonal antibody binds to p-40 subunit of both IL-12 and IL-23	PsO, PsA, IBD[64]	Known hypersensitivity to Ustekinumab[74]	B, II[65]	• Increased risk of infection including candidiasis, nasopharyngitis, UTIs[12]	• Dosed at 0.45–0.9 mg q1–3 months injections. (More frequent dosing and infusion approved for IBD pts)
Guselkumab/ p19 inhibitors	IgG1 monoclonal antibody that binds the P19 subunit of IL-23	PsO[64]	None[75]	C, III[76]	• Increased risk of skin infections including tinea, herpes[13]	• Dosed at 100 mg, loaded and then injected every 8 weeks
Secukinumab, Ixekizumab/ IL17 inhibitors	IgG1 monoclonal antibody that binds IL-17A	PsA[64]	Known hypersensitivity to Secukinumab, Ixekizumab; IBD[77]	C, III[78]	• Increased risk of infection • Flaring of IBD[15]	• Secukinumab: Dosed at 300 mg injection, loaded and then dosed every 4 weeks. Ixekizumab loaded and dosed 160 mg q4 weeks
Tofacitinib and janus kinase (JAK) inhibitors	JAK 3 inhibitor	RA, PsA, UC	Patients with severe hepatic impairment, known hypersensitivity	C, III[79]	• Cardiovascular events including venous clots • Increased risk of infection[80]	• Twice daily oral medication dosed at 5 or 10 mg. Increased risk of adverse events with higher dosing

Strength of Recommendation Taxonomy recommendation level: I, good-quality patient-oriented evidence; II, limited-quality patient-oriented evidence; and III, other evidence, including consensus guidelines, opinion, case studies, and disease-oriented evidence. Evidence grading level: A, recommendation based on consistent and good-quality patient-oriented evidence; B, recommendation based on inconsistent or limited-quality patient-oriented evidence; and C, recommendation based on consensus, opinion, case studies, or disease-oriented evidence.

AS, Ankylosing spondylitis; *CAPS,* Cryopyrin-Associated Periodic Syndromes; *CHF,* congestive heart failure; *FCAS,* Familial Cold Autoinflammatory Syndrome; *HS,* hidradenitis suppurativa; *IBD,* Crohn disease and ulcerative colitis; *MS,* multiple sclerosis; *MW,* Muckle-Wells; *PsA,* psoriatic arthritis; *PsO,* psoriasis; *RA,* rheumatoid arthritis; *SLE,* Lupus.

Weight-based dosing is a potential advantage of infliximab, as is the ability to titrate the dose to effect. In general, higher doses of the medication may be more effective for more severe, inflammatory HS. Published data support the need for dose escalation in most patients (64%; 34/52), with treatment response and achievement of stable dosing generally occurring at 10 mg/kg every 6 to 8 weeks.[10] Other data suggest most (71%; 17/24) patients receiving 7.5 mg/kg every 4 weeks (after loading) achieve a good (HS PGA 0 to 2) clinical response, while dose escalation to 10 mg/kg every 4 weeks is often (50%; 6/12) successful in those who do not.[11]

Other Anti-Tumor Necrosis Factor Therapies

Etanercept, 50 mg injected subcutaneously weekly or twice weekly, was studied in two small prospective studies versus placebo and failed to yield significant disease improvement. Based on available evidence, it is not recommended for treatment of HS.

Evidence for the use of golimumab in HS is limited to two case reports, one positive and one negative.[12,13] Use of certolizumab is anecdotal. Despite a lack of data, these agents may be useful in some cases, particularly in the setting of a comorbid condition (e.g., rheumatoid arthritis, IBD) or a prior intolerance of alternative therapies.

Adverse Reactions to Anti-Tumor Necrosis Factor Therapies

Injection Site Reactions

Injection site reactions are a common complication of adalimumab use, characterized by erythematous patches and plaques, generally round and edematous, arising minutes to hours following drug administration.[14] Reactions generally occur within the first month of treatment and last 3 to 5 days after each exposure.[12] They are thought to constitute a type I hypersensitivity reaction and should be treated as such.[13] Reactions can be treated with topical steroids, antihistamines, nonsteroidal antiinflammatory drugs (NSAIDs) or acetaminophen, and ice.[13] Some severe reactions cause significant pain and edema and may require medication discontinuation. In these cases, a switch to a citrate-free formula of adalimumab can help control injection site reactions while sparing the patient the need to switch to an alternative therapy.

Infusion Reactions

Infusion reactions (IR) to infliximab are well-documented given the drug's extensive use in other rheumatologic, dermatologic, and gastrointestinal conditions. IRs can be divided into early reactions, which occur peri-infusion, and late reactions, which occur 24 hours following infusion. Immediate IRs include symptoms such as pruritus, dyspnea, flushing, and headache, as well as anaphylaxis.[15] These reactions are thought to be mediated via host activation of complement, IgE, and mast-cell degranulation in the setting of the TNF immune globulin.[16,17] Mild infusion reactions such as transient flushing, myalgia, and pruritus are managed with attenuation of infusion rate, while moderate reactions such as fever, urticaria, and hypertension are treated with infusion interruption, oral antihistamine and acetaminophen therapy, and resumption of infusion at slower rates.[14] Severe IRs, including bronchospasm and hypotension, are managed promptly with typical anaphylaxis response and discontinuation of the infusion. Patients can be re-challenged with test doses and graded drug

infusion if infliximab is deemed warranted. Because immediate IRs are common, infliximab is generally ordered with as needed medication available and may be given following pre-medication with corticosteroids, antihistamines, and anti-pyretics. Montelukast may help prevent some respiratory symptoms.[18] In the case of severe IRs with intended re-challenge, input from allergy/immunology may help guide premedication protocols. While these premedication protocols are routinely employed in the setting of infliximab, evidence for their use is limited.[14]

Strategies for Addressing Human Anti-Chimeric Antibody Formation

Unlike immediate IRs, late IRs tend to develop as a result of immune complex deposition and develop in the setting of high human anti-chimeric antibodies (HACAs), prolonged drug-free intervals, and episodic treatment.[19–21] Because they impede the efficacy of infliximab (or adalimumab), preventing HACA development is critical. Therefore, missed doses and prolonged, drug-free intervals should be avoided to prevent development of HACAs. Low-dose methotrexate (MTX) (5 to 10 mg weekly), as well as azathioprine (50 mg daily), have been used in both the dermatologic and gastroenterologic contexts to prevent the development of HACAs.[22,23] Initiation of low-dose methotrexate *after* development of anti-chimeric antibodies is an alternative strategy which may successfully suppress HACAs and enable continued use of infliximab.[24] HACA formation should be suspected when a previously successful regimen ceases to be effective. In such instances, testing for antibody level and drug titer may be advised to guide next steps in management.

Infection and Cardiovascular Risk

The risk of serious infection is greater in patients treated with anti-TNF therapy as compared to those with the same condition treated with other, non-biologic therapies.[25] This includes bacterial infections (particularly pneumonia), tuberculosis and other mycobacterial infections, invasive fungal infections, as well as viral infections (namely, hepatitis B reactivation). Screening for latent tuberculosis and hepatitis B infection should occur before initiation of TNF-α inhibitor therapy; tuberculosis screening is generally repeated annually.

Some data resulting from randomized trials investigating TNF-α inhibitors as possible treatment for heart failure (HF) suggest they may be associated with HF exacerbation. Based on available evidence, patients with mild (New York Heart Association [NYHA] class I/II), stable HF may safely receive anti-TNF therapy. However, their use should be avoided in those with uncontrolled, symptomatic NYHA class III/IV disease.[25]

Other Biologic Therapies

The efficacy of anti-TNF therapy in patients with HS, along with elevated serum TNF levels, have highlighted the role of this pathway in the pathophysiology of HS.[4,5] However a significant number of patients with HS do not respond to anti-TNF therapy, suggesting the disease cannot be fully explained or controlled via a single inflammatory pathway alone. Research to date has demonstrated that Th17-associated cytokines are increased in HS, including IL-1, IL-17, and IL23. In kind, CD161, a marker of Th17 lineage T-cells, is significantly elevated in lesional skin (LS) and peri-lesional skin (PLS) in patients with HS, as compared to healthy controls. T-regulatory (Treg) cells are also elevated in

HS, LS, and PLS; however, the ratio of Th17 to Treg cells is highly skewed in HS tissue toward Th17 cells, suggesting immune dysregulation plays a significant role in HS inflammation.[6,7] IL-1β and TNF have themselves demonstrated differential concentrations in draining lesions, depending on the patient.[26]

IL-1 inhibitors, IL-17 inhibitors, and IL-23 inhibitors are generally the next rungs on the therapeutic ladder when patients fail anti-TNF therapy.[1] Oddly, many of these treatments can also paradoxically induce hidradenitis in certain patients and worsen the course for others.[27] The following section aims to review these therapies, their side effects, and the monitoring required.

Ustekinumab (Anti-12/23)

Ustekinumab is a monoclonal antibody which binds to the p40 subunit of IL-12 and IL-23 and is injected subcutaneously via a pre-filled syringe. Typical dosing for psoriasis or psoriatic arthritis is 45 mg for those weighing less than 100 kg and 90 mg for those weighing over 100 kg, administered as a loading dose at weeks 0 and 4, followed by maintenance dosing every 12 weeks after that. Ustekinumab is also used in treatment of Crohn's disease and ulcerative colitis, using a weight-based intravenous induction dose, followed by 90 mg injected subcutaneously every 8 weeks thereafter. Patients with severe Crohn's Disease may be dosed every 4 weeks thereafter.

Data supporting the use of ustekinumab for HS are limited to small (fewer than 20 patients), uncontrolled studies showing response to therapy by Hidradenitis Suppurativa Clinical Response (HiSCR) in roughly 50% of patients, along with improvement in measures of pain and quality of life.[28,29]

Little evidence is currently available to guide the dosing regimen for ustekinumab in HS. Anecdotally, higher dose and frequency of medication administration (e.g., a maintenance regimen of 90 mg every 6 to 8 weeks) may, in the authors' experience, be more effective. However, in general, patients with severe HS who have failed anti-TNF therapy frequently have an inadequate response to ustekinumab, regardless of dose. This option may be attractive in those patients with comorbid HS and IBD, in which case ustekinumab is reasonable for management of both diseases. The infrequency of dosing is also a relative advantage over other regimens. Medication monitoring consists of tuberculosis screening.

Guselkumab (Anti-IL-23)

Guselkumab is a monoclonal antibody which binds to the p-19 subunit of IL-23 and is delivered subcutaneously at a dose of 100 mg at weeks 0 and 4, then every 8 weeks after that. Its successful use has been reported in a handful of case reports.[30,31] A recent report of four cases and literature review suggests clinical benefit is modest, with fewer than half (7/16) of patients included in the review having clinical improvement (reduction of ≧ 1 point on HS-PGA or ≧ 2 points on DLQI or VAS for pain) at week 12.[32]

Anakinra (Anti-IL-1)

Anakinra is an injectable IL-1α and β inhibitor developed for use in patients with autoinflammatory diseases. Dosing is standardized at 100 mg administered as a once-daily subcutaneous injection. Case reports and series have suggested a beneficial effect for selected patient with HS.[27] One small randomized, controlled trial demonstrated decreased disease activity, with 78% (7 of 9) of those receiving anakinra achieving HiSCR at 12 weeks, compared to 30% (3 of 10) in the placebo arm. Circulating interferon-γ production was also decreased in the treatment arm. Other endpoints, however, including visual analogue scale (VAS) scores, pain scores, and Sartorius scores, were unchanged in both the treatment and placebo groups following 24 weeks of therapy.[28,33]

In practice, as with ustekinumab, those treated with anakinra frequently have severe HS unresponsive to TNF-inhibitors; thus, response rates may be lower than reported in the literature. Unfortunately, anakinra is not a good option for patients with comorbid IBD, since it is not an effective treatment for that indication. Compared to the dosing regimens of other biologics, the daily injections of anakinra are inconvenient and more frequently complicated by painful injection site reactions. General advice for preventing reactions includes warming the medication to room temperature before injection, cooling the injection site with an ice pack for a few minutes before and after injection, applying a topical steroid to the area, and rotating injection sites. Monitoring of the absolute neutrophil count should occur monthly for three months, then every three months for the first year. Unlike ustekinumab and the TNF inhibitors, anakinra should be adjusted for renal impairment.

Canakinumab (Anti-IL-1β)

Canakinumab is a long-acting anti-IL-1β monoclonal antibody, approved for various autoinflammatory syndromes. Unlike anakinra, the medication is typically dosed every 4 to 8 weeks subcutaneously by weight. Scant data are available, with a small number of case reports describing both response and non-response to therapy.[34-37]

Secukinumab (Anti-IL-17)

Secukinumab is an anti-IL-17 agent which has been investigated for management of hidradenitis suppurativa. Standard dosing is 300 mg injected subcutaneously weekly for 5 weeks, followed by 300 mg every 4 weeks after that. An open-label study and a retrospective review reported HiSCR of 70% (14/20) and 75% (15/20), respectively, in patients with moderate to severe HS receiving secukinumab, without comparison to a control group.[38,39]

Secukinumab monitoring includes screening for tuberculosis. Additionally, there is concern that use of IL-17 inhibitors may be associated with IBD. HS itself is associated with an increased prevalence of IBD.[40] Consequently, patients treated with secukinumab should be monitored for gastrointestinal symptoms. Secukinumab is not a good choice for management of coexisting HS and IBD.

Ixekizumab (Anti-IL-17)

Ixekizumab is another anti-IL-17 agent dosed subcutaneously every 4 weeks following an initial loading dose. Only two case reports describing the use of ixekizumab in HS are available, both demonstrating improvement in HS among patients with concomitant psoriasis.[41,42]

Apremilast (PDE4)

Apremilast is an oral phosphodiesterase 4 (PDE4) inhibitor which is dosed at 30 mg twice daily, following a 5-day titration period. The utility of apremilast for HS has been investigated in a case series and an open-label study,[43] which showed modest benefit in treating HS, which was relatively less severe. A small randomized controlled trial enrolled 20 patients with moderate HS, randomized 3:1 to apremilast versus placebo. Eight of 15 (53%) treated patients met the HiSCR at week 16, versus 0 of 5 (0%) of those receiving placebo ($P = .055$).[44]

Apremilast has been associated with gastrointestinal side effects such as diarrhea and nausea, weight loss, and depression. It appears to be only modestly effective for treatment of HS, and the cost of the medication may be prohibitive if insurance coverage cannot be obtained. Nevertheless, as an oral medication with a novel mechanism of action, it may be a potentially attractive option for some patients.

Tofacitinib (JAK Inhibitor)

Tofacitinib, generally dosed at either 5 mg or 10 mg orally, twice daily 5 mg orally, twice daily, is a Janus kinase (JAK) inhibitor which acts through the JAK-STAT pathway to suppress inflammatory cytokines, including IL-1β, IL-6, and TNF-α. A report of two patients with recalcitrant, ulcerative HS described response to tofacitinib dosed at 5 mg twice daily, in concert with other therapies, where prior treatment with other biologics had failed.[45]

Special Circumstances in the Use of Biologic Therapy for Hidradenitis Suppurativa

Pregnancy and Lactation

Not enough is known about the effects of pregnancy on HS, and vice versa. Despite being most common in women of child-bearing age, HS has not been systematically studied in the context of pregnancy and lactation.

Available data suggest HS may worsen during pregnancy in 61.9% (70/113), versus staying the same in 30.1% (34/113) or improving in 8.0% (9/113) of pregnancies; meanwhile, 66.1% (82/124) of pregnancies led to worsening HS in the postpartum period.[46] Despite this, many HS treatment options are contraindicated in pregnancy, and the minority of patients receive HS-specific therapy during pregnancy.[47,48] A registry has been created to help address knowledge gaps related to hidradenitis suppurativa and pregnancy.[49]

For patients with moderate or severe HS who have been stably managed on a biologic therapy or who meet criteria for initiation of a biologic may, in many cases, continue these needed therapies, similar to patients with other systemic inflammatory conditions like rheumatoid arthritis or IBD. The benefits of adalimumab and infliximab are felt to outweigh the risks in the first and second trimesters. Available data suggest exposure to TNF inhibitors *in utero* does not increase the risk of pregnancy-related complications.[50] During the third trimester, when the placenta is most permeable to transfer of maternal IgG antibodies, and translocation of the drug across the placenta could result in neonatal immunosuppression, the risks and benefits of anti-TNF therapy should be weighed.[51] Among TNF inhibitors, certolizumab is considered the safest during pregnancy. As a pegylated TNF inhibitor, its larger molecular size limits placental transfer, but there are no data to support its use in hidradenitis. Ustekinumab and secukinumab may be used

safely during pregnancy, but the use of anakinra and apremilast is discouraged given limited safety data.[52]

In general, the TNF-inhibitors and ustekinumab are considered safe during lactation, whereas caution is advised for anakinra, secukinumab, and apremilast. It is always safest to review the most up-to-date information on pregnancy and lactation in a drug reference guide before prescribing. Coordination of care between dermatology and obstetrics-gynecology is essential in these complex cases.[46,47] Special considerations for HS in women are further discussed in Chapter in 31.

Pediatric Population

Direct evidence for the use of biologic therapies for management of hidradenitis suppurativa in the pediatric population is limited. However, some assumptions can be made on the basis of efficacy data from the adult population and safety data derived from the use of biologics in children with other inflammatory diseases.

In 2016, adalimumab was approved by the FDA for use in adolescents with HS (age 12 years and older) using a model-informed drug development approach, extrapolated from the phase 3 studies performed in adult patients, population pharmacokinetic simulations, and long-term safety data.[53] As for adults, adalimumab and infliximab are recommended for pediatric patients with severe HS.[53–55]

Naturally, data guiding the use of other biologic therapies in the pediatric population are fewer. Successful use of ustekinumab has been reported, and the safe long-term use of anakinra for pediatric autoinflammatory diseases is well-established. Dosing of biologic agents in children should be adjusted according to weight.[56] Special considerations for HS in children are further discussed in Chapter in 29.

Use of Biologic Therapies in the Setting of Malignancy

Large pooled datasets looking specifically for an increased risk of lymphoma or malignancy have found no such risk in patients on long-term anti-TNF therapy as compared to patients with the same inflammatory condition on alternative drugs.[57–59] A meta-analysis of patients with rheumatoid arthritis and prior malignancy found no increased risk of new or recurrent cancer among those receiving biologic therapies (including TNF inhibitors, rituximab, or anakinra) compared to other disease-modifying antirheumatic drugs (DMARDs).[60] A large cohort study similarly found the risk of incident malignancy among rheumatoid arthritis patients receiving biologic therapies was no higher than for those receiving DMARDs or those in a general population comparator group.[61] A retrospective chart review of patients with psoriasis and history of malignancy similarly found no increased risk of recurrence or progression of cancer associated with use of biologic therapies, including among a small number of patients receiving concurrent cancer therapy.[62]

While these data are reassuring, caution is advised. In the setting of malignancy or a history of malignancy, it is important to consider carefully the risks and benefits of biologic therapy, including which biologic therapy, on an individual basis, with the help of the patient's oncologist and primary physician. In some cases, the prospect of improved control of severe and life-altering HS will outweigh potential risks. Dermatologic input may provide key perspective in guiding this medical decision making.

Conclusion

While adalimumab may help many patients with moderate-to-severe HS, the disease is often refractory, necessitating trials of other agents. High-dose infliximab is successful in many such patients. For those who cannot tolerate or fail to respond to anti-TNF therapy, other targeted therapies should be considered, depending on patient comorbidities. Additional options include anti-IL1 therapy and anti-IL12/23 inhibitors. Anti-IL17 therapies, JAK inhibitors, and PDE4 inhibitors have also been trialed. New medications are in development to help those patients who remain refractory to existing targeted therapies. The need for expanded treatment options for moderate-to-severe HS remains significant.

References

1. Alikhan A, Sayed C, Alavi A, et al. North American clinical management guidelines for hidradenitis suppurativa: a publication from the United States and Canadian Hidradenitis Suppurativa Foundations: Part I: Diagnosis, evaluation, and the use of complementary and procedural management. *J Am Acad Dermatol.* 2019;81(1):76–90. https://doi.org/10.1016/j.jaad.2019.02.06.
2. Alikhan A, Sayed C, Alavi A, et al. North American clinical management guidelines for hidradenitis suppurativa: a publication from the United States and Canadian Hidradenitis Suppurativa Foundations: Part II: Topical, intralesional, and systemic medical management. *Am Acad Dermatol.* 2019;81(1):76–90. https://doi.org/10.1016/j.jaad.2019.02.06.
3. Sotiriou E, Goussi C, Lallas A, et al. A prospective open-label clinical trial of efficacy of the every week administration of adalimumab in the treatment of hidradenitis suppurativa. *J Drugs Dermatol.* 2012;11(5)(suppl):s15–s20. suppl.
4. Kimball AB, Tzellos T, Calimlim BM, Teixeira HD et al. Achieving Hidradenitis Suppurativa Response Score is Associated with Significant Improvement in Clinical and Patient-reported Outcomes: Post Hoc Analysis of Pooled Data from Pioneer I and II. *Acta Derm Venereol.* 2018;Nov 5;98(10):932–937.
5. Jemec GBE, Okun MM, Forman SB, Gulliver WPF, et al. Adalimumab medium- term dosing strategy in moderate-to-severe hidradenitis suppurativa integrated results from the phase III randomized placebo-controlled PIONEER trials. *Br J Dermatol.* 2019;181(5):967–975.
6. Zouboulis CC, Desai N, Emtestam L, Hunger RE, et al. European S1 guideline for the treatment of hidradenitis suppurativa/acne inversa. *J Eur Acad Dermatol Venereol.* 2015 Apr;29(4):619–644.
7. Ingrham J. Interventions for Hidradenitis SuppurativaUpdated Summary of an Original Cochrane Review. *JAMA Dermatol.* 2017 May 1;153(5):458–459.
8. Grant A, Gonzalez T, Montgomery MO, et al. Infliximab therapy for patients with moderate to severe hidradenitis suppurativa: a randomized, double-blind, placebo-controlled crossover trial. *J Am Acad Dermatol.* 2010 Feb;62(2):205–217.
9. Paradela S, Rodriguez-lojo R, Fernandez-Torres R, et al. Long-term efficacy of infliximab in hidradenitis suppurativa. *J Dermatolog Treat.* 2012 Aug;23(4):278–283.
10. Oskardmay AN, Miles JA, Sayed CJ. Determining the optimal dose of infliximab for treatment of hidradenitis suppurativa. *J Am Acad Dermatol.* 2019 Sep;81(3):702–708.
11. Ghias MH, Johnston AD, Kutner AJ, et al. High-dose, high-frequency infliximab: a novel treatment paradigm for hidradenitis suppurativa. *J Am Acad Dermatol.* 2019 Oct 4. pii: S0190-9622(19)32820-8.
12. Tursi A. Concomitant hidradenitis suppurativa and pysotomatitis vegetans in silent ulcerative colitis successfully treated with golimumab. *Dig Liver Dis.* 2016 Dec;48(12):1511–1512.
13. Van der Zee HH, Prens EP. Failure of anti-interleukin-1 therapy in severe hidradenitis suppurativa: a case report. *Dermatology.* 2013;226(2):97–100.
14. Matsui T, Umetsu R, Kato Y, et al. Age related trends in injection site reaction incidence induced by the tumor necrosis factor-α (TNF α) inhibitors etanercept and adalimumab:the Food and Drug Administration adverse event reporting system, 2004–2015. *Int J Med Sci.* 2017 Jan 15;14(2):102–109.
15. Lichtenstein L, Ron Y, KIvity S, et al. Infliximab-Related Infusion Reactions: Systematic Review. *J Crohns Colitis.* 2015 Sep;9(9):806–815.
16. Heifetz A, Smedley M, Martin S, et al. The incidence and management of infusion reactions to infliximab: a large center experience. *Am J Gastroenterol.* 2003;98:1315–1324.
17. Vultaggio A, Matucci A, Nencini F, et al. Anti-infliximab IgE and non-IgE antibodies and induction of infusion-related severe anaphylactic reactions. *Allergy.* 2010;65:657–661.
18. Robert D. The Management of Recalcitrant Reactions utilizing a modified antibody infusion protocol. *Inflamm Bowel Dis.* 2014;1(20):1.
19. Hanauer S, Rutgeerts P, D'Haens G, Targan S. Delayed hypersensitivity to infliximab [Remicade] re-infusion after a 2–4 year interval without treatment. *Gastroenterology.* 1999;116:A731.
20. Grosen A, Julsgaard M, Christensen LA. Serum sickness-like reaction due to Infliximab reintroduction during pregnancy. *J Crohns Colitis.* 2013;7: e191.
21. Gamarra RM, McGraw SD, Drelichman VS, Maas LC. Serum sicknesslike reactions in patients receiving intravenous infliximab. *J Emerg Med.* 2006;30:41–44.
22. Baert F, Noman M, Vermiere S, et al. Influence of immunogenicity on the long-term efficacy of infliximab in Crohn's Disease. *N Engl J Med.* 2003;348(7):601–608.
23. Sandborn WJ. Optimizing anti-tumor necrosis factor strategies in inflammatory bowel disease. *Curr Gastroenterol Rep.* 2003 Dec;5(6):501–505.
24. Wang LL, Micheletti R. Low-dose methotrexate as rescue therapy in patients with hidradenitis suppurativa and pyoderma gangrenosum developing human antichimeric antibodies to infliximab: A retrospective chart review. *J Am Acad Dermatol.* 2020 Feb;82(2):507–510.
25. Solomon DH, Rassen JA, Kuriya B, Chen L et al. Heart Failure risk among patients with rheumatoid arthritis starting a TNF Antagonist. *Ann Rheum Dis.* 2013 Nov;72(11):1813–1818. Epub 2012 Nov 15.) (Circulation. 2003;107(25):3133.
26. Kanni T, Tzanetakou V, Savva A, et al. Compartmentalized cytokine responses in hidradenitis suppurativa. *PLoS One.* 2015;10(6): e0130522. https://doi.org/10.1371/journal.pone.0130522.
27. Russo V, Alikhan A. Failure of Anakinra in a case of severe hidradenitis Suppurativa. *J Drug Dermatol.* 2016 Jun 1;15(6):772–774.
28. Romani J, Vilarrasa E, Martorell A, et al. Ustekinumab with intravenous infusion: results in hidradenitis suppurativa. *Dermatology.* 2020;26(1):21–24.
29. Blok JL, Li K, Brodmerkel C, et al. Ustekinumab in hidradenitis suppurativa: clinical results and a search for potential biomarkers in serum. *Br J Dermatol.* 2016 Apr;174(4):839–846.
30. Kovacs M, Podda M. Guselkumab in the treatment of severe hidradenitis suppurativa. *Eur Acad Dermatol Venereol.* 2019 Mar;33(3): e140–e141.
31. Kearney N, Byrne N, Kirby B, et al. Successful use of guselkumab in the treatment of severe hidradenitis suppurativa. *Clin Exp Dermatol.* 2020 Jul;45(5):618–619.
32. Motero-Vilchez T, Martinez-Lopez A, Salvador-Rodriguez L, et al. The use of guselkumab 100 mg every 4 weeks on patients with hidradenitis suppurativa and a literature review. *Dermatol Ther.* 2020 May;33(3):e13456.
33. Leslie KS, Tripathi SV, Nguyen T, et al. An open-label study of anakinra for the treatment of moderate to severe hidradenitis suppurativa. *J Am Acad Dermatol.* 2014;70(2):243–251.

34. Sun NZ, Ro T, Jolly P, et al. Non-response to IL1 Canakinumab in two patients with refractory pyoderma gangrenosum and hidradenitis suppurativa. *J Clin Aesthet Dermatol.* 2017 Sep;10(9):36–38.

35. Houriet C, Jafari SM, Thomi T, et al. Canakinumab for severe hidradenitis suppurativa: preliminary experience in 2 cases. *JAMA Dermatol.* 2017 Nov 1;153(11):1195–1197.

36. Tekin B, Salman A, Ergun T. Hidradenitis suppurativa unresponsive to canakinumab treatment: a case report. *Indian J Dermatol Venereol Leprol.* 2017 Sep–Oct;83(5):615–617.

37. Jaeger T, Andres C, Grosber M, et al. Pydoerma gangrenosum and concomitant hidradenitis supprutiva—rapid response to canakinumab (anti-IL-1B). *Eur J Dermatol.* 2013 May–Jun;23(3):408–410.

38. Reguiai Z, Fougerousse AC, Maccari F, Becherel PA. Effectiveness of secukinumab in hidradenitis suppurativa: an open study (20 cases). *J Eur Acad Dermatol Venereol.* 2020 May 13. https://doi.org/10.1111/jdv.16605.

39. Casseres RG, Prussick L, Zancanaro P, et al. Secukinumab in the treatment of moderate to severe hidradenitis suppurativa: results of an open-label trial. *J Am Acad Dermatol.* 2020 Jun;82(6):1524–1526.

40. Deckers IE, Benhadou F, Koldijk MR, et al. Inflammatory bowel disease is associated with hidradenitis suppurativa. Results from a multicenter cross-sectional study. *J Am Acad Dermatol.* 2017;76:49–53.

41. Megna M, Ruggiero A, Guida AD, et al. Ixekizumab: an efficacious treatment for both psoriasis and hidradenitis suppurativa. *Dermatol Ther.* 2020 Jun;4:e13756.

42. Odorici G, Pellacani G, Conti A. Ixekizumab in hidradenitis suppurativa: a case report in a psoriatic patient. *G Ital Dermatol Venereol.* 2019 Jan 9. https://doi.org/10.23736/S0392-0488.18.06135-7.

43. Weber P, Jafari SMS, Yawalkar N, et al. Apremilast in the treatment of moderate to severe hidradenitis suppurativa: a case series of 9 patients. *J Am Acad Dermatol.* 2017 Jun;76(6):1189–1191.

44. Vossen AR, Doorn M, van der Zee H, Prens E. Apremilast for moderate hidradenitis suppurativa: results of a randomized controlled trial. *J Am Acad Dermatol.* 2019 Jan;80(1):80–88.

45. Savage KT, Santillan MR, Flood K, et al. Tofacitinib shows benefit in conjunction with other therapies in recalcitrant hidradenitis suppurativa patients. *JAAD Case Rep.* 2020 Jan 20;6(2):99–102.

46. Lyons AB, Peacock A, McKenzie S, et al. Evaluation of Hidradenitis Suppurativa Disease course during pregnancy and postpartum. *JAMA Dermatol.* 2020 Apr 29;156(6):1–5.

47. Lyons AB, Peacock A, McKenzie SA, et al. Retrospective cohort study of pregnancy outcomes in hidradenitis suppurativa. *Br J Dermatol.* 2020 Apr 25. https://doi.org/10.1111/bjd.19155.

48. Perng P, Zampella JG, Okoye GA. Considering the impact of pregnancy on the natural history of hidradenitis suppurativa. *Br J Dermatol.* 2018 Jan;178(1):e13–e14.

49. Adelekun AA, Micheletti RG, Hsiao JL. Creation of a registry to address knowledge gaps in hidradenitis suppurativa and pregnancy. *JAMA Dermatol.* 2020 Jan 1;156(3):353.

50. Perng P, Zampella JG, Okoye GA. Management of hidradenitis suppurativa in pregnancy. *J Am Acad Dermatol.* 2017 May;76(5):979–989.

51. Androulakis I, Zavos C, Christopoulos P, et al. Safety of anti-tumor necrosis factor therapy during pregnancy in patients with inflammatory bowel disease. *World J Gastroenterol.* 2015;21(47):13205–13211.

52. Mariette X, Forger F, Abraham B, Flynn AD. Lack of placental transfer of certolizumab pegol during pregnancy: results from CRIB, a prospective, postmarketing, pharmacokinetic study. *Ann Rheum Dis.* 2018 Feb;77(2):228–233.

53. Nguyen Qb, Starling CT, Hebert AA. The use of TNFα inhibitors in treating pediatric skin disorders. *Pediatr Drugs.* 2020;22:311–319.

54. Mikkelsen PR, Jemec GB. Hidradenitis suppurativa in children and adolescents: a review of treatment options. *Paediatr Drugs.* 2014 Dec;16(6):483–489.

55. Liy-Wong C, Pope E, Lara-Corrales I. Hidradenitis suppurativa in the pediatric population. *J Am Acad Dermatol.* 2015 Nov;73(5 suppl 1):S36–S41.

56. Provini LE, Stellar JJ, Stetzer MN, et al. Combination hyperbaric oxygen therapy and ustekinumab for severe hidradenitis suppurativa. *Pediatr Dermatol.* 2019 May;36(3):381–383.

57. Caspersen S, Elkjaer M, Riis L, et al. Infliximab for inflammatory bowel disease in Denmark 1999–2005: clinical outcome and follow-up evaluation of malignancy and mortality. *Clin Gastroenterol Hepatol.* 2008 Nov;6(11):1212–1217.

58. Hyams JS, Dubinsky MS, Baldassano RN, et al. Infliximab Is Not Associated With Increased Risk of Malignancy or Hemophagocytic Lymphohistiocytosis in Pediatric Patients With Inflammatory Bowel Disease. *Gastroenterology.* 2017 Jun;152(8):1901–1914.

59. Lichtenstein GR, Feagan BG, Cohen RD, et al. Infliximab for Crohn's Disease: More Than 13 Years of Real-world Experience. *Inflamm Bowel Dis.* 2018 Feb 15;24(3):490–501.

60. Xie W, Xiao S, Huang Y, et al. A meta-analysis of biologic therapies on risk of new or recurrent cancer in aptients with rheumatoid arthritis and a prior malignancy. *Rheumatology.* 2020 May;59(5):930–939.

61. Wadstrom H, Frisell T, Askling J, et al. Malignant neoplasm in patients with rheumatoid arthritis treated with tumor necrosis factor inhibitors, tocilizumab, abatacept, or rituximab in clinical practice: A Nationwide Cohort Study From Sweden. *JAMA Intern Med.* 2017;177(11):1605–1612.

62. Kahn JS, Casseres RG, Her MJ, et al. Treatment of psoriasis with biologics and apremilast in patients with history of malignancy: a retrospective chart review. *J Drugs Dermatol.* 2019;18(4):387–390.

63. Ebell MH, Siewk J, Weiss BD, et al. Strength of recommendation taxonomy (SORT): a patient-centered approach to grading evidence in the medical literature. *Am Fam Physician.* 2004;69(3):548–556.

64. Kaushik SB, Lebwohl MG. Psoriasis: which therapy for which patient: psoriasis comorbidities and preferred systemic agents. *J Am Acad Dermatol.* 2019 Jan;80(1):27–40.

65. Alikhan A, Sayed C, Alavi A, et al. North American clinical management guidelines for hidradenitis suppurativa: a publication from the United States and Canadian Hidradenitis Suppurativa Foundations. *J Am Acad Dermatol.* 2019 Jul;81(1):76–90.

66. Scheinfeld N. Adalimumab: a review of side effects. *Expert Opin Drug Saf.* 2005 Jul;4(4):637–641.

67. Hanauer SB. Review article: safety of infliximab in clinical trials. *Aliment Pharmacol Ther.* 2002. 999 Sep;13 Suppl 4:16–22.

68. Hsu L, Snodgrass BT, Armstrong AW. Antidrug antibodies in psoriasis: a systematic review. *Br J Dermatol.* 2014 Feb;170(2):261–267.

69. Cavalli G, Dinarello C. Anakinra Therapy for Non-cancer Inflammatory Diseases. *Front Pharmacol.* 2018 Nov 6;9:1157.

70. Ramirez J, Canete JD. Anakinra for the treatment of rheumatoid arthritis: a safety evaluation. *Expert Opin Drug Safe.* 2018 Jul;17(7):727–732.

71. Dhimolea E. Canakinumab. *MAbs.* Jan-Feb 2010;2(1):3–13.

72. Houriet C, Jafari SM, Thom R, et al. Canakinumab for Severe Hidradenitis Suppurativa: Preliminary Experience in 2 Cases. *JAMA Dermatol.* 2017 Nov 1;153(11):1195–1197.

73. Ridker P, Everett BM, Thuren T, et al. Anti-inflammatory therapy with canakinumab for atherosclerotic disease. *N Engl J Med.* 2017 Sep 21;377(12):1119–1131.

74. https://www.accessdata.fda.gov/drugsatfda_docs/label/2016/761044lbl.pdf (Date visited: 8/1/2020).

75. https://www.accessdata.fda.gov/drugsatfda_docs/label/2017/761061s000lbl.pdf (Date visited: 8/1/2020).

76. Kovacs M, Podda M. Guselkumab in the treatment of severe hidradenitis suppurativa. *J Eur Acad Dermatol Venereol.* 2019 Mar;33(3): e140–e141.

77. https://www.accessdata.fda.gov/drugsatfda_docs/label/2016/ 125504s001s002lbl.pdf (Date visited: 8/1/2020).

78. Casseres RG, Prussick L, Zancanaro P, et al. Secukinumab in the treatment of moderate to severe hidradenitis suppurativa: results of an open label trial. *J Am Acad Dermatol.* 2020 Jun;82(6): 1524–1526.

79. Savage KT, Santillan MR, Flood KS, et al. Tofacitinib shows benefit in conjunction with other therapies in recalcitrant hidradenitis suppurativa patients. *JAAD Case Rep.* 2020 Jan 20;6 (2):99–102.

80. Huang F, Luo ZC. Adverse drug events associated with 5 mg versus 10 mg Tofacitinib (Janus kinase inhibitor) twice daily for the treatment of autoimmune diseases: a systematic review and meta-analysis of randomized controlled trials. *Clin Rheumatol.* 2019;38: 523–534.

19

Pain and Itch Control

EMILY F. COLE, KEVIN T. SAVAGE, AND LAUREN A.V. ORENSTEIN

Introduction

Pain is the most burdensome symptom of hidradenitis suppurativa (HS), accounting for greater impairment in HS-related quality of life (QoL) than even disease severity.[1,2] Although it has received relatively less attention, pruritus is also common in HS and contributes to disability and poor health-related QoL among those living with HS. This chapter summarizes what is currently known about the epidemiology, clinical characteristics, and pathophysiology of HS-related pain and itch and synthesizes these data to suggest rational approaches to clinical management of these symptoms.

Pain in Hidradenitis Suppurativa

Epidemiology of Pain in Hidradenitis Suppurativa

Prevalence and Severity of Pain in Hidradenitis Suppurativa

Nearly all individuals living with HS experience lesion-associated pain during the disease course,[1] and a large proportion report pain that occurs on a weekly basis (77% to 91%).[1] In a cross-sectional study of 294 patients, the mean number of days with pain in the past month was 9.51 ± 9.67.[3] A prospective international study of 1299 HS patients found that the majority of patients (61.4%) rate their pain severity as ≥ 5 on a numeric rating scale (NRS) of 0 to 10 and that 4.5% rate their pain as the "worst possible" or 10/10.[4] When evaluating pain severity, other studies' findings have been comparable, with average weekly NRS pain scores ranging from 3.6 to 5.0.[1,4–6]

Compared to other painful dermatologic conditions such as blistering diseases, leg ulcers, atopic dermatitis, lichen sclerosis, and skin tumors, those with HS had more frequent and severe pain.[6–8] Individuals with HS are at increased risk for chronic opioid use[9] as well as other substance misuse[10] when compared to non-HS controls. Poorly controlled pain may contribute to this phenomenon, increasing the importance of recognizing and managing pain in patients with HS.

Risk Factors

Risk factors for HS pain include severe HS disease activity[1] and a higher number of anatomic regions involved.[8] Psychiatric comorbidities such as anxiety and depression further compound pain perception.[8,11] Physical factors such as friction and tight-fitting clothing have also been reported to exacerbate HS pain.[11]

Impact of Pain on Quality of Life

HS is highly debilitating, with worse patient-reported QoL than almost any other skin disease.[7,11–14] Pain has been identified as the major contributor to reduced QoL and disability in HS, even more so than HS severity.[1–3] Painful HS lesions directly impact physical function and daily activities. Individuals living with HS commonly report that HS lesional pain impacts mobility, participation in exercise and sports, work productivity, and sexual health.[15–18] HS pain is also associated with insomnia and poor sleep quality.[19] HS pain impacts psychological well-being, resulting in increased risks for depression, anxiety, and suicide among those living with HS.[20,21] The HS pain experience and the uncertainty of its course contribute to a sense of powerlessness and worsened emotional function.[17,22] Further, HS patients report feeling isolated and invalidated when others fail to understand and empathize with the severity of their pain.[22]

Clinical Characteristics of Hidradenitis Suppurativa Pain

The quality of HS pain may vary between patients and may also vary over time within the same individual. The timing of HS pain may be acute with associated flare or worsening inflammatory activity, or chronic in nature. HS pain has been described by patients as nociceptive and neuropathic in character.[8,17,23] Nociceptive pain results from a noxious stimulus that has potential for tissue damage, and is often described as "aching," "gnawing," or "throbbing."[8] In HS, nociceptive pain may result from direct inflammatory tissue damage (see Pathophysiology of Pain in HS). Neuropathic pain arises from damage to the somatosensory nervous system. Neuropathic pain is classically described as "burning," "stinging," or "stabbing," and these descriptors are common among HS patients experiencing pain.[8] In a study of 92 HS patients, 31.5% of patients reported symptoms suspicious for neuropathic pain, 41.3% had no neuropathic symptoms, and 27.2% had unclear results.[23] Those with neuropathic pain were more likely to experience moderate to severe pain and to report psychiatric comorbidities.[23]

Pathophysiology of Pain in Hidradenitis Suppurativa

Overview of Pain Response

The physiologic response to pain resulting from tissue injury is an important evolutionary strategy in withdrawal from and avoidance of harmful stimuli. This response, which is not specific to HS, involves four major components: (1) transduction, (2) transmission, (3) modulation or transformation, and (4) perception.[24] Transduction is the process by which primary afferent neurons or nociceptors convert noxious stimuli including chemical, mechanical, heat, and cold into nociceptive electrical signals. Pain, in addition to itch and temperature, are transmitted mainly by unmyelinated c-fibers and thinly myelinated Aδ fibers. If this electrical signal reaches the threshold for activation potential, transmission occurs, sending a nociceptive signal from peripheral nerve fibers to the central nervous system (CNS). Modulation or transformation modifies these signals at the level of the CNS. Perception is the final stage of the nociceptive process that integrates cognitive and affective responses, resulting in the subjective pain experience (Fig. 19.1). The sections that follow incorporate current knowledge of HS pathophysiology with clinical descriptions of HS pain to suggest mechanisms which may contribute to the pain response in HS.

Nociceptors, Signal Transduction, and Transmission in Hidradenitis Suppurativa

Inflammatory tissue damage likely plays a substantial role in generating the nociceptive signals that are the first step in the HS pain response pathway. HS is associated with a mixed inflammatory infiltrate including neutrophils, T-cells, B-cells, plasma cells, NK cells, mast cells, macrophages, and dendritic cells. These cells produce a variety of cytokines, chemokines, and growth factors which serve as stimuli to nociceptors. The role of inflammatory cells in causing HS pain is supported by the finding that anti-inflammatory therapies can produce an analgesic effect in HS.[25,26] Lifestyle factors and comorbid conditions, such as obesity, nicotine use, and metabolic syndrome, likely contribute to

the stress response and enhance recruitment of inflammatory cells. Additionally, inflammatory cells recruitment results in damage to peripheral tissue, inducing keratinocytes to release pro-inflammatory factors such as prostaglandins, substance P, and calcitonin gene-related peptide (CGRP). These mediators subsequently bind to nociceptors, resulting in a series of electrical impulses at the afferent nerve terminal.

Of particular note, tumour necrosis factor-α (TNF-α) is a pro-inflammatory cytokine that has been found in lesional skin[27] and serum[28,29] of individuals with HS. Pharmacologic neutralization of TNF-α was shown to block nociceptive activity in the thalamus, somatosensory cortex, and limbic system within the first 24 hours and prior to any anti-inflammatory effect in peripheral tissues, suggesting that this cytokine may play a role in nociception, both peripherally and centrally.[30]

Neuropathic Pain in Hidradenitis Suppurativa

Neuropathic pain arises from damage to the somatosensory nervous system, typically to peripheral fibers (Aβ, Aδ, and C-fibers) or central neurons. Studies of patient-reported pain descriptions suggest that neuropathic pain likely also plays a major role in pain in HS (see Clinical Characteristics of Pain).[8,17,23] The precise mechanism for neuropathic pain in HS has not been elucidated. However, one explanation is that the inflammatory infiltrate, including mast cells, may promote neurogenic inflammation through release of mediators including histamine, tryptase, interleukin (IL)-31, and Nerve growth factor (NGF) which activate nociceptors on pain-sending neurons.[31] Eosinophils and neutrophils may have similar, but less pronounced interactions with C-fibers. Additional studies are needed to fully understand the mechanism by which neuropathic pain occurs in HS.

Pain Perception in Hidradenitis Suppurativa

Pain experiences vary greatly between individuals. Differences in pain perception may in part be due to emotional distress, depression,[8] and even socioeconomic predictors of health. In HS, these differences have been attributed to multiple causes including alterations in descending modulatory pathways as well as an exaggerated stress response. Modulatory pathways represent a complex system of feedback loops in the CNS that mediate top-down regulation of nociceptive processing. Altered descending modulatory pathways resulting in maintenance or amplification of pain signaling is implicated in various chronic pain states.[32] Given that pain perception in HS does not necessarily correlate with disease severity, aberrant modulatory pathways may represent an important factor in HS pain.[33]

Additionally, an overactive stress response in HS may result in a generalized inflammatory state that promotes pro-inflammatory cytokines including TNF-α, IL-1, and IL-6.[34] Depression and anxiety are associated with higher serum levels of pro-inflammatory cytokines which may also contribute to a state of generalized inflammation.[35,36] This theory is supported by the observations of worsening of HS disease in the setting of increased psychological stress as well as improvement in pain and psychological symptoms following treatment with adalimumab.[37]

Pain Management in Hidradenitis Suppurativa

The pathophysiology of pain perception in HS is complex and closely linked with mental health. The most effective management strategies, therefore, likely require multimodal therapies that address nociceptive and neuropathic pain as well as the associated psychological distress. In other chronic pain syndromes, a multidisciplinary approach has been shown to yield superior pain outcomes.[38] We

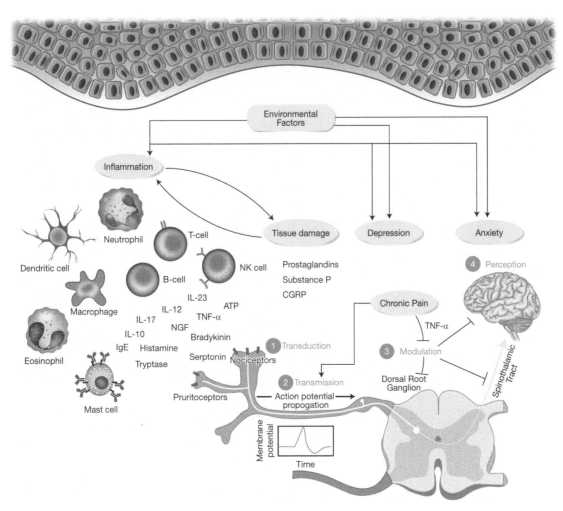

• **Fig. 19.1** Pathophysiology of pain and itch in hidradenitis suppurativa (HS). (1) Cutaneous sensory neurons are activated at the tissue level through various stimuli including mechanical stress, heat, cold, and inflammatory mediators (transduction); (2) This activation initiates an electrical impulse, called an action potential, to propagate along the nerve axon (transmission); (3) The action potential reaches the dorsal root ganglion, where the cell bodies of primary sensory neurons lie, and synapse with second order neurons in the dorsal horn of the spinal cord. Modulation modifies these signals at the level of the central nervous system; (4) Sensory information on pain and itch travels up to the thalamus and eventually cerebral cortex via the lateral spinothalamic tract, where conscious perception occurs. *IgE*, Immunoglobulin E, *IL*, interleukin, *TNF*, tumour necrosis factor-α, *ATP*, adenosine triphosphate, *NGF*, nerve growth factor.

therefore recommend early inclusion of non-pharmacologic treatments for HS pain such as physical therapy, appropriate wound care, and mental/behavioral health.

Overview of Evidence-Based Guidelines

Although multiple major international HS treatment guidelines have been published in recent years, few offer detailed guidance about management of HS pain.[39–42] Some common themes and recommendations from these guidelines are highlighted in Box 19.1.

Clinical Evaluation of Hidradenitis Suppurativa Pain

The best validated tools for evaluating pain severity across a wide spectrum of diseases include the Visual Analog Scale (VAS) and the Numeric Rating Scale (NRS). These are simple and practical for routine clinical use, making them a first choice for regular assessment of HS pain severity given the absence of HS-specific data currently. Pain was recently identified by the Hidradenitis SuppuraTiva cORe outcome set International Collaboration (HISTORIC) as one of six domains in the core outcome set for HS clinical trials. Additional effort is ongoing to determine the best measurement instrument and frequency evaluation for HS pain measurement in clinical trials.[43]

In addition to evaluating pain severity, assessing the quality of HS pain may help distinguish nociceptive and neuropathic pain and help direct selection of pharmacologic analgesia. The McGill Pain Questionnaire and painDETECT survey have been used to help characterize HS pain,[8,23] although neither has been specifically validated for use in HS. A patient interview including questions about the description of pain may be used to evaluate the pain character. Nociceptive pain is likely when the pain is localized to HS lesions and the patient describes pain as "aching," "gnawing," "pressure," "squeezing," or "throbbing." Nociceptive pain is suggested by distal radiation, sensory deficits, use of temperature descriptors, and exaggerated hypersensitivity to classically non-painful stimuli. Common descriptors of nociceptive pain include

---

• BOX 19.1 **Pain Management Recommendations Among International Hidradenitis Suppurativa Guidelines**

- Hidradenitis suppurativa (HS) pain should be acknowledged and treated.

- Patient-reported outcomes including pain assessment are recommended.
- HS disease control improves pain.
- Intralesional triamcinolone may reduce pain due to acutely inflamed HS lesion.
- Incision and drainage may temporarily relieve HS pain due to abscesses.

- Non-steroidal antiinflammatory drugs (NSAIDs) may be used to treat HS pain.
- Short-acting opioid analgesics should be used judiciously and for limited intervals.

See References 39–42, 65–69.

"lancinating," "shooting," "electricity," "tingling," and "itching." Clinically distinguishing nociceptive and neuropathic pain may have therapeutic implications, as many management guidelines for chronic non-cancer pain suggest different treatments for nociceptive and neuropathic pain.[44]

Hidradenitis Suppurativa Pain Treatment Algorithms

One set of pain management algorithms has been published to date and has been reproduced in Figs. 19.2 and 19.3. Although these algorithms provide a practical guide for healthcare providers in managing HS pain, improved knowledge of HS pain pathophysiology and effective therapies for HS pain management are critically needed. The strongest data for pain control in HS derive from clinical trials of HS disease-modifying therapies. First and foremost, HS pain control must begin with an appropriate medical management of the underlying disease.

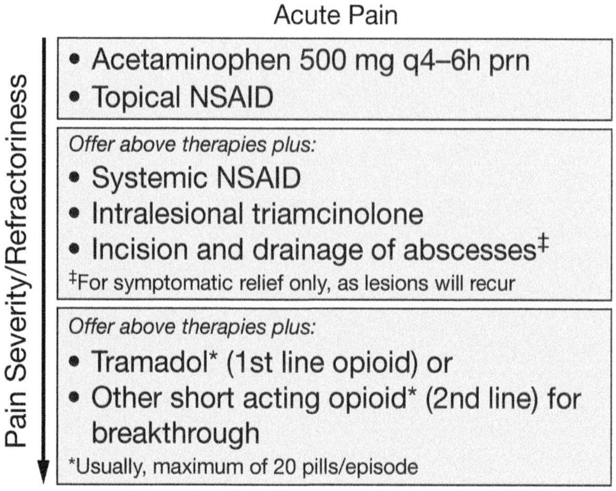

Pharmacologic Analgesia

Several reviews of the management of HS pain and chronic dermatologic pain provide comprehensive overviews of pharmacologic

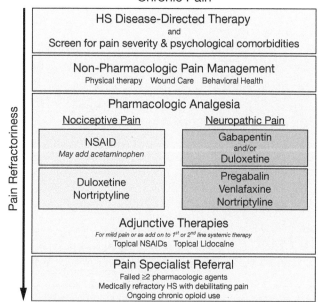

• Fig. 19.3 Algorithm for Treatment of Chronic Pain in Hidradenitis Suppurativa. As hidradenitis suppurativa (HS) pain is related to disease activity and impact, HS disease-directed therapy and assessment of pain severity and psychological comorbidities is critical to reduce chronic HS pain. Physical therapy, wound care, and behavioral health are non-pharmacologic chronic pain management tools. Understanding if the pain is nociceptive or neuropathic can guide the type of pharmacologic analgesia that may be most beneficial. For nociceptive pain (yellow boxes), first-line options include non-steroidal anti-inflammatory drugs (NSAIDs) or celecoxib (COX-2 inhibitor), and second-line options include duloxetine (SNRI) or nortriptyline (TCA). For neuropathic pain (blue boxes), first-line options include gabapentin (anticonvulsant) and duloxetine, and second line are pregabalin, venlafaxine (SNRI), and nortriptyline. Anticonvulsants and SNRIs may be safely combined, however SNRIs should not be combined with other serotonergic agents. Adjunctive therapies for all patients with chronic pain include topical NSAIDs and topical lidocaine. Some patients may also be interested in other complementary and alternative medicine (CAM) options such as turmeric (curcumin), α-lipoic acid, acupuncture, or medical cannabis. Referral to a pain specialist is recommended if the patient continues to experience chronic pain after utilizing these approaches, and before starting regular opioids. (From Savage KT, Singh V, Patel ZS, et al. Pain management in hidradenitis suppurativa and a proposed treatment algorithm. *J Am Acad Dermatol.* 2020 Sep 17:S0190-9622(20)32627-X. doi: 10.1016/j.jaad.2020.09.039. Epub ahead of print. PMID: 32950543.)

Acute Pain

(Pain Severity/Refractoriness)

- Acetaminophen 500 mg q4–6h prn
- Topical NSAID

Offer above therapies plus:
- Systemic NSAID
- Intralesional triamcinolone
- Incision and drainage of abscesses‡

‡For symptomatic relief only, as lesions will recur

Offer above therapies plus:
- Tramadol* (1st line opioid) or
- Other short acting opioid* (2nd line) for breakthrough

*Usually, maximum of 20 pills/episode

• Fig. 19.2 Algorithm for Treatment of Acute Pain in Hidradenitis Suppurativa. Acetaminophen and/or topical non-steroidal antiinflammatory drugs (NSAIDs) may be useful for mild acute pain, which is predominantly nociceptive. If acute pain persists, oral NSAIDs and/or intralesional triamcinolone may be helpful. If acute pain worsens or persists, first-line is tramadol or second-line oxycodone (both usually maximum of 20 pills/episode). Referral to a pain management specialist is recommended before starting regular opioids. (‡) For symptomatic relief of an acute painful abscess, incision and drainage may be indicated although lesions typically recur. (From Savage KT, Singh V, Patel ZS, et al. Pain management in hidradenitis suppurativa and a proposed treatment algorithm. *J Am Acad Dermatol.* 2020 Sep 17:S0190-9622(20)32627-X. doi: 10.1016/j.jaad.2020.09.039. Epub ahead of print. PMID: 32950543.)

analgesia treatment options.[25,45,46] Few disease-specific data in HS exist, and therefore pharmacologic therapies are often selected based on pain chronicity (acute vs. chronic) and character (nociceptive vs. neuropathic). Table 19.1 describes commonly employed analgesics, dosing guidelines, and risk profiles. Surgical management of HS including wide local excision and healing via secondary intent may result in increased acute pain symptoms. We recommend creating a pain management plan in advance for patients who are planning to undergo surgical management to ensure that pain is appropriately controlled in the pre- and post-operative periods.

Psychological Treatment Modalities

Depression and anxiety are common comorbidities of HS and strongly influence pain perception.[20] Although studies evaluating the effectiveness of psychological treatments in HS specifically are lacking, cognitive behavioral therapy (CBT) and acceptance and commitment

TABLE 19.1	Pharmacologic analgesia in Hidradenitis Suppurativa	
Medication	**Dose**	**Selected Risks**
Topical and Intralesional Therapies		
Intralesional triamcinolone	• 10–40 mg/mL	• Cutaneous atrophy and dyspigmentation • Systemic absorption at high doses
Topical diclofenac	• 1% gel: Apply 2 g 4 × daily prn • 1.3% patch: Apply one patch q12 h prn	• Application site reaction
Lidocaine topical	• 5% cream: Apply to intact skin q4h prn • 4% patch: Apply to intact skin for ≤12 h daily; may apply up to 3 patches simultaneously	• Application site reaction • Avoid application to large open wounds to reduce risk of systemic absorption and toxicity
Menthol topical	• 4% ointment/cream: Apply ≤4 × daily	• Application site reaction
Non-Steroidal Antiinflammatory Drugs and Acetaminophen		
Diclofenac sodium, delayed-release	• 50 mg q8h prn	• Elevated risk of CV events • Acute kidney injury • GI ulcers and bleeding
Ibuprofen	• 300–800 mg q8h prn; max 2400 mg daily	• Risks comparable to those of diclofenac
Naproxen	• Base: 250–500 mg q12h prn • Sodium: 275–550 mg q12h prn	• NSAID of choice in patients with CV risk factors • Otherwise, risks comparable to diclofenac
Celecoxib	• 100–200 mg q12–24h prn	• ↑ risk of CV events compared to other NSAIDs • Risk of GI bleed, but less compared to other NSAIDs
Acetaminophen	• 325–650 mg q4–6 prn	• Liver failure
Calcium Channel Alpha-2 Ligands		
Gabapentin	• Start 300 mg daily. Increase dose by 300 mg each day. • Max: 1200 mg TID	• Drowsiness
Pregabalin	• Start: 150 mg daily divided BID/TID; • Week 2: ↑ to 300 mg daily; Weeks 3–5 : ↑ to 300 mg daily • Max: 600 mg daily divided BID/TID	• Drowsiness • Crosses blood brain barrier, causing euphoria and ↑ addiction potential
Serotonin-Norepinephrine Reuptake Inhibitors		
Duloxetine	• Start: 30 mg daily • Titration: After 1 week, ↑ to 60 mg daily. • Max: 120 mg daily (60 mg daily is usually equally effective)	• GI intolerance; Sexual dysfunction • Serotonin syndrome, especially if combined with other serotonergic agents • Black Box warning for suicidality if ≤24 years old
Venlafaxine	• Start: 37.5–75 mg daily • Titration: Each week, may ↑ by up to 75 mg daily • Max: 225 mg daily	• QTc prolongation • Other risks comparable to duloxetine
Tricyclic Antidepressants		
Desipramine and Nortriptyline	• Start 25 mg nightly. Every 3–7 days, ↑ by up to 25 mg daily. • Max: 150 mg daily	• QTc prolongation • Anticholinergic effects (nortriptyline > desipramine) and weight gain
Amitriptyline	• Same as desipramine and nortriptyline above	• Much higher risk of anticholinergic effects compared to other TCAs

BID, Two times daily; *CV*, cardiovascular; *div*, divided; *GI*, gastrointestinal; *h*, hour; *NSAIDs*, nonsteroidal anti-inflammatory drugs; *prn*, as needed; *q*, every; *TCA*, tricyclic antidepressant; *TID*, three times daily.

therapy (ACT) are evidence-based interventions for chronic pain.[47–49] CBT aims to reduce pain through cognitive restructuring, relaxation techniques, and activities. ACT, by contrast, aims to reduce suffering due to pain even when the elimination of pain is not feasible.

Pruritus in Hidradenitis Suppurativa

Previously, most studies assessing symptom experience in HS focused on pain as this is the predominant symptom reported by patients with HS. However, pruritus has recently started to receive recognition as an important symptom in HS. The epidemiology, quality-of-life impact, potential pathomechanisms, and treatment options are described below.

Epidemiology of Pruritus in Hidradenitis Suppurativa

Prevalence and Severity of Itch in Hidradenitis Suppurativa

Pruritus is a common symptom in HS, with reported prevalence varying from 41.7%[1] to 67.3%.[50] In the largest cross-sectional study on pruritus in Spanish patients with HS, 61.8% of patients reported a numeric rating score greater than 3 for pruritus, compared to 65.2% reporting an NRS greater than 3 for pain.[5] In another large cross-sectional study in Denmark, 67.3% of patients reported a NRS for itch ≥1, and 57.3% reported a score ≥3.[50]

Although the degree of HS-associated pruritus is usually less severe than pain, pruritus nonetheless represents an important symptom in HS. Although most studies assessing itch severity in HS have used numerical rating scales (NRS) or visual analog scales (VAS), the timeframe for assessing itch severity varied. Four cross-sectional studies totaling 841 patients reported the highest intensity pruritus over the past 7 days to range from 3.7 to 5.5.[1,3,5,6] In a cross-sectional study of 294 patients with HS from Denmark, pruritus VAS was 3.72 ± 3.17, compared to 3.91 ± 3.18 for pain and 2.87 ± 3.34 for malodor.[3] Notably, none of the available studies assessing pruritus have utilized validated itch-specific measures other than NRS or VAS. This represents an important gap in our knowledge of pruritus in HS.

Risk Factors

Several risk factors have been identified for pruritus in HS. In multivariable regression, a Danish study of 211 patients identified clinical severity (Hurley III—OR 7.73, 95% CI 2.01 to 2.27) and pain (OR 1.34 95% CI 1.18 to 1.52) as independent risk factors for pruritus as indicated by Pruritus NRS ≥3, in HS.[50] Although current affected body site (OR 1.70, CI 1.32 to 2.19) and smoking status (OR 2.27, CI 1.08 to 1.76) were associated with pruritus in univariate models, they did not remain significant when adjusting for other covariates. Another study totaling 103 patients reported that itch was predominantly associated with buttock and axillary disease, whereas pain was equally distributed among all anatomic sites.[1] Similar to the Danish study, smokers and patients with Hurley stage III disease experienced more severe pruritus, although this did not reach statistical significance. A Spanish study of 233 patients with HS identified a positive correlation between pruritus intensity and female sex, number of affected body regions, intensity of suppuration, and presence of comorbid Crohn disease.[5] Additional studies are needed to fully elucidate risk factors for pruritus in HS and may also provide valuable insight into pathophysiology.

Impact of Itch on Quality of Life

Similar to other inflammatory dermatoses, itch in HS has a major negative impact on QoL. Studies evaluating QoL and disability using the DLQI[5,6] and EuroQoL-5D instrument[3] have consistently demonstrated worse outcomes among HS patients experiencing pruritus. Qualitative studies have also suggested that both itch and pain are sources of psychosocial distress, leading to poorer QoL outcomes.[51] Further, itch in HS has also been shown to negatively impact sleep.[19,50]

Clinical Characteristics of Itch in Hidradenitis Suppurativa

The clinical characteristics of itch in HS do not differ greatly from those of other pruritic inflammatory skin diseases. Itch descriptors reported in HS, including burning, stinging, tickling, and prickling, suggest neuropathic and pruritoceptive components to itch.[1] Additionally, itch prior to the onset of an HS flare is the third most common localized symptom (20%) behind erythema (75%) and paresthesia (63%).[52] The factor most frequently associated with aggravation of itch in HS is sweating, followed by heat, physical activity, and hot water.[1]

Pathophysiology of Itch in Hidradenitis Suppurativa

Historically, the sensations of itch and pain have been considered related but antagonistic. For example, the response to itch is scratching, which may cause pain, and opioid analgesics designed to treat pain cause itch. However, as the neurobiology of these symptoms is becoming clearer, striking similarities between these two symptoms become more apparent. Itch is transduced at the level of the skin to electrical impulses, which are subsequently transmitted as action potentials through the dorsal horn of the spinal cord and to the CNS. Similar to pain, itch can also undergo modulation at multiple levels of the itch pathway. However, there are several key mediators that are specific to itch rather than pain, outlined below.

Eosinophils, Mast Cells, and Immunoglobulin E

Eosinophilia (both systemic and tissue-specific) is commonly seen in pruritic skin conditions such as atopic dermatitis. Eosinophils promote pruritus through several mechanisms, including recruitment of inflammatory cells, production of reactive oxygen species, and production of enzymes, growth factors, and additional Th2 cells. Eosinophils may directly interact with C-fibers, and this is supported by the observations that in murine models, eosinophils in the skin localize to areas of increased nerve density and that eosinophils in culture with nerve fibers cause increased branching of sensory neurons.[53] Although not a predominate cell type in HS, eosinophils have been identified in both perilesional and lesional skin. In one cross-sectional study, hematoxylin and eosin (H&E) staining was performed on 24 specimens obtained from large radical excisions of chronically inflamed HS skin. Eosinophils were observed in 25% of perilesional skin biopsies and 62.5% of lesion skin biopsies, supporting a role as mediator of pruritus rather than an incidental finding.[50]

Eosinophils also promote pruritus through interactions with mast cells. In many allergic disorders, eosinophils and mast cells are found in close proximity (deemed the "allergic effector unit"), and physical interaction between eosinophils and mast cells produces a hyperactive state through release of various chemical mediators. There is also evidence for a strong relationship between mast cells and C-fibers through release of chemical mediators. These interactions can result in direct stimulation of C-fibers, resulting in the sensation of itch.

Tryptase-positive mast cells have been identified in all stages of HS, including in perilesional skin.[54] Although presence of mast cells was correlated with HS disease severity, no correlation was identified between mast cell count and the maximum 7 days itch severity. Increased serum immunoglobulin E (IgE) has also been reported in some patients with HS, suggesting HS itch may be at least partially mediated by cross-linking of IgE with its high-affinity receptor (FcεRI) on the surface of mast cells. IgE levels were even higher in smokers, men, and those with HS lesions outside of the groin.[55] An association between smoking and itch in HS has been reported, and although this association did not reach statistical significance,[1] these results suggest a potential mechanism for the influence of environmental factors on itch. These authors also hypothesized that elevated IL-10 in tissue promotes B-cell differentiation to plasma cells, therefore increasing production of IgE.

Neutrophils

Neutrophils release mediators which may also be implicated in HS. Mediators released by neutrophils which may be implicated in itch include histamine, tryptase, leukotriene B4 (LTB4), and various chemokines such as neutrophil-dependent C-X-C motif chemokine 10 (CXCL10). Neutrophils may also recruit inflammatory cells to the site.[56] Neutrophils are one of the primary cell types in the inflammatory infiltrate of HS,[57] and recent data suggest that enhanced formation of neutrophil extracellular traps (NET) as well as immune responses to neutrophil and NET-related antigens may promote immune dysregulation. NETs have been hypothesized to play a role in pruritus in other inflammatory skin diseases and investigation into the association between itch and HS represents an important direction for future studies.[58]

Other Factors Potentially Implicated in Hidradenitis Suppurativa Itch

In addition to the factors listed above, other factors may contribute to itch in HS. Th17-associated cytokines, such as IL-17, IL-12, IL-23, and complement may promote the innate immune response and recruit additional inflammatory mediators. IL-31 may act on sensory C-fibers to initiate itch signals, as has been described in other pruritic skin conditions such as atopic dermatitis.[59] Toll-like receptors (TLRs), a type of pattern recognition receptor, are crucial for inducing immune responses. Although increased expression of TLR2 by macrophages and dendritic cells is the main finding described in HS,[60] other TLRs play an important role in mediating itch in other pruritic skin conditions.[61,62] The mammalian target of rapamycin (mTOR) has been identified as a potential factor in the regulation of primary afferent nerve homeostasis, particularly in the settings of chronic pain and itch.[63] Upregulation of the mTORC1 pathway has been observed in multiple inflammatory dermatoses including HS,[64] suggesting another potential therapeutic target in the treatment of itch in HS. Finally, recurrent and chronic

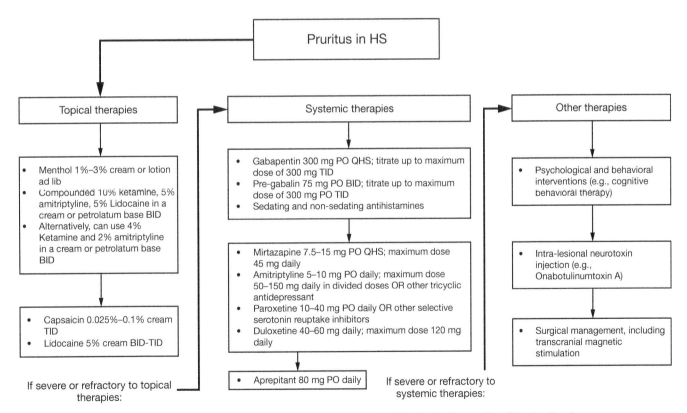

• **Fig. 19.4** Proposed Algorithm for Management in Pruritus in Hidradenitis Suppurativa. This algorithm is based on expert opinion and evidence in other pruritic disease states,[70-77] as there exist no studies of therapies for HS itch management. Initial therapy for mild-moderate pruritus in hidradenitis suppurativa (HS) should focus on skin-directed topical therapies. If adequate relief of pruritus is not achieved with topical therapies, systemic therapies including gabapentinoids or antidepressants should be utilized. Invasive or experimental therapies, including psychological interventions and invasive procedures, should only be attempted as a last resort in cases of severe, refractory HS pruritus.

inflammation may cause a small fiber neuropathy due to destruction of C-fibers, scar formation, and nerve fiber regrowth along with neovascularization, resulting in enduring neuropathic itch.

Treatment of Itch in Hidradenitis Suppurativa

Given the complex etiology of itch in HS, a multi-modal treatment approach is likely necessary. Like pain, the treatment of itch is focused on several targets: (1) Decreasing inflammation that promotes mediators of pruritus and (2) Treating the neuropathic component to itch. There is currently a paucity of data for treatment of itch in HS. Therefore, the suggestions found in this section are based on experience in other pruritic diseases and author opinion.

Decreasing the innate inflammatory response can be accomplished through several therapeutic strategies, including systemic antibiotics and targeted biologic therapies including TNF-α, IL-12/IL-23, and components of the complement cascade (e.g., C5). Treatments for neuropathic itch, like neuropathic pain, may include topical therapies such as capsaicin or lidocaine, gabapentin, pregabalin, tricyclic antidepressants, selective serotonin reuptake inhibitors (SSRIs), carbamazepine, duloxetine, and psychological and behavioral interventions (Fig. 19.4). Refractory cases may be amenable to more invasive procedures such as transcranial magnetic stimulation. Opioids in the management of HS-related pain should be avoided given their effect on central opioid receptors and accompanying strong association with pruritus.

Conclusion

Pain and itch are major causes of QoL impairment in HS. Much remains to be learned about the underlying pathophysiology of these symptoms in HS. Future elucidation of the mechanisms for pain and itch in HS is critical in order to define therapeutic targets and ultimately develop evidence-based therapies that can increase quality of life among individuals living with HS.

References

1. Matusiak Ł, Szczęch J, Kaaz K, et al. Clinical Characteristics of Pruritus and Pain in Patients with Hidradenitis Suppurativa. *Acta Derm Venereol.* 2018;98(2):191–194.
2. Patel Zarine S, Hoffman LK, Buse DC, et al. Pain, Psychological Comorbidities, Disability and Impaired Qualify of Life in Hidradenitis Suppurativa HHS Public Access. *Curr Pain Headache Rep.* 2017;21(12):49.
3. Riis PT, Vinding GR, Ring HC, Jemec GBE. Disutility in Patients with Hidradenitis Suppurativa: A Crosssectional Study Using EuroQoL-5D. *Acta Derm Venereol.* 2016;96(2):222–226.
4. Garg A, Neuren E, Cha D, et al. Evaluating patients' unmet needs in hidradenitis Suppurativa: results from the Global Survey Of Impact and Healthcare Needs (VOICE) Project. *J Am Acad Dermatol.* 2020;82(2):366–376.
5. Molina-Leyva A, Cuenca-Barrales C. Pruritus and Malodour in Patients with Hidradenitis Suppurativa: Impact on Quality of Life and Clinical Features Associated with Symptom Severity. *Dermatology (Basel, Switzerland).* 2020;236(1):59–65.
6. Onderdijk AJ, van der Zee HH, Esmann S, et al. Depression in patients with hidradenitis suppurativa. *J Eur Acad Dermatol Venereol.* 2013;27(4):473–478.
7. Balieva F, Kupfer J, Lien L, et al. The burden of common skin diseases assessed with the EQ5D™: a European multicentre study in 13 countries. *Br J Dermatol.* 2017;176(5):1170–1178.
8. Nielsen RM, Lindsø Andersen P, Sigsgaard V, Theut Riis P, Jemec GB. Pain perception in patients with hidradenitis suppurativa. *Br J Dermatol.* 2020 Jan;182(1):166–174. https://doi.org/10.1111/bjd.17935. Epub 2019 Jul 8. PMID: 30919930.
9. Reddy S, Orenstein LAV, Strunk A, Garg A. Incidence of Long-Term Opioid Use among Opioid-Naive Patients with Hidradenitis Suppurativa in the United States. *JAMA Dermatol.* 2019;155(11):1284–1290.
10. Garg A, Papagermanos V, Midura M, et al. Opioid, alcohol, and cannabis misuse among patients with hidradenitis suppurativa: a population-based analysis in the United States. *J Am Acad Dermatol.* 2018;79(3):495–500.
11. Ring HC, Riis PT, Miller IM, et al. Self-reported pain management in hidradenitis suppurativa. *Br J Dermatol.* 2016;174(4):909–911.
12. Matusiak Ł, Andrzej B, Jacek CS. Hidradenitis Suppurativa Markedly Decreases Quality of Life and Professional Activity. *J Am Acad Dermatol.* 2010;62(4):706–708.
13. Storer MA, Danesh MJ, Sandhu ME, et al. An assessment of the relative impact of hidradenitis suppurativa, psoriasis, and obesity on quality of life. *Int J Womens Dermatol.* 2018;4:198–202.
14. Wolkenstein P, Loundou A, Barrau K, et al. Quality of life impairment in hidradenitis suppurativa: a study of 61 cases. *J Am Acad Dermatol.* 2007;56:621–623.
15. Alavi A, Farzanfar D, Rogalska T, et al. Quality of life and sexual health in patients with hidradenitis suppurativa. *Int J Womens Dermatol.* 2018;4(2):74–79.
16. Deckers IE, Alexa BK. The Handicap of Hidradenitis Suppurativa. *Dermatol Clin.* 2016;34(1):17–22.
17. Patel ZS, Hoffman LK, Sutton L, Cohen SR, Lowes MA, Seng EK. The patient experience of pain in hidradenitis suppurativa. *Br J Dermatol.* 2020 Aug;183(2):401–402. https://doi.org/10.1111/bjd.19016. Epub 2020 May 26. PMID: 32134499.
18. Yao Y, Astrid-Helene RJ, Simon FT. Work productivity and activity impairment in patients with hidradenitis suppurativa: A Cross-Sectional Study. *Int J Dermatol.* 2020;59(3):333–340.
19. Kaaz K, Szepietowski JC, Matusiak Ł. Influence of Itch and Pain on Sleep Quality in Patients with Hidradenitis Suppurativa. *Acta Derm Venereol.* 2018;98:757–761.
20. Machado MO, Stergiopoulos V, Maes M, et al. Depression and Anxiety in Adults with Hidradenitis Suppurativa: A Systematic Review and Meta-Analysis. *JAMA Dermatol.* 2019;155(8):939–945.
21. Thorlacius L, Cohen AD, Gislason GH, et al. Increased Suicide Risk in Patients with Hidradenitis Suppurativa. *J Invest Dermatol.* 2018;138:52–57.
22. Keary E, Hevey D, Tobin AM. A Qualitative Analysis of Psychological Distress in Hidradenitis Suppurativa. *Br J Dermatol.* 2019;0–3.
23. Huilaja L, Hirvonen MJ, Lipitsä T, Vihervaara A, Harvima R, Sintonen H, Kouri JP, Ranta M, Pasternack R. Patients with hidradenitis suppurativa may suffer from neuropathic pain: A Finnish multicenter study. *J Am Acad Dermatol.* 2020 May;82(5):1232–1234. https://doi.org/10.1016/j.jaad.2019.11.016. Epub 2019 Nov 12. PMID: 31730843.
24. Cohen SP, Jianren M. Neuropathic pain: mechanisms and their clinical implications. *BMJ (Online).* 2014;348:1–12.
25. Horváth B, Janse IC, Sibbald GR. Pain management in patients with hidradenitis suppurativa. *J Am Acad Dermatol.* 2015;73(5 suppl 1):S47–S51.
26. Kimball AB, Sundaram M, Shields AL, et al. Adalimumab alleviates skin pain in patients with moderate-to-severe hidradenitis suppurativa: secondary efficacy results from the PIONEER I and PIONEER II randomized controlled trials. *J Am Dermatol.* 2018;79:1141–1143.
27. Kelly G, Hughes R, McGarry T, et al. Dysregulated cytokine expression in lesional and nonlesional skin in hidradenitis suppurativa. *Br J Dermatol.* 2015;173(6):1431–1439.
28. Frew JW, Jason E, James G. A systematic review and critical evaluation of inflammatory cytokine associations in hidradenitis suppurativa. *F1000Research.* 2018;7:1930.

29. van der Zee HH, de Ruiter L, van den Broecke DG, et al. Elevated levels of tumour necrosis factor (TNF)-α, interleukin (IL)-1β and IL-10 in hidradenitis suppurativa skin: a rationale for targeting TNF-α and IL-1β. *Br J Dermatol.* 2011;164(6):1292–1298.

30. Hess A, Axmann R, Rech J, et al. Blockade of TNF-α rapidly inhibits pain responses in the central nervous system. *Proc Natl Acad Sci U S A.* 2011;108(9):3731–3736.

31. Siiskonen H, Ilkka H. Mast Cells and Sensory Nerves Contribute to Neurogenic Inflammation and Pruritus in Chronic Skin Inflammation. *Front Cell Neurosci.* 2019;13:422.

32. Gruener H, Zeilig G, Laufer Y, et al. Differential pain modulation properties in central neuropathic pain after spinal cord injury. *Pain.* 2016;157(7):1415–1424.

33. van Straalen KR. Chronic Pain in Hidradenitis Suppurativa Explained Through the Process of Central Sensitization. *JAMA Dermatol.* 2020;156(6):615–616.

34. Farzanfar D, Dowlati Y, French LE, et al. Inflammation: A Contributor to Depressive Comorbidity in Inflammatory Skin Disease. *Skin Pharmacol Physiol.* 2018;31(5):246–251.

35. Dowlati Y, Herrmann N, Swardfager W, et al. A meta-analysis of cytokines in major depression. *Biol Psychiatry.* 2010;67(5):446–457.

36. Rosenblat JD, Danielle SC, Rodrigo BM, Roger SM. Inflamed moods: a review of the interactions between inflammation and mood disorders. *Prog Neuropsychopharmacol Biol Psychiatry.* 2014;53:23–34.

37. Scheinfeld N, Sundaram M, Teixeira H, et al. Reduction in pain scores and improvement in depressive symptoms in patients with hidradenitis suppurativa treated with adalimumab in a phase 2, randomized, placebo-controlled trial. *Dermatol Online J.* 2016;22(3). 13030/qt38x5922j.

38. Kamper SJ, Apeldoorn AT, Chiarotto A, et al. Multidisciplinary biopsychosocial rehabilitation for chronic low back pain: Cochrane systematic review and meta-analysis. *BMJ (Online).* 2015;350. h444.

39. Alikhan A, Sayed C, Alavi A, et al. North American clinical management guidelines for hidradenitis suppurativa: a publication from the United States and Canadian Hidradenitis Suppurativa Foundations: Part I: Diagnosis, evaluation, and the use of complementary and procedural management. *J Am Acad Dermatol.* 2019;81(1):76–90.

40. Ingram JR, Collier F, Brown D, et al. British Association of Dermatologists guidelines for the management of hidradenitis suppurativa (acne inversa) 2018. *Br J Dermatol.* 2019;180(5):1009–1017.

41. Zouboulis CC, Bechara FG, Dickinson-Blok JL, et al. Hidradenitis suppurativa/acne inversa: a practical framework for treatment optimization—systematic review and recommendations from the HS ALLIANCE working group. *J Eur Acad Dermatol Venereol.* 2019;33(1):19–31.

42. Zouboulis CC, Desai N, Emtestam L, et al. European S1 guideline for the treatment of hidradenitis suppurativa/acne inversa. *J Eur Acad Dermatol Venereol.* 2015;29(4):619–644.

43. Thorlacius L, Ingram JR, Villumsen B, et al. A core domain set for hidradenitis suppurativa trial outcomes: an international Delphi process. *Br J Dermatol.* 2018;179(3):642–650.

44. Turk DC, Hilary DW, Alex C. Treatment of chronic non-cancer pain. *Lancet (London, England).* 2011;377(9784):2226–2235.

45. Enamandram M, James PR, Alexandra BK. Chronic pain management in dermatology a guide to assessment and nonopioid pharmacotherapy. *J Am Acad Dermatol.* 2015;73(4):563–573.

46. Enamandram M, James PR, Alexandra BK. Chronic pain management in dermatology pharmacotherapy and therapeutic monitoring with opioid analgesia. 2015;73(4):575–582.

47. Ehde DM, Tiara MD, Judith AT. Cognitive-behavioral therapy for individuals with chronic pain: efficacy, innovations, and directions for research. *Am Psychol.* 2014;69(2):153–166.

48. Lin J, Laura IK, Lance MM, Harald B. Psychological flexibility mediates the effect of an online-based acceptance and commitment therapy for chronic pain: an investigation of change processes. *Pain.* 2018;159(4):663–672.

49. Veehof MM, Maarten JO, Karlein MGS, Ernst TB. Acceptance-based interventions for the treatment of chronic pain: a systematic review and meta-analysis. *Pain.* 2011;152(3):533–542.

50. Vossen ARJV, Schoenmakers A, van Straalen KR, et al. Assessing Pruritus in Hidradenitis Suppurativa: A Cross-Sectional Study. *Am J Clin Dermatol.* 2017;18(5):687–695.

51. Esmann S, Gregor BEJ. Psychosocial impact of hidradenitis suppurativa: a qualitative study. *Acta Derm Venereol.* 2011;91(3):328–332.

52. Ring HC, Riis TP, Zarchi K, et al. Prodromal symptoms in hidradenitis suppurativa. *Clin Exp Dermatol.* 2017;42(3):261–265.

53. Lee JJ, Protheroe CA, Luo H, et al. Eosinophil-dependent skin innervation and itching following contact toxicant exposure in mice. *J Allergy Clin Immunol.* 2015;135(2):477–487.

54. Van Der Zee HH, de Ruiter L, Boer J, et al. Alterations in leucocyte subsets and histomorphology in normal-appearing perilesional skin and early and chronic hidradenitis suppurativa lesions. *Br J Dermatol.* 2012;166(1):98–106.

55. Pascual JC, García-Martínez FJ, Martorell A, et al. Increased total serum IgE levels in moderate-to-severe hidradenitis suppurativa. *Br J Dermatol.* 2016;175(5):1101–1102.

56. Lima AL, Karl I, Giner T, et al. Keratinocytes and neutrophils are important sources of proinflammatory molecules in hidradenitis suppurativa. *Br J Dermatol.* 2016;174(3):514–521.

57. Miller IM, Ring HC, Prens EP, et al. Leukocyte Profile in Peripheral Blood and Neutrophil-Lymphocyte Ratio in HS. *Dermatology.* 2016;232(4):511–519.

58. Hashimoto T, Jordan DR, Kristen MS, Gil Y. Possible Role of Neutrophils in Itch. *Itch.* 2018;3(4), e17.

59. Fung-Yi Cheung P, Wong CK, Wing-Yin Ho A, et al. Activation of human eosinophils and epidermal keratinocytes by Th2 cytokine IL-31: implication for the immunopathogenesis of atopic dermatitis. *Int Immunol.* 22(6):453–467.

60. Hunger RE, Surovy AM, Hassan AS, et al. Toll-like receptor 2 is highly expressed in lesions of acne inversa and colocalizes with C-type lectin receptor. *Br J Dermatol.* 2008;158(4):691–697.

61. Liu T, Xu ZZ, Park CK, et al. Toll-like receptor 7 mediates pruritus. *Nat Neurosci.* 2010;13(12):1460–1462.

62. Liu T, Berta T, Xu ZZ, et al. TLR3 deficiency impairs spinal cord synaptic transmission, central sensitization, and pruritus in mice. *J Clin Invest.* 2012;122(6):2195–2207.

63. Obara I, Medrano MC, Signoret-Genest J, et al. Inhibition of the mammalian target of rapamycin complex 1 signaling pathway reduces itch behaviour in mice. *Pain.* 2015;156(8):1519–1529.

64. Monfrecola G, Balato A, Caiazzo G, et al. Mammalian target of rapamycin, insulin resistance and hidradenitis suppurativa: a possible metabolic loop. *J Eur Acad Dermatol Venereol.* 2016;30(9):1631–1633.

65. Alavi A, Lynde C, Alhusayen R, et al. Approach to the Management of Patients with Hidradenitis Suppurativa: A Consensus Document. *J Cutan Med Surg.* 2017;21(6):513–524.

66. Gulliver W, Zouboulis CC, Prens E, et al. Evidence-based approach to the treatment of hidradenitis suppurativa/acne inversa, based on the European guidelines for hidradenitis suppurativa. *Rev Endocr Metab Disord.* 2016;17(3):343–351.

67. Gulliver W, Ian DRL, David M, Syed P. Hidradenitis Suppurativa: A Novel Model of Care and an Integrative Strategy to Adopt an Orphan Disease. *J Cutan Med Surg.* 2018;22(1):71–77.

68. Hunger RE, Laffitte E, Läuchli S, et al. Swiss Practice Recommendations for the Management of Hidradenitis Suppurativa/Acne Inversa. *Dermatology.* 2017;233(2–3):113–119.

69. Magalhães RF, Rivitti-Machado MC, Duarte GV, et al. Consensus on the treatment of hidradenitis suppurativa—Brazilian Society of Dermatology. *An Bras Dermatol.* 2019;94:7–19.

70. Heckmann M, Gisela H, Birgit B, Gerd P. Botulinum toxin type A injection in the treatment of lichen simplex: an open pilot study. *J Am Acad Dermatol.* 2002;46(4):617–619.

71. Jones O, Igor S, Henning H. Transcranial magnetic stimulation over contralateral primary somatosensory cortex disrupts perception of itch intensity. *Exp Dermatol.* 2019;28(12):1380–1384.

72. Kaur R, Sinha VR. Antidepressants as antipruritic agents: a review. *Eur Neuropsychopharmacol.* 2018;28(3):341–352.

73. Lee HG, Grossman SK, Valdes-Rodriguez R, et al. Topical ketamine-amitriptyline-lidocaine for chronic pruritus: a retrospective study assessing efficacy and tolerability. *J Am Acad Dermatol.* 2017;76 (4):760–761.

74. Matsuda KM, Divya S, Ariel RS, Shawn GK. Gabapentin and pregabalin for the treatment of chronic pruritus. *J Am Acad Dermatol.* 2016;75(3):619–625.e6.

75. Schut C, Mollanazar NK, Kupfer J, et al. Psychological Interventions in the Treatment of Chronic Itch. *Acta Derm Venereol.* 2016;96(2):157–161.

76. Ständer S, Siepmann D, Herrgott I, et al. Targeting the neurokinin receptor 1 with aprepitant: a novel antipruritic strategy. *PLoS ONE.* 2010;5(6), e10968.

77. Weisshaar E, Nadine D, Harald G. Topical capsaicin therapy in humans with hemodialysis-related pruritus. *Neurosci Lett.* 2003;345(3):192–194.

20

Dressings and Wound Care Supplies for Hidradenitis Suppurativa

MAXIMILLIAN A. WEIGELT, DANIELA P. SANCHEZ, AND HADAR LEV-TOV

CHAPTER OUTLINE

Introduction to Wound Care in Hidradenitis Suppurativa

The most important step in managing hidradenitis suppurativa (HS)-related wounds is to treat the underlying disease with appropriate medical and surgical approaches. Even so, proper local wound care is a key cornerstone of management for patients with HS, especially in those with advanced disease.[1] Clinicians will encounter two types of wounds: typical or lesional HS wounds, and post-surgical wounds. The former can be further sub-divided into draining nodules and abscesses, draining tunnels, pyogenic granuloma-like lesions, and frank ulcerations (e.g., knife-like ulcers, pyoderma gangrenosum-like ulcers). Local wound care is instrumental to suppress potential triggers of immune dysfunction, manage exudate, reduce maceration, and decrease the likelihood of secondary infection.[1,2] The benefits of such an approach include accelerated healing, decreased pain, optimized cosmesis, and improved quality of life.[3-5] Lesional HS wounds cause pain, produce exudate and odor, and thus have significant and typically underappreciated effects on patients' quality of life.[6] Social embarrassment, decreased work productivity, and missed employment opportunities are commonly reported.[7] Indeed, many patients with HS live with dressings that require frequent, cumbersome changes that further interfere with everyday activities.[8]

Standard post-surgical wound care is well-established[9]; however, selection of an effective and comfortable dressing for typical HS lesions is often an overlooked dimension of care with immense potential to improve quality of life. Currently, there are no HS-specific dressings, which is a significant limitation especially with regard to the anatomical location of typical wounds in HS (i.e., skin folds). Therefore, when choosing a dressing for HS-specific lesions, clinicians should take into account the location and morphology of lesions, the degree of pain and inflammation, amount of exudate, odor, and the cost and availability of the product. The ideal dressing for HS-specific lesions should: appropriately absorb exudate to maintain healthy moisture balance, protect the skin from external trauma and infection; promote collagen synthesis and re-epithelialization; stay in place to avoid friction; and be appropriately shaped to fit curved locations if necessary.[1,8] Selecting the optimal dressing for a given patient is challenging given that HS classically involves difficult anatomic areas (e.g., groin, axillae) and is characterized by fluctuating disease activity.

Evidence to support optimal choice of dressings for HS is scarce and limited to few small studies.[1,6,8] Current knowledge is primarily derived from expert opinion and studies on acute wounds and other types of chronic wounds. Recommendations herein are thus based on synthesis of this available data by experts in HS and wound care.

Given lack of evidence and the heterogenous nature of the disease, it is unlikely that one dressing will fit the needs of all patients or lesions at all times. Therefore, clinicians must become familiar with the fundamental properties of the dressings available on the market and together with their patients build a regimen that will address the patients' needs, dynamic as they may be. Key to a successful wound care regimen is the realization that typically, wound care is delivered by the patient on a daily basis, at home. Therefore, treatment planning should always begin with listening to the patient's needs (e.g., work schedule, access to supplies and home care), assessing their health literacy and ability to care for their disease, and ensuring that the final treatment plan is practical. Clinicians should demonstrate dressing changes for the patients and provide written instructions, as well as other resources, in order to ensure the success of the wound care plan.

In this chapter, a lesion-based clinical approach is proposed for each type of HS wound. For clarity, the discussion is divided into management of typical lesions (e.g., nodules, abscesses, etc.) and post-surgical wounds. For each of these broad categories, descriptions and evidence levels for each type of dressing are provided, where applicable. All HS dressing discussed herein, their characteristics, and utility are summarized in Table 20.1. Finally, an overarching algorithm for dressing selection in HS patients is outlined.

Dressings for Typical Hidradenitis Suppurativa Lesions

Typical HS lesions to consider include acute inflammatory nodules and tunnels both acute (flared) and chronic. Acute HS nodules tend to be painful and have minimal to no drainage.[8,10] Given these characteristics, acute nodules would most benefit from non-adherent dressings with cooling effect such as hydrogel or hydrocolloid dressings.[8] These atraumatic dressings will limit skin damage and minimize trauma and pain with dressing changes.[1,8] In case drainage occurs from a nodule, foams may serve as an added padded layer on the affected skin, further aiding with pain management and providing excellent absorption.[8]

Flaring tunnels are often associated with pain and heavy drainage.[10] Dressings of choice for these lesions therefore include absorbent and superabsorbent dressings (see section "Absorbent Dressings for Typical HS Lesions"). Chronic tunnels, that is, those which have failed to heal by approximately 40% within 4 weeks, ought to be treated as chronic wounds.[11] Chronic wounds typically exhibit increased fibrinogen and fibrin, which are thought to impair the wound healing process. Chronic wounds are also at risk of infection, and may require debridement.[12] Depending on the amount of drainage, hydrocolloid dressings (see section "Superabsorbent Dressings for Typical HS Lesions") or foams (see section "Foam Dressings for Typical HS Lesions") can be beneficial for these, as they can facilitate wound healing by assisting with autolytic debridement.[13,14]

Absorbent Dressings for Typical Hidradenitis Suppurativa Lesions

The 2008 consensus on wound exudate management per the World Union of Wound Healing Societies recommends absorbent dressings for heavily exudating wounds. These include foams, gelling fibers, and super-absorbent polymers. These dressings will be discussed in the sections below. Additionally, hydrocolloid dressings and over-the-counter absorbents are discussed. Overall, data on absorbent dressings for typical HS lesions is limited. Data on the use of absorptive dressing for primary HS lesions is critically

needed to guide clinicians. In the interim, clinical judgement should be practiced for dressing selection. Close follow-up is advised in order to understand the amount of dressings used by the patient over the course of an average week in order to ensure adequate supply is available.

Foam Dressings for Typical Hidradenitis Suppurativa Lesions

Foam dressings are composed of semipermeable materials that aid in managing wound exudate. The absorptive capacity of foams depends on the thickness of the dressing. The contact area of foam dressings is non-adherent, making these dressings easily removable, thus preventing dressing-related trauma and minimizing discomfort and pain at the wound site.[8] Additionally, foams can be impregnated with anti-microbial agents such as silver or honey (see section "Contact Layers for Typical HS Lesions"). Foams are flexible and can be molded or cut to fit different body parts, making them particularly useful in HS. Studies that have attempted to establish optimal wound care for HS have favored foam dressings for these reasons.[10] Finally, foam dressings have increased capacity for autolytic debridement, which may be a useful property in tunnels and frank ulcerations when appropriate.

Superabsorbent Dressings for Typical Hidradenitis Suppurativa Lesions

Superabsorbent dressings are multilayered with highly absorptive materials, such as cotton, rayon, or cellulose, designed to manage highly exudative wounds. These can be used as primary or secondary dressings. A prospective observational study done on 15 patients with highly exudating wounds demonstrated that these dressings reduced maceration as well as the number of dressing changes required from once daily to twice weekly. Superabsorbent dressings were found to overall reduce complications associated with exudate production, save time and cost for caregivers, and increase patient comfort.[15] This is significant in HS, where exudate management has a large impact on quality of life.

Hydrocolloid and Hydrofiber Dressings for Typical Hidradenitis Suppurativa Lesions

Hydrocolloid dressings are composed of gelatin, carboxymethylcellulose, pectins, and an occlusive backing. The occlusive backing is typically in the form of a film or foam and serves to protect the wound from the environment. This allows patients to maintain their daily activities, such as showering, with more ease. Hydrocolloids form a gel when in contact with exudate. This gel helps to protect wounds by maintaining wound moisture, temperature, and facilitating autolytic debridement. Hydrocolloid fiber (Hydrofiber) dressings build upon the gel-forming properties of hydrocolloids and boast an increased absorptive capacity.[16] Notably, available data on hydrocolloids and hydrofibers relates to post-surgical wounds while data on their use in primary lesions of HS is lacking. Nonetheless, these dressings are useful for typical HS lesions exhibiting mild-to-moderate levels of exudate.

Over-the-Counter Absorbent Dressings for Typical Hidradenitis Suppurativa Lesions

Other relatively cost-effective and simple dressings that can be used to treat typical HS lesions include infant diapers, adult briefs, and

TABLE 20.1   Summary of Available Dressings for Hidradenitis Suppurativa: Strengths, Weaknesses, and Utility in Hidradenitis Suppurativa

Type	Subtype	Strengths	Weaknesses	Utility in HS
Moist	Hydrogel	Maintain moist environment Cools and soothes skin Facilitate autolytic debridement	Poor absorptive capacity	Dry to minimally exudative Acute nodules Simple post-surgical
Absorbent	Gauze	Low cost Easy to acquire	Requires tape which may be irritating May be painful to remove	Mild-to-moderately exudative (non-adherent gauze)
Absorbent	Abdominal Pads	Absorbent	Expensive Bulky	As cost/coverage necessitates
Absorbent	Infant Diapers/Adult Briefs/Sanitary Napkins	Highly absorbent Can be bought in bulk Wick away moisture	Bulky May be uncomfortable	Cost-effective solution
Absorbent	Foams	Easily removable Impregnable with antimicrobials Flexible, pliable High absorptive capacity	Expensive	Moderately exudative Nodules Chronic Tunnels Post-surgical (simple or complex)
Absorbent	Hydrocolloid	Maintain moist environment Temperature regulation Facilitate autolytic debridement	Unpleasant odor/color changes	Mild-to-moderately exudative Chronic Tunnels
Absorbent	Hydrofiber	Higher absorptive capacity than hydrocolloids May be less painful to remove	Not compatible with oil-based products, e.g., petroleum jelly	Mild-to-moderately exudative Simple post-surgical
Absorbent	Alginate	Highly absorbent Hemostatic properties Reduce bacterial infections Long wear-time	Expensive Distinctive odor May disintegrate quickly	Moderately exudative Deroofed nodules Post-surgical (simple or complex)
Absorbent	Superabsorbent	Highest absorptive capacity	Expensive	Highly exudative Acute Tunnels Post-surgical (simple or complex)
Antimicrobial	Silver	Bactericidal May control odor	May inhibit acute wound healing	Clinical signs of infection
Antimicrobial	Iodine	Bactericidal Does not impede healing	May irritate skin	Clinical signs of infection
Antimicrobial	Honey	Bactericidal Relieves pain and inflammation in acute wounds	No evidence for efficacy in chronic wounds	Clinical signs of infection
Antimicrobial	Topical Antiseptics	Reduces development of bacterial antibiotic resistance	Effects attenuated by biofilms	Clinical signs of infection Often recommended as maintenance therapy
Contact Layers	Contact Layers	Easy to remove Will not disrupt wound bed	Requires secondary dressing	

sanitary napkins. These are highly absorbent, can be bought in bulk, and are designed to wick away moisture. However, they can be bulky and uncomfortable compared to the other dressings discussed in this chapter. Abdominal pads are very effective for exudative wounds but are even more expensive (albeit often covered by health insurance policies) and bulky than the aforementioned options.[10]

Topical Antiseptics for Typical Hidradenitis Suppurativa Lesions

The role of cutaneous flora in the pathogenesis of HS is becoming increasingly recognized.[17,18] Dysregulation of normal skin flora and secondary infection of active HS lesions are significant drivers of disease activity.[17] Additionally, biofilms (extracellular polymeric matrices secreted by bacteria which grant protection against host defenses and conventional therapies) may contribute to the pathology seen in HS, though their exact role remains unclear.[19] Accordingly, topical antimicrobial therapy is a mainstay of therapy for patients with HS and topical antiseptics and cleaning solutions are commonly employed for this purpose in the management of HS. Therefore, when considering wound care for typical HS lesions, topical antiseptics are essential for a comprehensive approach. Chlorhexidine, a broad-spectrum biocide, is used to reduce the stimulation of the immune response by resident bacteria. However, the effects of chlorhexidine are greatly impaired in the presence of biofilms. Although it is commonly recommended by clinicians, clinical evidence for the use of chlorhexidine in HS is low, and its benefits lie mainly in the reduction of bacterial resistance compared with oral antibiotic therapy alone.[20]

Contact Layers for Typical Hidradenitis Suppurativa Lesions

Contact layers are designed to lie directly on the wound bed and protect wound bed tissue as well as the surrounding skin during healing.[21] They are generally non-adherent or lightly adherent and, while not highly absorbent themselves, are designed to allow upward drainage of fluids into a secondary dressing.[21] Contact layer dressings have been shown to promote granulation and epithelialization in non-HS related wounds.[21,22] These dressings are easy and painless to remove and will not disrupt the wound bed during dressing changes.[8] In HS patients, using a contact layer as a primary dressing that can stay on the wound for 2 to 3 days will allow for more frequent secondary absorbent dressing changes (e.g., alginate) without trauma to the wound.

Moist Dressings for Typical Hidradenitis Suppurativa Lesions

Hydrogel dressings are semi-occlusive, gel-based products with a high (90%) water content that protects the wound bed and provides a moist wound-healing environment. In addition to rehydrating wounds and eschars, hydrogels are also designed to aid in autolytic debridement without harming epithelial cells or granulation tissue. Hydrogels have a cooling and soothing effect on the skin, which is particularly useful in HS-specific lesions. Hydrogels work by expanding when in contact with water, or fluids such as wound exudate. These types of dressings are recommended for typical HS lesions that dry or are mildly exudative and can remain in place for up to 3 days.[23]

Odor control for Typical Hidradenitis Suppurativa Lesions

Slough, bacteria, and exudate release volatile organic compounds that are processed as odor by the olfactory apparatus.[24] Malodor is a significant driver of decreased quality of life for patients with HS as it contributes to embarrassment, stigma, and poor self-image, increasing the barrier to interpersonal relationships.[25] A high level of odor has been linked to a greater degree of social isolation as well as more significant quality-of-life impairment as measured by the Skindex-29.[25] Odor in HS is thought to be a marker of bacterial colonization, and it has been suggested that antiseptic dressings may help in this regard by destroying surface bacteria.[25] Dressings containing charcoal may be useful in absorbing wound-associated odors.[26] There are many purported treatments for

wound odor; however, few are well-studied in high-quality randomized-controlled trials.[24] Silver dressings and metronidazole gel have the best evidence to support efficacy in combating chronic wound odors, but HS-specific data is currently lacking.[24]

Post-surgical wounds

Post-surgical wounds can be closed primarily, left for secondary intention healing, or grafted. Management of post-surgical wounds in HS is generally similar to other post-surgical wounds.[1] A comprehensive discussion of post-surgical wound care is beyond the scope of this chapter. Generally, the astute surgeon should follow current surgical guidelines.[9] A summary of the existing evidence for post-surgical wounds after HS-related surgery is presented herein. Current guidelines cite minimal evidence to support any specific dressing for post-surgical wounds in HS.[8] Complex post-surgical HS wounds that have become infected or otherwise failed to follow an appropriate healing trajectory may require additional attention.[8] Absorbent dressings (i.e., foams, alginates, hydrofibers, etc.) or negative-pressure wound therapy (NPWT) may be useful for such slow-healing wounds. Post-surgical wounds should be closely monitored for infection and cultured appropriately if necessary. Antimicrobial dressings can be used in the event of an infected wound.

Absorbent Dressings for Post-Surgical Wounds in Hidradenitis Suppurativa

Alginates for Post-Surgical Wounds in Hidradenitis Suppurativa

Alginate dressings are light, nonwoven fabrics derived from algae or seaweed.[13] Designed for moderately to heavily exudating wounds, they are highly absorbent, have mild hemostatic properties, reduce bacterial infections, and can stay on the wound bed for days.[13,16,27] Alginates have been used in combination with silicone dressings for post-surgical wound care of surgically deroofed HS cysts and sinuses,[28] as well as for Skin Tissue-Sparing Excision with Electrosurgical Peeling (STEEP) procedures for patients in advanced stages of HS.[29] Alginate dressings tend to fall apart faster than other dressings, which may present a significant limitation in use for primary HS lesions, as parts of the dressing may lodge in sinuses. Use of a contact layer as a primary dressing may improve the overall performance of an alginate dressing.

Hydrocolloids and Hydrofibers for Post-Surgical Wounds in Hidradenitis Suppurativa

The use of these dressings has specifically been described in HS. One study described the use of hydrocolloid dressings for 2 days in addition to polymyxin B ointment and bacitracin on 61 HS patients who underwent CO_2 laser excision. All patients in this study healed with excellent cosmetic outcomes and comfort.[30] Hydrofibers have been used for postoperative care of HS patients undergoing CO_2 laser surgery. A retrospective analysis of 35 patients treated with hydrofibers for CO_2 laser surgical wounds of different sizes and anatomic locations, left to heal by secondary intention, found a mean healing time of 4 weeks.[31] A second cohort of nine patients, some healed by first intention and others by second, found a mean healing time of 2 weeks.[30] It has been suggested that hydrofiber dressings may be less painful to remove than other dressings for these post-surgical wounds, however these claims have not yet been studied in a controlled manner.[31]

Antimicrobial Dressings for Post-Surgical Wounds in Hidradenitis Suppurativa

Silver for Post-Surgical Wounds in Hidradenitis Suppurativa

The antimicrobial properties of silver have been known for centuries.[32] Ionized silver (Ag^{2+}) is toxic to a wide variety of pathogenic organisms commonly found in wounds.[32] Accordingly, silver has been incorporated into a variety of dressings which vary in the types of material used, formulation of the silver compound, location of compound in the dressing, and total silver content released into the wound.[32] Although some studies have found silver to have beneficial effects on healing outcomes in chronic wounds, others have failed to observe any differences between silver and non-silver dressings.[33] Studies focusing on silver dressings in the context of HS are limited. Silver dressings should be used judiciously as they are not intended to be used for extended periods, particularly if there is no infection.[32] Additionally, *in vitro* and *in vivo* studies have found that silver is toxic to fibroblasts and keratinocytes and thus inhibits acute wound healing by slowing re-epithelialization.[34]

Iodine For Post-Surgical Wounds in Hidradenitis Suppurativa

Iodine is another agent with broad-spectrum antimicrobial activity, boasting anti-inflammatory properties and an excellent safety profile.[35] It has not been found to disturb wound healing.[35] In a study where 44 HS patients with various stages of disease activity underwent deroofing of lesions, postoperative wound care was achieved with 5 days of mupirocin, with wedging to keep the wound open, followed by once-daily dressing changes with iodine-ointment-containing gauzes. The surgical defects were found to generally heal with cosmetically acceptable scars.[36] However, the small number of patients and lack of control arm limits the applicability of these data for treating people with HS related wounds, except to suggest an acceptable safety profile for both silver and iodine. Although less likely with modern iodine formulations (e.g., iodophors), iodine-containing compounds may cause skin irritation.[37]

Honey for Post-Surgical Wounds in Hidradenitis Suppurativa

Honey has antibacterial, anti-inflammatory, and antioxidant properties that can be harnessed and incorporated into a dressing in order to promote wound healing.[38] Honey's antibacterial effects are due to its high acidity, osmotic effect, and hydrogen peroxide content. The usage of honey in the setting of wound healing has been associated with pain relief and a decreased inflammatory response.[38] However, these effects have only been demonstrated in acute wounds such as acute burns and postoperative wounds.[32] Honey has not been found to be effective in chronic wounds such as chronic leg ulcers.[38] The use of honey-impregnated dressings may therefore be limited to acute HS wounds, and postoperative wounds in particular.

Negative-Pressure Wound Therapy for Post-Surgical Wounds in Hidradenitis Suppurativa

NPWT may also be considered for complex wounds, heavily exudating wounds, those not closed primarily, or those with significant depth.[1,8] NPWT helps by increasing oxygen tension, decreasing bacterial load, stimulating cellular activity, and promoting granulation tissue and also serves to prepare the wound bed for grafting if necessary.[1]

Gauze Dressings for Post-Surgical Wounds in Hidradenitis Suppurativa

Gauze has historically been ubiquitous in wound care and may still play a role in the treatment of patients with HS despite the availability of modern dressings. Its low cost and accessibility can make it an attractive choice, although it requires the use of tape to adhere to the skin, which may be irritating and cause pain during dressing changes. Gauze also tends to stick to wounds when exudate dries which may further increase pain.[10] Non-adherent gauze may serve similar purposes without the pain and disruption of the wound bed associated with changing a dry gauze. In a cohort of 185 patients undergoing CO_2 laser excision for HS lesions, patients received postoperative wound care with antibacterial ointment and hydrocolloid dressing for 2 days, followed by daily warm water compresses, petroleum jelly, and a non-adherent gauze dressing until healing. All patients healed with acceptable-to-excellent cosmetic and recurrence outcomes during a follow-up period ranging from 1 to 19 years.[14]

Summary

Selection of an effective dressing for HS is challenging due to the inherently fluctuant nature of the disease and diverse array of lesions that may be present. Many factors must be taken into account during dressing selection, namely: the location and morphology of lesions, the extent of disease activity, amount of exudate, odor, and the cost and availability of the product. A summarized approach to dressing selection for HS based on wound type and characteristics can be found in Table 20.2.

A challenge that may arise when caring for patients with HS is the cost of dressings; insurance coverage for dressings frequently comes up short and patients might be left with fewer supplies than necessary. Reimbursement for dressings is often based on wound size area, which is not an accurate representation of disease burden for HS. Strategies to overcome this include marking the entire affected area (e.g., the axilla) as the wounded area if disease activity is sufficiently severe.

Although beyond the scope of this chapter, cellular- and tissue-based products (CTPs) represent a novel technology for the treatment of wounds which continue to increase in popularity. Various products have been studied and received FDA approval for other types of wounds such as venous leg ulcers, diabetic foot ulcers, and burns.[39] There is not yet any evidence to support the use of CTPs for wounds in HS; however, it stands to reason that they would be effective in specific circumstances that are similar to the other types of wounds studied (e.g., post-surgical wounds and chronic tunnels). As more of these products continue to be developed, they may find a role in the treatment of patients with HS.

Finally, a significant consideration should be made regarding the lack of data to support evidence-based practice for wound care in people with HS. Many questions remain; it is unclear if HS patients lack the ability to heal normally. As demonstrated above, there are virtually no controlled studies regarding wound care in HS and therefore conclusions drawn from the studies presented are limited. Ultimately, clinicians should develop sound knowledge of dressing types, gain clinical experience in managing HS patients, and have open discussion with their patients who, until

<table>
<tr><th colspan="2">TABLE 20.2</th><th colspan="2">Suggested Dressing Selection in Hidradenitis Suppurativa</th></tr>
</table>

Wound Type	Wound Characteristics/ Lesion Type		Suggested Dressings
Post-Surgical	Simple		Absorbent, superabsorbent Foams, hydrofibers, alginates Non-adherent Gel-based
	Complex or Non-Healing		Absorbent, superabsorbent Foams, hydrofibers, alginates Antimicrobial
Non-Surgical	Exudate	Heavy	Absorbent, superabsorbent
		Moderate	Foams, hydrofibers, alginates Non-adherent
		Mild	Non-adherent
	Clinical Signs of Infection		Antimicrobial
	Odor		Silver-impregnated Metronidazole gel Charcoal
	Nodules		Foams, alginates, hydrogel, hydrocolloid
	Tunnels		Acute: Absorbent, superabsorbent Chronic: Hydrocolloid, foam
	Erosive Pyoderma Gangrenosum		Hydrogels, hydrofibers

When dressings are listed as a class (e.g., absorbent), refer to Table 2.1 and text for specifications.

controlled data becomes available, remain our best wound care experts.

The authors of this chapter would like to acknowledge the following guest editor:

Robert S. Kirsner, MD, PhD
Chairman & Harvey Blank Professor
Dr. Phillip Frost Department of Dermatology & Cutaneous Surgery
Professor of Public Health Sciences
Director, University of Miami Hospital and Clinics Wound Center
University of Miami Miller School of Medicine
Miami, FL, USA

References

1. Alavi A, Kirsner RS. Local wound care and topical management of hidradenitis suppurativa. *J Am Acad Dermatol.* 2015;73(5 Suppl 1):S55–S61.
2. Shi C, Wang C, Liu H, et al. Selection of Appropriate Wound Dressing for Various Wounds. *Front Bioeng Biotechnol.* 2020;8:182.
3. Sood A, Granick MS, Tomaselli NL. Wound Dressings and Comparative Effectiveness Data. *Adv Wound Care (New Rochelle).* 2014;3(8):511–529.
4. Jourdan M, Madfes DC, Lima E, Tian Y, Seite S. Skin Care Management For Medical And Aesthetic Procedures To Prevent Scarring. *Clin Cosmet Investig Dermatol.* 2019;12:799–804.
5. Olsson M, Jarbrink K, Divakar U, et al. The humanistic and economic burden of chronic wounds: A systematic review. *Wound Repair Regen.* 2019;27(1):114–125.
6. Antia C, Alavi A, Alikhan A. Topical management and wound care approaches for hidradenitis suppurativa. *Semin Cutan Med Surg.* 2017;36(2):58–61.
7. Alavi A, Anooshirvani N, Kim WB, Coutts P, Sibbald RG. Quality-of-life impairment in patients with hidradenitis suppurativa: a Canadian study. *Am J Clin Dermatol.* 2015;16(1):61–65.
8. Braunberger TL, Fatima S, Vellaichamy G, Nahhas AF, Parks-Miller A, Hamzavi IH. Dress for Success: a Review of Dressings and Wound Care in Hidradenitis Suppurativa. *Current Dermatology Reports.* 2018;7(4):269–277.
9. Ubbink DT, Brolmann FE, Go PM, Vermeulen H. Evidence-Based Care of Acute Wounds: A Perspective. *Adv Wound Care (New Rochelle).* 2015;4(5):286–294.
10. Kazemi A, Carnaggio K, Clark M, Shephard C, Okoye GA. Optimal wound care management in hidradenitis suppurativa. *J Dermatolog Treat.* 2018;29(2):165–167.
11. Lazarus GS, Cooper DM, Knighton DR, et al. *Definitions and Guidelines for the Assessment of Wounds and Evaluation of Healing*; 1994.
12. Liu W-L, Jiang Y-L, Wang Y-Q, Li Y-X, Liu Y-X. Combined debridement in chronic wounds: A literature review. *Chinese Nursing Research.* 2017;4(1):5–8.
13. Dini V, Oranges T, Rotella L, Romanelli M. Hidradenitis Suppurativa and Wound Management. *Int J Low Extrem Wounds.* 2015;14(3):236–244.
14. Hazen PG, Hazen BP. Hidradenitis suppurativa: successful treatment using carbon dioxide laser excision and marsupialization. *Dermatol Surg.* 2010;36(2):208–213.
15. Faucher N, Safar H, Baret M, Phillippe A, Farid R. Superabsorbent dressings for copiously exuding wounds. *Br J Nursing.* 2012;21(12):S22. S24, S26028.
16. Harding KG, Price P, Robinson B, Thomas SS, Hofman D. Cost and Dressing Evaluation of Hydrofiber and Alginate Dressings in the Management of Community-Based Patients with Chronic Leg Ulceration. *WOUNDS.* 2001;13(6):229–236.
17. Ring HC, Bay L, Kallenbach K, et al. Normal Skin Microbiota is Altered in Pre-clinical Hidradenitis Suppurativa. *Acta Derm Venereol.* 2017;97(2):208–213.
18. Naik H, Jo J, Paul M, Kong H. Skin Microbiota Perturbations Are Distinct and DIsease Severity-Dependent in Hidradenitis Suppurativa. *J Invest Dermatol.* 2020;140(4).
19. Kjaersgaard Andersen R, Ring HC, Kallenbach K, Eriksen JO, Jemec GBE. Bacterial biofilm is associated with higher levels of regulatory T cells in unaffected hidradenitis suppurativa skin. *Exp Dermatol.* 2019;28(3):312–316.
20. Frew JW, Hawkes JE, Krueger JG. Topical, systemic and biologic therapies in hidradenitis suppurativa: pathogenic insights by examining therapeutic mechanisms. *Ther Adv Chronic Dis.* 2019;10. 2040622319830646.
21. David F, Wurtz JL, Breton N, et al. A randomised, controlled, non-inferiority trial comparing the performance of a soft silicone-coated wound contact layer (Mepitel One) with a lipidocolloid wound contact layer (UrgoTul) in the treatment of acute wounds. *Int Wound J.* 2018;15(1):159–169.
22. EG P, AL B. *Epidermolysis Bullosa Simplex.* Seattle (WA): GeneReviews [Internet]; 1998 [Updated 2016].
23. Weller C. Interactive dressings and their role in moist wound management. In: Rajendran S, ed. *Advances Textiles for Wound Care.* 2nd ed. Elsevier; 2009:97–113.

24. Darwin ES, Thaler ER, Lev-Tov HA. Wound odor: current methods of treatment and need for objective measures. *G Ital Dermatol Venereol.* 2019;154(2):127–136.

25. Alavi A, Farzanfar D, Lee RK, Almutairi D. The Contribution of Malodour in Quality of Life of Patients With Hidradenitis Suppurativa. *J Cutan Med Surg.* 2018;22(2):166–174.

26. Folestad A, Gilchrist B. Wound Exudate and the Role of Dressings. *Int Wound J.* 2008;5:iii–12.

27. Aderibigbe BA, Buyana B. Alginate in Wound Dressings. *Pharmaceutics.* 2018;10(42):1–19.

28. Mandal A, Watson J. Experience with different treatment modules in hidradenitis suppurativa: A study of 106 cases. *Surgeon.* 2005;3(1):23–25.

29. Blok JL, Spoo JR, Leeman FW, Jonkman MF, Horvath B. Skin-Tissue-sparing Excision with Electrosurgical Peeling (STEEP): a surgical treatment option for severe hidradenitis suppurativa Hurley stage II/III. *J Eur Acad Dermatol Venereol.* 2015;29(2):379–382.

30. Madan V, Hindle E, Hussain W, August PJ. Outcomes of treatment of nine cases of recalcitrant severe hidradenitis suppurativa with carbon dioxide laser. *Br J Dermatol.* 2008;159(6):1309–1314.

31. Lapins J, Sartorius K, Emtestam L. Scanner-assisted carbon dioxide laser surgery: a retrospective follow-up study of patients with hidradenitis suppurativa. *J Am Acad Dermatol.* 2002;47(2):280–285.

32. Davies P, McCarty S, Hamberg K. Silver-containing foam dressings with Safetac: a review of the scientific and clinical data. *J Wound Care.* 2017;26(6):S1–S31.

33. Rodriguez-Arguello J, Lienhard K, Patel P, et al. A Scoping Review of the Use of Silver Impregnated Dressings for the Treatment of Chronic Wounds. *Wound Management and Prevention.* 2018;64(3):14–31.

34. Barnea Y, Weiss J, Gur E. A review of the applications of hydrofiber dressing with silver (Aquacel Ag) in wound care. *Therapeutics and Clinical Risk Management.* 2010;6:21–27.

35. Gwak HC, Han SH, Lee J, et al. Efficacy of a povidone-iodine foam dressing (Betafoam) on diabetic foot ulcer. *Int Wound J.* 2020;17(1):91–99.

36. van der Zee HH, Prens EP, Boer J. Deroofing: a tissue-saving surgical technique for the treatment of mild to moderate hidradenitis suppurativa lesions. *J Am Acad Dermatol.* 2010;63(3):475–480.

37. MB. M, B. K. Severe irritant contact dermatitis induced by povidone iodine solution. *Indian J Pharmacology.* 2009;41(4):199–200.

38. Yaghoobi R, Kazerouni A, Kazerouni O. Evidence for Clinical Use of Honey in Wound Healing as an Anti-bacterial, Anti-inflammatory Anti-oxidant and Anti-viral Agent: A Review. *Jundishapur Journal of Natural Pharmaceutical Products.* 2013;8(3):100–104.

39. Liu Y, Panayi AC, Bayer LR, Orgill DP. Current Available Cellular and Tissue-Based Products for Treatment of Skin Defects. *Advances in Skin and Wound Care.* 2019;32(1):19–25.

21

Quality of Life

JOSEPH R. WALSH, ZARINE S. PATEL, AND TIEN VIET NGUYEN

Introduction

Hidradenitis suppurativa (HS) is characterized by relapsing, painful, suppurating, bleeding nodules, abscesses, and sinus tracts that primarily affect intertriginous skin. Aside from its debilitating physical manifestations, the disease carries a profound psychological burden and socioeconomic impact. These factors contribute to a significantly impaired quality of life (QoL) for patients with HS. In this chapter, we will cover a broad range of factors that impact QoL in HS patients, including physical symptoms, mental health disorders, substance use disorders, sexual health, and daily and work functions. We also provide recommendations for clinicians on how to mitigate these contributing factors (Table 21.1). Finally, we will end the chapter with a discussion of the high HS-related costs incurred by individual patients and society as a whole.

Quality of Life Comparisons to Other Dermatologic Diseases

The impact of HS on patients' QoL has been compared to that of other chronic dermatoses. There are a few publications in the literature that shed light on this topic, with the majority utilizing patient-level data (e.g., self-reported questionnaires). A French study conducted in a hospital-based setting ($n = 61$) found HS to have a more debilitating effect on QoL than neurofibromatosis type 1 (NF1), chronic urticaria, psoriasis, or atopic dermatitis.[1] The authors found significantly higher mean Skindex-France index scores, indicating a stronger impact on QoL in the HS cohort versus the NF1 cohort.[1] HS patients also fared worse in several dimensions of the VQ-Dermato index (a French-language dermatology-specific QoL instrument), with significantly higher mean scores than patients with chronic urticaria, psoriasis, and atopic dermatitis.[1]

Psoriasis is often chosen as a comparator disease due to an abundance of data and shared similarities with HS (i.e., disease chronicity and psychosocial burden). Published data from international clinical trials for adalimumab revealed that HS patients reported significantly higher scores than patients with plaque-type psoriasis in several important QoL metrics (Visual Analog Scale [VAS] pain: 54.3 vs. 36.1; Dermatology Life Quality Index [DLQI]: 15.3 vs. 11.3; EuroQoL 5D VAS 58.8 vs. 50.8).[2] In a study conducted in an Italian outpatient dermatology clinic ($n = 69$), similar results were reported in a patient-level assessment of how HS impacts QoL.[3] Compared with psoriasis patients, HS patients in this study reported a higher mean symptom score (69.4 vs. 53.7) and psychosocial score (56.1 vs. 32.7), indicating worse QoL than their psoriasis counterparts.[3]

Despite the higher reported QoL burden of HS than psoriasis, there are currently many more systemic treatment options for psoriasis than HS. We hope that this will change in the near future with increased investigation of potential therapeutic modalities for HS. A discussion of pipeline therapeutics can be found in Chapter 34.

Physical Symptoms and Disease Severity

Physical symptoms of HS include pain, pruritus, exudation, bleeding, and malodor. Given the chronicity of HS, these symptoms may lead to physical and psychosocial suffering or even disability.[4–7] A Polish observational study ($n = 103$) found that patients identified pain as the most troublesome symptom of their disease.[6] Nearly all of the study participants (97.1%) reported pain during the course of their disease, and 77.5% reported pain in the last 7 days.[6] In comparison, 62.1% reported pruritus over the course of their disease, and 41.7% reported pruritus within the last 7 days.[6] Pain has been described as interfering with activities of daily life, work, personal relationships, and sleep for patients with HS.[6,8,9] The pathophysiology and management of pain in HS are discussed in detail in Chapter 19.

TABLE 21.1 Recommendations to Help Mitigate Factors Impacting Quality of Life in Hidradenitis Suppurativa Patients

Quality of Life Factor	Recommendations for Clinicians
Physical Symptoms	
Pain	• Optimize pain management, see Chapter 19
Pruritus	• Optimize pruritus management, see Chapter 19
Drainage	• Implement wound care, see Chapter 20
Odor	• Optimize disease control to reduce malodorous discharge • Counsel patients about wound dressings, clothing choices, and other methods of odor control[5]
Mental Health	
Depression	• Screen for depressive symptoms (e.g., sadness, hopelessness, lack of interest in usual activities, reduced appetite, poor concentration) • Optimize disease control to reduce impact on mood • Ensure patient has a primary care provider • Refer to a mental health specialist as needed
Risk of suicide	• Screen depressed patients for suicidality • If risk of suicide suspected, follow institutional/facility protocol to ensure immediate patient safety • Follow up closely and collaborate with mental health specialists for long-term care
Anxiety	• Assess patients for signs and symptoms of anxiety • Optimize disease control to reduce severity and frequency of flares • Provide patients with a written home-management action plan that provides instructions on flare recognition and steps for treatment • If an anxiety disorder is suspected, refer to a mental health specialist
Substance Use Disorders (SUD)	
Alcohol, opioids, cannabinoids	• Screen all patients for use of alcohol, opioids, or cannabinoids • Screen habitual users for substance misuse and/or dependence • Refer patients with SUD to mental health specialists or treatment centers as needed • Provide patients with information regarding substance-specific support networks • Monitor patients long-term for SUD relapse
Sexual Health	
Sexual distress and dysfunction	• Elicit patient concerns regarding sexual health • Optimize disease control to minimize pain, inflammation, and discharge • Ask patients for permission to involve their partners in disease education and expectation management • Educate patients and their partners that hidradenitis suppurativa (HS) is not contagious • Privately screen patients for intimate partner violence; if suspected, follow protocols to ensure patient safety
Daily and Work Functions	
Sleep disturbance	• Assess for sleep disturbance or insomnia in patients struggling with daily life and work functioning • Control physical symptoms of HS and associated psychological components • Encourage good sleep hygiene practices • Use caution when prescribing sleep pharmacotherapy in patients using alcohol, sleep aids, opioids, or any other substances or medications with central nervous system-depression properties
Work disability	• Screen for reduced or loss of work productivity and income due to HS-related disability • Advocate for work conditions that accommodate patient needs related to HS (e.g., cooler temperatures, appropriate work uniforms, adequate break periods for wound care, etc.) • Assist patients in obtaining disability benefits due to debilitating effects of HS when needed

Although pain is the predominantly reported symptom, itch and malodor also impact QoL. A Spanish cross-sectional study involving 233 HS patients revealed statistically significant correlations between DLQI scores and respective Numerical Rating Scale (NRS) values for pain, pruritus, and malodor.[10] The authors found that pruritus intensity was associated with female sex, number of anatomic regions affected, intensity of suppuration, and concomitant Crohn's Disease.[10] Meanwhile, malodor intensity was positively correlated with body mass index, disease duration, number of affected regions, intensity of suppuration, and Hurley stage classification.[10]

With respect to malodor alone, a Canadian cross-sectional study ($n = 51$) found that 88% of the study participants experienced malodorous discharge in affected skin regions.[5] Even though the authors did not find any significant difference in mean DLQI scores between the high-odor and low-odor groups, total and emotions-related mean Skindex-29 scores demonstrated a statistically significant difference between these comparator groups.[5] Patients in this study reported a wide spectrum of management strategies; the most commonly reported ones were wearing loose-fitting clothes, bandaging of malodorous areas, utilizing warm compresses, reducing weight, and using anti-perspirant/deodorants.[5]

Aside from the physical symptoms related to HS, disease severity can also impact QoL profoundly. Studies have shown a significant association between clinical stages of HS and measures on the DLQI.[11–13] In turn, higher DLQI scores, indicating a greater impact on QoL, correlated with worsening severity of depression, anxiety, and loneliness.[8,14]

Mental Health

Depression

Depressive disorders are marked by sadness, emptiness, irritability, somatic (e.g., poor sleep and appetite) and cognitive (e.g., poor concentration) features that interfere with an individual's ability to function.[15] Specifically, major depressive disorder (MDD) as a psychiatric diagnosis is characterized by at least 2 weeks of changes in affect, cognition, and neurovegetative functions.[15] In the United States, the 12-month prevalence of MDD is approximately 7%, and MDD is an established comorbidity of chronic pain.[16]

To date, studies examining the psychiatric burden of HS have primarily focused on the prevalence of depression, and less on anxiety or other psychiatric disorders. Depression has been identified as an important comorbidity of HS in a number of studies, but results of studies examining the prevalence of depressive symptoms have been mixed.[17–20] A recent meta-analysis of 28 studies of depression in HS found a prevalence of 21% and that HS patients were twice as likely to have depression compared to controls.[21] In a retrospective analysis of new-onset depression in HS patients based on electronic health records data ($n = 49,280$ for adult HS patients and 3,042 for pediatric HS patients), depression incident rates of 4.8 per 100 person-years in the adult population and 3.0 per 100 person-years in the pediatric population were reported.[22]

Research has confirmed that feelings of shame, stigma, embarrassment, social isolation, and pain can contribute to depressive symptoms in HS.[14,23–25] Since HS patients experience at least one, and often several, of these factors on a daily basis, it is not difficult to understand how depressive symptoms may evolve and intensify over the course of the disease. For instance, in one study ($n = 94$), HS patients demonstrated significantly higher scores than healthy controls with respect to depression (5.45 vs. 4.16) and loneliness (UCLA Loneliness Scale: 42.8 vs. 35.57), as well as significantly lower self-esteem (Rosenberg Self-Esteem Scale: 18.91 vs. 19.77).[14]

Suicide

In general, thoughts of death, suicidal ideation, and suicide attempts are common in individuals suffering from MDD.[15] Given that depressive symptoms disproportionately affect HS patients as previously discussed, the risk of suicide for those suffering from this chronic inflammatory disease merits attention. Furthermore, chronic pain, a clinical hallmark of HS, can compound the suicide risk in HS.[26]

A population-based study in the United States ($n = 49,380$ HS patients and approximately 23 million non-HS controls) found the absolute risk of completed suicide to be 0.8% in HS compared with 0.3% in the control population.[27] After adjusting for age, gender, and race, the authors reported that HS patients had a significantly increased risk of suicide compared to those without HS (OR: 2.88).[27] The risk of suicide in HS correlated with advancing age, and was the highest in individuals aged 60 or older (OR: 3.62).[27]

A Danish cohort and cross-sectional study ($n = 7,732$ HS patients and 4,354,137 background population) corroborated the above findings from the U.S. study regarding the risk of completed suicide in HS.[20] They found a significantly increased risk of completed suicide (adjusted hazard ratio [HR]: 2.42) and antidepressant use (adjusted HR: 1.30) in the HS cohort compared to the background population.[20] Suicidality might not always be apparent, so we recommend screening as appropriate by all members of the interdisciplinary HS care team.

Anxiety

A small number of studies have examined anxiety as an associated psychiatric comorbidity of HS.[18,19] Anxiety disorders are defined by excessive fear and anxiety along with related behavioral disturbances.[15] They can be further categorized as panic disorder, social anxiety disorder, agoraphobia, or generalized anxiety disorder.[15] Fear of disease flare-ups, malodourous discharge, soiling of clothing from bleeding/exudation, and financial distress have been postulated to exacerbate symptoms of anxiety in HS.[14,28] In a recently published meta-analysis of 12 studies, the authors found a prevalence of 12% and a nearly two-fold risk of anxiety among HS patients relative to controls.[21]

Bipolar Disorder, Psychosis, and Personality Disorders

Few studies have examined the prevalence of other psychiatric diagnoses, such as bipolar disorder, schizophrenia, or personality disorders. An Israeli cross-sectional study ($n = 4,191$ HS patients and 20,941 matched controls) found a significantly higher prevalence of schizophrenia in the HS cohort than the control group (1.4% vs. 0.4%).[29] Analysis of a Finnish registry found that HS patients have a significantly increased risk of being diagnosed with at least one psychiatric comorbidity compared to psoriasis (PSO) patients (OR: 1.34) or those with melanocytic nevi (MN) (OR: 2.04).[30] Respectively, the authors found a significantly higher prevalence of schizophrenia, bipolar disorder, and personality disorders in the Finnish HS population relative to their matched psoriasis and MN controls.[30]

These findings do not indicate causality and need to be further explored. We encourage dermatologists to assess patients for mental health disorders, including those on the psychosis spectrum, as early diagnosis and referral to treatment can be life-changing. They may even enhance adherence to medical therapy and thus affect treatment outcomes for HS patients.

Substance Use Disorders

Several studies have demonstrated an increased prevalence of substance abuse disorders (SUD) in HS patients.[31–33] One US cross-sectional analysis ($n = 32,625$) found a statistically significant difference between the prevalence of SUD among HS patients compared to their non-HS counterparts (4.0% vs. 2.0%; $P < .001$).[31] Of the HS patients affected by SUD, the three most commonly reported substances are alcohol, opioids, and cannabinoids.[31] While HS patients demonstrate higher instances of SUD, it remains unclear if such behaviors evolved to help them cope with the chronic inflammation and pain of the disease, or if they are more closely tied to the psychosocial burden of living with HS.

Interestingly, the authors found that the likelihood of developing SUD was higher in HS patients who were *not* diagnosed with depression or anxiety.[31] The authors postulated that chronic pain issues and overall QoL impairment might play a larger role in the development of SUD in HS than the presence of comorbid psychiatric conditions. We recommend a comprehensive approach to managing HS patients affected by SUD. This includes ensuring that the patient has a primary care provider, referring the patient to mental health specialists, as well as addressing the patient's disease symptoms, psychiatric burden, and other associated comorbidities.

Alcohol

The proportion of SUD cases among HS patients that are attributed to alcohol abuse was reported to be as high as 47.9% in the aforementioned U.S. cross-sectional study.[31] In another study, 27,725 blood donors from Denmark were queried about their drinking habits.[34] Significantly greater proportions of participants with HS reported wine and spirits consumption relative to non-HS participants.[34] There was no significant difference in beer consumption habits between those with and without HS.[34] The authors did not control for psychiatric comorbidities, such as depression, or socioeconomic factors. Moderate depression was found to be significantly more prominent in the HS group (3.2%) than the non-HS group (0.7%), which could have contributed to increased alcohol consumption by HS patients.[34]

A single-center study reported an increased risk of alcohol dependence among HS patients; however, after adjusting for psychiatric comorbidities and other confounding variables, HS patients actually had smaller odds of alcohol dependence compared with the control group.[32] Two case-control studies relying on patient-level data were not able to demonstrate any association between HS and alcohol dependence.[35] Future research with large and well-controlled studies on alcohol dependence and HS is warranted.

Opioids

The Diagnostic and Statistical Manual of Mental Disorder (DSM)-5 publication characterizes opioid use disorder (OUD) along a mild-moderate-severe spectrum, on which a patient's seeking behavior progresses despite multiple deleterious consequences to their personal and professional lives.[15] In determining whether HS patients are at an inherent risk for OUD, several confounding factors must be taken into account. Given that pain is a hallmark feature of HS, opioids and other forms of pain control have been prescribed to patients suffering from the disease.[36–38]

Few studies have addressed the incidence and management strategies of OUD in HS. The proportion of SUD cases attributable to opioids has been reported as 32.7% in the US-based cross-sectional analysis.[31] In addition, a separate retrospective cohort study involving over 20,000 HS patients found them to be at a significantly increased risk (adjusted OR: 1.53) of developing new

long-term opioid use relative to controls.[38] Certain risk factors, such as advancing age, ever smoking, history of depression, and baseline Charlson comorbidity index score, were correlated with higher odds of OUD development in HS.[38]

We recommend thorough screening for SUD in HS patients and paying special attention to pain management. Over-prescribing opioids to appease patients without adequately assessing their pain control needs could lead to opioid tolerance and dependence in HS. Undertreating pain for fear of inducing opioid addiction can create a cycle of uncontrolled pain, which in turns exacerbates opioid-seeking behavior. Early referral of patients with chronic or recalcitrant pain to pain management specialists is recommended. A mental health specialist may need to be involved to address any underlying psychosocial component that may predispose a patient to opioid misuse. A multi-disciplinary strategy to address OUD may help preserve physician-patient rapport and improve patient adherence to medical therapy.

Cannabinoids

Few studies have shown increased cannabis use among patients with HS.[31,33] Cannabis accounted for up to 29.7% of SUD cases in the above-referenced US cross-sectional study.[31] A retrospective French study reported a significant difference between the prevalence of cannabis use in the HS cohort (34.0%) during the past 12 months compared to the psoriasis cohort (11.6%).[33] The cannabis users in this study consisted mostly of young men with lower body mass indexes.[33] Of note, both HS and psoriasis participants reported pleasure as the first motivation for cannabis use, not pain control, and the majority of the HS group (69.4%) had begun using cannabis prior to disease onset.[33] Within the HS group, the researchers found no significant differences in Hurley stage, DLQI scores, or disease course between cannabis users and nonusers. Interestingly, cannabis users reported a significantly higher VAS pain score during disease remission periods than nonusers (1.7 vs. 1.1), while there was no statistically significant difference in pain scores between the two groups during disease flares.[33] The level of addiction to cannabis was significantly higher in the HS group compared with the psoriasis group (Cannabis Abuse Testing Score: 8.4 vs. 4.1).[33] These studies highlight the need for further research on cannabis use in HS patients.

Sexual Health

There is limited evidence regarding the impact of HS on sexual health.[13,39,40] However, a correlation between sexual distress/dysfunction and decreased QoL in HS patients has been found.[11,13,39] Some studies suggest that female HS patients tend to be disproportionately affected by sexual distress compared with their male counterparts.[11,13]

A Danish study on the psychosocial impact of HS reported descriptive data on intimate relations from 12 participants at a single HS clinic.[23] Patients described finding a partner as challenging due to "disgusting lesions too complicated and too difficult to explain."[23] Those who were in a relationship found it burdensome to disclose and explain the nature of their HS, and avoided showing their skin to their partners if draining lesions were present.[23] Some of the study participants reported that their sexual life had stopped due to HS.[23]

The impact of HS on sexual health and partner intimacy extends beyond emotional health to encompass safety concerns. A Canadian cross-sectional study with 128 HS patients and 115 acne patients found that HS patients are at a significantly increased risk (OR: 2.35) for intimate partner violence (IPV) compared to the acne control group.[41] Research has uniformly underscored the importance of assessing sexual health during routine clinic visits and as an outcome measure in HS trials. Providers should also have a heightened awareness regarding the risk of IPV among their HS patients and should consider screening for IPV with a validated screening tool.

Daily and Work Functions

The physical symptoms and psychosocial burden associated with HS can interfere with daily life/work functioning and thus further impact patients' QoL. In this section, we will discuss specific lifestyle and vocational issues experienced by HS patients. These include sleep disturbance, disutility (i.e., disability due to a chronic disease) and loss of work productivity, as well as challenges to implementing recommended lifestyle modifications.

Sleep Disturbance and Daytime Somnolence

In the literature and our clinical experience, HS patients often report sleep disturbance and daytime somnolence. Recent studies have shown that pain and pruritus are major contributors to poor sleep quality.[7,42] Components of sleep that are affected in HS patients include sleep latency, duration, and disturbance.[42] The authors of a cross-sectional Polish study with over 100 HS patients and 50 healthy controls found that HS patients had a significantly more impaired sleep quality score relative to healthy controls.[42] Severities of pruritus and pain as measured by VAS scores were positively correlated with insomnia scores.[42] These findings are in line with what we have learned from other skin conditions (e.g., atopic dermatitis), where pruritus can lead to disrupted sleep patterns. Activities of daily life may be impacted by two independent factors: pruritus alone, or daytime somnolence as a result of insomnia.

Disutility and Loss of Work Productivity

HS patients often face challenges involving disutility and loss of work productivity.[4,12] HS typically appears during the second and third decades of life and thus has the potential to negatively impact patients' early career trajectories.[43,44] Studies have shown that HS patients missed more workdays than the general public, with one study reporting up to an average work loss of 33.6 days per year.[12] At 2-year follow-up, 23% of the study participants believed that HS negatively impacted their chance for a promotion, and 10% reported losing their jobs due to HS.[12]

A retrospective study investigated a claims database of employed HS patients in the United States.[45] The researchers found that newly diagnosed HS patients experienced a slower income growth and were significantly more likely to leave the work force than controls.[45] HS patients demonstrated statistically significant differences compared to controls in the following metrics: more work loss days (18.4 vs. 7.7), higher annual indirect costs ($2,925 vs. $1,483), and lower annual income ($54,925 vs. $62,357).[45]

Challenges to Implementing Lifestyle Modifications

HS patients often face physical and social barriers, which may hinder their ability to implement positive lifestyle changes. HS has been linked to obesity and active smoking.[46] Despite their deleterious health effects, tobacco usage and overeating are ways in which some patients cope with the stress associated with HS.[17] In a qualitative Danish focus-group study, patients reported feeling that HS and its symptoms are outside their control.[23] As such, they considered any long-term lifestyle modifications as futile.[23]

Studies have shown that appropriate weight loss and smoking cessation can improve the overall health of HS patients.[47–49] However, in addition to feeling a lack of control over their health, chronic pain often prevents patients from engaging in activities that can help promote weight loss, such as exercising or participating in sports.[17] Moreover, embarrassment and fear of judgment could prevent HS patients from forming healthy social interactions.[17] The aforementioned qualitative study also found that HS patients reported feeling alone regarding their disease and would like the opportunity to meet or have online contact with other HS patients.[23]

Empowering patients to be partners in managing their HS disease may lead to enhanced care outcomes. In addition, encouraging HS patients to explore patient-led groups for social support and sharing of resources may promote a sense of community among them. HS support groups are discussed in detail in Chapter 33.

Healthcare Costs Related to Hidradenitis Suppurativa

HS places a large socioeconomic burden upon individual patients and society as a whole. First and foremost, the financial consequences of HS rest on the shoulders of each patient. As previously mentioned, HS patients reported more work day loss, lower annual income, and higher total indirect costs compared to the general public.[45] This does not factor in the expenses associated with medical/hygiene supplies (e.g., wound dressings and bandages) and the time dedicated to taking care of HS lesions on a daily basis.[23]

Second, HS-related care can inflict disproportionately high costs on the healthcare system.[50–55] A 3-year claims data analysis in the United States with over 150,000 patients found that HS patients had a significantly higher rate of inpatient hospitalization (15.8%) than psoriasis patients (10.8%) and healthy controls (8.6%).[50] Similarly, emergency department (ED) utilization was significantly higher in the HS cohort (27.1%) than the psoriasis cohort (17.4%) or the control group (17.2%).[50] The mean outpatient cost was significantly higher among HS patients ($6,863) compared to psoriasis patients ($6,267) and healthy controls ($4,071).[50]

Another U.S.-based cohort study reflected similar findings as above: the HS cohort utilized high-cost healthcare settings significantly more than the psoriasis cohort (hospitalization: 5.1% vs. 1.6%; ED admission: 7.4% vs. 2.6%).[51] Based on data from the US National Inpatient Sample between 2002 and 2012, a separate group of researchers found that HS accounted for greater than $38 million of excess mean costs of mental health-related hospitalizations per year.[55]

The high use of acute care settings likely stems from multiple factors, including delayed or misdiagnosis, poor access to HS treatment centers, and a limited armamentarium of effective and lasting therapy for this disease.[56] Research has shown that patients receive more appropriate and cost-effective care at outpatient dermatology clinics than from non-dermatologists or from ED visits.[50,52,56,57] Increasing awareness of HS among front-line providers to reduce delay in diagnosis, encouraging earlier referrals to dermatology to establish a "home" for HS, and providing patients with written home-management action plans are steps to decreasing acute care setting utilization.

Conclusion

The debilitation and devastation that HS brings to patients' lives are often widespread. With this chapter, we aimed to paint a more complete picture of the challenges that HS patients face on a daily basis and raise awareness about the profound impact the disease has on patients' QoL. Most importantly, we hope that this awareness can translate into continued and heightened efforts to improve disease education and research, optimize medical treatments, and expand psychological/social/financial support for HS patients.

References

1. Wolkenstein P, Loundou A, Barrau K, et al. Quality of life impairment in hidradenitis suppurativa: a study of 61 cases. *J Am Acad Dermatol.* 2007;56(4):621–623. https://doi.org/10.1016/j.jaad.2006.08.061.
2. Hamzavi IH, Sundaram M, Nicholson C, et al. Uncovering burden disparity: a comparative analysis of the impact of moderate-to-severe psoriasis and hidradenitis suppurativa. *J Am Acad Dermatol.* 2017;77(6):1038–1046. https://doi.org/10.1016/j.jaad.2017.07.027.
3. Sampogna F, Fania L, Mazzanti C, et al. The Broad-Spectrum Impact of Hidradenitis Suppurativa on Quality of Life: A Comparison with Psoriasis. *Dermatology.* 2019;235(4):308–314. https://doi.org/10.1159/000496604.
4. Riis P, Vinding G, Ring H, Jemec G. Disutility in Patients with Hidradenitis Suppurativa: A Cross-sectional Study Using EuroQoL-5D. *Acta Derm Venereol.* 2016;96(2):222–226. https://doi.org/10.2340/00015555-2129.
5. Alavi A, Farzanfar D, Lee RK, Almutairi D. The Contribution of Malodour in Quality of Life of Patients With Hidradenitis Suppurativa. *J Cutan Med Surg.* 2018;22(2):166–174. https://doi.org/10.1177/1203475417745826.
6. Matusiak Ł, Szczęch J, Kaaz K, et al. Clinical Characteristics of Pruritus and Pain in Patients with Hidradenitis Suppurativa. *Acta Derm Venereol.* 2018;98(2):191–194. https://doi.org/10.2340/00015555-2815.
7. Vossen ARJV, Schoenmakers A, van Straalen KR, et al. Assessing Pruritus in Hidradenitis Suppurativa: A Cross-Sectional Study. *Am J Clin Dermatol.* 2017;18(5):687–695. https://doi.org/10.1007/s40257-017-0280-2.
8. Onderdijk AJ, van der Zee HH, Esmann S, et al. Depression in patients with hidradenitis suppurativa: depression in HS patients. *J Eur Acad Dermatol Venereol.* 2013;27(4):473–478. https://doi.org/10.1111/j.1468-3083.2012.04468.x.
9. Ring H, Sørensen H, Miller I, et al. Pain in Hidradenitis Suppurativa: A Pilot Study. *Acta Derm Venereol.* 2016;96(4):554–556. https://doi.org/10.2340/00015555-2308.
10. Molina-Leyva A, Cuenca-Barrales C. Pruritus and Malodour in Patients with Hidradenitis Suppurativa. Impact on Quality of Life

11. Janse IC, Deckers IE, van der Maten AD, et al. Sexual health and quality of life are impaired in hidradenitis suppurativa: a multicentre cross-sectional study. *Br J Dermatol.* 2017;176(4):1042–1047. https://doi.org/10.1111/bjd.14975.
12. Matusiak Ł, Bieniek A, Szepietowski JC. Hidradenitis suppurativa markedly decreases quality of life and professional activity. *J Am Acad Dermatol.* 2010;62(4):706–708.e1. https://doi.org/10.1016/j.jaad.2009.09.021.
13. Kurek A, Peters EMJ, Chanwangpong A, et al. Profound disturbances of sexual health in patients with acne inversa. *J Am Acad Dermatol.* 2012;67(3):422–428.e1. https://doi.org/10.1016/j.jaad.2011.10.024.
14. Kouris A, Platsidaki E, Christodoulou C, et al. Quality of Life and Psychosocial Implications in Patients with Hidradenitis Suppurativa. *Dermatology.* 2016;232(6):687–691. https://doi.org/10.1159/000453355.
15. American Psychiatric Association: *Diagnostic and Statistical Manual of Mental Disorders : DSM-5.* 5th ed. Washington, D.C.: American Psychiatric Association; 2013.
16. Bair MJ, Robinson RL, Katon W, Kroenke K. Depression and Pain Comorbidity: A Literature Review. *Arch Intern Med.* 2003;163(20):2433. https://doi.org/10.1001/archinte.163.20.2433.
17. Deckers IE, Kimball AB. The Handicap of Hidradenitis Suppurativa. *Dermatol Clin.* 2016;34(1):17–22. https://doi.org/10.1016/j.det.2015.07.003.
18. Machado MO, Stergiopoulos V, Maes M, et al. Depression and Anxiety in Adults With Hidradenitis Suppurativa: A Systematic Review and Meta-analysis. *JAMA Dermatol.* 2019;155(8):939. https://doi.org/10.1001/jamadermatol.2019.0759.
19. Patel KR, Lee HH, Rastogi S, et al. Association between hidradenitis suppurativa, depression, anxiety, and suicidality: a systematic review and meta-analysis. *J Am Acad Dermatol.* 2019. https://doi.org/10.1016/j.jaad.2019.11.068. Published online December. S0190962219332992.
20. Thorlacius L, Cohen AD, Gislason GH, et al. Increased Suicide Risk in Patients with Hidradenitis Suppurativa. *J Invest Dermatol.* 2018;138(1):52–57. https://doi.org/10.1016/j.jid.2017.09.008.
21. Jalenques I, Ciortianu L, Pereira B, et al. The prevalence and odds of anxiety and depression in children and adults with hidradenitis suppurativa: systematic review and meta-analysis. *J Am Acad Dermatol.* 2020;83(2):542–553. https://doi.org/10.1016/j.jaad.2020.03.041.
22. Wright S, Strunk A, Garg A. New-onset depression among children, adolescents, and adults with hidradenitis suppurativa. *J Am Acad Dermatol.* 2020. https://doi.org/10.1016/j.jaad.2020.05.090. Published online May. S0190962220309609.
23. Esmann S, Jemec G. Psychosocial Impact of Hidradenitis Suppurativa: A Qualitative Study. *Acta Derm Venereol.* 2011;91(3):328–332. https://doi.org/10.2340/00015555-1082.
24. Ingram JR, Jenkins-Jones S, Knipe DW, et al. Population-based Clinical Practice Research Datalink study using algorithm modelling to identify the true burden of hidradenitis suppurativa. *Br J Dermatol.* 2018;178(4):917–924. https://doi.org/10.1111/bjd.16101.
25. Kimball AB, Jemec GB. *Hidradenitis Suppurativa: A Disease Primer.* Springer Nature; 2017. https://doi.org/10.1007/978-3-319-50594-7.
26. Ilgen MA, Zivin K, McCammon RJ, Valenstein M. Pain and suicidal thoughts, plans and attempts in the United States. *Gen Hosp Psychiatry.* 2008;30(6):521–527. https://doi.org/10.1016/j.genhosppsych.2008.09.003.
27. Garg A, Pomerantz H, Midura M, et al. Completed suicide in patients with hidradenitis suppurativa: a population analysis in the United States. *J Invest Dermatol.* 2017;137(5):S38. https://doi.org/10.1016/j.jid.2017.02.237.
28. Shavit E, Dreiher J, Freud T, et al. Psychiatric comorbidities in 3207 patients with hidradenitis suppurativa. *J Eur Acad Dermatol Venereol.* 2015;29(2):371–376. https://doi.org/10.1111/jdv.12567.

29. Tzur Bitan D, Berzin D, Cohen AD. Hidradenitis suppurativa and schizophrenia: a nationwide cohort study. *J Eur Acad Dermatol Venereol.* 2020;34(3):574–579. https://doi.org/10.1111/jdv.15997.

30. Huilaja L, Tiri H, Jokelainen J, et al. Patients with Hidradenitis Suppurativa Have a High Psychiatric Disease Burden: A Finnish Nationwide Registry Study. *J Invest Dermatol.* 2018;138(1):46–51. https://doi.org/10.1016/j.jid.2017.06.020.

31. Garg A, Papagermanos V, Midura M, et al. Opioid, alcohol, and cannabis misuse among patients with hidradenitis suppurativa: a population-based analysis in the United States. *J Am Acad Dermatol.* 2018;79(3):495–500.e1. https://doi.org/10.1016/j.jaad.2018.02.053.

32. Shlyankevich J, Chen AJ, Kim GE, Kimball AB. Hidradenitis suppurativa is a systemic disease with substantial comorbidity burden: a chart-verified case-control analysis. *J Am Acad Dermatol.* 2014;71(6):1144–1150. https://doi.org/10.1016/j.jaad.2014.09.012.

33. Lesort C, Villani AP, Giai J, et al. High prevalence of cannabis use among patients with hidradenitis suppurativa: results from the VERADDICT survey. *Br J Dermatol.* 2019;181(4):839–841. https://doi.org/10.1111/bjd.17930.

34. Theut Riis P, Pedersen OB, Sigsgaard V, et al. Prevalence of patients with self-reported hidradenitis suppurativa in a cohort of Danish blood donors: a cross-sectional study. *Br J Dermatol.* 2019;180(4):774–781. https://doi.org/10.1111/bjd.16998.

35. Revuz JE, Canoui-Poitrine F, Wolkenstein P, et al. Prevalence and factors associated with hidradenitis suppurativa: results from two case-control studies. *J Am Acad Dermatol.* 2008;59(4):596–601. https://doi.org/10.1016/j.jaad.2008.06.020.

36. Davis SA, Lin H-C, Balkrishnan R, Feldman SR. Hidradenitis Suppurativa Management in the United States: An Analysis of the National Ambulatory Medical Care Survey and MarketScan Medicaid Databases. *Skin Appendage Disord.* 2015;1(2):65–73. https://doi.org/10.1159/000431037.

37. Puza CJ, Wolfe SA, Jaleel T. Pain Management in Patients With Hidradenitis Suppurativa Requiring Surgery:. *Dermatol Surg.* 2019;45(10):1327–1330. https://doi.org/10.1097/DSS.0000000000001693.

38. Reddy S, Orenstein LAV, Strunk A, Garg A. Incidence of Long-term Opioid Use Among Opioid-Naive Patients With Hidradenitis Suppurativa in the United States. *JAMA Dermatol.* 2019;155(11):1284. https://doi.org/10.1001/jamadermatol.2019.2610.

39. Alavi A, Farzanfar D, Rogalska T, et al. Quality of life and sexual health in patients with hidradenitis suppurativa. *Int J Womens Dermatol.* 2018;4(2):74–79. https://doi.org/10.1016/j.ijwd.2017.10.007.

40. Sampogna F, Abeni D, Gieler U, et al. Impairment of Sexual Life in 3,485 Dermatological Outpatients From a Multicentre Study in 13 European Countries. *Acta Derm Venereol.* 2017;97(4):478–482. https://doi.org/10.2340/00015555-2561.

41. Sisic M, Tan J, Lafreniere KD. Hidradenitis Suppurativa, Intimate Partner Violence, and Sexual Assault. *J Cutan Med Surg.* 2017;21(5):383–387. https://doi.org/10.1177/1203475417708167.

42. Kaaz K, Szepietowski J, Matusiak Ł. Influence of Itch and Pain on Sleep Quality in Patients with Hidradenitis Suppurativa. *Acta Derm Venereol.* 2018;98(8):757–761. https://doi.org/10.2340/00015555-2967.

43. Garg A, Lavian J, Lin G, et al. Incidence of hidradenitis suppurativa in the United States: a sex- and age-adjusted population analysis. *J Am Acad Dermatol.* 2017;77(1):118–122. https://doi.org/10.1016/j.jaad.2017.02.005.

44. Dufour DN, Emtestam L, Jemec GB. Hidradenitis suppurativa: a common and burdensome, yet under-recognised, inflammatory skin disease. *Postgrad Med J.* 2014;90(1062):216–221. https://doi.org/10.1136/postgradmedj-2013-131994.

45. Tzellos T, Yang H, Mu F, et al. Impact of hidradenitis suppurativa on work loss, indirect costs and income. *Br J Dermatol.* 2019;181(1):147–154. https://doi.org/10.1111/bjd.17101.

46. Sartorius K, Emtestam L, Jemec GBE, Lapins J. Objective scoring of hidradenitis suppurativa reflecting the role of tobacco smoking and obesity. *Br J Dermatol.* 2009;161(4):831–839. https://doi.org/10.1111/j.1365-2133.2009.09198.x.

47. Ring HC, Theut Riis P, Miller IM, et al. Self-reported pain management in hidradenitis suppurativa. *Br J Dermatol.* 2016;174(4):909–911. https://doi.org/10.1111/bjd.14266.

48. Saunte DM, Boer J, Stratigos A, et al. Diagnostic delay in hidradenitis suppurativa is a global problem. *Br J Dermatol.* 2015;173(6):1546–1549. https://doi.org/10.1111/bjd.14038.

49. Jemec GBE, Heidenheim M, Nielsen NH. The prevalence of hidradenitis suppurativa and its potential precursor lesions. *J Am Acad Dermatol.* 1996;35(2):191–194. https://doi.org/10.1016/S0190-9622(96)90321-7.

50. Kirby JS, Miller JJ, Adams DR, Leslie D. Health Care Utilization Patterns and Costs for Patients With Hidradenitis Suppurativa. *JAMA Dermatol.* 2014;150(9):937. https://doi.org/10.1001/jamadermatol.2014.691.

51. Khalsa A, Liu G, Kirby JS. Increased utilization of emergency department and inpatient care by patients with hidradenitis suppurativa. *J Am Acad Dermatol.* 2015;73(4):609–614. https://doi.org/10.1016/j.jaad.2015.06.053.

52. Marvel J, Vlahiotis A, Sainski-Nguyen A, et al. Disease burden and cost of hidradenitis suppurativa: a retrospective examination of US administrative claims data. *BMJ Open.* 2019;9(9). https://doi.org/10.1136/bmjopen-2019-030579, e030579.

53. Desai N, Shah P. High burden of hospital resource utilization in patients with hidradenitis suppurativa in England: a retrospective cohort study using hospital episode statistics. *Br J Dermatol.* 2017;176(4):1048–1055. https://doi.org/10.1111/bjd.14976.

54. Mehdizadeh A, Rosella L, Alavi A, et al. A Canadian Population-Based Cohort to the Study Cost and Burden of Surgically Resected Hidradenitis Suppurativa. *J Cutan Med Surg.* 2018;22(3):312–317. https://doi.org/10.1177/1203475418763536.

55. Patel KR, Rastogi S, Singam V, et al. Association between hidradenitis suppurativa and hospitalization for psychiatric disorders: a cross-sectional analysis of the National Inpatient Sample. *Br J Dermatol.* 2019;181(2):275–281. https://doi.org/10.1111/bjd.17416.

56. Jemec GBE, Guérin A, Kaminsky M, et al. What happens after a single surgical intervention for hidradenitis suppurativa? A retrospective claims-based analysis. *J Med Econ.* 2016;19(7):710–717. https://doi.org/10.3111/13696998.2016.1161636.

57. Garg A, Lavian J, Strunk A. Low Utilization of the Dermatology Ambulatory Encounter among Patients with Hidradenitis Suppurativa: A Population-Based Retrospective Cohort Analysis in the USA. *Dermatology.* 2017;233(5):396–398. https://doi.org/10.1159/000480379.

22
Office-Based Non-Excision Procedures

CHRIS SAYED, RON BIRNBAUM, AND JAN SMOGORZEWSKI

It is worth mentioning that the patients were extremely grateful.
Fred Mullens (1959)[1]

Treatment of Chronic Hidradenitis Suppurativa; Surgical Modification
(Reported in 1959 as the first "exteriorization" or deroofing procedure for hidradenitis suppurativa)

CHAPTER OUTLINE

Introduction

In the last few decades, surgical interventions for hidradenitis suppurativa (HS) have expanded well beyond traditional excisional approaches with the popularization of deroofing, the use of electrosurgical and laser-based excisions, and combined approaches that take both medical and surgical management into account. Equally important has been the motivation to move some procedures out of operating rooms with general anesthesia and into a clinic-based approach that makes surgical treatment more accessible and safer for many patients. With this movement comes important considerations regarding how to approach procedures in the outpatient setting. This chapter will explore frequently used clinic-based procedures and describe the appropriate way to plan for, perform, and postoperatively care for patients that choose these procedures as part of their care.

General Approach to Procedures

HS is a follicular disorder characterized by follicular rupture and chronic inflammation with terrible consequences in predictable anatomic areas in susceptible patients. The body's disordered attempt to re-epithelialize the exposed surfaces under the skin results in the formation of sinus tracts filled with a semi-solid substance, a disease-specific bacterial microbiome (heavy in anaerobes and organized in biofilms),[2] and related inflammatory elements collectively designated by Danby as the "invasive proliferative gelatinous mass"[3] or IPGM of HS. This trapped mass of sinus tracts and the IPGM are responsible for the enduring or episodic inflammatory symptoms in patients with the disease: pain, suppuration and purulent drainage, odors, scar-formation, overall debility, and sexual dysfunction. Late sequela of the disease may include lymphedema and squamous cell carcinoma. A discussion about complications from HS disease can be found in Chapter 9.

The optimal treatment of HS includes three broad categories of intervention: (1) prevention of new lesion formation, (2) palliation of suffering from existing lesions, and (3) the extirpation/destruction of established lesions which, when left alone, continue to drive inflammation and suffering. Resolution of HS is achieved when there is complete prevention of new lesions and all existing lesions have either been extirpated, "burnt out," or are otherwise eliminated. Medical strategies, including lifestyle modifications and topical and systemic agents, have considerable value in minimizing new lesions and disease progression, but physical remodeling of tissues and some degree of inflammation typically persist where sinuses have formed. Symptoms in these areas often last for years or even indefinitely, so surgical interventions that remove or resolve the tunneling are critical for relieving long-term symptoms.

Office procedures play a central role in all three treatment categories and are the focus of this chapter (Table 22.1). There are many choices, but we stress the importance of the deroofing technique as *the central and most essential office-based technique in the care of these patients.* Deroofing is safe and effective, it can be done with simple tools readily available in any office that regularly performs other procedures like excisions, and involves application of skills that essentially all dermatologists and other surgically trained physicians acquire in the course of their residency training. Deroofing is also an inexpensive procedure.

TABLE 22.1 Categorization of Office Procedures by Intent and Purpose

Office Procedures Intended to Prevent New Hidradenitis Suppurativa Lesion Formation	Office Procedures Intended to Mitigate Inflammation and Pain in Established Lesions	Office Procedures Intended to Resolve Chronic or Recurrent Lesions
Chemical Peels **Radiation** **Neurotoxins** Laser and light epilation (see Chapter 25) Photodynamic therapy (see Chapter 25)	**Intralesional Triamcinolone** **Incision and Drainage** **Radiation** Photodynamic therapy (see Chapter 25)	**Deroofing** Local Excision (see Chapter 23 and 24) Laser Destruction (see Chapter 25 and 26) Cryoinsufflation (see Chapter 26)

Procedures in bold are examined in detail in this chapter.

In considering the appropriateness of office-based procedural interventions (indeed, all interventions), clinicians must proceed from history and physical examination and categorization of the extent and complexity of individual foci of the disease. The most useful classification schema for this purpose was defined by Hurley and is widely known as Hurley Staging[4]:

Hurley Stage I: Abscess formation, single or multiple, without sinus tracts and cicatrization

Hurley Stage II: Recurrent abscesses with tract formation and cicatrization; single or multiple widely separated lesions

Hurley Stage III: Diffuse or near diffuse involvement, or multiple interconnected tracts and abscesses across entire area

In this chapter, we consider several treatments which have varying efficacy and make more sense when applied to the correct clinical stage of a given focus of the disease and for the correct purpose (Table 22.2). Educating the patient on the nature of the disease and the purpose of any given procedure is vital to the success of these endeavors. For example, laser epilation is intended to destroy hair follicles in HS-prone areas in a predisposed patient; each destroyed follicle is one less potential site of inflammation and follicular rupture. However, laser epilation may have no effect on longstanding lesions. Intralesional injections of triamcinolone or incision and drainage of individual lesions may have valuable palliative effect on treated lesions for a few to several weeks. However, if the patient believes that these treatments were intended to "cure" the lesion, then those procedures may be considered failures after symptoms return. The deroofing technique and its variants can reliably resolve specific sinuses but have no specific impact on preventing new disease. Thus, office procedures must fit into a well-conceived program of multi-modal medical and surgical care. Starting with patient education, small procedural interventions and building trust in the patient-physician relationship is an optimal way to care for the patient with HS.

Preoperative Anesthesia/Anxiolytics

HS is painful, and its lesions are tender. In nearly all cases, office procedures are also painful. Compassionate procedural care of non-sedated patients with HS requires careful consideration of acute intra-procedural pain and anticipatory anxiety. Failure to address these may convince patients that procedures that would otherwise help them are intolerable, thereby unnecessarily narrowing the therapeutic armamentarium. Certain patients may benefit from a pre-procedure oral anxiolytic with a single dose of a benzodiazepine, such as 1 to 2 mg lorazepam or 10 mg of diazepam given 30 to 60 minutes prior to the procedure. Pretreating areas with topical anesthetics, such as commercially available eutectic mixture of local anesthetics (e.g., 2.5% lidocaine and 2.5% prilocaine applied for at least 1 hour) under occlusion or compounded high-concentration anesthetic creams (e.g., lidocaine 23% and tetracaine 7%),[5] may facilitate the tolerability of definitive local anesthesia (via injection) for deroofing or before injection of intralesional triamcinolone, neurotoxins, or laser treatments. Skin cooling with 10 to 15 seconds of ice pack application or similar methods can also help ease injection pain.

Direct injection of local anesthetics is the principal approach to eliminating procedural pain and limiting procedural blood loss during office procedures like deroofing. The commonly used amine is lidocaine with epinephrine. A rule of thumb is that 0.5 to 1 mL of lidocaine 1% with epinephrine 1:100,000 per square centimeter of planned treatment area will suffice, modified for lesional thickness as indicated. Warming anesthetics, high gauge (i.e., small) needles, slow injection, buffering with 1:10 dilution of sodium bicarbonate and topical pre-treatments may lessen the pain associated with local anesthesia. The approach of the authors is to start with a ½-inch 30-gauge needle to create a small area for

TABLE 22.2 Utility of Selected Office Procedures by Hurley Stage, Based on Practical Applicability and Evidence of Efficacy

Hurley Stage	Intralesional Triamcinolone	Incision and Drainage	Deroofing	Local Excision	Neurotoxins	Chemical Peels	Radiation
Stage I	++	++	+	-	+	++	-
Stage II	++	++	+++	++	+	+	+
Stage III	+	++	+++[a]	-	-	-	+

[a]For practical reasons, i.e., limitations of time and local anesthetic toxicity limits, deroofing is sometimes performed in a staged manner or limited to one body site for each surgical episode in Hurley Stage III disease. These patients may prefer procedures performed with general anesthesia in an operating room, but based on patient preference, in-office deroofing or excisions have value as time permits and may be achieved by use of more dilute concentrations of anesthetics or with tumescent anesthesia for extensive areas.

−, No utility.

+, Limited utility.

++, Useful in many selected cases.

+++, Indicated and nearly always useful.

anesthesia through which a 1.5 inch 25- or 27-gauge needle can be introduced. Using a fanning technique, large areas can be anesthetized with relatively few individual injections sites, and this also allows for deeper anesthesia when needed.

The proceduralist can begin by injecting anesthetic in a ring at the periphery of the lesion. Then, a small amount of anesthetic can be introduced directly into sinus tracts with the twin benefits of dilating those tracts to facilitate the probing step of deroofing and distributing anesthetic throughout the lesion. Finally, the rest of the lesion is injected. Starting in a superficial subcutaneous plane is often well-tolerated and makes the subsequent anesthesia of the dermis less painful. Awareness of the systemic toxicity from lidocaine overload (limit to 7 mg/kg when using lidocaine with epinephrine) is essential given the size of lesions treated in office settings. Indeed, lidocaine toxicity limits are one of the key parameters limiting the size of office-setting deroofing procedures. Diluting the lidocaine component to 0.5% or 0.25% can greatly expand the area that can be safely treated. Performing serial deroofing procedures in smaller stages or using tumescent anesthesia are additional strategies for treating larger lesions.

Intralesional Triamcinolone

Intralesional triamcinolone has been used frequently in the management of HS for many years. Despite this, little data exists that supports efficacy and provides guidance on the optimal concentration, volume, and clinical context for its use. An uncontrolled retrospective study using average volumes of 0.75 mL of triamcinolone 10 mg/kg demonstrated improved pain and physician-reported outcomes over a 7-day period, but lacked a control group for comparison.[6] Another prospective study using ultrasound to identify and follow small (mean 5 to 17 mm) fistulous tracts found that nearly half resolved at 90 days after treatment with a mean of 0.5 mL of triamcinolone 10 mg/mL.[7] While promising, this study similarly lacks a control group and there is uncertainty regarding the typical natural history of relatively small fistulous tracts as determined by ultrasound.

A recent randomized controlled trial evaluated 0.1 mL of intralesional triamcinolone 10 mg/mL, 40 mg/mL versus non-bacteriostatic normal saline for the treatment of isolated nodules or abscesses less than 2 cm in size. Fifty-eight lesions had outcome data. Similar improvements in pain visual analog scale change, days to lesions resolution as determined by patients, and patient satisfaction were found across all three groups throughout a 14-day follow-up period.[8] While the lack of improvement compared to the normal saline control is discouraging, the overall volume of triamcinolone used in this study was lower than in the previous uncontrolled studies. Of great interest is the finding that even patients receiving normal saline injections consistently reported benefit. While a placebo effect is possible, it is also possible that puncturing a lesion and instilling an external solution alone is helpful.

While the current data on the efficacy of triamcinolone is mixed, many patients report benefit and request treatment in clinical practice. Given the low overall risk, it is reasonable to offer treatment and discuss the available evidence regarding efficacy. In some patients that are hesitant to undergo injections due to pain, the limitations of this treatment and alternatives should be considered. For patients with widespread disease, it is also important to consider systemic absorption and potential side effects, which, while uncommon, do sometimes occur with repeated doses of 60 mg or more.[9,10] Doses in the 30 to 60 mg range have been

found to induce slight changes in the hypothalamic pituitary axis but generally do not result in symptomatic effects.[11] Doses under 20 mg generally have negligible systemic effect.[12] Future studies evaluating a range of doses and concentrations with appropriate control groups are needed to determine the optimal way to utilize intralesional steroids for acute HS flares.

From a practical standpoint, use of intralesional triamcinolone is straightforward. Use of skin cooling and topical anesthetics can reduce injection pain but are not frequently required. The skin is cleaned with alcohol, taking care to avoid ulcerated skin in which this would be more painful. Quick introduction of the needle, aiming for the dermal component of a nodule or into an inflamed sinus is ideal, followed by slow injection. In darker-skinned patients, care should be taken to minimize superficial infiltration that may lead to hypopigmentation. In some cases, introducing the needle directly through the opening of a sinus may be less painful than the surrounding skin. A concentration of 10 mg/mL should be used when treating many lesions, while fewer may be treated with 40 mg/mL to help minimize the overall dose administered. The dose of 0.1 to 1 mL may be administered in one or multiple injection sites depending on lesion size, typically with 0.1 to 0.2 mL per square centimeter of affected tissue. Aftercare is typically not required.

Incision and Drainage

The conflation of HS with simple bacterial abscesses is perhaps the single biggest cause of delayed diagnosis (averaging 7 to 10 years),[13] mistreatment, and physician contribution to patient suffering in the care of this disease. The most frequently misapplied procedure in this context is incision and drainage, which has great value in the cure of bacterial abscess or pain relief for an acute HS abscess, but limited value for definitively resolving chronic or recurrent lesions. In bacterial abscesses, incision and drainage eliminates the motherlode of etiopathogenic material—the stew of bacteria and pus. However, in HS, the ongoing driver of inflammatory symptoms—the trapped epithelial elements and the IPGM—remain in part or in whole after incision and drainage attempts. For lesions that are already persistently draining, incision and drainage typically serves little purpose. Deroofing is often indicated instead.

Appropriate Use of Incision and Drainage

When does it make sense to incise and drain an HS lesion? Danby describes the specific indication that justifies it as follows. "A tense abscess that is too painful to bear should be incised after wide circumferential local anesthesia... The actively growing IPGM is not eliminated. An alternative surgical approach is indicated."[14] In the case of small, early abscesses, intralesional triamcinolone may achieve the same effect both through the introduction of the corticosteroid and puncturing, but abscesses larger than 2 cm may ultimately require surgical or spontaneous drainage before improving. When incision and drainage is appropriately chosen, a technique familiar to the proceduralist for abscess drainage will generally suffice. However, packing is generally not needed as it often results in increased morbidity and has not been shown to improve outcomes in comparative studies.[15,16]

In the experience of the authors, anesthesia can typically be limited to a focal area of the abscess that looks and feels most superficial. A 6-mm punch tool can be used to incise the lesion and can be used in telescoping fashion if needed to access the abscess cavity (Video 22.1). This typically allows for rapid drainage without the need for intense pressure or pain once anesthesia is achieved for the incision. Care should be taken to cover the punch tool with gauze as pus may be rapidly propelled through the hub of the instrument on initial incision. The punch site can be covered with a simple bandage and left to heal by secondary intention, allowing the area to continue to drain for a few days if needed.

Deroofing

Deroofing (alternatively called unroofing or sinus tract exteriorization)[17–20] is a simple technique, first described by Mullins et al.[1] Table 22.3 and Figs. 22.1 and 22.2 summarize a practical approach to the procedure, and video is available online (Video 22.2). Most typically, a sinus is marked and completely anesthetized. A blunt probe is gently passed into a sinus tract until resistance is encountered. The tract's roof is cut open over the probe using sharp scissors, a scalpel, cutting electrical current, or ablative laser. The roof flaps are reflected and trimmed off at the hinge. Any newly exposed sinus tracts are probed and likewise treated. The exposed "floors" are optionally treated with sharp curettage and/or by raking them with coarse gauze applied with downward pressure to increase frictional forces; a maneuver termed "grattage." The sum effect of this is to eliminate the gelatinous content of the sinus tract—the IPGM—without further tissue

TABLE 22.3	Stepwise Guide to Deroofing Procedures	
	Standard Approach	**Alternatives and Comments**
Supplies	• Consent form • Marking pen • Alcohol pads • Gauze (include coarse) • Nonsterile gloves/face shield • Lidocaine 0.25 to 1% with 1:100,000 epinephrine • Syringes and needles for local anesthesia • ½ inch 30-gauge and 1–½ inch, 27-gauge for large areas • Probes (ideally double-ended malleable steel probe or simple cotton-tipped applicator) • Sharp tissue scissors • Toothed forceps • #15 scalpel • 4 mm curette (disposable) • Aluminum Chloride in alcohol • Electrocautery device and tips • Petrolatum/non-stick gauze/ordinary gauze/tape for dressing wounds	See individual steps for alternative supplies
Patient Selection	Hurley Stage II and III patients, in most typical locations whether inflamed or not	Pilonidal cyst/sinus is a distinct entity and requires other techniques
Marking and Skin Preparation	• Clean involved area with alcohol. • Carefully palpate for firmness/induration and mark by circling the visibly and palpably involved skin (whether inflamed or not) and circle sinus tract openings.	Betadine or chlorhexidine may be used to clean the surgical area
Anesthesia	• Instill a ring of anesthetic around the periphery of the marked lesion starting in superficial subcutaneous plane prior to dermal infiltration. • Directly introduce anesthetic into sinus tracts which helps dilate and defines them. • Inject the rest of the marked lesion. • Inject a 1 cm margin around the marked lesion	Pre-treat with topical anesthetic (e.g., lidocaine 2.5% and prilocaine 2.5%) • Start with ½-inch 30-gauge needle for small area and then use 1–½ inch 27-gauge needle in fanning technique for larger areas • Tumescent anesthesia for large lesions.
Probing and Opening the Roof	• Introduce the blunt metal probe into the biggest or most accessible sinus tract. • Advance steadily until it stops or comes out another opening. Care is taken to avoid creating false tracts by using excessive force into healthy subcutaneous fat. • Cut the roof skin with tissue scissors (or scalpel) over the probe. • Carefully examine for any nearby comedones that may connect to the larger sinus and investigate with probe or sharp-tipped scissor.	• The wooden end of disposable cotton-tipped applicators may also be used as a probe • Occasionally, ostia of sinus tracts have closed and need gentle force with a probe at sites of erythema and atrophy or a small snip or cut to access the tunnel • Small recurrent lesions can be opened with a punch ("mini-unroofing") • Alternatives for opening the roof: scalpel, hyfrecator/Bovie/CO_2 laser
"Excising at Hinge"	• With roof opened, reflect back the roof and then trim it off at the hinge (either with scissors or scalpel, assisted by forceps). • Sloped edges are acceptable and preferred.	Trimmings can be sent to a pathologist for histologic confirmation. They should be sent if verrucous or nodular change is apparent to rule out a complicating squamous cell carcinoma.

TABLE 22.3	Stepwise Guide to Deroofing Procedures—cont'd	
	Standard Approach	**Alternatives and Comments**
Final Probing	• Follow all sinus tracts until all roofs open • Always reprobe after trimming off roof, as that action exposes new tracts • Probing is complete when it reveals no more tracts	
Treating the "Floor"	• Curette and/or use firm pressure and coarse gauze to generate friction, and rake the floor ("coarse gauze grattage") to remove gelatinous content	Areas where gelatinous material does not easily come free at an edge may indicate disease extension and should be carefully explored.
Hemostasis (3 P's)	• Point cautery of vessels bleeding profusely • Pressure applied with aluminum chloride-soaked gauze or cotton-tipped applicators • Point cautery of any residual bleeding vessels, after assuring aluminum chloride has fully dried due to fire hazard of cautery	Ferric chloride or ferric subsulfate (Monsel's solution) may be used instead of aluminum chloride for broad area hemostasis.
Repair	None (secondary intent)	If repair is desired, a full thickness excision is generally first performed around and deep in to the unroofed area to avoid trapping epithelialized elements deep to the repair.
Dressing	• Fill space with petrolatum • Apply a non-stick gauze • Standard absorbent gauze placed on top • Tape completely (pressure dressing technique)	Xeroform or other petrolatum-impregnated gauze is an alternative
Wound Care and Analgesia	• For many inflamed patients, the procedure takes away more pain than it causes • Non-opioid analgesia, opioids in select cases • Remove dressing in 24 hours • Wash with soap and water • Apply petrolatum (or xeroform) • Cover to keep wound moist and petrolatum off clothes	Patients with HS are usually wound care experts by the time they have their first deroofing
Follow-up	• 1–2 weeks for first time patients who often need reassurance when they see big granulating wounds • In 6–8 weeks or when desired otherwise	

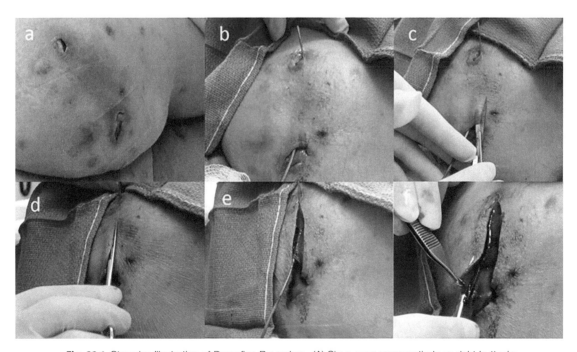

• **Fig. 22.1** Stepwise Illustration of Deroofing Procedure. (A) Sinus seen preoperatively on right buttocks, (B) double-ended fistula probe inserted in one ostia and exiting another, (C) iris scissor used to begin opening the tunnel, (D) further sharp dissection of the roof of the tunnel over the probe, (E) tunnel opened with probe in inflammatory proliferative gelatinous mass (IPGM), and (F) reflection and excising at the hinge of the overlying skin.

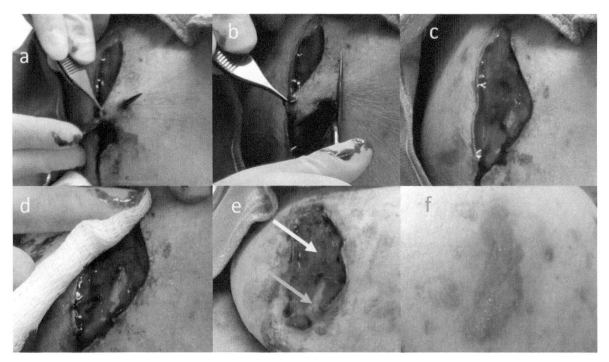

• **Fig. 22.2** Stepwise Illustration of Deroofing Procedure. (A) Iris scissor used to probe extension of sinus through additional ostia, and (B) excision of additional overlying tissue, (C) deroofed sinus with IPGM covering the floor, (D) firm gauze grattage to remove IPGM revealing, (E) a floor composed of scar/dermis (yellow arrow) and epithelialized lining (blue arrow), (F) healed scar at 3.5 months follow-up. (Courtesy Dr. Sayed).

disruption. Hemostasis is achieved via ordinary methods and the wound is dressed and allowed to heal by secondary intent. Painful suppurating scarred lesions are replaced with quiescent soft scars, often much smaller than the area deroofed. Because hidradenitis is confined to the dermis and subcutis, the discipline of treating only probed tracts prevents surgical damage to deep structures like the brachial plexus in the axilla, and reduces risk of blind excisions. Hurley Stage I lesions, essentially furuncle-like abscesses occurring within a single folliculo-pilosebaceous unit and without sinus tract formation, can be treated with a modified version of deroofing known as "mini-unroofing." Instead of probing and cutting into the roof of a sinus tract, a punch biopsy tool (between 5 and 8 mm in diameter) is used to open the cystic space. Table 22.3 provides a stepwise guide to the deroofing procedure and common variants. Hurley Stage III lesions may also be treated using deroofing and are often aided by some modifications: moving care to an operating room and using general anesthesia, using tumescent or more dilute anesthesia in the clinic setting, or by executing serial small deroofings in which each episode of care is limited to a portion of a lesion. Lesions 20 to 40 cm^2 are relatively straightforward and quick to treat, though areas over 100 cm^2 can be treated if the situation requires immediate attention, the patient prefers an outpatient setting, and if the practitioner's time permits. In particular, patients with comorbidities that restrict access to general anesthesia may find the outpatient setting as their only avenue for surgical treatment.

Deroofing: Efficacy, Safety, Recurrence, and Patient Reception

Overall, patient satisfaction rates with surgical procedures for HS are high, which is also true of office deroofing.[21] Secondary intent healing rates are generally superior to primarily closed wounds and approximate those seen with flap and graft repairs, with lower complication rates.[22–25] Healing occurs between 2 and 8 weeks depending on wound size and location. Complications other than postoperative pain (which is often less than pain stemming from acute disease) are rare. Bleeding is an uncommon but occasional problem in the early postoperative period. Review of literature and the authors' experience do not identify a single case of infection after a deroofing procedure, suggesting this is an exceedingly rare complication. Recurrence rates range from 4% to 27%,[18,21,26–29] but should in no way be equated with "treatment failure." None of these studies distinguishes between recurrence due to incomplete lesion extirpation and the appearance of new lesions in a disease prone area. The symptom-free interval between surgical healing and the reappearance of any disease may represent a significant benefit to the patient despite the recurrence, and even patients with recurrence generally report high satisfaction with treatment.[21]

Radiation

Radiotherapy for HS dates back to 1950, with the first reported use of x-rays as a primary therapy conducted on 54 patients who achieved improvement in axillary lesions without recurrence.[30] As the pathophysiology of HS became more fully understood, x-ray therapy fell out of favor for several decades until the largest retrospective study of 231 patients treated with orthovoltage therapy was conducted (superficial x-rays penetrating only skin and superficial tissue) in Germany in 2000. Patients were treated with single doses ranging from 0.5 to 1.5 Gy with total series doses reaching 3.0 to 8.0 Gy with complete relief in 89 (38%) patients, and improvement in 92 (40%).[31] More recent case reports and series recommend radiotherapy as a viable treatment option for patients who have exhausted topical and systemic therapies and may not be candidates for larger excisions. Advances in technology have expanded radiotherapy modalities and now include electron beam radiation composed of electrons, as opposed to the photons that make up x-ray beams. Electron beams only penetrate the superficial skin. The largest retrospective study of patients receiving electron beam radiation therapy involved five patients with Hurley Stage II or III and showed promising results 2 months after treatment, particularly in the axillae, although the degree of improvement was not reported. Treatment of the groin and perineum in the same patients produced less satisfying improvement; this is theorized to have been due to more extensive scarring in these areas, resulting in impaired electron beam penetration.[32] The most frequently reported treatment dose per location is 7.5 Gy in 2.5 Gy fractions.[32,33] Theoretically, radiotherapy acts through depilation and destruction of the follicular unit. Positioning and dosing of patients depends on locations of involvement and requires consultation with radiation oncology colleagues.

As opposed to external beam radiation therapy described above, brachytherapy is a type of radiation therapy that involves the placement of a radiation source directly adjacent to the target with a probe; in the case of HS, directly on the skin. One patient with severe HS of the neck and groin along with significant acne conglobata of the chest and dissecting cellulitis of the scalp, was successfully treated with a 10 Gy protocol given at 2.5 Gy fractions over 4 days to both the groin and scalp. He tolerated the treatment well with no toxic skin reaction and no recurrence. Interestingly, the patient also had significant improvement of distant lesions not directly treated with brachytherapy, a phenomenon similar to the abscopal effect whereby radiation of a primary tumor results in shrinkage of distant metastases.[34]

Microwave ablation (MiraDry) targeting eccrine and apocrine sweat glands along with hair follicles through thermolysis has not been shown to be effective, and in fact may worsen mild HS in some patients.[35] A split-body study involving microwave ablation of only one axilla was terminated early because five of eight patients experienced worsened lesion formation compared to the contralateral axilla. The adverse effect was long lasting with lesions persisting for a median of 43 days compared to 5.5 days for the untreated axilla.[35]

Patients tolerate radiation therapy with only mild cutaneous side effects, though there is potential carcinogenic risk. One study, based on average doses and locations of treatment of HS, estimates a risk of inducing a fatal tumor at 2 per 1000 treated female patients, although this is not based on patient data and represents a theoretical calculation.[36]

Of note, there exist several reports of HS worsening or becoming induced after radiation therapy for unrelated breast or uterine malignancies, even in patients who did not previously exhibit lesions of HS. One case involved treatment of ductal carcinoma in situ of the breast in a patient with a known history of HS who developed open and closed comedones with sinus tracts and inflammatory nodules limited to a well demarcated area of radiation that was previously clear. Another patient who had no history of HS, but did have a risk factor of smoking, developed inflammatory nodules and sinus tracts of the groin and inguinal folds three weeks after external beam radiotherapy for uterine adenocarcinoma.[37]

The authors speculate that radiation-induced apoptosis and subsequent inflammatory response lead to manifestations of HS. The radiotherapy doses utilized in patients who experienced flare-ups were significantly higher (~50 GY) than in patients who received radiotherapy as treatment (3 to 7 GY), lending credence to the idea that significant tissue destruction in certain patients results in a regional immune dysregulation termed an "iso-radiotopic" response.[38]

In summary, referral for radiation therapy does represent a treatment option that may be safe and effective, but precise dosages and the overall treatment course are yet to be determined and require further study.

Chemical Peels

Resorcinol is a phenol derivative with keratolytic properties directed at hydrogen bonds in keratin and is the only chemical peel with case series and uncontrolled clinical trials supporting its use in HS at a concentration of 15%. At higher concentrations (>20%), systemic toxicity has been reported, including cold sweats, dizziness, and clinical signs of hyperthyroidism.[39]

In an uncontrolled clinical trial involving 32 patients who were classified as Hurley Stage I and II, resorcinol 15% was applied twice daily for 30 days to single non-fistulous lesions less than 2 cm in size with no other therapies. Lesions decreased significantly at day 7 and 30 with corresponding reduction in size on ultrasound. Pain was also significantly decreased.[40] In an earlier open trial, 12 patients with Hurley Stage I and II disease self-treated with daily application of resorcinol 15% in an oil/water cream with emulsifying waxes to flaring lesions in the groin and axillae. Patients noted reductions in duration of painful abscesses from their typical average of 5 to 3.7 days. The authors emphasized the rapid reduction in pain with topical resorcinol and patient satisfaction with self-application of medication at the first sign of new lesion formation. Side effects included desquamation and irritation in the area of application, which was mitigated with moisturizers, as well as a reversible brown discoloration in 4 out of 12 patients.[39]

Limitations to topical resorcinol include lack of easy access to the medication, the need for compounding pharmacies, and lack of third-party coverage of medication. Caution should be taken when combining resorcinol with other potentially irritating treatment modalities. Treatment with intense pulsed light therapy for hair reduction in patients using concomitant resorcinol resulted in significant adverse effects of erythema, minor infection, minor burn, and worsening of HS.[41]

Theoretically, other chemical peel modalities (glycolic, salicylic acid, Jessner's) may be helpful secondary to their keratolytic properties, but this has not been adequately studied.

Neurotoxins

Botulinum toxin A in the form of abobotulinum toxin A (Dysport) and onabotulinotoxin A (Botox) has been successfully utilized both in the axillae and the inguinal folds. Remissions range from 6 months to 3 years. One of the cases involved the treatment of a 7-year-old female (see table 22.4). The positive treatment response of HS to botulinum toxin may in part be related to a reduction in sweat with resultant decrease in maceration, or the prevention of follicular rupture and inflammatory sinus tract formation. Outcome measurements in these studies were varied and poorly defined. The small numbers of patients treated without larger studies verifying the benefits of botulinum toxin in HS make this treatment modality difficult to recommend. The cost, lack of availability to many patients, and short duration of benefit with need for repeat treatments also limit the utility of botulinum toxin therapy. Further larger studies will help elucidate the scenarios and patients that may benefit from botulinum toxin injections (Table 22.4).

TABLE 22.4 Summary of Studies Using Botulinum Toxin A for Hidradenitis Suppurativa

First Author (Year)[ref.]	n	Hurley Stage (I, II, III, or N/A)/Patient Characteristics, If Mentioned	Botulinum A Dosage	Frequency of Administration	Technique Utilized	Regions Treated	Remission Time
O'Reilly (2005)[45]	1	N/A "pustular eruptions...and secondary scarring"	250 U of Dysport	Once	"Intradermal blebs throughout the axillae"	Axillae	10 months
Feito-Rodriguez (2009)[46]	1	N/A "Moderate" 7 year old pediatric patient	40 U total	Twice, repeated after 6 months	"Injected intradermally at 10 to 12 points over the elliptical area on each side" Performed with topical anesthesia and inhalation of nitrous oxide.	Groin/Inguinal	6 months
Khoo (2014)[47]	3	II, N/A, N/A	50 U per axillae	Four treatments over 3 years in one patient, not stated for other two patients	Not stated	Axillae	5 months to 1 year
Campanati (2019)[48]	2	II, II	Patient 1: 50 U Vistabex diluted in 2.5 mL 0.9% preservative free sterile saline per axilla, 4 U in each square of 1.5 cm^2 limited to hairy area; Patient 2: 100 U Botox per axilla	Patient 1: Once Patient 2: Repeated after 10 months	"Using a 27/30 G needle, each square was injected with 0.1 mL in the center point intradermal to a depth of 2 mm and at a 45° angle to the skin surface."	Axillae	6–12 months
Shi (2019)[49]	1	III	50–100 U in 2 mL normal saline, 400 U maximum per treatment	Five treatments	"Injected intradermally in 1-inch linear parallel track about 1 cm apart with 30-gauge 1 inch needle, 5 units in 0.1 mL each injection, about 20 injections in one area...For papules or any inflammatory areas, we injected around them and literally blanched the erythematous areas"	Axillae, inframammary folds, groin, perineum, post-auricularly	N/A

Postoperative Considerations

Given the range of procedures used in the care of patients with HS, there are a variety of wound types and postoperative care regimens to consider. More extensive procedures performed in the operative setting may require more complex approaches discussed in Chapter 23 and 24; and the focus in this section will be on wounds created by incision and drainage, deroofing, and local excisions.

Across the range of wounds created in the outpatient setting, the risk of postoperative infection and most other complications is notably low. In a variety of operative settings and techniques for 590 patients reported by Kohorst et al., an infection rate of 1.5% was noted and a single hematoma occurred.[29] In another series specifically focused on deroofing in the clinic setting, van der Zee et al. reported no infections and only a single episode of postoperative bleeding.[17] Given that more than 40% of these procedures were performed in the groin and many additional procedures on the buttocks, there is no clear indication that these areas present higher risk for infection. Local excisions with closure may result in higher overall complication rates based on a series of 92 patients treated in the outpatient setting that found 5% of patients experienced postoperative infection. Bleeding was also encountered postoperatively in 8% of these patients, and 22% experienced wound dehiscence.[42] Given the low overall risk of infection, the use of prophylactic perioperative antibiotics is not indicated in the large majority of circumstances.

Pain management following surgery for HS has not yet been systematically studied. Pain control following most dermatologic procedures can be adequately achieved with the use of acetaminophen and ibuprofen, though consensus guidelines suggest that the addition of opioid analgesics is warranted for certain procedure types.[43] In the experience of the authors, many patients do require opioid analgesics for postoperative days 1 to 3 for procedures involving lesions larger than 2 to 3 cm or in locations such as buttocks and groin. In this instance, 50 to 100 mg tramadol every 6 hours or 5 mg hydrocodone every 6 hours can be taken, in addition to 800 mg ibuprofen every 8 hours and 650 mg acetaminophen every 6 hours, as needed.

Care following local excisions and deroofing are relatively similar and are adapted to body location. A thick layer of petrolatum to the sutured wound or base of the deroofed area is typically soothing and prevents adhesion of the non-stick contact layer to the wound that can result in pain with bandage changes. Wet-to-dry dressings are also recommended by some providers, though the authors typically avoid these due to discomfort with this type of bandage change and lack of clear benefit. For axillary wounds, the use of adherent dressings can lead to irritant reactions and skin tearing of adjacent skin with daily changes due to the need for movement of the shoulder and requirement for extensive adhesive layers to keep the bandage in place. Anecdotally, Hypafix tape, a self-adhesive with non-woven fabric material, is well-liked by patients, though individual patient preference should be taken into account. Options that avoid adhesives altogether in this location are limited, but a garment for bandaging axillary HS wounds without adhesives has recently been made available.[44]

For wounds in the groin, perianal area, and buttocks, similar nonstick contact layers and petrolatum can be applied. Depending on location, adhesive tape or bandages may be used to secure dressings in place, or the use of compressive undergarments may be adequate and obviate the need for adhesives. Disposable mesh underwear can be provided at low cost to patients immediately following procedures for this purpose as well. Abdominal pads are often helpful for fresh or highly exudative wounds, though thinner, non-adherent dressings or even menstrual pads that can be held in place in undergarments by an adhesive backing are often preferable and inexpensive.

Patients with HS often bring their own practical experience in self-care of wounds to their first procedure. That experience is valuable and should be discussed, honored, and validated, unless specifically understood by the provider to be harmful to healing. A further discussion on HS wound care can be found in Chapter 20.

Conclusion

In summary, clinic-based procedures are vitally important in both the acute and chronic management of HS, though the level of evidence supporting treatment types varies considerably (Table 22.5). In-office procedures such as intralesional triamcinolone injections and incision and drainage have the potential to provide rapid relief for localized flares when utilized appropriately. In areas of chronic involvement, the option to avoid general anesthesia for local excisions and deroofings allows much greater access to surgical care for many patients, and allows for a wider range of patient choice and involvement in care decisions during procedure planning.

Of course, situations do exist in which clinic-based procedures may not be suitable for extensive disease; however, for a large proportion of patients, it is a valuable option that can reduce procedural morbidity and inconvenience. There are substantial gaps in our current knowledge of the efficacy of other clinic-based procedural approaches including neurotoxins, chemical peels, and radiation, but each is promising and can be considered in the appropriate context. Further study is needed to rigorously measure and help compare outcomes for the procedures described in this chapter and to characterize and contrast the patient experience with these procedures in the clinic versus operative setting.

TABLE 22.5 Level of Evidence and Recommendations for Outpatient Procedural Management of Hidradenitis Suppurativa

Recommendations	Strength of Recommendation	Level of Evidence	References
Intralesional triamcinolone	C	II	6–8
Incision and drainage	C	II	25, 26, 29
Unroofing/deroofing	B	II	18, 21, 26, 27, 29
External beam radiation therapy	C	III	30–33
Microwave ablation	Not recommended	II	35
Resorcinol peels	C	II	39, 40
Botulinum toxin	C	III	45–49

Strength of Recommendation Taxonomy (SORT) recommendation level: I. Good-quality patient-oriented evidence; II. Limited-quality patient-oriented evidence; III. Other evidence, including consensus guidelines, opinion, case studies, or disease-oriented evidence.
Evidence grading level: A. Recommendation based on consistent and good-quality patient-oriented evidence; B. Recommendation based on inconsistent or limited-quality patient-oriented evidence; C. Recommendation based on consensus, opinion, case studies, or disease-oriented evidence.[50]

References

1. Mullins JF, McCash WB, Boudreau RF. Treatment of chronic hidradenitis suppurativa: surgical modification. *Postgrad Med.* 1959;26:805–808.

2. Ring HC, Sigsgaard V, Thorsen J, et al. The microbiome of tunnels in hidradenitis suppurativa patients. *J Eur Acad Dermatol Venereol.* 2019;33(9):1775–1780.

3. Kidacki M, Cong Z, Flamm A, et al. "Invasive proliferative gelatinous mass" of hidradenitis suppurativa contains distinct inflammatory components. *Br J Dermatol.* 2019 Jul;181(1):192–193.

4. Hurley HJ. Axillary hyperhidrosis, apocrine bromhidrosis, hidradenitis suppurativa, and familial benign pemphigus: surgical approach. In: Roenigk RK, Roenigk HH Jr, eds. *Roenigk and Roenigk's Dermatologic Surgery: Principles and Practice.* 2nd ed. New York, NY: Marcel Dekker; 1996:623–645.

5. Willey A, Lee PK. WAaL. Cutaneous anesthesia. In: Ratz JL, Roenigk RK, Roenigk HH eds. *Roenigk's Dermatologic Surgery.* Boca Raton: Taylor & Francis Group; 2007;86.

6. Riis PT, Boer J, Prens EP, et al. Intralesional triamcinolone for flares of hidradenitis suppurativa (HS): a case series. *J Am Acad Dermatol.* 2016;75:1151–1155.

7. Alvarez P, Garcia-Martinez FJ, Poveda I, Pascual JC. Intralesional Triamcinolone for Fistulous Tracts in Hidradenitis Suppurativa: An Uncontrolled Prospective Trial with Clinical and Ultrasonographic Follow-Up. *Dermatology.* 2020;236:46–51.

8. Fajgenbaum K, Crouse L, Dong L, et al. Intralesion triamcinolone may not be beneficial for treating acute Hidradenitis Suppurativa lesions: A double-blind, randomized, placebo-controlled trial. *Dermatol Surg.* 2020;46(5):685–689.

9. Goldzweig O, Carrasco R, Hashkes PJ. Systemic adverse events following intraarticular corticosteroid injections for the treatment of juvenile idiopathic arthritis: two patients with dermatologic adverse events and review of the literature. *Semin Arthritis Rheum.* 2013;43:71–76.

10. Fredman R, Tenenhaus M. Cushing's syndrome after intralesional triamcinolone acetonide: a systematic review of the literature and multinational survey. *Burns.* 2013;39:549–557.

11. Reddy S, Ananthakrishnan S, Garg A. A prospective observational study evaluating hypothalamic-pituitary-adrenal axis alteration and efficacy of intramuscular triamcinolone acetonide for steroid-responsive dermatologic disease. *J Am Acad Dermatol.* 2013;69:226–231.

12. Jarratt MT, Spark RF, Arndt KA. The effects of intradermal steroids on the pituitary-adrenal axis and the skin. *J Invest Dermatol.* 1974;62:463–466.

13. Garg A, Neuren E, Cha D, et al. Evaluating patients' unmet needs in hidradenitis suppurativa: Results from the Global Survey Of Impact and Healthcare Needs (VOICE) Project. *J Am Acad Dermatol.* 2020 Feb;82(2):366–376.

14. Danby FW, Hazen PG, Boer J. New and traditional surgical approaches to hidradenitis suppurativa. *J Am Acad Dermatol.* 2015;73:S62–S65.

15. O'Malley GF, Dominici P, Giraldo P, et al. Routine packing of simple cutaneous abscesses is painful and probably unnecessary. *Acad Emerg Med.* 2009;16:470–473.

16. Kessler DO, Krantz A, Mojica M. Randomized trial comparing wound packing to no wound packing following incision and drainage of superficial skin abscesses in the pediatric emergency department. *Pediatr Emerg Care.* 2012;28:514–517.

17. van der Zee HH, Prens EP, Boer J. Deroofing: a tissue-saving surgical technique for the treatment of mild to moderate hidradenitis suppurativa lesions. *J Am Acad Dermatol.* 2010;63:475–480.

18. van Hattem S, Spoo JR, Horvath B, et al. Surgical treatment of sinuses by deroofing in hidradenitis suppurativa. *Dermatol Surg.* 2012;38:494–497.

19. Lin CH, Chang KP, Huang SH. Deroofing: An Effective Method for Treating Chronic Diffuse Hidradenitis Suppurativa. *Dermatol Surg.* 2016;42:273–275.

20. Danby FW. Commentary: unroofing for hidradenitis suppurativa, why and how. *J Am Acad Dermatol.* 2010;63(481):e1–e3.

21. Kohorst JJ, Baum CL, Otley CC, et al. Patient Satisfaction and Quality of Life Following Surgery for Hidradenitis Suppurativa. *Dermatol Surg.* 2017;43:125–133.

22. Worden A, Yoho DJ, Houin H, et al. Factors Affecting Healing in the Treatment of Hidradenitis Suppurativa. *Ann Plast Surg.* 2020; 84:436–440.

23. Fertitta L, Hotz C, Wolkenstein P, et al. Efficacy and satisfaction of surgical treatment for hidradenitis suppurativa. *J Eur Acad Dermatol Venereol.* 2020;34:839–845.

24. Shavit E, Pawliwec A, Alavi A, George R. The surgeon's perspective: a retrospective study of wide local excisions taken to healthy subcutaneous fat in the management of advanced hidradenitis suppurativa. *Can J Surg.* 2020;63:E94–E99.

25. Janse I, Bieniek A, Horvath B, Matusiak L. Surgical Procedures in Hidradenitis Suppurativa. *Dermatol Clin.* 2016;34:97–109.

26. Mehdizadeh A, Hazen PG, Bechara FG, et al. Recurrence of hidradenitis suppurativa after surgical management: a systematic review and meta-analysis. *J Am Acad Dermatol.* 2015;73:S70–S77.

27. Janse IC, Hellinga J, Blok JL, et al. Skin-Tissue-sparing Excision with Electrosurgical Peeling: A Case Series in Hidradenitis Suppurativa. *Acta Derm Venereol.* 2016;96:390–391.

28. Deckers IE, Dahi Y, van der Zee HH, Prens EP. Hidradenitis suppurativa treated with wide excision and second intention healing: a meaningful local cure rate after 253 procedures. *J Eur Acad Dermatol Venereol.* 2018;32:459–462.

29. Kohorst JJ, Baum CL, Otley CC, et al. Surgical Management of Hidradenitis Suppurativa: Outcomes of 590 Consecutive Patients. *Dermatol Surg.* 2016;42:1030–1040.

30. Schenck SG. Hidradenitis suppurativa axillaris; an analysis of 54 cases treated with roentgen rays. *Radiology.* 1950;54:74–77. illust.

31. Frohlich D, Baaske D, Glatzel M. Radiotherapy of hidradenitis suppurativa—still valid today? *Strahlenther Onkol.* 2000;176:286–289.

32. Patel SH, Robbins J, Hamzavi I. Radiation Therapy for Chronic Hidradenitis Suppurativa. *J Nucl Med Radiat Ther.* 2013;4:1–3.

33. Trombetta M, Werts ED, Parda D. The role of radiotherapy in the treatment of hidradenitis suppurativa: case report and review of the literature. *Dermatol Online J.* 2010;16:16.

34. Paul S, Bach D, LeBoeuf NR, et al. Successful use of brachytherapy for a severe hidradenitis suppurativa variant. *Dermatol Ther.* 2016;29:455–458.

35. Vossen A, van Huijkelom M, Nijsten TEC, et al. Aggravation of mild axillary hidradenitis suppurativa by microwave ablation: results of a randomized intrapatient-controlled trial. *J Am Acad Dermatol.* 2019;80:777–779.

36. Jansen JT, Broerse JJ, Zoetelief J, et al. Estimation of the carcinogenic risk of radiotherapy of benign diseases from shoulder to heel. *Radiother Oncol.* 2005;76:270–277.

37. Haber R, Gottlieb J, Zagdanski AM, et al. Radiation-induced hidradenitis suppurativa: a case report. *JAAD Case Rep.* 2017;3:182–184.

38. De Vita V, Ruocco E. Hidradenitis suppurativa after radiotherapy for uterine adenocarcinoma: a typical example of an isoradiotopic response. *JAAD Case Rep.* 2017;3:570–571.

39. Boer J, Jemec GB. Resorcinol peels as a possible self-treatment of painful nodules in hidradenitis suppurativa. *Clin Exp Dermatol.* 2010;35:36–40.

40. Pascual JC, Encabo B, Ruiz de Apodaca RF, et al. Topical 15% resorcinol for hidradenitis suppurativa: an uncontrolled prospective trial with clinical and ultrasonographic follow-up. *J Am Acad Dermatol.* 2017;77:1175–1178.

41. Theut Riis P, Saunte DM, Sigsgaard V, et al. Intense pulsed light treatment for patients with hidradenitis suppurativa: beware treatment with resorcinol. *J Dermatolog Treat.* 2018;29:385–387.

42. van Rappard DC, Mooij JE, Mekkes JR. Mild to moderate hidradenitis suppurativa treated with local excision and primary closure. *J Eur Acad Dermatol Venereol.* 2012;26:898–902.

43. McLawhorn JM, Stephany MP, Bruhn WE, et al. An expert panel consensus on opioid-prescribing guidelines for dermatologic procedures. *J Am Acad Dermatol.* 2020;82:700–708.
44. Khoo AB, Burova EP. Hidradenitis suppurativa treated with Clostridium botulinum toxin A. *Clin Exp Dermatol.* 2014;39(6):749–750.
45. O'Reilly DJ, Pleat JM, Richards AM. Treatment of hidradenitis suppurativa with botulinum toxin A. *Plast Reconstr Surg.* 2005;116:1575–1576.
46. Feito-Rodriguez M, Sendagorta-Cudos E, Herranz-Pinto P, de Lucas-Laguna R. Prepubertal hidradenitis suppurativa successfully treated with botulinum toxin A. *Dermatol Surg.* 2009;35:1300–1302.
47. Khoo AB, Burova EP. Hidradenitis suppurativa treated with Clostridium botulinum toxin A. *Clin Exp Dermatol.* 2014;39:749–750.
48. Campanati A, Martina E, Giuliodori K, et al. Two cases of Hidradenitis suppurativa and botulinum toxin type a therapy: a novel approach for a pathology that is still difficult to manage. *Dermatol Ther.* 2019;32(3), e12841.
49. Shi W, Schultz S, Strouse A, Gater DR. Successful treatment of stage III hidradenitis suppurativa with botulinum toxin A. *BMJ Case Rep.* 2019;12(1), e226064.
50. Ebell MH, Siwek J, Weiss BD, et al. Strength of recommendation taxonomy (SORT): a patient-centered approach to grading evidence in the medical literature. *Am Fam Physician.* 2004;69:548–556.

23

Operative Techniques for Hidradenitis Suppurativa

STEPHANIE R. GOLDBERG, RALPH GEORGE, AND FALK G. BECHARA

"Confusion, conservatism, credulity, and can't have permeated physicians attitudes towards hidradenitis suppurativa."

Dr. William Pollock[1]

CHAPTER OUTLINE

History of Surgery in Hidradenitis Suppurativa

Hidradenitis suppurativa (HS) was first described by two surgeons in the 1800s, Velpeau[2] and Verneuil.[3] There was much debate surrounding whether HS was primarily a venereal disease, tumor, or abscess. In the 1890s, Barthelemy suggested HS was a folliculitis that led to increased dermatologic interest in HS as a skin disease. For the next 60 years, treatment was largely targeted at medical therapy until the 1950s when Greely proposed the role of excision of chronic disease in the small percentage of cases that evolved beyond the acute setting.[4] The following 60 years focused largely on techniques for excision and reconstruction. In the surgical world, HS was considered primarily as a sweat gland disease that was treated with excision. The most widely popularized operative procedure, the Pollock procedure, focused on primary axillary excision with immediate closure.[5] This chapter will discuss the role of surgery and surgical goals of care in HS, operative techniques for diseased tissue, reconstruction, patient optimization preoperatively, and the role of interdisciplinary care.

Setting Goals for Surgery

Historically, surgery was indicated largely for chronic disease. As our knowledge of HS pathogenesis has evolved, the role for surgical management of HS has also evolved, as has the timing of surgery for acute and chronic lesions. Surgery may be indicated for mild to severe disease and in both the acute and chronic settings, if goals of surgery are established. Surgical management should be viewed as an integral aspect of an HS treatment plan.

Surgery can take on many forms, including incision and drainage, deroofing, and excision with reconstruction when indicated. In the past, surgical management of HS has been met with skepticism stemming from reported high recurrence and postoperative infection rates. However, most of the studies focused on "recurrence" as the primary outcome measure in a disease where surgery should be considered an adjunctive therapy combined with medical therapy rather than a cure.[59] Moving forward, it is important that we define the goal of any surgical intervention in HS. This should be addressed during the initial surgical evaluation. In some patients with focal and limited disease, surgery may provide more definitive therapy for HS lesions. However, in patients with more diffuse disease, surgery may be indicated for symptomatic control of areas that repeatedly flare with the goal of decreasing inflammation and disease burden. In these situations, recurrences would be expected to occur, but hopefully with less frequency, drainage, inflammation, and pain. Surgery in HS has been suggested to work synergistically with medical treatments for HS by decreasing inflammation to allow medications to penetrate more effectively. Surgeons should have preoperative discussions with patients and dermatologists to define the goals of care in each HS patient with the goal of improved outcomes and patient satisfaction.

Operative Techniques

Deroofing

Deroofing is a technique for the management of HS tracts in which the anterior wall of an HS tunnel is removed using a probe to identify the entirety of the tract.[6,7] This can be used for an abscess, cyst, or tract. Once the probe is inserted, the tunnel is opened, and the anterior wall of the tunnel is removed using scissors, a scalpel, or an electrocautery device. This allows for an open cavity without the risk of the skin edges closing together before the wound has been able to heal by secondary intention. The lining of the tunnel, often the gelatinous material, is removed using a curette and another form of debridement to the level of the epithelial lining of the cavity. The wound is covered with a moist dressing, changed daily, until the wound has completely healed by secondary intention. Techniques can be utilized to fully identify the extent of the tract, including filling the cavity of the tract with methylene blue dye before the tract is open. Once the tract is open and the anterior wall is removed, the tunnel will appear blue and serve as a guide for debridement to ensure the extent of the tunnel has been deroofed and may minimize recurrences from partially unroofed tracts. The benefit of the deroofing technique is that it is a tissue-sparing technique that can be used in the office on small HS lesions or in the operating room on larger or more complex tunnels. Patients do not require inpatient hospitalization, although skilled nursing may be helpful for wound care in more complex cases. Deroofing can be performed in lesions on all anatomic areas of the body.

Most patients heal rapidly with good cosmetic outcomes from deroofing techniques if the tract has been fully identified and deroofed. Deroofed wounds may experience a delay in wound healing if they develop a significant biofilm and bioburden but respond well to mechanical in-office debridement and silver-impregnated dressings. In general, scarring is minimal, and wounds are less noticeable compared to other surgical techniques, such as …. Patients may experience flares within the scar if the extent of the tract has not been fully identified at the time of deroofing or if disease develops adjacent to the deroofed area. There also may be microscopic tunnels forming adjacent to the tunnels that are not identifiable at the time of procedure, which then develop into more prominent and symptomatic disease. These focal areas of recurrence respond well to additional focal deroofing procedures or excision with healing by secondary intention, but for these reasons, it is important that patients undergo concomitant medical therapy to suppress ongoing disease and minimize disease progression. Other complications include bleeding, which responds well to pressure or chemical cauterization. In a study of 88 deroofed lesions, recurrence rates were reported as 17% after a 4.6-month median

follow-up. Patient satisfaction was reported as 90%, including patients who experienced a recurrence.[7]

Deroofing has been used to approach more complex wounds in a staged fashion, which would ordinarily require extensive wide excision with reconstruction. Deroofing procedures are performed at approximately 8-week intervals in large tunnels to allow wounds to heal completely prior to additional procedures and are often performed with excisions at the lateral margins of the wound. This approach allows for a series of outpatient procedures, less pain, small open wounds at a given time, and allows patients to return to their daily activities and responsibilities much sooner. Per our experiences, patients who undergo deroofing have less overall cosmetic disfigurement than with wide excision.

Deroofing has been combined with subsequent excision to remove fibrotic tissue that remains once the wound has healed from the initial procedure in patients with moderate to severe hidradenitis. This modified two-staged approach has been postulated to decrease recurrence rates based on the assumption that recurrence originates from epithelialized tracts that may become hidden in the fibrous tissue.[8] It was also hypothesized that recurrence following simple deroofing could arise from baseline progression of disease in adjacent tissue.

Excision

Excision has been considered the gold standard for surgical management of HS. Past recurrence rates, which were considered to be relatively high, were thought to result from incomplete resection of diseased tissue.[5,9] We now understand that HS is a systemic disease; therefore, excision is not curative. However, excision is an excellent technique to remove isolated areas of active disease. The procedure may be performed under local or tumescent anesthesia in the clinic setting, while larger areas may require sedation or general anesthesia. Active disease should be excised down to the level of subcutaneous tissue to remove all visible tunnels and disease tissue. This can be performed using a variety of devices, including scalpels, CO_2 lasers, or electrocautery devices. There is not enough data to suggest that one tool is superior to the other in terms of excision and recurrence rates, but the use of electrocautery or CO_2 laser may help to facilitate hemostasis during the procedure. It is important to counsel patients that disease recurrence may occur in the postoperative wound adjacent to the scar. This can either be explained by incomplete resection of diseased tissue or the natural progression of HS in surrounding tissue.

Staged Techniques

Patients with diffuse disease may benefit from multiple staged operative procedures. Staged deroofing techniques have been shown to decrease overall inflammation. As each wound heals, there appears to be a decrease in surrounding inflammation, which facilitates control of surrounding HS disease and allows for a targeted, skin-preserving approach requiring less reconstruction. Subsequent deroofings heal with ease, given the decreased inflammation. Patients do not require inpatient hospitalization. Staged excisions can also be utilized and are encouraged in large anatomic areas to allow for manageable wound care, to minimize inpatient hospitalization, and to avoid fluid losses that can occur with loss of skin as a protective barrier. Staged excisions are also useful in perianal HS to minimize anal retraction and stenosis.

Options for Wound Closure and Reconstruction in Hidradenitis Suppurativa

A variety of different closure techniques have been described in the literature. Aside from primary closure, other common reconstruction techniques include secondary intention healing, vacuum-assisted closure, skin grafts, and various types of flaps. The choice for a specific technique depends on multiple variables such as size and location of the defect, existing perioperative structures within the surgical center (e.g., physiotherapy, wound care), patient compliance, and the surgeon's preference and training. General guidelines are missing and individual approaches are necessary.

Primary Closure

Primary closure can be useful after small excisions, especially in Hurley stage II patients.[9] Some authors have described shorter inpatient stay, lower morbidity, and fewer postoperative complaints about the mentioned technique.[5,10,11] The most important limitation for primary closure is the size of the defect (Fig. 23.1). Moreover, immobilization can be necessary, and the risk for wound dehiscence and infection must be discussed. In some situations, partial primary closure with the usage of a drain may be useful to speed up wound healing and reduce the risk for contraction.

Secondary Intention Healing

Some surgeons prefer secondary intention healing in the inguinal, anogenital, and the lower abdominal areas (Fig. 23.2).[12] Advantages are immediate mobilization, acceptable scar formation, early reintegration into daily life and occupation, and a low risk for complications and recurrence of HS.[12–19] These wounds can require complex wound care to be performed by a patient family member or a skilled nurse. Limitations include prolonged wound healing, painful changing of wound dressings, and a risk for contraction, especially in the axillary region.[13,15,20,21] During secondary intention healing, adequate wound care and physiotherapeutic support to prevent prolonged wound healing, contraction, and the risk of restriction of movement are mandatory. Additionally, in the author's view, the experience-dependent preoperative assessment of risk for contraction is crucial and depends on localization and size of the defect.

Negative Pressure Wound Therapy

Negative pressure wound therapy (NPWT) has been reported to be associated with faster wound granulation and re-epithelialization, reduction of bacterial load, and increased tissue oxygenation.[22] A small case series illustrated that the combination of NPWT and skin grafting was associated with a higher rate of graft-take and faster wound healing (Fig. 23.3).[23–25] Additional advantages include added fixation of skin grafts, a drainage of wound secretion, and a reduced number of wound dressings.[24,26] However, existing data does not allow a final evaluation of NPWT in HS surgery.

Skin Grafting

Most commonly, split-thickness skin grafts (STSGs) are used for skin grafting in HS surgery. STSGs are able to be meshed if larger defects must be covered. Skin grafting can be performed primarily after excision in a one-stage procedure or secondary after wound conditioning (Fig. 23.4).[21,27] Skin grafting after granulation of the wound to the level of adjacent skin seems to be associated with more favorable aesthetic outcomes (GrDIN ZOTERO_IT). Additionally, the wound contraction leads to smaller graft sizes in the secondary two-stage procedure.

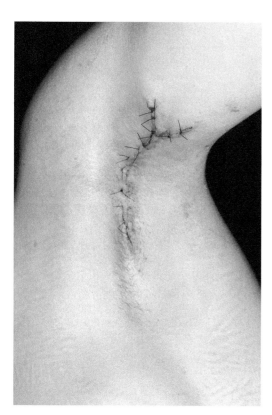

• **Fig. 23.1** Primary Excision With Immediate Closure in Axillary Hidradenitis. (Photograph courtesy Dr. Falk G. Bechara.)

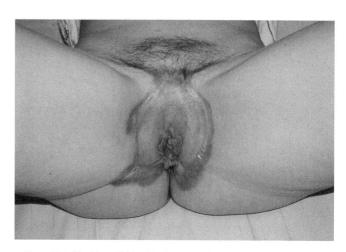

• **Fig. 23.2** Excision With Healing by Secondary Intention in the Pubic Area. (Photograph courtesy Dr. Falk G. Bechara.)

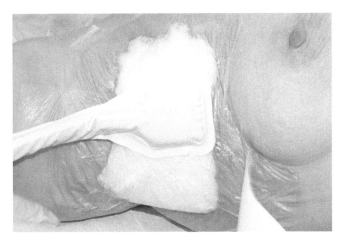

• **Fig. 23.3** Axillary Excision With Negative Pressure Vacuum Therapy. (Photograph courtesy Dr. Falk G. Bechara.)

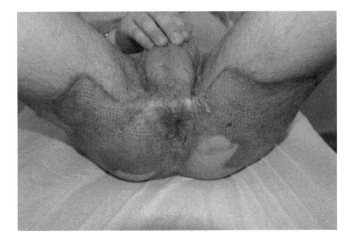

• **Fig. 23.4** Surgical Excision With Split-Thickness Skin Graft for Reconstruction. (Photograph courtesy Dr. Falk G. Bechara.)

Generally, skin grafts can be applied to defects on all anatomic areas. The most frequently grafted sites are the perianal, gluteal, genital, and inguinal regions.[28] Some authors prefer skin grafting due to low recurrence rates and a favorable cosmetic outcome.[a] Reported limitations include possible risk of contractures and the morbidity of donor sites, especially pain.[29] Successful graft acceptance depends on postoperative wound management with special regard to moisture control and bacterial colonization. After stable graft acceptance, a physiotherapeutic support and scar massage can influence the functional and aesthetic outcome.

Based on prior experience, scrotal and penile defects should be covered primarily in a one-stage procedure to prevent deviation. All other locations (e.g., reconstruction of the gluteal area) can be covered after wound conditioning in a second step operation.

A modification of the classic STSG, the "reused skin graft technique," has been described by Kuo and colleagues. The STSG is taken with an electrical dermatome from the area to be excised; it is then meshed and finally "reused" for coverage of the defect.[30] With this procedure, a classical donor site is avoided. Some reports

describe the use of dermal regeneration templates for axillary defects in combination with NPWT and subsequent STSG[31] (ADDIN Ztary: two-stage surgery for hidradenitis suppurativa: staged artificial dermis and skin grafting—PubMed—NCBI,o-stage).

Flaps

A variety of different flaps have been reported for defect reconstruction in HS.[5,11,15,16,32–41] In most cases, local flaps are used for coverage of axillary defects, with the intention to reduce the risk of contractions in the shoulder joint—thereby avoiding long-lasting wound healing—or to cover exposed vessels (Fig. 23.5).[11,32,42–48] The advantages of local flaps include shorter healing time, fewer painful dressing changes, shorter inpatient stay and immobilization, reduced risk for contractures, and in some cases, a more favorable aesthetic outcome.[42,48,49] Limitations include more difficult application for very large defects, complex surgical techniques, and prolonged surgery times.[50] Janse and colleagues propose the use of flaps for large defects in the axillary and genital region; however, they do not see them as the first option in other locations.[51]

Summary Reconstruction Techniques

Due to a lack of missing evidence-based data, no general recommendations for specific reconstruction are available in HS. Complete resection of an irreversibly destructed area or lesion is necessary before any reconstruction. The choice for a specific technique does not only depend on the size and location of the defect, but notably also on the patient's compliance, the individual clinical findings, and the surgeon's experience. The available postoperative wound care and physiotherapy in each HS center have to be

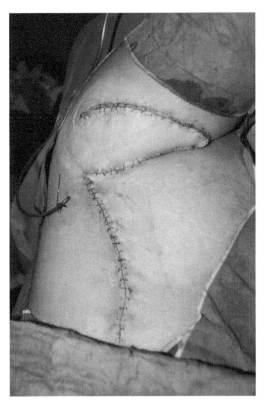

• **Fig. 23.5** Primary Axillary Excision With Transposition Artery Flap. (Photograph courtesy Dr. Falk G. Bechara.)

considered. The mentioned concerns underline that an optimal surgical plan is still an individual decision in each HS patient.

Postoperative Wound Healing After Reconstruction

Postoperative wound healing time and immobility are of crucial importance for the patient. Inconsistent definitions for postoperative wound healing make it difficult to evaluate existing data for various reconstruction techniques. In the literature, postoperative wound healing is often described for various time periods without taking defect size and localization into account. The time needed to complete healing ranges from 2 weeks to 5 months.[9,52]

The shortest time to complete healing was reported with flaps (2 to 4 weeks) and deroofing (2 to 6 weeks).[14–18] Obviously, the longest time to healing is reported for secondary intention healing with 3.5 weeks and 5 months.[14,15,17,19,53] After skin grafting, 2 to 8 weeks were observed for complete healing.[14,15,19,28,53–57] Two studies reported a significantly shorter healing time in the axillary region for flaps compared to STTG (5 vs. 14 weeks).[18,58]

How to Optimize the Surgical Patient

Timing of Operative Intervention

Wide surgical excision in HS addresses areas of persistent or recurring disease, removing heaped scarring, and tunnels resistant to medical therapy. As it does not address the primary biological phenomenon of follicular occlusion, surgical effectiveness relies on initial medical therapy to demonstrate recalcitrant disease and ongoing medical care to control new or recurrent eruptions. Control in the area treated by wide excision is predicted by the adequacy of the resection.[59–61]

In the case series, Alharbi et al. advocated for the control of acute inflammation medically, including deroofing persistent abscesses to optimize the surgical site for later wide excision.[32] Slade et al. emphasized interdisciplinary input into the timing and planning of major surgery.[62] The randomized adalimumab trials, Pioneer I and II, showed significant patient response compared to placebo at 3 months.[63] A randomized study of pre- and perioperative adalimumab chose 12 weeks of preoperative therapy and demonstrated no increase of adverse events in the treatment arm compared to placebo.[64] In the setting of biologic therapy, these studies suggest at least a 3-month interval between the initiation of therapy and the timing of surgery to ensure an adequate preoperative medical response. Most antibiotic regimens are also for several months and fit into this same time frame when used preoperatively.[65]

Careful timing of operative intervention can also allow comorbidities to be addressed. Smoking, obesity, and diabetes all influence the disease severity of HS[66] and are known to impact wound healing. Smoking affects wound healing and infection rates, and even a 4-week cessation can have a positive impact on surgical outcomes (SDDIN ZOTERO_IT). Diabetic management can be optimized preoperatively in affected patients. It can be difficult to address obesity preoperatively, but both bariatric surgery and weight loss are shown to reduce HS disease activity[67] and need to be part of the adjunctive care offered to HS patients. Anesthetic planning to assess potential airway difficulty and address any obstructive sleep apnea should be part of a comprehensive approach to planning surgery in obese HS patients.[68]

Nutrition

Malnutrition has a negative impact on wound healing and surgical outcomes and needs to be addressed if present. Wound healing requires adequate protein and specific vitamins and micronutrients (calcium, zinc, Vitamins C, A, B, and D).[69] A nutritionist's input should be sought in patients with inadequate intake and diet.

Newer research suggests that diet has a significant effect on HS disease severity. Diet can also impact surgical outcomes. Danby recommends a non-dairy and low glycemic diet in addition to surgical intervention. Cannistra has published reports of improved surgical outcomes in a brewer's yeast and wheat restricted diet (CannistrTERO_ITEM CSL_C).[70]

Antibiotics and Infection

Bacteria are not thought to be the initiating event in HS, but bacterial presence and alterations in the microbiome play a role in ongoing inflammation.[71] Appropriate antibiotic therapy, usually guided by dermatological or infectious disease input, is advocated in surgical series by Alharbi[32] and Slade[62] and combined with biologics for especially severe cases in preparation for wide surgical excision.[72] Locally applied antibiotics were not as effective in surgical cases demonstrated by a randomized study of HS wounds closed with an absorbable gentamicin collagen sponge. The investigators showed reduced complications at one week but no differences at 3 months and no effect on postoperative recurrence rates.[73]

Wound Healing Adjuncts

Many wound care products and devices are being used in practice. Randomized studies and a Cochrane review found inconsistent differences in healing. Dressings help to keep wounds moist, absorb exudate, control odor, and provide a barrier to bacteria. A variety of foam, gel, and colloidal products are available and can be tailored to individual needs. Gauze alone increases discomfort and patient dissatisfaction.[74]

NPWT has been shown to improve granulation in secondary intention and delayed primary closure wounds after wide excision.[75] A large European randomized trial of open abdominal wounds showed a faster time to closure (36 vs. 39 days), but an increased relative risk of wound-related adverse events (RR = 1.51).[76] A Cochrane review suggests more studies to determine the overall benefit in secondary closure wounds.[77] NPWT is used selectively by the chapter's authors in large wounds healing by secondary intention or delayed primary healing.

Adjuncts to Surgical Management (Combined Medical and Surgical Management)

Biologics

Biologics have become an important part of HS medical care. Their use in conjunction with surgical management is recommended for severe cases (SDDIN ZOTERO_IT). The SHARPS study, which included preoperative adalimumab, settled concerns about anti-TNF agents increasing postoperative infections and complication rates.[64] Several surgical series now show decreased recurrence and reduction in new disease combined with wide surgical excisions and targeted biologic therapy.[32,61]

Ertapenem

A pilot study of 30 HS patients treated with intravenous ertapenem demonstrated remarkably favorable response rates.[78] Ertapenem has become a rescue treatment for severe HS. Unfortunately, ertapenem withdrawal can be associated with a rapid resurgence of disease. It is currently used to gain disease control while biologics are initiated, and as a bridge to surgical resection in severely inflamed patients with poor response to other therapies (SDDIN ZOTERO_IT).

Role for Interdisciplinary Care and Collaboration

Modern care for HS has become interdisciplinary. Medical treatments help to resolve inflammation and reveal recalcitrant disease. Surgical interventions act upon resistant pockets, removing heaped scarring, and tunnels. Ongoing medical management appears to reduce both local recurrence and new disease. Earlier and aggressive medical and local surgical treatment for HS has shown promise in reducing patients' need for wide surgical excisions (SDDIN ZOTERO_IT).

References

1. William Pollock, 1971.
2. Velpeau: Dictionnaire de médicine, un Repertoire...—Google Scholar [WWW Document], n.d. https://scholar.google.com/scholar_lookup?title=Dictionnaire+de+m%C3%A9decine,+un+repertoire+g%C3%A9n%C3%A9rale+des+Sciences+Medicals+sous+le+rapport+theorique+et+pratique&author=A+Velpeau&publication_year=1839& (accessed May 14, 2020).
3. Verneuil: Etudes sur les tumeurs de la peau; de quelques...—Google Scholar [WWW Document], n.d. https://scholar.google.com/scholar_lookup?journal=Arch+Gen+Med&title=Etudes+sur+les+tumeurs+de+la+peau;+de+quelques+maladies+des+glandes+sudoripares&author=A+Verneuil&volume=4&publication_year=1854&pages=447-468& (accessed May 14, 2020).
4. Greeley PW. Surgical treatment of chronic suppurative hidradenitis. *Arch Surg.* 1950;61:193–198.
5. Pollock WJ, Virnelli FR, Ryan RF. Axillary hidradenitis suppurativa. A simple and effective surgical technique. *Plast Reconstr Surg.* 1972;49:22–27.
6. Mullins JF, Mccash WB, Boudreau RF. Treatment of chronic hidradenitis suppurativa: surgical modification. *Postgrad Med.* 1959;26:805–808.
7. van der Zee HH, Prens EP, Boer J. Deroofing: a tissue-saving surgical technique for the treatment of mild to moderate hidradenitis suppurativa lesions. *J Am Acad Dermatol.* 2010;63:475–480.
8. Dahmen RA, Gkalpakiotis S, Mardesicova L, et al. Deroofing followed by thorough sinus tract excision: a modified surgical approach for hidradenitis suppurativa. *J Dtsch Dermatol Ges.* 2019;17:698–702.
9. van Rappard DC, Mooij JE, Mekkes JR. Mild to moderate hidradenitis suppurativa treated with local excision and primary closure. *J Eur Acad Dermatol Venereol.* 2012;26:898–902. https://doi.org/10.1111/j.1468-3083.2011.04203.x.
10. Greeley PW. Plastic surgical treatment of chronic suppurative hidradenitis. *Plast Reconstr Surg (1946).* 1951;1946:143–146.
11. Paletta FX. Hidradenitis suppurativa: pathologic study and use of skin flaps. *Plast Reconstr Surg.* 1963;31:307–315.
12. Ariyan S, Krizek TJ. Hidradenitis suppurativa of the groin, treated by excision and spontaneous healing. *Plast Reconstr Surg.* 1976;58:44–47.
13. Ather S, Chan DSY, Leaper DJ, et al. Surgical treatment of hidradenitis suppurativa: case series and review of the literature. *Int Wound J.* 2006;3:159–169.
14. Balik E, Eren T, Bulut T, et al. Surgical approach to extensive hidradenitis suppurativa in the perineal/perianal and gluteal regions. *World J Surg.* 2009;33:481–487.
15. Harrison BJ, Mudge M, Hughes LE. Recurrence after surgical treatment of hidradenitis suppurativa. *Br Med J Clin Res Ed.* 1987;294:487–489.
16. Morgan WP, Harding KG, Hughes LE. A comparison of skin grafting and healing by granulation, following axillary excision for hidradenitis suppurativa. *Ann R Coll Surg Engl.* 1983;65:235–236.
17. Parks RW, Parks TG, Hughes LE. Pathogenesis, clinical features and management of hidradenitis suppurativa. *Ann R Coll Surg Engl.* 1997;79:309–310.
18. Rompel R, Petres J. Long-term results of wide surgical excision in 106 patients with hidradenitis suppurativa. *Dermatol Surg.* 2000;26(7):638–643.
19. Silverberg B, Smoot CE, Landa SJ, et al. Hidradenitis suppurativa: patient satisfaction with wound healing by secondary intention. *Plast Reconstr Surg.* 1987;79:555–559.
20. Banerjee AK. Surgical treatment of hidradenitis suppurativa. *Br J Surg.* 1992;79:863–866.
21. Bieniek A, Matusiak L, Okulewicz-Gojlik D, Szepietowski JC. Surgical treatment of hidradenitis suppurativa: experiences and recommendations. *Dermatol Surg.* 2010;36(12):1998–2004.
22. Morykwas MJ, Argenta LC, Shelton-Brown EI, et al. Vacuum-assisted closure: a new method for wound control and treatment: animal studies and basic foundation. *Ann Plast Surg.* 1997;38:553–562.
23. Elwood ET, Bolitho DG. Negative-pressure dressings in the treatment of hidradenitis suppurativa. *Ann Plast Surg.* 2001;46:49–51.
24. Hynes PJ, Earley MJ, Lawlor D. Split-thickness skin grafts and negative-pressure dressings in the treatment of axillary hidradenitis suppurativa. *Br J Plast Surg.* 2002;55:507–509.
25. Jianbing T, Biao C, Qin L, et al. Topical negative pressure coupled with split-thickness skin grafting for the treatment of hidradenitis suppurativa: a case report. *Int Wound J.* 2015;12:334–337.
26. Blackburn JH, Boemi L, Hall WW, et al. Negative-pressure dressings as a bolster for skin grafts. *Ann Plast Surg.* 1998;40:453–457.
27. Ching CC, Stahlgren LH. Clinical review of hidradenitis suppurativa: management of cases with severe perianal involvement. *Dis Colon Rectum.* 1965;8:349–352.
28. Anderson BB, Cadogan CA, Gangadharam D. Hidradenitis suppurativa of the perineum, scrotum, and gluteal area: presentation, complications, and treatment. *J Natl Med Assoc.* 1982;74:999–1003.
29. Menderes A, Sunay O, Vayvada H, et al. Surgical management of hidradenitis suppurativa. *Int J MedSci.* 2010;7:240–247.
30. Kuo HW, Ohara K. Surgical treatment of chronic gluteal hidradenitis suppurativa: reused skin graft technique. *Dermatol Surg.* 2003;29(2):173–178.
31. Gonzaga TA, Endorf FW, Mohr WJ, et al. Novel surgical approach for axillary hidradenitis suppurativa using a bilayer dermal regeneration template: a retrospective case study. *J Burn Care Res.* 2013;34:51–57.
32. Alharbi Z, Kauczok J, Pallua N. A review of wide surgical excision of hidradenitis suppurativa. *BMC Dermatol.* 2012;12:9. https://doi.org/10.1186/1471-5945-12-9.
33. Anderson MJ, Dockerty MB. Perianal hidradenitis suppurativa; a clinical and pathologic study. *Dis Colon Rectum.* 1958;1:23–31.
34. Bell BA, Ellis H. Hydradenitis suppurativa. *J R Soc Med.* 1978;71:511–515.
35. Broadwater JR, Bryant RL, Petrino RA, et al. Advanced hidradenitis suppurativa. Review of surgical treatment in 23 patients. *Am J Surg.* 1982;144:668–670.
36. Harrison SH. Axillary hidradenitis. *Br J Plast Surg.* 1964;17:95–98.
37. Hartwell SW. Surgical treatment of hidradenitis suppurativa. *Surg Clin N Am.* 1975;55:1107–1109.

38. Knaysi GA, Cosman B, Crikelair GF. Hidradenitis suppurativa. *JAMA*. 1968;203:19–22.
39. Masson JK. Surgical treatment for hidradenitis suppurativa. *Surg Clin N Am*. 1969;49:1043–1052.
40. O'Brien J, Wysocki J, Anastasi G. Limberg flap coverage for axillary defects resulting from excision of hidradenitis suppurativa. *Plast Reconstr Surg*. 1976;58:354–358.
41. Tasche C, Angelats J, Jayaram B. Surgical treatment of hidradenitis suppurativa of the axilla. *Plast Reconstr Surg*. 1975;55:559–562.
42. Altmann S, Fansa H, Schneider W. Surgical treatment of axillary hidradenitis suppurativa. *Chirurg*. 2001;72:1413–1416.
43. Amarante J, Reis J, Santa Comba A, et al. A new approach in axillary hidradenitis treatment: the scapular island flap. *Aesthetic Plast Surg*. 1996;20:443–446.
44. Büyükaşik O, Hasdemir AO, Kahramansoy N, et al. Surgical approach to extensive hidradenitis suppurativa. *Dermatol Surg*. 2011;37(6):835–842.
45. Chuang CJ, Lee CH, Chen TM, et al. Use of a versatile transpositional flap in the surgical treatment of axillary hidradenitis suppurativa. *J Formos Med Assoc*. 2004;103:644–647.
46. Civelek B, Aksoy K, Bilgen E, et al. Reconstructive options in severe cases of Hidradenitis suppurativa. *Open Med*. 2010;5. https://doi.org/10.2478/s11536-009-0126-2. Commentary: two-stage surgery for hidradenitis suppurativa: staged artificial dermis and skin grafting.—PubMed—NCBI [WWW Document], n.d. https://www.ncbi.nlm.nih.gov/pubmed/24490984. Accessed 14 May 2020.
47. Rehman N, Kannan RY, Hassan S, et al. Thoracodorsal artery perforator (TAP) type I V-Y advancement flap in axillary hidradenitis suppurativa. *Br J Plast Surg*. 2005;58:441–444.
48. Weyandt G. Surgical management of acne inversa. *Hautarzt*. 2005;56(11):1033–1039.
49. Soldin MG, Tulley P, Kaplan H, et al. Chronic axillary hidradenitis–the efficacy of wide excision and flap coverage. *Br J Plast Surg*. 2000;53:434–436.
50. Tanaka A, Hatoko M, Tada H, et al. Experience with surgical treatment of hidradenitis suppurativa. *Ann Plast Surg*. 2001;47:636–642.
51. Janse I, Bieniek A, Horváth B, et al. Surgical Procedures in Hidradenitis Suppurativa. *Dermatol Clin*. 2016;34:97–109.
52. Wiltz O, Schoetz DJ, Murray JJ, et al. Perianal hidradenitis suppurativa. The Lahey Clinic experience. *Dis Colon Rectum*. 1990;33:731–734.
53. Morgan WP, Harding KG, Hughes LE. A comparison of skin grafting and healing by granulation, following axillary excision for hidradenitis suppurativa. *Ann R Coll Surg Engl*. 1983;65:235–236.
54. Mandal A, Watson J. Experience with different treatment modules in hidradenitis suppuritiva: a study of 106 cases. *Surgeon*. 2005;3:23–26.
55. Rosenfeld N, Babar A. Hidradenitis suppurativa of the perineal and gluteal regions, treated by excision and skin grafting. Case report. *Plast Reconstr Surg*. 1976;58:98–99.
56. Bohn J, Svensson H. Surgical treatment of hidradenitis suppurativa. *Scand J Plast Reconstr Surg Hand Surg*. 2001;35(3):305–309.
57. Watson JD. Hidradenitis suppurativa—a clinical review. *Br J Plast Surg*. 1985;38:567–569. https://doi.org/10.1016/0007-1226(85)90022-0.
58. Hudson DA, Krige JEJ. Axillary hidradenitis suppurativa: wide excision and flap coverage is best. *Eur J Plast Surg*. 1993;16. https://doi.org/10.1007/BF00196440.
59. Mehdizadeh A, Hazen PG, Bechara FG, et al. Recurrence of hidradenitis suppurativa after surgical management: A systematic review and meta-analysis. *J Am Acad Dermatol*. 2015;73:S70–S77.
60. DeFazio MV, Economides JM, King KS, et al. Outcomes After Combined Radical Resection and Targeted Biologic Therapy for the Management of Recalcitrant Hidradenitis Suppurativa. *Ann Plast Surg*. 2016;77:217–222.
61. Shanmugam VK, Mulani S, McNish S, et al. Longitudinal observational study of hidradenitis suppurativa: impact of surgical intervention with adjunctive biologic therapy. *Int J Dermatol*. 2018;57:62–69.
62. Slade DEM, Powell BW, Mortimer PS. Hidradenitis suppurativa: pathogenesis and management. *Br J Plast Surg*. 2003;56:451–461.
63. Kimball AB, Okun MM, Williams DA, et al. Two Phase 3 Trials of Adalimumab for Hidradenitis Suppurativa. *N Engl J Med*. 2016;375:422–434.
64. Bechara FG, Podda M, Prens EP, et al. Efficacy and Safety of Adalimumab in Conjunction With Surgery in Moderate to Severe Hidradenitis Suppurativa: The SHARPS Randomized Clinical Trial. *JAMA Surg*. 2021 Aug 18:e213655. https://doi.org/10.1001/jamasurg.2021.3655.
65. Alikhan A, Sayed C, Alavi A, et al. North American clinical management guidelines for hidradenitis suppurativa: a publication from the United States and Canadian Hidradenitis Suppurativa Foundations: Part I: Diagnosis, evaluation, and the use of complementary and procedural management. *J Am Acad Dermatol*. 2019;81:76–90.
66. Sartorius K, Emtestam L, Jemec GBE, et al. Objective scoring of hidradenitis suppurativa reflecting the role of tobacco smoking and obesity. *Br J Dermatol*. 2009;161:831–839.
67. Sivanand A, Gulliver WP, Josan CK, et al. Weight Loss and Dietary Interventions for Hidradenitis Suppurativa: A Systematic Review. *J Cutan Med Surg*. 2020;24:64–72.
68. Benumof JL. Obesity, sleep apnea, the airway and anesthesia. *Curr Opin Anaesthesiol*. 2004;17:21–30.
69. Kavalukas SL, Barbul A. Nutrition and wound healing: an update. *Plast Reconstr Surg*. 2011;127(Suppl 1):38S–43S.
70. Aboud C, Zamaria N, Cannistrà C. Treatment of hidradenitis suppurativa: surgery and yeast (Saccharomyces cerevisiae)-exclusion diet. Results after 6 years. *Surgery*. 2020;167(6):1012–1015.
71. Frew JW, Hawkes JE, Krueger JG. Topical, systemic and biologic therapies in hidradenitis suppurativa: pathogenic insights by examining therapeutic mechanisms. *Ther Adv Chronic Dis*. 2019;10. 2040622319830646 https://doi.org/10.1177/2040622319830646.
72. Shavit E, Pawliwec A, Alavi A, et al. The surgeon's perspective: a retrospective study of wide local excisions taken to healthy subcutaneous fat in the management of advanced hidradenitis suppurativa. *Can J Surg*. 2020;63:E94–E99.
73. Buimer MG, Ankersmit MFP, Wobbes T, Klinkenbijl JH. Surgical treatment of hidradenitis suppurativa with gentamicin sulfate: a prospective randomized study. *Dermatol Surg*. 2008;34(2):224–227.
74. Vermeulen H, Ubbink DT, Goossens A, et al. Systematic review of dressings and topical agents for surgical wounds healing by secondary intention. *Br J Surg*. 2005;92:665–672. https://doi.org/10.1002/bjs.5055.
75. Ge S, Orbay H, Silverman RP, et al. Negative Pressure Wound Therapy with Instillation and Dwell Time in the Surgical Management of Severe Hidradenitis Suppurativa. *Cureus*. 2018;10, e3319. https://doi.org/10.7759/cureus.3319.
76. Seidel D, Diedrich S, Herrle F, et al. Negative Pressure Wound Therapy vs. Conventional Wound Treatment in Subcutaneous Abdominal Wound Healing Impairment: The SAWHI Randomized Clinical Trial. *JAMA Surg*. 2020. https://doi.org/10.1001/jamasurg.2020.0414.
77. Dumville JC, Owens GL, Crosbie EJ, et al. Negative pressure wound therapy for treating surgical wounds healing by secondary intention. *Cochrane Database Syst Rev*. 2015;CD011278. https://doi.org/10.1002/14651858.CD011278.pub2.
78. Join-Lambert O, Coignard-Biehler H, Jais JP, et al. Efficacy of ertapenem in severe hidradenitis suppurativa: a pilot study in a cohort of 30 consecutive patients. *J Antimicrob Chemother*. 2016;71: 513–520.

24

Office-Based Excision for Hidradenitis Suppurativa: A Surgeon's Decades-Long Experience

RICHARD G. BENNETT

CHAPTER OUTLINE

Introduction

Every patient with hidradenitis suppurativa (HS) has a unique story to tell. All too often this story is a long one that includes numerous treatments, frustration, pain, and social embarrassment. By the time I see the patient, he or she has a skeptical feeling toward–if not frank distrust of–physicians. Fortunately for most patients, HS can be regionally cured if an adequate surgical excision is performed. This chapter will explore the literature regarding surgery for HS and my own perspective after personally performing more than 200 HS operative procedures, mostly in the past 10 years at the University of California, Los Angeles (UCLA).

I was fortunate to train in dermatology at the University of Pennsylvania under Drs. Walter Shelley and Harry Hurley.[1] Both of these physicians had a great interest in apocrine gland diseases and sparked my interest in HS. It was Dr. Hurley who first showed me how to unroof HS (in those days we called it "marsupialization"). Early in my career, I subsequently wrote about this technique and demonstrated it to plastic surgeons in the operating room.[2]

Over the years, my career has been mainly devoted to Mohs micrographic surgery. As my surgical ability increased, I began to operate on more extensive and difficult HS cases. This interest led to the development of an HS Clinic at UCLA. Mohs micrographic surgery and HS excisions have a lot in common. Both techniques are used to spare normal tissue, try to fully extirpate the disease process, involve management of healing wounds, and are sensitive to the complexities of histologic examination. We now examine frozen sections on all HS patients—not to examine for

excision margins, but rather to gain a new perspective on HS pathology by careful orientation of the excised specimens to visualize the relationship between the skin, sinus tracts, and inflammation. My experiences and clinical pearls regarding surgical excisions in HS patients are shared in this chapter.

Historical Perspective

Although HS was first described in the 19th century by Velpeau[3] and Verneuil,[4] adequate treatment was not available until the mid-20th century. Initially, hot packs,[5] incision and drainage, or even x-rays,[6,7] were recommended. It should be noted that x-rays were also recommended in HS for epilation,[8] similar to laser hair removal today. Around 1950, general surgeons and plastic surgeons began recommending large excisions that were repaired with split thickness skin grafts.[9] Slightly later, in the 1960s and 1970s, excision with skin flaps was advised. Since then, numerous skin flap techniques have been described for both the axilla and inguinal areas. More recently, microvascular free flaps have also been reported.[10] Along the way, healing by granulation was mentioned, especially in the axilla, groin, buttock, and perianal areas.

Dermatologists working independently from surgeons came up with the idea of unroofing HS lesions. Although this technique was first described in 1959 by J. Fred Mullins,[11] it was largely overlooked until recently, when it was again popularized by Bill Danby.[12-14] However, this technique is useful mainly on small superficial HS lesions.

Surgical Approaches

There are several surgical approaches that can be used to excise HS, ranging from conservative to radical. Almost all these procedures can be performed safely and conveniently under local anesthesia in an office setting with the exception of large flaps or in patients with extensive HS. Since each patient presents with a unique problem, the choice of surgical treatment depends upon the disease stage and when the patient appears. Incision and drainage, deroofing, and lasers are discussed in detail in other chapters (see below).

HIDRADENITIS SUPPURATIVA SURGICAL APPROACHES

- Incision and Drainage
- Unroofing
- Electrocutting
- Laser
- Excision and First Intention Healing
  - Side-to-Side Repair
  - Excision and Split Thickness Skin Graft
  - Excision and Skin Flap
    - Random
    - Axial
    - Fasciocutaneous
    - Microvascular
- Excision and Second Intention Healing
- Excision and Third Intention Healing

Incision and Drainage (see Chapter 22)

Incising and draining small, painful, fluctuant HS abscesses is commonly done, especially by primary care or emergency room physicians. Although this procedure produces dramatic and immediate pain relief, the result is only temporary and there is almost a 100% chance of recurrence if no future excision is done.[15-19] Occasionally, in my own practice, when a patient has a very large and tense abscess associated with HS, an I&D may be necessary for immediate pain reduction with the understanding that once the abscess is quiescent, more definitive surgery may need to be done.

Unroofing (see Chapter 22)

This technique has gone by a variety of names, including deroofing,[12,13,20] exteriorization,[21-23] and marsupialization.[2] For patients with mild disease with very superficial abscesses and tracts, removing the overlying skin to expose the disease process below can be very helpful.[11,24,25] Once the skin has been widely removed either with a scalpel blade or scissors, the underlying tortuous tracts are explored with a probe, such as the 6-inch non-malleable probe with eye (Miltex Inc, York, PA) or hemostat to detect and delineate the extent of the fistulous tracts and the hidden margins of the disease. The probe or hemostat needs to be inserted with minimal force; otherwise, false tunnels can be created. Any gelatinous material found is curetted and the base and sides of the resultant wound electrocoagulated. It is important to remove all the gelatinous material to prevent progression of gelatinous invasion and further sinus tract formation.

Danby et al.[13] entitled the rather characteristic gelatinous or jelly-like mass "invasive proliferative gelatinous mass" (IPGM) and described it as a clear gel with a cloudy pink consistency similar to granulation tissue or more fibrous material (see Figs. 24.2C,

24.5C and F). As pointed out by Danby,[13] the unroofing procedure destroys less normal tissue and places less stress on the healing process. The electrocoagulation is bactericidal, hemostatic, and destroys sinus tract linings. The resultant wound is always allowed to heal by second intention (granulation, contraction, epidermization). If this technique is applied to small, superficial lesions, the cure rate is high. The advantages of deroofing are that it is easy, fast, and can be done in the office. This technique works well in all areas where HS occurs, especially in the axilla and buttocks.[11,26,27] The disadvantage is that it is insufficient for very deep and large HS lesions.

Electrocutting[28,29]

Electrocutting utilizes the loop electrode with the cutting current on an electrosurgical device to peel away layers of tissue involved by HS. This technique is also called "skin-tissue-saving excision with electrosurgical peeling" (STEEP).[30] Its advantage is that little bleeding occurs. Other advantages are that minimal tissue is resected and the tissue heat from the electrosurgical device helps to seal any inapparent tracts. Therefore, quick wound healing occurs with a good cosmetic result. Although some published cure rates are promising (Blok[30] reports a relapse rate of 29.2%), I suspect that lesion selection is important to achieve a high cure rate.

Lasers (see Chapter 25)

Lasers can be used as cutting and coagulation instruments for excision of HS.[31] As with electrosurgery, patient and lesion selection are important for success. The lasers mentioned frequently for HS include the CO_2 ablative laser[22,31-33] and the neodymium-doped yttrium aluminum garnet (Nd:YAG) laser. Tissue is vaporized by laser light-heating tissue; the laser is used to peel away layers of skin. The advantage of the laser for HS excision is its precision and it helps to seal inapparent sinus tracts. The CO_2 laser can also be defocused to coagulate bleeding areas with minimal tissue destruction. Wounds are allowed to heal by second intention after laser excision.

Excision and First Intention Healing (per primam intentionem)

Excision of an affected HS area is most often done for deep lesions (see Video 24.1). If the wound edges are brought together side-to-side or if the wound is closed with a flap or graft, the closure is considered a first intention closure. This method is generally used to speed up wound healing.

a. *Side-to-Side Repair.* Side-to-side repairs can be done on relatively small lesions. However, margins may be compromised depending upon the surgeon's ability to excise and suture wounds. In one series by Jemec,[34] 72 patients underwent HS excisions and primary repair. The cure rate was only 14.7% but there was a high patient satisfaction rate of 68%. Some physicians advocate for side-to-side closure of a very large excision, especially in the axilla. This technique was popularized by Pollock[35] and became known as the Pollock procedure.[36] It relies on mobilization of the abundant loose tissue surrounding the axilla. However, the technique as described by Pollock[35] is complicated and involves numerous (8-16) holding sutures and no arm abduction until the 17th or 18th postoperative day. In one series of 47 axillae closed with this technique, 8 (17%) had wound separation.[37] In another searies,[38] 54% of sutured large axillary excisions (perhaps not done by the Pollock technique) required re-excision.

b. *Excision With Split Thickness Skin Graft (STSG).* Split thickness skin graft, especially in the axilla, has been used for over 70 years.[9] It became popular once skin graft harvesting machines (dermatomes) became available. Prior to that time, split thickness grafts needed to be cut by hand which was difficult to do consistently. Sometimes, the technique utilizes fenestrating or meshing the STSG, so it allows the underlying wound to drain easily; a meshed STSG covers a larger surface area than the initial size of the cut graft and thus avoids a large donor site excision.[39,40]

It is usually recommended that all hear-bearing skin be excised if a STSG is used in the axilla.[37] The advantage of excision with STSG repair is that a large area of skin and underlying tissue can be excised and repaired. This affords the patient fast wound healing[40] and perhaps a great chance for cure in the operated area, especially if the area had been operated on previously. Advocates of STSGs state that there is a high cure rate[18,23] and a high patient satisfaction rate.[41] The disadvantage of an excision with STSG is that special equipment is necessary, and the patient has a donor site wound that takes time to heal and is often bothersome to the patient. Furthermore, the skin graft must be carefully fixed to underlying tissue; otherwise, partial or complete necrosis will occur. To maintain this fixation usually requires immobilizing the patient for a week or more. STSGs are often applied 3-4 days after excision.[42] (This delay in graft application is known as healing by third intention, discussed later.) Another rarely mentioned disadvantage of using a STSG is that the feel of the skin, especially in the axilla, is abnormal.

c. *Excision With Skin Flap.* The last half of the 20th century saw the development and description of different types of skin flaps for HS.[43] Random pattern (rhombic,[44,45,46] z-plasty[9,42,47]), axial (propeller[48]), fasciocutaneous (V to Y subcutaneous island pedicle flap[49]), musculocutaneous, and even microvascular flaps[10] have been described. The most commonly used flaps for HS are the z-plasty and rhombic flap. These are random pattern flaps from adjacent skin. The advantages are that the closure is immediate and flap survival is usually better and more predictable than STSGs.[50] In the axilla, flap repair is advised to protect the axillary vessels and brachial plexus if exposed.[51] The disadvantage is that the overall cosmetic result can be less than ideal[47] (Fig. 24.1). The worst results from flaps I have seen in HS patients are in the groin and buttocks. Flaps in these areas cause unsightly tissue distortion. Furthermore, flaps can dehisce or become necrotic. To preserve function, lessen contracture, and provide a good cosmetic result, STSGs appear to offer a better long-term solution in these areas if wound repair is necessary. Furthermore, there is more likelihood of recurrence when skin flaps are used compared to STSGs.[52] This is probably due to the fact that the HS excision is sized for the flap rather than the flap being sized for the excision's size.

d. *Excision and Second Intention Healing (per secundam intentionem).*[52-56] Healing by second intention involves three overlapping phases: granulation, contraction, and epidermization. In areas where the skin surface is concave, second intention healing is optimal because greater contraction can occur further than that which will occur on convex surfaces.[57] Thus, in the axilla, which is concave, healing by second intention works very well (Fig. 24.2). With second intention healing, the resultant scar is always smaller than the defect. Other sites where second intention healing works well is in the inguinal, perineum, gluteal cleft areas,[51,58] and the posterior neck[42,59] (Figs. 24.3 and 24.4).

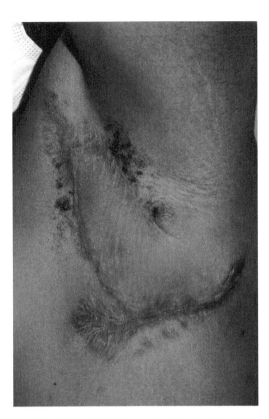

• **Fig. 24.1** Axillary Hidradenitis Suppurativa Treated Elsewhere by Excision and Closure With Rhombic Flap. Note remaining hair and noticeable scars, some of which are hypertrophic. The rhombic flap had dehisced at the point of maximum tension; a wound VAC was used to complete wound healing.

Another method described is a partial wound closure. In this technique, radial excisions with closures are done around a wound to reduce the wound size, leaving a central but reduced wound in the center; this smaller wound is allowed to heal by second intention.[17,60]

The advantages of second intention wound healing are the lack of sutures, avoidance of a secondary donor site, and minimally disfiguring scars. Patients are ambulatory immediately after surgery and thus have an increased sense of well-being. In a split HS axillary study, a greater number (70%) of patients preferred second intention wound healing compared to STSG (20%).[52] The main disadvantage is the long wound-healing time required (usually 4-12 weeks) for complete healing and the dressing changes required. Also, contracture may occur over flexion areas. The healing time will depend upon the wound size. For very large wounds, the healing time may be several months.[61] However, HS patients are usually experts at dressing changes by the time they require surgery.

e. *Excision and Third Intention Healing (per tertiam intentionem).* Third intention healing occurs when there is a repair delay after excision. The delay is usually 10 to 14 days,[62,63] but may occur sooner. This delay is sometimes recommended when an HS excision is complicated and deep. The delay allows for the formation of healthy granulation tissue in the wound. The repair is usually performed using a STSG. Delay of applying a STSG to a granulating wound is often more successful than applying a STSG immediately after excision, especially in the buttocks.[6,64] However, when reconstruction is delayed, further excision of skin margins is performed to freshen the edges.

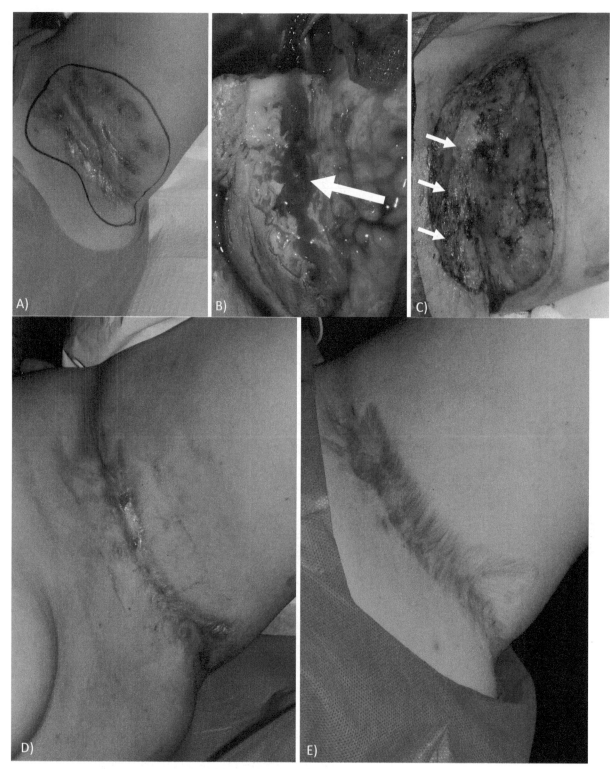

• **Fig. 24.2** Excision and Granulation of Left Axillary Hidradenitis Suppurativa. (A) Preoperative disease outlined by gentian violet. (B) Intraoperative view that shows gelatinous mass (arrow). (C) Intraoperative view after complete excision. The deep fascia was plicated (3 arrows) to protect underlying nerves and blood vessels uncovered during surgery. (D) Postoperative view of almost completely healed wound at 12 weeks. (E) Healed wound appearance 3 years postoperatively. Patient had full range of arm motion.

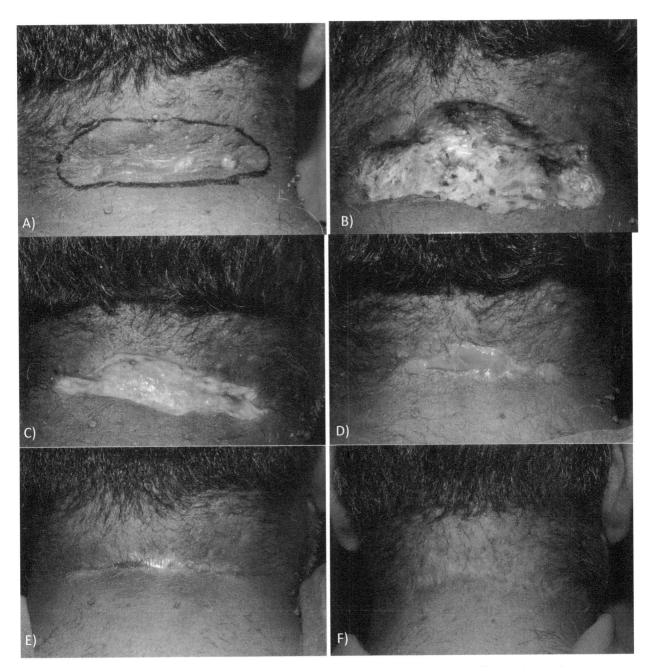

• **Fig. 24.3** Hidradenitis Suppurativa of Posterior Neck. (A) Preoperative appearance with general extent of excision marked with gentian violet. (B) Immediate postoperative appearance. Note excision extended in depth to deep fascia and superiorly and laterally beyond the marked border in A. Postoperative appearance at 1 week (C), 4 weeks (D), 8 weeks (E), and 3.5 years (F).

Cure Rates With Hidradenitis Suppurativa Excision

Multiple studies exist reporting cure rates for HS excision with or without repair. These cure rates range from 15%[34] to 100%[65] and vary depending on location and how the wound was managed. Although many prospective and retrospective cohort studies and case series exist, randomized, controlled trials for HS surgery are lacking.[66] Nevertheless, excision with or without repair results in high patient satisfaction rates.[67] One also must keep in mind that HS excisions change the course of the disease only in operated-on areas. Some of the variables within and between these studies that make assessment difficult are listed in the box and discussed below.

HIDRADENITIS SUPPURATIVA SURGERY CURE RATES UNDER SCRUTINY

1. Different Surgeons
2. Different Peripheral Margins
3. Different Depths
4. Selection Bias
5. How Recurrence Is Defined
6. How Patients Are Staged
7. Prior Surgical Treatment
8. Activity of Disease at Time of Excision

Continued

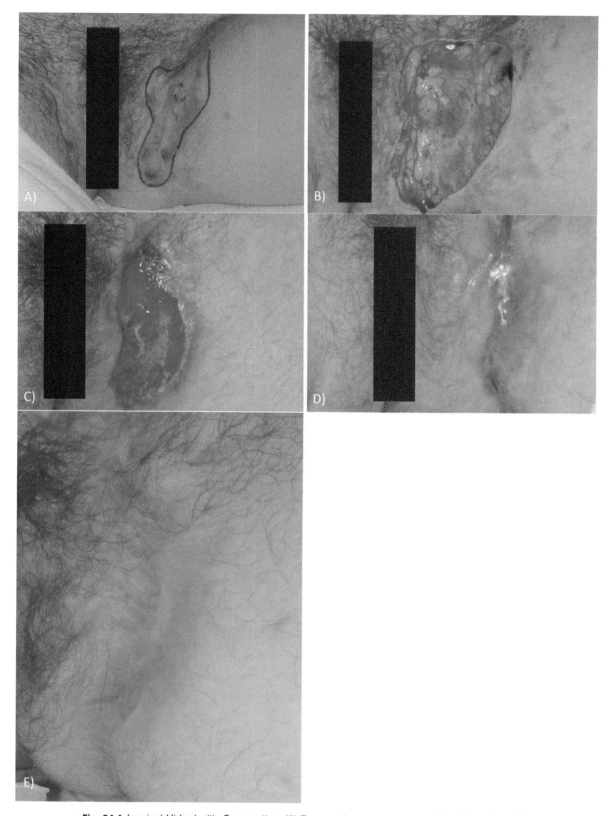

• **Fig. 24.4** Inguinal Hidradenitis Suppurativa. (A) Preoperative appearance marked with gentian violet. (B) Postoperative view immediately after excision. Note variable depth of excision with fascia exposed near upper center of wound base. Postoperative views at 3 weeks (C), 7 weeks (D), 1.5 years (E).

1. *Different Surgeons.* Different surgeons performed the operations. Usually, reports of case series are institutionally based—for instance, the Mayo Clinic[68] or the Lahey Clinic "experience."[69] Since no two surgeons operate in the same way, conclusions regarding cure rates are limited.

2. *Different Peripheral Margins.* Margins of surrounding normal appearing skin excised. Various recommendations regarding excision size of normal appearing skin surrounding HS necessary to remove for cure are suggested. Recommendations include the following: 1.5 cm,[55] 1-2 cm,[60,70] 2 cm,[67] 1 cm,[71] 0.5-1cm (axilla),[72] 1-1.5 cm (gluteal).[55] In addition, other poorly defined terms are used for excision margins such as, "beyond the borders of activity,"[73] "radical,"[19,41,55] "wide,"[24,55,74] "entire involved area,"[75] or "removal of all hair-bearing areas."[73] Saldin et al.[76] report no recurrences in 29 axillary excisions in which all hair-bearing skin was removed plus 2 cm additional normal appearing marginal skin. There is in fact little basis for these suggestions. Some feel the risk of HS recurrence is related more to the width or the "adequacy" of the excision rather than to the closure technique.[19,60,68,74,77] One report[15] states a 22% recurrence rate even with an "aggressive excision"; another report[19] states a 27% recurrence rate with a radical excision. Rompel and Petres[78] report a 6-month recurrence rate of only 2.5% within the operative field after "radical" excisions.

3. *Different Depths of Excision.* Often, the depth of excision is not stated. Vague statements are made, such as that excision is carried to deep subcutaneous fat or deep fascia,[65] which could mean different things depending upon the anatomic location. Also, sometimes stated is that the depth of the lesion depends upon completely excising the whole disease. That is, one adjusts the excision to the depth and breadth of the disease. Unnecessary overzealous excisions should be avoided so as not to damage neurovascular bundles in the axillary and inguinal areas. In the axilla, some authors warn not to transgress the deep axillary fascia so as not to expose vital arteries and nerves. However, if the disease process does involve the axillary fascia, it may be necessary to remove it. In one series of 47 axillae, complete excision of HS required violation of the axillary fascia in 3 cases.[37] Terms like "radical"[78] or "en-bloc"[67] are sometimes used. Anderson and Perry[37] advise removal of all indurated tissue with a cushion of normal appearing fat.

4. *Selection Bias.* Cases sent to plastic surgeons or general surgeons are usually more extensive than those sent to dermatologists. Thus, recurrence rates would be expected to be higher with more complex cases.

5. *How Recurrence Is Defined.* In some series, recurrence is defined as reappearance of HS within the operative scar whereas in other series it is defined as within 0.5–1 cm from the operative site.[54] As pointed out by Lapins,[22] new individual abscesses in a previously operated area cannot be prevented by any surgical method. These abscesses should be considered an outward manifestation of underlying HS disease activity rather than a fault of any particular surgical method.

6. *How Patients Are Staged.* For those case series performed by dermatologists, Hurley Stage[79] is often used. However, this staging system is rarely used by non-dermatologists, making it difficult to compare one study to another.[2] Furthermore, in many studies using the Hurley Staging System, the stages are lumped together (e.g., Hurley Stages II/III).

7. *Prior Surgical Treatment.* Those patients who were treated in the same area with excision prior to another HS excision are usually not identified. Perhaps these patients are more prone to recurrence.

8. *Activity of Disease at Time of Excision.* Little attention is paid to whether or not it is preferable to minimize disease activity prior to excision. Preoperative antibiotics or immunomodulators are rarely mentioned.[74] Although a few physicians advise preoperative or perioperative antibiotics,[37,60,68,72] most others do not state whether this was done. Some researchers[80,81] suggest that pre- and post-treatment with biologic therapy may lead to a lower recurrence rate and longer disease-free interval. I feel strongly that the patient needs to have either no or minimal activity at the time of HS excision as this leads to less chance of recurrence.

9. *Number of Diseased Regions Present.* As the number of HS locations increases, the likelihood of complete improvement decreases.[60] Some surgeons recommend removing multiple affected areas by separate operations.[9]

10. *Disease Location.* Usually, the general locations of the excision are given. However, this is not always the case when calculating overall cure rates. Recurrence tends to be more common in the inguinal-genital area.[54] In the inguinal, perineal, and perianal areas, radial excision is difficult and leads to a greater number of recurrences in those areas than in the axilla.[82,83]

11. *Length of Follow-Up.* Generally, a mean or median follow-up period in months is provided. However, this type of calculation can skew the data, particularly if a few patients have very long follow-up periods.

12. *Length of Time Patient Has Had Disease.* Most physicians believe that early recognition and early treatment of HS (especially surgery)[17] is important in keeping the disease from spreading. However, how long the patients have had their disease is often not mentioned in surgical case series.

13. *Local Versus General Anesthesia.* It may be that a larger amount of diseased tissue can be excised with a margin of normal skin under general anesthesia than under local anesthesia. In one study,[82] there was a 28.8% recurrence rate if the HS was excised under general anesthesia compared to a 40.6% recurrence rate under local anesthesia.

My Technique

Patient Preparation

A. *Preoperative Surgical Consultation.* Almost all HS patients come with a certain amount of distrust and frustration with physicians. This trust needs to be reestablished by listening to the patients and bringing their disease under control medically before operating. We have the patient complete an extensive questionnaire that extensively details symptoms and the prior history of treatments. I project a positive attitude regarding local cure as I go over the details of prior treatment. A physical exam is performed that grades each anatomic region involved by HS with the Hurley Stage.[79] I have found it useful to modify the Hurley Staging System as follows:

Stage		Description
I	a	1 abscess
	b	2–3 abscesses
	c	4 or more abscesses
II	a	1 tract between abscesses and fistulae
	b	2 tracts between abscesses and fistulae
	c	3 or more tracts between abscesses and fistulae
III	a	Multiple interconnecting tracts or abscesses
	b	Multiple interconnecting tracts plus hyperbolic or indurated scarring

B. *Drainage Reduction.* It is preferable that wound drainage is eliminated prior to surgery by use of oral antibiotic combinations. This is because surgery may spread any bacteria present and wound healing is facilitated when inflammation is eliminated or minimized. Another reason for giving antibiotics prior to surgery is that once the antibiotics calm down the HS, the patient is more trusting that their condition will now be well managed.

The preoperative antibiotic selection is important. I have found that giving two antibiotics simultaneously is optimal to eliminate drainage. One antibiotic is active against gram (+) organisms, and the other antibiotic is active against gram (−) organisms.. I prefer cephalexin and sulfamethoxazole-trimethoprim, although other combinations to consider are cephalexin and ciprofloxacin, cephalexin and doxycycline, or rifampin and clindamycin. In my experience, the combination of cephalexin and sulfamethoxazole-trimethoprim works in more than 90% of cases. The patient is seen back monthly to see how much drainage reduction has occurred. Usually, significant reduction in drainage will be noticed by the patient in 3 to 6 weeks. Concomitant with drainage reduction is a decrease in pain and new lesions. Patients may be switched from one antibiotic combination to another combination if the drainage does not decrease in a few months or if other problems with antibiotics occur, such as an allergic reaction or upset stomach.

C. *Preoperative Imaging.* Although some authors[70] suggest ultrasound or magnetic resonance imaging (MRI) prior to surgery, especially if the surgeon is uncertain about the disease extent, I have no experience with these techniques. However, imaging may be of value in the buttocks and perianal area where it may visualize fistulas into the rectum.[17]

Day of Surgery

Positioning the Patient: For axillary and pubic excisions, the patient is placed in the supine position on the operating table. For excisions in the posterior neck, the patient is placed prone. For excisions in the inguinal, scrotal, or vaginal areas, the patient is placed supine with his or her legs elevated in stirrups or leg rests. For lesions on the buttocks and perianal area, the patient is placed prone in the jack-knife Trendelenburg position with knees bent.

Site Preparation. The area to be operated on is photographed. Surrounding hair is clipped mainly so that there will be less irritation with future bandage changes. The area is then swabbed with povidine-iodine or chlorhexidine and the approximate area to be excised is marked with a gentian violet pen.

Anesthesia. If patients are particularly anxious and request some sedation, we use 5 to 10 mg of diazepam sublingually for fast absorption. Field block local anesthesia is obtained with 1% lidocaine with epinephrine 1:100,000. Prior to local anesthesia

in the axilla or inguinal area, topical anesthetic cream (e.g., EMLA) may be used 15 to 30 minutes prior to injection.[17,25] It is important to infiltrate anesthetic solution slowly using a 30 g needle. Be mindful that it is difficult to push anesthesia into scar tissue. Also, one must anesthetize at different tissue depths because HS may extend deeply. Maximum safe dose is 30 to 40 cc of 1% xylocaine for a 70kg person.

Occasionally, for a very large, complicated HS lesion in one anatomic area, the maximum safe dose of anesthetic solution may be exceeded. In those cases, I have opted to excise half the area at one operation and the other half a few weeks later. Staging large excisions allows one to excise very large lesions under local anesthesia in the office setting.

Some authors have suggested tumescent anesthesia because it provides less bleeding and anesthetic pain.[17,60] Tumescent anesthesia was developed for liposuction on the basis of slow absorption from fat tissue. It is unknown what the timing of serum absorption would be with tumescent anesthesia given in vascular areas such as the axilla or groin. In one study of 57 patients in whom tumescent anesthesia was used for HS excisions, 3 (5.3%) developed bleeding with hypovolemia.[60] Fluid shift problems have previously been described with tumescent anesthesia depending upon the volume of anesthetic given and the amount of tissue excised; this situation usually arises when the patient is under general anesthesia. Another problem with tumescent anesthesia is that the palpable induration I find valuable as a guide for excision size may be blunted by fluid expansion in the area.

Operative Approaches Based on Lesion Types

A. *Individual abscesses* are unroofed and any abnormal tissue below excised. Gelatinous tissue is sometimes seen below the abscess roof. This must be curetted out prior to excision of the surrounding tissue. The wound is generally allowed to heal by second intention, although I have occasionally sutured side-to-side if the excision is small and in an area that can be easily sutured.

B. *Multiple abscesses* are treated like individual abscesses. However, if multiple, would be more likely to allow the excisions to heal by second intention.

C. *Superficial tracts* can be "deroofed." I usually use a probe to locate the presence and direction of the tracts. Once identified, the tract roof is split open with scissors. The edges of the tract roof are further excised. Any gelatinous material in the base of the tract is curetted and the remaining tissue is electrocoagulated to destroy any small tracts that may be overlooked. The wound is allowed to heal by second intention.[2]

D. *Deep tracts* are the most common HS lesions excised in the office. The tract is palpated to get its general direction and depth. To open the tract, a 15-scalpel blade incises the lesion along the direction of the tract. Once the blade descends into the tract cavity, the edges of the tract are excised either with the scalpel blade or tenotomy scissors. Oftentimes one encounters gelatinous material that must also be excised. It is important when excising tracts that all scar tissue, both below and to the sides, be removed. A probe or hemostat may be useful to delineate and follow deep tracts (Fig. 24.5). This scar tissue can harbor additional tract extensions. The adequacy of excision is determined by palpation of the deep and lateral tissue. If the excision is adequate, one can sense by touch the normal non-scarred tissue on all sides and depth of the wound. If there is any question as to whether tissue is scarred or abnormal in appearance, it is excised. For multiple interconnecting tracts,

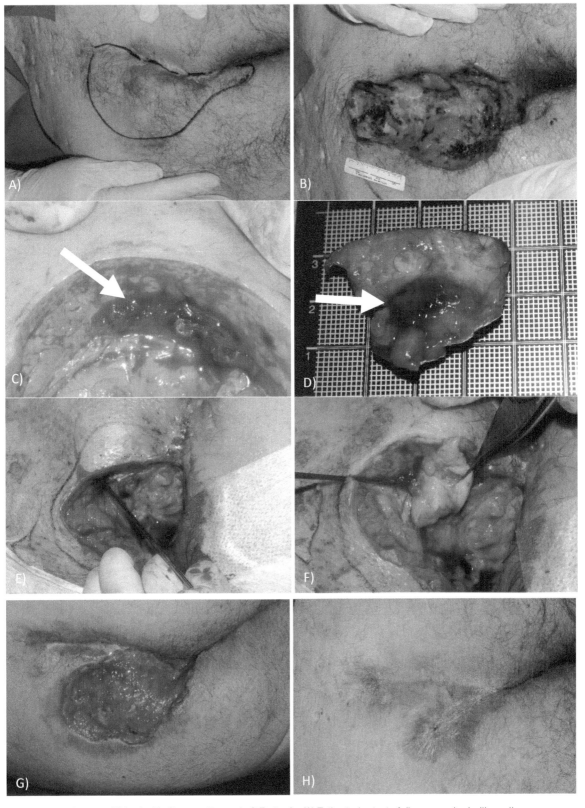

• **Fig. 23.5** Hidradenitis Suppurativa on Left Buttock. (A) Estimated extent of disease marked with gentian violet. (B) Intraoperative view. Note extension onto sacrum. (C) Close up view of gelatinous mass (arrow) in subcutaneous tissue. (D) Excised specimen. Note deep gelatinous mass (arrow). (E and F) Additional staged excision 2 months later. Using probe to determine extent. (G) Wound granulating 2 weeks postoperatively. (H) Healed scar at 5 months postoperatively.

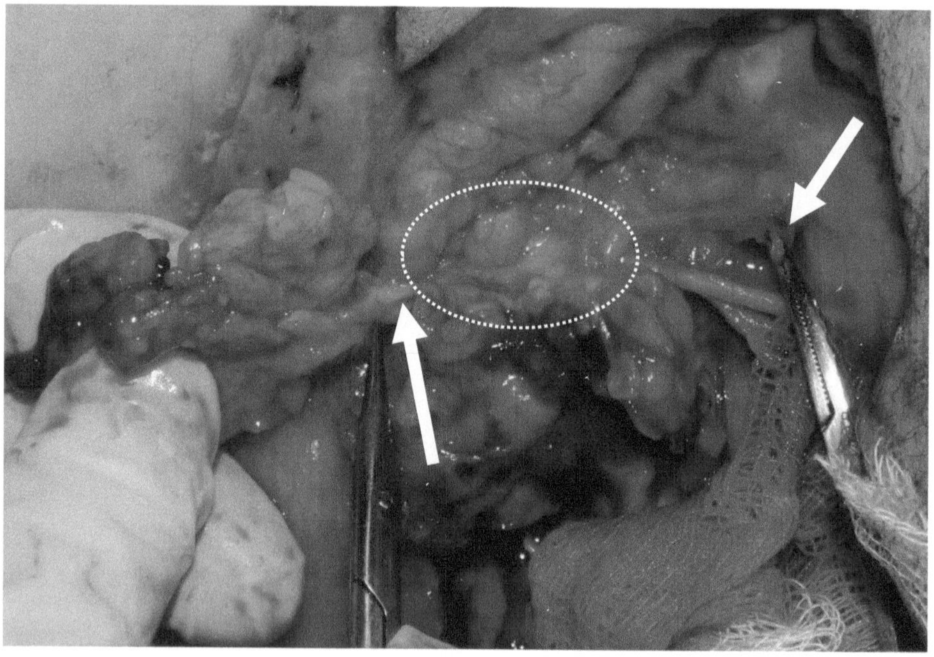

• **Fig. 24.6** Intraoperative dissection in an axilla with considerable fibrous tissue (*dotted circle* in center). Vessel ligated with hemostat on the right side (*right arrow*). Fibrous tissue carefully dissected off nerve using tenotomy scissors (*left arrow*). After dissection and excision of fibrous tissue complete, lateral fatty tissue and remaining fascia plicated over nerve to protect it during granulation (see Fig. 24.2C).

the surgery is the same as for one deep-seated tract. However, the resultant surgical wound size will be larger and complicated to close primarily. I am more likely to allow a large and deep wound to close by second intention.

Surgical Dissection. When dissecting deep in the axilla, one must keep in mind that the axillary vessels and brachial plexus are only millimeters away. Occasionally, during removal of scar tissue (especially in the axilla), important nerves and blood vessels are uncovered. These structures are preserved as much as possible by peeling or dissecting away surrounding scar tissue (Fig. 24.6). To protect these structures during second intention wound healing, I have found that the remaining fascia at the sides of the wound can be plicated with absorbable suture over the nerves and blood vessels (see Fig. 24.2C).

Hemostasis. One must be meticulous about stopping bleeding with large wounds. All bleeding vessels are clamped with a hemostat and ligated, usually with 4-0 or 5-0 polyglactin 910 (Vicryl®). The remaining tissue is electrocoagulated extensively. I prefer a "scorched earth policy," especially on the wound edges. Once the tract and any scarred tissue is excised, one decides between closure or granulation. I have found that granulation generally works better than immediate closure. Wound closure has more complications, such as hematoma and dehiscence. However, granulation will take longer (usually 6-8 weeks) than the time it takes for a sutured wound to heal (2 weeks).

Staged Excision for Very Large Lesions. When HS in one region involves an enormous area, one may "stage" the excision.[77] By this, I mean that one may excise half the lesion at one setting and the other half at a later time, usually 2 to 3 weeks later. This partial excision is usually done because one would exceed the upper safe limit of local anesthetic. However, I have not noticed a decrease in the cure rate removing lesions by staged excisions over time. The disadvantage of this approach is that

there will be additional normal tissue excised because, there is some overlap in the two excisions to completely remove the HS lesion.

Dressings. Dressings are done once or twice daily, depending upon how much drainage occurs in the wound. The wound is lightly cleaned with hydrogen peroxide on a cotton tipped applicator or gauze, and then an antibiotic ointment (e.g., bacitracin, zinc, and polymyxin B sulfate ointment [Polysporin®]) is applied, followed by a non-stick bandage (e.g., Telfa®), then gauze and paper tape. For the first dressing, a very sticky, slightly expandable bandage is used (e.g., adhesive non-woven fabric [Hypafix®]). If left to heal by granulation, drainage will be copious for 7 to 10 days. I usually see the patient back in two weeks to check on wound healing, and then monthly thereafter. Occasionally, the patient will develop an allergy to the antibiotic ointment or be irritated by tape being constantly applied to the surrounding skin. If so, Vaseline jelly is substituted for the antibacterial ointment. The irritation from the paper tape can be mitigated by slight rotation of the paper tape application. All wounds can get wet in the shower after 24 hours. For open wounds in the inguinal or buttock area, I have the patient do a sitz bath for 15 minutes each day.[59,61,84] Soaking in warm water stimulates wound healing and helps to keep the wound clean.

Surgical Challenges

Both immediate and long-term complications may be seen following surgery. There are also unique challenges based on the anatomic location of the patient's HS lesions. These situations are discussed in the following section.

Problems After Surgery

A. *Bleeding.* Once the local anesthesia has worn off and epinephrine is no longer present to constrict blood vessels, bleeding can occur. A hematoma may develop if the wound has been closed primarily. It is best to evacuate the blood as soon as possible and locate any arterial bleeders, which are then ligated. The wound is then re-sutured. If the wound has been left to heal by second intention, the wound is undressed, the bleeding located, and either electrocoagulated or ligated. If extensive, bleeding postoperatively can cause a significant fall in serum hemoglobin levels that might require transfusion. This situation has occurred when the patient has a low hemoglobin level preoperatively (around 10 gram per deciliter) and is prone to bleeding due to medications or underlying medical conditions.

A large wound closed primarily is more likely to dehisce or to develop a hematoma. Such wounds are therefore allowed to heal by granulation.

B. *Pain.* Pain is an individual phenomenon. Most patients after HS excision rarely need prescribed pain medication, especially if their wound is allowed to heal by second intention. Plain Tylenol is usually sufficient. Patients occasionally request something stronger. If so, I prescribe Tylenol #3 or Norco 5/325. Usually 10 to 15 tablets will be enough.

C. *Infection.* True infection (redness, pain, swelling, and growth of pathogenic bacteria on culture) is rare in my experience after HS excisions. Generally, patients are on antibiotics pre- and postoperatively. Also, granulating wounds are difficult to infect. Nevertheless, if the patient has increasing pain, one should suspect infection and do a wound culture.

D. *Hypergranulation Tissue.* Hypergranulation tissue (also known as proud flesh) occasionally occurs on wounds that heal by second intention.[30,59] Wounds in the inguinal creases are most prone to this problem. Hypergranulation can be left alone if small. If large, it can be curetted off, or silver nitrate 40% on sticks can be applied. By scraping or chemically cauterizing the hypergranulation tissue, the new epidermis will resurface over the granulation tissue quickly.

E. *Tape Irritation.* The daily removal of tape can irritate the skin. Usually paper tape is not as irritating as other types of tape. The patient can get some relief by changing the direction of tape application daily.

F. *Contact Dermatitis to Antibiotic Ointments.* Rarely a patient may develop an allergy to a component of an antibiotic ointment. This phenomenon is rare with HS patients. However, if this does occur, usually just switching to Vaseline® petroleum jelly solves the problem. If the patient has an extensive pruritic dermatitis, I prescribe a topical corticosteroid (e.g., triamcinolone acetonide cream 0.1%).

Long-Term Problems

A. *Tented Bands.* Small, tented bands can occur for wounds allowed to heal by second intention, especially in the axilla, where the skin is thin and loose. Usually, these small bands do not cause a significant problem for the patient. To remove the bands requires a z-plasty to be performed.[59]

B. *Scar Contracture.* Occasionally, if a very large wound is allowed to heal, especially in the axilla, a contracture might result that limits the arm range of motion. To prevent this problem, the patient can do stretching exercises prior to and immediately after wound healing. I usually recommend the patient walk

his or her arm along a wall. A physical therapist may also be useful.

If simple exercises fail to maintain or increase the range of motion, corticosteroid (e.g., triamcinolone acetonide, 10mg/cc) injection may be considered. This injection will not be effective if the contracture is significant. The solution then becomes surgical. Excision with a flap repair is usually the best solution (Fig. 24.7).

C. *Hypertrophic Scars and Keloids.* Although mentioned by some authors,[59] I have not seen these from surgery I have done. I have seen hypertrophic scars from skin flaps done elsewhere (see Fig. 24.1).

D. *Recurrence.* Probably the worst problem postoperatively is recurrence of HS. Usually, this occurs at the edge of the operated area, and rarely in the center. To treat the recurrence requires additional excision; however, this second excision is almost always smaller than the initial excisions.

Problems Associated With Various Sites

Axilla—The main problems long term are contracture bands and numbness. Contracture bands–if small–are not usually a problem, especially if the patient has full range of motion in the arm. However, contraction bands can limit range of motion. Occasionally, a V- to Y-, Z-plasty, or excisions and skin flap may be required to alleviate the contracture (see Fig. 24.7). Persistent anesthesia can occasionally occur on the upper posterior arm if a branch of the axillary nerve is cut during surgery.

Inframammary Area—HS in this area is difficult to control, even with "radical excision."[53]

Inguinal Area—Contractures and complications are extremely rare in this area.

Gluteal Cleft, Buttocks, Perineum, and Perianal Area—The main problem in this area is extension of the HS into the rectum or vagina. This may be apparent during excision of the HS via a fistula or may express itself by early recurrence HS. In one study,[63] anal fistulas occurred in about 10% of perianal HS. Anal fistulas associated with HS can be the most difficult to cure.[63] If this occurs, I usually refer the patient to a colorectal surgeon for definitive localization and treatment of the fistula. Preservation of the anal sphincter is important and can be challenging. Rarely, if HS is very extensive in these areas, a diverting colostomy may be necessary.[64]

Squamous cell carcinoma can occasionally occur in long standing HS in the buttocks, perianal, or labial areas.[85-88] Usually there is a delay in diagnosis of several years, oftentimes because initially, the squamous cell carcinoma is so well differentiated that the tissue is interpreted by the pathologist as reactive epidermal proliferation or pseudoepitheliomatous hyperplasia rather than squamous cell carcinoma. Although development of SCC with HS in the buttocks is unusual, all excised tissue in this area should be carefully and completely examined pathologically. In one series by Balik et al.,[64] one of 15 cases developed SCC (6.6%) and another study by Jackman[63] found 4 of 125 cases (3.2%) developed SCC. When SCC develops, it has a high rate of mortality despite measures to control its growth.[88]

Tissue Examination of HS. It is important that excised HS be sent for pathologic examination. Around the buttocks and rectum there is rarely degeneration to squamous cell carcinoma. In those instances, the diagnosis may be overlooked early on

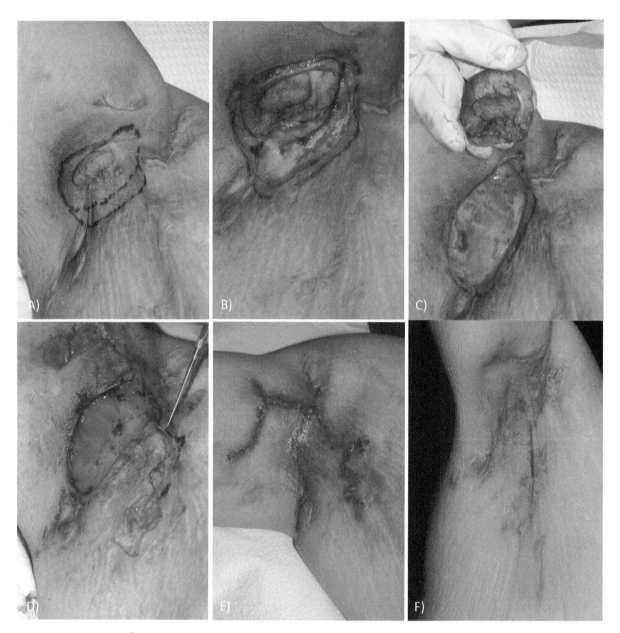

• **Fig. 24.7** Contracture in Axilla Causing Inability to Fully Raise Arm. (A) Proposed excision. (B) Initial incision. Note how wound edges enlarge. (C) Size of excised scar smaller than wound defect due to wound edge retraction. (D) Development of two rhombic flaps to close wound, a rhombic with two Z-plasties inferiorly and a rhombic flap superiorly. (E) Sutured flaps. (F) Appearance 2 years postoperatively. Note ability to fully raise arm.

because the tumor at first is so well differentiated as to be interpreted as epitheliomatous reactive hyperplasia.

I feel that HS tissue examination is ideally done first by frozen sections prior to being submitted for permanent sections (Fig. 24.8). The reason for this is that the surgeon can pick out critical areas to examine and orient the tissue prior to the tissue being cut on the microtome. Histopathological examination of these critical areas help in the understanding of HS pathogenesis. If tissue is submitted to pathology directly for paraffin sections, the laboratory often receives a mass of tissue from which random sectioning is done. The subsequent pathologic diagnosis, "consistent with hidradenitis suppurativa," is not very helpful.

Reimbursement

A subject infrequently discussed regarding HS surgery is the financial reimbursement from medical insurance companies in the United States. Generally, for the time spent, the reimbursement is quite low. Chapman[59] states that although he can complete a radical mastectomy in under two hours, an axillary HS dissection with a flap takes a minimum of three to four hours. Poor reimbursement has led to difficulty in referring patients to general surgeons or plastic surgeons. In other countries with completely nationalized medical systems, reimbursement is probably not a problem.

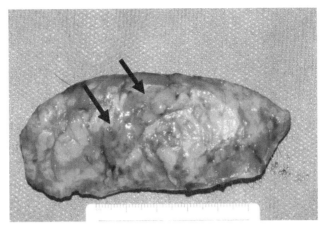

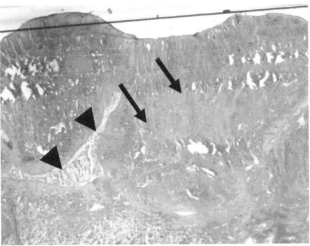

• **Fig. 24.8** Excised HS Specimen. *Top*: Tissue oriented to show location of gelatinous mass (*arrows*) relative to surface epidermis and subcutaneous tissue. Note its deep extension. *Bottom*: Corresponding frozen section of same tissue as in top oriented and cut to show histopathology of the gelatinous mass (*arrows*) and sinus tract (*arrowheads*). Note sinus tract shows keratinous debris and little or no inflammation.

Conclusion

As dermatologists gain extensive experience with skin surgery, extensive HS lesions are excised in the office under local anesthesia. These procedures are convenient for the patient, less expensive than those done in an operating room, and produce a minimal scar with little likelihood of recurrence. However, some experience is necessary, and we have taught and incorporated my excision technique into the dermatology residencies at UCLA and USC.

My experience with HS is that total surgical excision will result in a regional cure. Total excision is best obtained by manually feeling the excision wound for remaining scar and taking time to ensure that all abnormal tissue felt is excised. Probing for connections between the main excision and surrounding abscesses is also important. Almost all wounds from HS excisions I perform are allowed to heal by second intention. Patients with more than one region involved with HS are operated on at separate times. Once the disease is regionally removed, any new lesions in that area can be treated quickly and easily by excision. Most patients are grateful and pleased with this approach.

References

1. Hurley HJ, Shelley WB. *The Human Apocrine Sweat Gland in Health and Disease.* Springfield, IL: *Charles C Thomas*; 1960.
2. Bennett RG. *Treatment of Hidradenitis Suppurativa in Skin Surgery 5th Edition (Epstein E, Epstein Jr. E, Eds).* Springfield, IL: Charles C. Thomas; 1982:1127–1136.
3. Velpeau A. *Dictionnaire de Medicine, un Repertoire General des Sciences Medicales Sous la Rapport Theorique et Pratique.* 2nd Edition; 1839-1845. Aiselle, Vol. 2 p. 91. Anus. Vol. 3 p. 304. Mamelles, Vol. 19, p.1 Bechet Jeunc.
4. Verneuil A. Etudes sur les tumeurs de la peau: de quelques maladies des glandes sudoripares. *Arch Gen Med.* 1854;4(447-468):693–705.
5. Lane JE. Hidrosadenitis axillaris of verneuil. *Arch Derm Syphilol.* 1933;28(5):609–614. https://doi.org/10.1001/archderm.1933.01460050003001.
6. Conway H, Stark RB, Climo S, Weeter JC, Garcia FA. The surgical treatment of chronic hidradenitis suppurativa. *Surg Gynecol Obstet.* 1952;95(4):455–464.
7. Tachau P. Abcesses of the sweat glands in adults. *Arch Derm Syph.* 1939;40:595–600.
8. Zeligman L. Temporary X-ray epilation therapy of chronic axillary hidradenitis suppurativa. *Arch Dermat.* 1965;92:690–694.

9. Greeley PW. Surgical treatment of chronic suppurative hidradenitis. *Arch Surg.* 1950;61(2):193–198. https://doi.org/10.1001/archsurg.1950.01250020197001.

10. Tanaka A, Hatoko M, Tada H, Kuwahara M, Mashiba K, Yurugi S. Experience with surgical treatment of hidradenitis suppurativa. *Ann Plast Surg.* 2001;47(6):636–642. https://doi.org/10.1097/00000637-200112000-00010.

11. Mullins JF, McCash WB, Bourdeau RF. Treatment of chronic hidradenitis suppurativa: surgical modification. *Postgrad Med.* 1959;26:805–808. https://doi.org/10.1080/00325481.1959.11712723.

12. Danby FW. Commentary: unroofing for hidradenitis suppurativa, why and how. *J Am Acad Dermatol.* 2010;63(3):481.e1–481.e4813. https://doi.org/10.1016/j.jaad.2010.01.033.

13. Danby FW, Hazen PG, Boer J. New and traditional surgical approaches to hidradenitis suppurativa. *J Am Acad Dermatol.* 2015;73(5 Suppl 1):S62–S65. https://doi.org/10.1016/j.jaad.2015.07.043.

14. Margesson LJ, Danby FW. Hidradenitis suppurativa. *Best Pract Res Clin Obstet Gynaecol.* 2014;28(7):1013–1027.

15. Broadwater JR, Bryant RL, Petrino RA, Mabry CD, Westbrook KC, Casali RE. Advanced hidradenitis suppurativa. Review of surgical treatment in 23 patients. *Am J Surg.* 1982;144(6):668–670. https://doi.org/10.1016/0002-9610(82)90547-5.

16. Ellis LZ. Hidradenitis suppurativa: surgical and other management techniques. *Dermatol Surg.* 2012;38(4):517–536. https://doi.org/10.1111/j.1524-4725.2011.02186.x.

17. Janse I, Bieniek A, Horváth B, Matusiak Ł. Surgical Procedures in Hidradenitis Suppurativa. *Dermatol Clin.* 2016;34(1):97–109. https://doi.org/10.1016/j.det.2015.08.007.

18. Knaysi Jr GA, Cosman B, Crikelair GF. Hidradenitis suppurativa. *JAMA.* 1968;203(1):19–22.

19. Ritz JP, Runkel N, Haier J, Buhr HJ. Extent of surgery and recurrence rate of hidradenitis suppurativa. *Int J Colorectal Dis.* 1998;13(4):164–168. https://doi.org/10.1007/s003840050159.

20. van Hattem S, Spoo JR, Horvath B, Jonkman MF, Leeman FW. Surgical treatment of sinuses by deroofing in hidradenitis suppurativa. *Dermatol Surg.* 2012;38:494–497.

21. Culp CE. Chronic hidradenitis suppurativa of the anal canal. A surgical skin disease. *Dis Colon Rectum.* 1983;26(10):669–676. https://doi.org/10.1007/BF02553341.

22. Lapins J, Emtestam L. *Surgery in Hidradenitis Suppuraitva (Jemec, GBE., Revuz, J., Leyden, JJ., Eds.).* Berlin: Springer-Verlag; 2006:161–173.

23. Newell GB. Treatment of hidradenitis suppurativa. *JAMA.* 1973;223. 556-7.

24. Goldburg SR, Strober BE, Payette MJ. Hidradenitis suppurativa: Current and emerging treatments. *J Am Acad Dermatol.* 2020;82(5):1061–1082. https://doi.org/10.1016/j.jaad.2019.08.089.

25. van der Zee HH, Prens EP, Boer J. Deroofing: a tissue-saving surgical technique for the treatment of mild to moderate hidradenitis suppurativa lesions. *J Am Acad Dermatol.* 2010;63(3):475–480. https://doi.org/10.1016/j.jaad.2009.12.018.

26. Barron J. The surgical treatment of perianal hidradenitis suppurativa. *Dis Colon Rectum.* 1970;13(6):441–443. https://doi.org/10.1007/BF02616789.

27. Chernosky ME. *Scalpel and Scissors Surgery as seen by the Dermatologist in Skin Surgery (Epstein, E and Epstein Jr, E, eds).* Springfield: Charles C. Thomas; 1977:132–135.

28. Aksakal AB, Adisen E. Hidradenitis suppurativa: importance of early treatment with electrosurgery. *Dermatologic Surgery.* 2008;34(2):228–231.

29. Duncan WC. Surgical treatment of hidradenitis suppurativa. *J Dermatol Surg.* 1976;2(2):153–157. https://doi.org/10.1111/j.1524-4725.1976.tb00171.x.

30. Blok JL, Boersma M, Terra JB, et al. Surgery under general anaesthesia in severe hidradenitis suppurativa: a study of 363 primary operations in 113 patients. *J Eur Acad Dermatol Venereol.* 2015;29(8):1590–1597. https://doi.org/10.1111/jdv.12952.

31. Finley EM, Ratz JL. Treatment of hidradenitis suppurativa with carbon dioxide laser excision and second-intention healing. *J Am Acad Dermatol.* 1996;34(3):465–469. https://doi.org/10.1016/s0190-9622(96)90441-7.

32. Lapins J, Sartorius K, Emtestam L. Scanner-assisted carbon dioxide laser surgery: a retrospective follow-up study of patients with hidradenitis suppurativa. *J Am Acad Dermatol.* 2002;47(2):280–285. https://doi.org/10.1067/mjd.2002.124601.

33. Mikkelsen PR, Dufour DN, Zarchi K, Jemec GB. Recurrence rate and patient satisfaction of CO2 laser evaporation of lesions in patients with hidradenitis suppurativa: a retrospective study. *Dermatol Surg.* 2015;41(2):255–260.

34. Jemec GB. Effect of localized surgical excisions in hidradenitis suppurativa. *J Am Acad Dermatol.* 1988;18(5 Pt 1):1103–1107.

35. Pollock WJ, Virnelli FR, Ryan RF. Axillary hidradenitis suppurativa. A simple and effective surgical technique. *Plast Reconstr Surg.* 1982;49(1):22–27.

36. Tasche C, Angelats J, Jayaram B. Surgical treatment of hidradenitis suppurativa of the axilla. *Plast Reconstr Surg.* 1975;55(5):559–562. https://doi.org/10.1097/00006534-197505000-00005.

37. Anderson DK, Perry AW. Axillary hidradenitis. *Arch Surg.* 1975;110(1):69–72. https://doi.org/10.1001/archsurg.1975.01360070069012.

38. Watson JD. Hidradenitis suppurativa- -a clinical review. *Br J Plast Surg.* 1985;38(4):567–569. https://doi.org/10.1016/0007-1226(85)90022-0.

39. Kuo HW, Ohara K. Surgical treatment of chronic gluteal hidradenitis suppurativa: reused skin graft technique. *Dermatol Surg.* 2003;29(2):173–178. https://doi.org/10.1046/j.1524-4725.2003.29044.x.

40. Pittam MR, Ellis H. A comparison of skin grafting and healing by granulation following axillary excision for hidradenitis suppurativa. *Annals of the Royal College of Surgeons of England.* 1984;66(1):73.

41. Bohn J, Svensson H. Surgical treatment of hidradenitis suppurativa. *Scand J Plast Reconstr Surg Hand Surg.* 2001;35(3):305–309. https://doi.org/10.1080/028443101750523230.

42. Letterman G, Schurter M. Surgical treatment of hyperhidrosis and chronic hidradenitis suppurativa. *J Invest Dermatol.* 1974;63(1):174–182.

43. Paletta FX. Hidradenitis suppurativa: pathologic study and use of skin flaps. *Plast Reconstr Surg.* 1963;31:307–315.

44. Hermanson A. Surgical treatment of axillary hidradenitis suppurativa. *Scand J Plast Reconstr Surg.* 1982;16(2):163–165.

45. O'Brien J, Wysocki J, Anastasi G. Limberg flap coverage for axillary defects resulting from excision of hidradenitis suppurativa. *Plast Reconstr Surg.* 1976;58(3):354–358. https://doi.org/10.1097/00006534-197609000-00017.

46. Altmann S, Fansa H, Schneider W. Axillary hidradenitis suppurativa: a further option for surgical treatment. *J Cutan Med Surg.* 2004;8(1):6–10. https://doi.org/10.1007/s10227-003-0162-5.

47. Snyder CC, Farrell JJ. Hydradenitis suppurativa. *Plast Reconstr Surg (1946).* 1957;19(6):502–508. https://doi.org/10.1097/00006534-195706000-00006.

48. Elboraey MA, Alali AB, Alkandari QA. Immediate and Delayed Reconstruction after Excision of Axillary Hidradenitis Suppurativa Using a Propeller Flap. *Plast Reconstr Surg Glob Open.* 2019;7(8):e2387. Published 2019 Aug 12 https://doi.org/10.1097/GOX.0000000000002387.

49. Rieger UM, Erba P, Pierer G, Kalbermatten DF. Hidradenitis suppurativa of the groin treated by radical excision and defect closure by medial thigh lift: aesthetic surgery meets reconstructive surgery. *J Plast Reconstr Aesthet Surg.* 2009;62(10):1355–1360. https://doi.org/10.1016/j.bjps.2008.04.035.

50. Harrison SH. Axillary hidradenitis. *Br J Plast Surg.* 1964;17:95–98.

51. Armstrong DP, Pickrell KL, Giblin TR, Miller F. Axillary Hidradenitis Suppurativa. *Plast Reconstr Surg.* 1965;36:200–206. https://doi.org/10.1097/00006534-196508000-00007.

52. Morgan WP, Harding KG, Hughes LE. A comparison of skin grafting and healing by granulation, following axillary excision for hidradenitis suppurativa. *Ann R Coll Surg Engl.* 1983;65(4):235–236.

53. Banerjee AK. Surgical treatment of hidradenitis suppurativa. *Br J Surg.* 1992;79(9):863–866. https://doi.org/10.1002/bjs.1800790905.
54. Deckers IE, Dahi Y, van der Zee HH, Prens EP. Hidradenitis suppurativa treated with wide excision and second intention healing: a meaningful local cure rate after 253 procedures. *J Eur Acad Dermatol Venereol.* 2018;32(3):459–462. https://doi.org/10.1111/jdv.14770.
55. Harrison BJ, Mudge M, Hughes LE. Recurrence after surgical treatment of hidradenitis suppurativa. *Br Med J (Clin Res Ed).* 1987;294 (6570):487–489. https://doi.org/10.1136/bmj.294.6570.487.
56. Vellaichamy G, Braunberger TL, Nahhas AF, Hamzavi IH. Surgical procedures for hidradenitis suppurativa. *Cutis.* 2018;102(1):13–16.
57. Zitelli JA. Wound healing by secondary intention. A cosmetic appraisal. *J Am Acad Dermatol.* 1983;9(3):407–415. https://doi.org/10.1016/s0190-9622(83)70150-7.
58. Ariyan S, Krizek TJ. Hidradenitis suppurativa of the groin, treated by excision and spontaneous healing. *Plast Reconstr Surg.* 1976;58 (1):44–47. https://doi.org/10.1097/00006534-197607000-00007.
59. Chapman J. The surgical treatment of hidradenitis suppurativa. *J Natl Med Assoc.* 1972;64(4):328–330.
60. Bieniek A, Matusiak L, Okulewicz-Gojlik D, Szepietowski JC. Surgical treatment of hidradenitis suppurativa: experiences and recommendations. *Dermatol Surg.* 2010;36(12):1998–2004. https://doi.org/10.1111/j.1524-4725.2010.01763.x.
61. Silverberg B, Smoot CE, Landa SJ, Parsons RW. Hidradenitis suppurativa: patient satisfaction with wound healing by secondary intention. *Plast Reconstr Surg.* 1987;79(4):555–559.
62. Greeley PW. Plastic surgical treatment of chronic suppurative hidradenitis. *Plast Reconstr Surg.* 1951;7(2):143–146. https://doi.org/10.1097/00006534-195102000-00007.
63. Jackman RJ. Hidradenitis suppurativa: diagnosis and surgical management of perianal manifestations. *Proc R Soc Med.* 1959;52(Suppl 1):110–112. Suppl.
64. Balik E, Eren T, Bulut T, Büyükuncu Y, Bugra D, Yamaner S. Surgical approach to extensive hidradenitis suppurativa in the perineal/perianal and gluteal regions. *World J Surg.* 2009;33(3):481–487. https://doi.org/10.1007/s00268-008-9845-9.
65. Kagan RJ, Yakuboff KP, Warner P, Warden GD. Surgical treatment of hidradenitis suppurativa: a 10-year experience. *Surgery.* 2005;138 (4):734–741. https://doi.org/10.1016/j.surg.2005.06.053.
66. Zouboulis CC, Bechara FG, Dickinson-Blok JL, et al. Hidradenitis suppurativa/acne inversa: a practical framework for treatment optimization - systematic review and recommendations from the HS ALLIANCE working group. *J Eur Acad Dermatol Venereol.* 2019;33(1):19–31.
67. Posch C, Monshi B, Quint T, Vujic I, Lilgcnau N, Rappersberger K. The role of wide local excision for the treatment of severe hidradenitis suppurativa (Hurley grade III): Retrospective analysis of 74 patients. *J Am Acad Dermatol.* 2017;77(1). https://doi.org/10.1016/j.jaad.2017.01.055. 123-129.e5.
68. Kohorst JJ, Baum CL, Otley CC, et al. Surgical Management of Hidradenitis Suppurativa: Outcomes of 590 Consecutive Patients. *Dermatol Surg.* 2016;42(9):1030–1040. https://doi.org/10.1097/DSS.0000000000000806.
69. Wiltz O, Schoetz Jr DJ, Murray JJ, et al. Perianal hidradenitis suppurativa, The Lahey Clinic experience. *Dis Colon Rectum.* 1990;33:731–734.
70. Büyükaşik O, Hasdemir AO, Kahramansoy N, Çöl C, Erkol H. Surgical approach to extensive hidradenitis suppurativa. *Dermatol Surg.* 2011;37 (6):835–842. https://doi.org/10.1111/j.1524-4725.2011.01961.x.
71. Weyandt G. Operative therapie der acne inversa. *Hautarzt.* 2005;56: 1033–1039.
72. Menderes A, Sunay O, Vayvada H, Yilmaz M. Surgical management of hidradenitis suppurativa. *Int J Med Sci.* 2010;7(4):240–247.
73. Van Rappard DC, Mooji JE, Mekkes JR. Mild to moderate hidradenitis suppurativa treated with local excision and primary closure. *J Eur Acad Dermatol Venereol.* 2012;26:898–902.
74. Mehdizadeh A, Hazen PG, Bechara FG, et al. Recurrence of hidradenitis suppurativa after surgical management: A systematic review and meta-analysis. *J Am Acad Dermatol.* 2015;73(5 Suppl 1):S70–S77.
75. Alharbi Z, Kauczok J, Pallua N. A review of wide surgical excision of hidradenitis suppurativa. *BMC Dermatol.* 2012;12:9. Published 2012 Jun 26 https://doi.org/10.1186/1471-5945-12-9.
76. Soldin MG, Tulley P, Kaplan H, Hudson DA, Grobbelaar AO. Chronic axillary hidradenitis- -the efficacy of wide excision and flap coverage. *Br J Plast Surg.* 2000;53(5):434–436. https://doi.org/10.1054/bjps.1999.3285.
77. Mitchell KM, Beck DE. Hidradenitis suppurativa. *Surg Clin North Am.* 2002;82(6):1187–1197. https://doi.org/10.1016/s0039-6109 (02)00060-9.
78. Rompel R, Petres J. Long-Term Results of Wide Surgical Excision in 106 Patients with Hidradenitis Suppurativa. *Dermatologic Surgery.* 2000;26:638–643.
79. Hurley, H.J. Axillary hyperhidrosis, apocrine bromhidrosis, hidradenitis suppurativa and familial benign pemphigus: surgical approach. In. Roenighk RK, Roenigk HH, editios. Dermatologic surgery. *Marcel Dekker*, New York, 1989, p.729-39.
80. DeFazio MV, Economides JM, King KS, et al. Outcomes After Combined Radical Resection and Targeted Biologic Therapy for the Management of Recalcitrant Hidradenitis Suppurativa. *Ann Plast Surg.* 2016;77(2):217–222. https://doi.org/10.1097/SAP.0000000000000584.
81. Van Rappard DC, Mekkes JR. Treatment of severe hidradenitis suppurativa with infliximab in combination with surgical interventions. *Br J Dermatol.* 2012;167(1):206–208. https://doi.org/10.1111/j.1365-2133.2012.10807.x.
82. Walter AC, Meissner M, Kaufmann R, Valesky E, Pinter A. Hidradenitis Suppurativa After Radical Surgery-Long-Term Follow-up for Recurrences and Associated Factors. *Dermatol Surg.* 2018;44 (10):1323–1331. https://doi.org/10.1097/DSS.0000000000001668.
83. Anderson Jr MJ, Dockerty MB. Perianal hidradenitis suppurativa; a clinical and pathologic study. *Dis Colon Rectum.* 1958;1(1):23–31. https://doi.org/10.1007/BF02616510.
84. Thornton JP, Abcarian H. Surgical treatment of perianal and perineal hidradenitis suppurativa. *Dis Colon Rectum.* 1978;21(8):573–577.
85. Humphrey LJ, Playforth H, Leavell Jr UW. Squamous cell carcinoma arising in hidradenitis suppurativum. *Arch Dermatol.* 1969;100 (1):59–62.
86. Rosser C. The etiology of anal cancer. *The American Journal of Surgery.* 1931;11(2):328–333.
87. Zachary LS, Robson MC, Rachmaninoff N. Squamous cell carcinoma occurring in hidradenitis suppurativa. *Ann Plast Surg.* 1987;18:71–73.
88. Bennett RG. Commentary on Squamous Cell Carcinoma in Perineal, Perianal and Gluteal Hidradenitis Suppurativa. *Dermatol Surg.* 2019;45(4):527–528.

25

Laser and Light Treatments for Hidradenitis Suppurativa

ALEXIS B. LYONS AND ILTEFAT H. HAMZAVI

CHAPTER OUTLINE

ABBREVIATIONS:

hidradenitis suppurativa (HS), carbon dioxide (CO_2), neodymium-doped yttrium aluminum garnet (Nd:YAG), Hidradenitis Suppurativa Clinical Response (HiSCR), Dermatology Life Quality Index (DLQI), photodynamic therapy (PDT), methyl aminolevulinate (MAL), 5-aminolevulinic acid (ALA), methylene blue (MB)

Introduction

In additional to traditional topical, medical, and surgical modalities, hidradenitis suppurativa (HS) can also be managed with laser and light-based treatments. These methods have the advantage of targeting affected areas with little to no systemic side effects. They can be used as monotherapy or combined with other treatments. These work by selective photothermolysis to target specific components of the skin and work via several mechanisms, including: debulking lesions, stimulating wound healing, improving scarring, decreasing inflammation, destroying hair follicles, targeting sebaceous glands, and killing bacteria (Fig. 25.1).[1] Energy-based treatments are important options in the HS management ladder with different lasers recommended for various stages of severity (Table 25.1). They are often used in conjunction with medical, surgical, and lifestyle modifications as part of comprehensive care for HS patients.

Carbon Dioxide Laser

The carbon dioxide (CO_2) laser (10,600 nm) is used to treat active HS areas as well as for scarring secondary to HS itself or previous HS surgery. Use of CO_2 to vaporize sinus tracts was first described in 1987 by Dalrymple and Monighan,[2] and methods for CO_2 laser excision have evolved from there.

Ablative

The CO_2 laser can be used in the ablative setting to selectively excise HS affected areas while sparing unaffected tissue. It is recommended for patients with Hurley stage II and III HS who have fibrotic sinus tracts.[3] This laser can be used on patients under local anesthesia (with or without tumescent anesthesia) in an outpatient office setting. This results in a decreased risk compared to traditional wide local excision under general anesthesia. Treatment settings include a fluence of 55 W with a 0.2 to 1 mm spot size.[1] The hemostatic properties of the laser allow for excellent visualization of the operative field and accurate assessment of the excised area for residual sinus tracts.[4] The resultant wound is typically left to heal via secondary intention (Fig. 25.2). Thus, appropriate wound care is needed until healing occurs.

Patient satisfaction after CO_2 excision is generally high, with one study reporting 95% of patients having some or great improvement, with 91% recommending the surgery to others.[5] Recurrence rates after CO_2 excision range from 1% to 29%, and infection rates range from 1.6% to 4.9%.[5–8] Variations in recurrence rates are thought to be due to operator technique, severity and location of disease, and duration of follow-up.

To decrease the risk for recurrence, CO_2 ablation is sometimes used in conjunction with other treatment modalities. In one study, CO_2 laser excision with marsupialization (suturing edges of an abscess) resulted in a recurrence rate of only 1%.[6] Another study found that neodymium-doped yttrium aluminum garnet (Nd:YAG) treatment followed by deroofing sinus tracts with CO_2 laser resulted in lower recurrence than with CO_2 deroofing alone.[9]

TABLE 25.1 Summary of Laser and Light-based Treatment Modalities

Treatment Modality	Level of Evidence	Mechanism of Action	Patient Selection	Pre- and Post-Procedure Care	Complications, Barriers, and Limitations
Ablative CO_2	C	Tissue debulking or destruction	Patients with Hurley stage II or III disease with sinus tracts	Intralesional anesthesia pre-procedure, wound is typically left to heal via secondary intention-wound care needed until healing occurs	Patient discomfort, wound care necessary, risk of infection, nerve damage, and recurrence
Fractionated CO_2	C	Improve scarring and stimulate wound healing	Patients with contracture from scarring	Petroleum jelly to the area post-procedure	Patient discomfort
Nd:YAG	B	Follicular destruction	All Fitzpatrick skin phototypes and all Hurley stages	None	• Patient discomfort • Requires more than one treatment
Alexandrite	C	Follicular destruction	All Hurley stages	None	• Patient discomfort • Requires more than one treatment
Diode	C	Follicular destruction	All Hurley stages	None	• Patient discomfort • Requires more than one treatment
Topical PDT	C	Tissue debulking or destruction and kill bacteria	Patients with superficial lesions	Incubation period of photosensitizer	• Patient discomfort • Requires more than one treatment
Intralesional PDT	C	Tissue debulking or destruction and kill bacteria	Patients with deep sinus tracts	Incubation period of photosensitizer	Patient discomfort, risk of infection
Nonablative Radiofrequency	C	Decrease sebaceous gland activity	All Hurley stages	None	Patient discomfort
Ablative Radiofrequency	C	Tissue debulking or destruction	Patients with deep sinus tracts	Intralesional anesthesia pre-procedure	Patient discomfort, risk of infection and burn
IPL	C	Follicular destruction and decrease inflammation	All Hurley stages	None	Patient discomfort
External Beam Radiation	C	Tissue destruction	Patients who have failed other treatments	None	Patient discomfort, risk of secondary malignancy

CO_2, Carbon dioxide; *IPL,* intense pulsed light; *Nd:YAG,* neodymium-doped yttrium aluminum garnet laser; *PDT,* photodynamic therapy.

Fractionated

CO_2 laser can also be used in a fractionated setting to help improve disease severity and to loosen contractures secondary to scarring from HS or previous HS surgery. The fractionated setting involves creating many small microbeams with normal skin intervening, allowing for more rapid wound healing and less downtime. Several case studies have shown improvement in number and severity of HS lesions, chronic ulceration with granulation tissue, and scar contracture/mobility.[10–13]

Neodymium-doped Yttrium Aluminum Garnet Laser

The Nd:YAG laser is another modality that works by emitting wavelengths of light using crystals to generate heat and destroy cells.[1] In dermatology, this laser is typically used for laser hair removal or for the treatment of vascular lesions. For HS, this laser works by selective photothermolysis to target hair follicles, using melanin and water as a chromophore.[14] Because melanin and water both serve as chromophores, this treatment modality is recommended for patients of all Fitzpatrick skin phototypes and all Hurley stages.[14] A physician performing Nd:YAG on the axilla of a patient with Hurley stage 1 HS is shown in Video 25.1. Settings should be guided by the endpoint of delayed post-treatment perifollicular erythema or vaporization of hairs.[15] Several studies have demonstrated the effectiveness of Nd:YAG for the treatment of HS. A study of 22 patients with HS showed that 3 to 4 monthly 1064 nm Nd:YAG treatments led to clinical improvement and remission of disease for up to 2 months after treatments, and demonstrated that histologically, decreased inflammation and fibrosis were seen after 1 and 2 months, respectively.[14,16] Another study

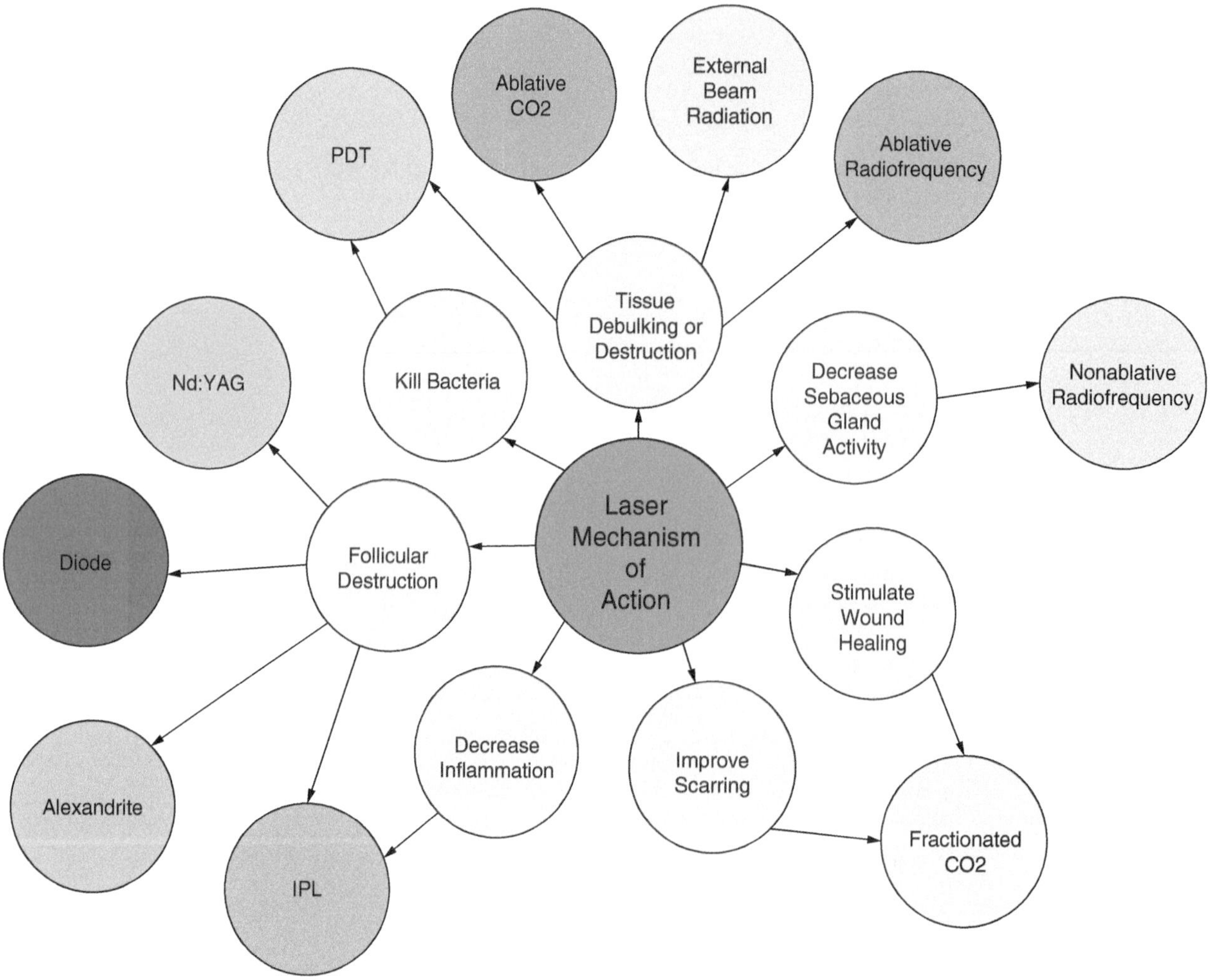

• **Fig. 25.1** Various Mechanism of Actions of Lasers and Light Treatments for Hidradenitis Suppurativa. *IPL*, Intense pulsed light; *Nd:YAG*, neodymium-doped yttrium aluminum garnet laser; *PDT*, photodynamic therapy.

examined the role of Nd:YAG to see if it could alter the course of the disease and found that when treating patients with Hurley stage I, the number of monthly flares and disease severity were reduced.[17]

Nd:YAG has also been used with CO_2 for refractory cases. A case series of four patients who underwent CO_2 deroofing alone had recurrence, but subsequently when Nd:YAG followed by CO_2 deroofing was performed, there was no recurrence for up to 3 years.[5] Another study found that combining fractional CO_2 laser with Nd:YAG was superior to Nd:YAG alone for improving HS symptoms, perhaps due to the increased depth of penetration of the Nd:YAG following fractional CO_2 treatment.[10]

Alexandrite Laser

Similar to Nd:YAG, alexandrite lasers (755 nm) use crystals to generate energy, have been used for laser hair removal, have little to no downtime, and have also been trialed for the treatment of HS through the mechanism of follicular destruction.[18] The 755 nm wavelength does have a higher degree of absorption by melanin

than 1064 nm devices. This may increase efficacy in skin phototypes 1 to 3 but also increases side effects in skin phototypes 4 to 6. Several case reports have reported improvement in HS severity using a variety of number of alexandrite laser treatments (1 to 11 sessions).[19-21] Due to increased depth of penetration of Nd:YAG compared to alexandrite, as well as randomized trials demonstrating effectiveness with Nd:YAG,[14] the authors prefer Nd:YAG over alexandrite for treatment of patients with HS.

Diode Laser

Diode lasers use diodes rather than crystals to generate various wavelengths and have been used in small case series and case reports for the treatment of HS by way of follicular destruction.[22] Case reports have reported HS improvement using diode lasers (800 to 1450 nm) after four to six treatments.[23,24] Diode lasers have also been trialed intralesionally for HS. In a study of 20 patients who received intralesional 1064 nm diode laser treatment every 2 weeks for four treatments, 65% of patients achieved Hidradenitis Suppurativa Clinical Response (HiSCR).[22]

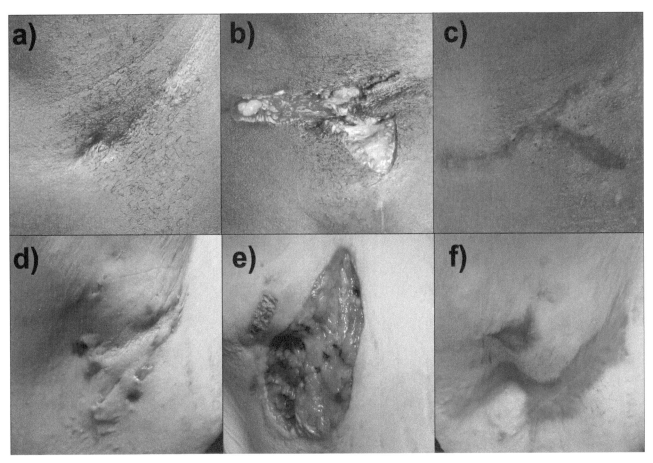

• **Fig. 25.2** (A) African American patient's axilla with sinus tract before, (B) immediately after, (C) 6 months postoperatively with scar formation after CO_2 surgery, and (D) Caucasian patient's axilla with sinus tracts before, (E) immediately after, and (F) 5 months postoperatively with scar formation after CO_2 surgery.

Photodynamic Therapy

Photodynamic therapy (PDT) is a light treatment in which a photosensitizer is applied to the skin, followed by exposure to a light source. This produces reactive oxygen species and subsequent cell death. In HS, this causes destruction of HS lesions and kills bacteria/biofilms.[25] Methyl aminolevulinate (MAL) and 5-aminolevulinic acid (ALA) are the most common photosensitizers used in the United States and have been trialed topically as well as intralesionally for HS.

Topical

Topical PDT studies for HS have yielded variable results. Topical PDT has been successful in small case series and case reports at reducing severity of HS in terms of lesion counts, Dermatology Life Quality Index (DLQI), and pain in some patients.[26–31] For topical PDT for HS, 4% to 25% ALA can be applied for 45 minutes to 4 hours prior to irradiation with either a red or blue light source at 1 to 2 week intervals for a total of two to nine treatments.[26–31] In contrast, other studies have reported no clinical improvement, and patients reported intense pain during treatment.[32–34]

Intralesional

Intralesional PDT allows for deeper penetration of the photosensitizer and has shown more promising results. This modality is best when used for deeper sinus tracts and involves insertion of a fiber optic probe into the tract. In one study, 29/38 patients achieved complete response to intralesional 5% ALA-PDT (delivered via an injection into solitary nodules or through a plastic cannula into sinus tracts) incubated for 2 hours and then irradiated through a fiber optic probe of 400 μm inserted within a centimeter marked needle after only 1 treatment, with an average DLQI improvement of 10 points.[35] Another study of patients who underwent intralesional 1% ALA-PDT incubated for 3 hours prior to irradiation found that 26/27 had at least a partial improvement.[36] A similar study with methylene blue (MB)-PDT had 5/7 patients achieving remission in the treated area at 6 months.[37] Reported side effects to intralesional PDT included pain, erythema, and edema.

Radiofrequency

Nonablative

Nonablative radiofrequency has been shown to improve acne severity in previous studies by decreasing sebaceous gland activity and volume.[38] Because of this, radiofrequency has also been tried for HS. A patient with HS who underwent nonablative radiofrequency treatment every 2 months for a total of three treatments reported significant improvement in symptoms after the first treatment with no new lesions developing during that time.[39]

Ablative

Radiofrequency ablation has been used to treat varicose veins, as well as benign and malignant tumors, and has also been tried for

HS. Intralesional ablative radiofrequency involves inserting an insulated probe into the deep dermal or subcutaneous lesions for direct destruction and tissue necrosis. In a case of one patient with HS who underwent one ablative radiofrequency treatment, the patient reported "complete improvement" at a 5-month follow-up.[40]

Intense Pulse Light

Intense pulse light (IPL) uses a broad spectrum pulsed light source to emit wavelengths that are absorbed by various chromophores including hemoglobin, melanin, and water.[41] It is typically used to treat dermatologic vascular lesions, acne, conditions with irregular pigmentation, and hypertrichosis. Because IPL has anti-inflammatory effects and causes follicular destruction, it has been used as a potential treatment modality for HS.

A prospective study of 18 patients had a 33% reduction in Sartorius score after IPL (420 nm) two times per week for 4 weeks.[42] An additional case series of two patients had complete resolution of inflammation and pain after four sessions of IPL (500 nm) at 15 to 20 days intervals.[43] The combination of IPL with radiofrequency has also been trialed. A recent prospective study of 47 patients found that the combination of IPL plus radiofrequency was better than radiofrequency or IPL alone when it came to DLQI and active lesion numbers.[44]

External Beam Radiation

External beam radiation works by damaging DNA and thus results in local destruction of tissue.[45] External beam radiation has been used in select cases for treatment refractory cases for destruction of HS affected tissue. Doses from studies and case series range from 3 to 8 Gy with improvement in some patients and treatment sites, but not in others.[46–48] In one study of 231 patients, 38% had complete symptom relief, while 40% had partial improvement.[46] However, this modality is not recommended as a first line treatment due to the potential for development of secondary malignancies.

Conclusion

Laser and light treatments are a viable option as a single treatment or adjunct to topical, intralesional, systemic, or surgical treatments. Often, incorporation of these energy-based modalities along with other treatments in a multimodality approach is recommended. Laser/light treatments have the advantage of no systemic side effects and require less downtime compared to surgery. Because most information is gleaned from case reports and case series, larger, randomized controlled trials are warranted. In addition, outcome measures vary greatly between trials, with some documenting lesion counts while others grade overall severity, making comparisons between treatments difficult. An individualized treatment approach to each patient is needed to come up with an ideal management plan.

References

1. Hamzavi IH, Griffith JL, Riyaz F, et al. Laser and light-based treatment options for hidradenitis suppurativa. *J Am Acad Dermatol.* 2015;73(5 Suppl 1):S78–S81. https://doi.org/10.1016/j.jaad.2015.07.050.

2. Dalrymple J, Monaghan J. Treatment of hidradenitis suppurativa with the carbon dioxide laser. *Br J Surg.* 1987;74(5):420.

3. Alikhan A, Sayed C, Alavi A, et al. North American clinical management guidelines for hidradenitis suppurativa: a publication from the United States and Canadian Hidradenitis Suppurativa Foundations: Part I: Diagnosis, evaluation, and the use of complementary and procedural management. *J Am Acad Dermatol.* 2019;81(1):76–90. https://doi.org/10.1016/j.jaad.2019.02.067.

4. Madan V, Hindle E, Hussain W, August P. Outcomes of treatment of nine cases of recalcitrant severe hidradenitis suppurativa with carbon dioxide laser. *Br J Dermatol.* 2008;159(6):1309–1314.

5. Mikkelsen PR, Dufour DN, Zarchi K, Jemec GB. Recurrence rate and patient satisfaction of CO_2 laser evaporation of lesions in patients with hidradenitis suppurativa: a retrospective study. *Dermatol Surg.* 2015;41(2):255–260.

6. Hazen PG, Hazen BP. Hidradenitis suppurativa: successful treatment using carbon dioxide laser excision and marsupialization. *Dermatol Surg.* 2010;36(2):208–213.

7. Lapins J, Marcusson J, Emtestam L. Surgical treatment of chronic hidradenitis suppurativa: CO_2 laser stripping-secondary intention technique. *Br J Dermatol.* 1994;131(4):551–556.

8. Lapins J, Sartorius K, Emtestam L. Scanner-assisted carbon dioxide laser surgery: a retrospective follow-up study of patients with hidradenitis suppurativa. *J Am Acad Dermatol.* 2002;47(2):280–285.

9. Jain V, Jain A. Use of lasers for the management of refractory cases of hidradenitis suppurativa and pilonidal sinus. *J Cutan Aesthet Surg.* 2012;5(3):190–192. https://doi.org/10.4103/0974-2077.101377.

10. Abdel Azim AA, Salem RT, Abdelghani R. Combined fractional carbon dioxide laser and long-pulsed neodymium: yttrium-aluminium-garnet (1064 nm) laser in treatment of hidradenitis suppurativa; a prospective randomized intra-individual controlled study. *Int J Dermatol.* 2018;57(9):1135–1144. https://doi.org/10.1111/ijd.14075.

11. Cho SB, Jung JY, Ryu DJ, et al. Effects of ablative 10,600-nm carbon dioxide fractional laser therapy on suppurative diseases of the skin: a case series of 12 patients. *Lasers Surg Med.* 2009;41(8):550–554.

12. Krakowski AC, Admani S, Uebelhoer NS, et al. Residual scarring from hidradenitis suppurativa: fractionated CO_2 laser as a novel and noninvasive approach. *Pediatrics.* 2014;133(1):e248–e251.

13. Nicholson CL, Hamzavi I, Ozog DM. Rapid healing of chronic ulcerations and improvement in range of motion after fractional carbon dioxide (CO_2) treatment after CO_2 excision of hidradenitis suppurativa axillary lesions: a case report. *JAAD Case Rep.* 2016;2(1):4–6.

14. Xu LY, Wright DR, Mahmoud BH, et al. Histopathologic study of hidradenitis suppurativa following long-pulsed 1064-nm Nd:YAG laser treatment. *Arch Dermatol.* 2011;147(1):21–28. https://doi.org/10.1001/archdermatol.2010.245.

15. Tierney E, Mahmoud BH, Hexsel C, et al. Randomized control trial for the treatment of hidradenitis suppurativa with a neodymium-doped yttrium aluminium garnet laser. *Dermatol Surg.* 2009;35(8):1188–1198. https://doi.org/10.1111/j.1524-4725.2009.01214.x.

16. Mahmoud BH, Tierney E, Hexsel CL, et al. Prospective controlled clinical and histopathologic study of hidradenitis suppurativa treated with the long-pulsed neodymium:yttrium-aluminium-garnet laser. *J Am Acad Dermatol.* 2010;62(4):637–645. https://doi.org/10.1016/j.jaad.2009.07.048.

17. Vossen A, van der Zee HH, Terian M, et al. Laser hair removal alters the disease course in mild hidradenitis suppurativa. *J Dtsch Dermatol Ges.* 2018;16(7):901–903. https://doi.org/10.1111/ddg.13563.

18. Nistico SP, Del Duca E, Farnetani F, et al. Removal of unwanted hair: efficacy, tolerability, and safety of long-pulsed 755-nm alexandrite laser equipped with a sapphire handpiece. *Lasers Med Sci.* 2018;33(7):1479–1483. https://doi.org/10.1007/s10103-018-2503-z.

19. Chan JY. Long-pulsed alexandrite laser for treatment of hidradenitis suppurativa. *J Am Acad Dermatol.* 2013;68(4).

20. Koch D, Pratsou P, Szczecinska W, et al. The diverse application of laser hair removal therapy: a tertiary laser unit's experience with less common indications and a literature overview. *Lasers Med Sci.* 2015;30(1):453–467. https://doi.org/10.1007/s10103-013-1464-5.

21. Pratsou P, Koch D, Szczecinska W, et al. The diverse application of laser hair removal: experience from a single laser unit. *Br J Dermatol.* 2012;167:94–95.

22. Fabbrocini G, Franca K, Lotti T, et al. Intralesional Diode Laser 1064 nm for the Treatment of Hidradenitis Suppurativa: A Report of Twenty Patients. *Open Access Maced J Med Sci.* 2018;6(1):31–34. https://doi.org/10.3889/oamjms.2018.045.

23. Downs A. Smoothbeam laser treatment may help improve hidradenitis suppurativa but not Hailey-Hailey disease. *J Cosmet Laser Ther.* 2004;6(3):163–164. https://doi.org/10.1080/14764170410003002.

24. Sehgal VN, Verma P, Sawant S, Paul M. Contemporary surgical treatment of hidradenitis suppurativa (HS) with a focus on the use of the diode hair laser in a case. *J Cosmet Laser Ther.* 2011;13(4):180–190. https://doi.org/10.3109/14764172.2011.594066.

25. Tricarico PM, Zupin L, Ottaviani G, et al. Photobiomodulation as potential novel third line tool for non-invasive treatment of Hidradenitis Suppurativa. *G Ital Dermatol Venereol.* 2020;155(1):88–98. https://doi.org/10.23736/s0392-0488.19.06247-3.

26. Andino Navarrete R, Hasson Nisis A, Parra Cares J. (2014). Effectiveness of 5-aminolevulinic acid photodynamic therapy in the treatment of hidradenitis suppurativa: a report of 5 cases. *Actas Dermosifiliogr.* 2015;105(6):614–617. https://doi.org/10.1016/j.ad.2013.10.016.

27. Gold M, Bridges TM, Bradshaw VL, Boring M. ALA-PDT and blue light therapy for hidradenitis suppurativa. *J Drugs Dermatol.* 2004;3(1 Suppl):S32–S35.

28. Guglielmetti A, Bedoya J, Acuna M, et al. Successful aminolevulinic acid photodynamic therapy for recalcitrant severe hidradenitis suppurativa. *Photodermatol Photoimmunol Photomed.* 2010;26(2):110–111. https://doi.org/10.1111/j.1600-0781.2010.00499.x.

29. Saraceno R, Teoli M, Casciello C, Chimenti S. Methyl aminolaevulinate photodynamic therapy for the treatment of hidradenitis suppurativa and pilonidal cysts. *Photodermatol Photoimmunol Photomed.* 2009;25(3):164–165. https://doi.org/10.1111/j.1600-0781.2009.00428.x.

30. Schweiger ES, Riddle CC, Aires DJ. Treatment of hidradenitis suppurativa by photodynamic therapy with aminolevulinic acid: preliminary results. *J Drugs Dermatol.* 2011;10(4):381–386.

31. Zhang Y, Yang Y, Zou X. Photodynamic therapy for Hidradenitis Suppurativa/acne inversa: Case report. *Photodiagnosis Photodyn Ther.* 2018;22:251–252. https://doi.org/10.1016/j.pdpdt.2018.04.014.

32. Passeron T, Khemis A, Ortonne JP. Pulsed dye laser-mediated photodynamic therapy for acne inversa is not successful: a pilot study on four cases. *J Dermatolog Treat.* 2009;20(5):297–298. https://doi.org/10.1080/09546630902882063.

33. Sotiriou E, Apalla Z, Maliamani F, Ioannides D. Treatment of recalcitrant hidradenitis suppurativa with photodynamic therapy: report of five cases. *Clin Exp Dermatol.* 2009;34(7):e235–e236. https://doi.org/10.1111/j.1365-2230.2008.03094.x.

34. Strauss RM, Pollock B, Stables GI, Goulden V, Cunliffe WJ. Photodynamic therapy using aminolaevulinic acid does not lead to clinical improvement in hidradenitis suppurativa. *Br J Dermatol.* 2005;152(4):803–804. https://doi.org/10.1111/j.1365-2133.2005.06475.x.

35. Suarez Valladares MJ, Eiris Salvado N, Rodriguez Prieto MA. Treatment of hidradenitis suppurativa with intralesional photodynamic therapy with 5-aminolevulinic acid and 630nm laser beam. *J Dermatol Sci.* 2017;5(3):241–246. https://doi.org/10.1016/j.jdermsci.2016.12.014.

36. Valladares-Narganes LM, Rodriguez-Prieto MA, Blanco-Suarez MD, et al. Treatment of hidradenitis suppurativa with intralesional photodynamic therapy using a laser diode attached to an optical cable: a promising new approach. *Br J Dermatol.* 2015;172(4):1136–1139. https://doi.org/10.1111/bjd.13385.

37. Agut-Busquet E, Romani J, Gilaberte Y, et al. Photodynamic therapy with intralesional methylene blue and a 635 nm light-emitting diode lamp in hidradenitis suppurativa: a retrospective follow-up study in 7 patients and a review of the literature. *Photochem Photobiol Sci.* 2016;15(8):1020–1028. https://doi.org/10.1039/c6pp00082g.

38. Ruiz-Esparza J, Gomez JB. Nonablative radiofrequency for active acne vulgaris: the use of deep dermal heat in the treatment of moderate to severe active acne vulgaris (thermotherapy): a report of 22 patients. *Dermatol Surg.* 2003;29(4):333–339. discussion 339.

39. Iwasaki J, Marra DE, Fincher EF, Moy RL. Treatment of hidradenitis suppurativa with a nonablative radiofrequency device. *Dermatol Surg.* 2008;34(1):114–117. https://doi.org/10.1111/j.1524-4725.2007.34025.x.

40. Subhadarshani S, Gupta V, Taneja N, et al. Efficacy and Safety of a Novel Method of Insulated Intralesional Radiofrequency Ablation for Deep Dermal and Subcutaneous Lesions: A 3-Year Institutional Experience. *Dermatol Surg.* 2018;44(5):714–720. https://doi.org/10.1097/dss.0000000000001437.

41. Ciocon DH, Boker A, Goldberg DJ. Intense pulsed light: what works, what's new, what's next. *Facial Plast Surg.* 2009;25(5):290–300.

42. Highton L, Chan WY, Khwaja N, Laitung J. Treatment of hidradenitis suppurativa with intense pulsed light: a prospective study. *Plast Reconstr Surg.* 2011;128(2):459–466.

43. Piccolo D, Di Marcantonio D, Crisman G, et al. Unconventional use of intense pulsed light. *Biomed Res Int.* 2014;2014:618206.

44. Wilden S, Friis M, Tuettenberg A, et al. Combined treatment of hidradenitis suppurativa with intense pulsed light (IPL) and radiofrequency (RF). *J Dermatolog Treat.* 2019;1–8. https://doi.org/10.1080/09546634.2019.1677842.

45. Myers JN, Mason AR, Gillespie LK, Salkey KS. Treatment of acne conglobata with modern external beam radiation. *J Am Acad Dermatol.* 2010;62(5):861–863. https://doi.org/10.1016/j.jaad.2009.06.031.

46. Frohlich D, Baaske D, Glatzel M. Radiotherapy of hidradenitis suppurativa—still valid today? *Strahlenther Onkol.* 2000;176(6):286–289.

47. Patel SH, Robbins JR, Hamzavi I. Radiation therapy for chronic hidradenitis suppurativa. *J Nuc Med Radiat Ther.* 2013;4:146.

48. Trombetta M, Werts ED, Parda D. The role of radiotherapy in the treatment of hidradenitis suppurativa: case report and review of the literature. *Dermatol Online J.* 2010;16(2):16.

26

Hidradenitis Suppurativa—Other Procedural Treatments

BARRY I. RESNIK AND PAUL G. HAZEN

CHAPTER OUTLINE

Introduction

The treatments for hidradenitis suppurativa (HS) can generally be divided into those with pharmacologic focus, and those that are procedural. For milder Hurley stage I disease, management is usually medication-focused, and designed to control or prevent the inflammatory events. For more severe disease, the physical signs of scars, acute or persistent abscesses, nodules, and sinus tracts may be accompanied by symptoms of ongoing or acute pain, drainage, itching, and odor. It is therefore in the setting of incomplete control of either signs or symptoms of the disease that procedural management becomes an important option.

Procedural Options

Procedures may be categorized by their applications in (1) the acute manifestations of the disease, or (2) for chronic, persistent disease. When treating acute lesions, it is helpful to note that the intensity of inflammation alters the pH of the perifollicular dermis, leading to blunting of the effectiveness of local anesthetics. It is, therefore necessary to often administer a "ring" of anesthesia outside the inflamed lesion. Additionally, the presence of scarring, multilocular abscesses, or sinus tracts may limit anesthetic dispersal, and thereby reduce the effectiveness of anesthetic agents.

Treatment of the Acute Lesion

Management of the acute lesion can be pharmacologic, destructive, or ablative in nature.

Acute flares may be initially managed with medications, with treatment options including oral or intralesional anti-inflammatory agents, antibiotics with anti-inflammatory properties, or analgesics. The question of superinfection with bacterial pathogens should be considered; this may be suggested by the presence of prominent erythema and warmth surrounding the primary process, and/or increasing malodor. Culture, and treatment with appropriate antibacterial agents, may be warranted.

Procedural treatments may be considered for those lesions that might be uncontrolled with pharmacologic agents alone. Large abscesses, or lesions comprised of sinus tracts and/or scars, are especially not likely to be successfully managed with only pharmacologic therapy. Intralesional corticosteroids may help to reduce acute pain in the short term, but are often ineffective in acute, larger cavitary lesions.

Unroofing/Deroofing, Incision, and Drainage

Unroofing and incision and drainage (I&D) are most beneficial for the solitary abscess or tract; they are less effective in the more chronic lesions where there may be scarring, nodules, and sinus tracts. For management of larger, acute lesions, a procedure to facilitate release of the purulent material within an abscess is often associated with almost-immediate symptom improvement. I&D is usually effective in reducing acute pain, but is associated with significant risk of recurrence.[1] Unroofing, also known as deroofing, is generally more effective than I&D, and results in less risk of recurrent abscess formation. It may be helpful especially where there is a single cavitary abscess.[2] Unroofing/deroofing and I&D are discussed in detail in Chapters 22-24.

Other options for procedural treatment of HS lesions may be broadly categorized into two general choices: (1) destruction/ablation, or (2) removal. Destruction may be defined as the ablation of the inflammatory process, without physically removing tissue. Alternatively, physical removal of affected skin may be employed, with various options for wound-healing. Local anesthesia is appropriate for all these procedures.

Destruction

Destruction of the acute lesion attempts to produce controlled injury to the tissue, followed by healing with lesion resolution. Multiple approaches have been evaluated, including carbon dioxide laser ablation, radiotherapy, peeling agents, cryoinsufflation, and neurotoxins. Each of these will be reviewed, with strength of recommendations as noted in Table 26.1.

Treatment of the Chronic Lesions

Carbon Dioxide (CO_2) Laser Ablation

Laser ablation has the same goals as that noted with cryo- or electro- surgical approaches; that is, the destruction of the inflammatory process. Although potentially able to treat acute lesions, the treatment is largely reserved for Hurley stage II to III patients with chronic disease.

The principle of such treatment relies on the laser energy absorption by the moisture of skin, with the resultant thermal effects causing destruction of the targeted lesion. The technique is usually performed using local anesthesia. Patients may continue pharmacologic therapy without interruption.

In 1987, Darlymple and Monaghan described the use of CO_2 laser to ablate HS lesions in six patients with a variety of sites.[3] Subsequently, in 1991, Sherman and Reid reported using the CO_2 laser to treat large areas of the vulva in 11 patients, employing a combination of laser ablation and focal areas of laser excision.[4]

The technique is performed as follows. The visible and palpable margins of the lesion to be treated are identified. The laser parameters are set for scanning/defocused mode, to make repeated passes over the HS lesion. Treatment is continued until the delivery has reached the pre-set depth and margins of the affected lesion(s). All

elements of HS, including abscesses, nodules, scars and sinus tracts may be treated. Healing takes place by secondary intention.[5] The presence of thickened scars and/or extensive epithelial-lined sinus tracts may blunt the effects of the scanning laser.

The technique has been associated with good patient acceptance, acceptable qualities of healing, and improved comfort of treated areas.[6] However, recurrence rates approach 30%. A potential side effect is a post-operative flare of other involved areas.[5] Laser treatments for HS, including Nd:YAG, are further discussed in chapter 25.

Radiotherapy

Superficial x-ray therapy has been used for over 75 years to treat numerous dermatologic diseases. It was used to successfully treat dissecting cellulitis of the scalp[7,8] as well as axillary HS.[9–11] While superficial x-ray therapy fell out of favor in the 1970s, superficial radiotherapy is valuable for the subset of HS patients who have severe disease and have failed all other therapies. Today, electron beam therapy is the source of superficial radiotherapy, and has been used to successfully treat acne conglobata, axillary HS, and dissecting cellulitis of the scalp.[12,13]

Treatment of chronic lesions of HS with ionizing radiation has been suggested for recalcitrant lesions or for patients who may not be surgical candidates. X-ray therapy has been used to *treat areas* of variable size when such circumstances exist.[10,14,15] In 1950, Schenck reported a series of 54 patients treated three times per week for 5 to 10 treatments, with virtually all patients showing clinical improvement.[9] However, there is little published data in the recent literature addressing this modality, and older reports detail the results from treatment using orthovoltage.

Fröhlich et al. treated 231 HS patients with orthovoltage therapy using multiple fractionation regimens.[14] Of the total treated, complete amelioration of symptoms was seen in 38%, with an additional 40% seeing improvement. No side effects were noted. They felt their results warranted more attention to superficial radiotherapy as an effective treatment for severe HS.

Dissecting cellulitis of the scalp is quite difficult to treat. Chinnaiyan et al. treated four patients with electron beam and/or photon therapy.[13] All patients experienced significant pain reduction as well as decrease in drainage and nodule size. Because these patients already had significant hair loss secondary to scarring, dosing was selected not only to treat the inflammatory element but to also ensure as little residual hair growth as possible.

Myers et al. treated a 53-year-old man with long-standing severe acne conglobata and HS after the patient had failed multiple therapies.[12] The patient underwent several sessions of electron beam radiation to large plaques on the cheeks. At 3 weeks, cyst size, drainage, pain, and self-esteem were all improved. No dryness or pigmentary changes were noted. These changes persisted to the 5-month follow-up visit.

Trombetta et al. treated one patient with stage III HS, refractory to all other therapies.[16] Significant improvement was seen 3 weeks after treatment and was proven to be a durable change. Small persistent lesions were treated with additional fractions.

Patel et al. treated five patients suffering from severe refractory HS with various fractions of electron beam therapy to multiple areas.[17] Some response was noted in all patients 2 months after treatment, but only in the axillary region. No response was noted in the perineal areas. The authors suggest that the significant scarring in these areas was deeper than the radiotherapy could penetrate, thus compromising the effect. Prolonged follow-up was noted to be difficult, as all patients went on to receive different additional treatments for their HS.

TABLE 26-1 Procedural Modalities for Management of Acute and Chronic Lesions of Hidradenitis Suppurativa: Literature Review, to Determine Strength of Recommendation, Level of Evidence

Modality	Strength of Recommendation	Level of Evidence
Incision & Drainage	C	III
Unroofing/Deroofing	B	II
Cryosurgery	C	III
Cryoinsufflation	E	III
Peeling Agents	B	II
Neurotoxins	D	III
CO_2 Laser Excision	C	II
CO_2 Laser ablation	C	II
Staged CO_2 Laser Excision/ Marsupialization	C	II
Radiation	C	II

One case report detailed radiation treatment induction of HS.[18] The patient, a 52-year-old woman with axillary, inframammary fold and groin involvement, underwent 6 weeks of radiation therapy for breast ductal carcinoma in-situ (DCIS). She developed an HS flare only in the window of her radiation treatment. The authors post that the significantly higher dosing for DCIS induced a greater immune response leading to the flare. As a cautionary note, it is recognized that the clinical findings of HS may mimic clinical findings of metastatic breast cancer. Inflammatory lesions should have diagnostic pathologic findings before being considered for radiotherapy.

Superficial radiotherapy has played an important role in the treatment of HS for many years. There are few studies looking at large numbers of patients, and a long-term follow-up is not available for any of these patients. Most of the literature details treatment, specifically in severe refractory cases of HS. In 1965, Zeligman detailed his experience with a single dose of superficial x-ray therapy, which he felt would provide temporary epilation.[10] In his hands, this dose resulted in long-term resolution of chronic HS.

Unfortunately, there is a great deal of concern evinced by patients when superficial radiation treatment is offered as a treatment, whether for skin cancer or HS. This could be a reason why it is not offered or performed more often. There is a need for better optimization of regimens, which will be difficult to achieve because of such concerns. Patel et al. and Trombetta et al. both used similar regimens to effect change, which appears to have been efficacious.

The authors feel that superficial radiotherapy should be considered when the following criteria are observed: contraindication or failure of systemic therapy; significant and ongoing debilitation; age greater than 60; areas of involvement are so large and/or comorbidities preclude or mitigate against successful surgical therapy. One of us (BR) has used superficial radiotherapy to treat two patients, both with significant buttock and perirectal disease. Both patients were over the age of 60, had failed multiple therapies including several biologics, and their disease was not controllable with standard therapy. It was felt that the benefits of the therapy outweighed the short and long-term risks. In both cases, significant decrease in discharge and pain were noted within 2 weeks of treatment and persisted after treatment for at least 1.5 years. One patient refused additional treatment but offered no criticism of the superficial radiotherapy he had previously received. The other patient's treated disease remained in remission but the patient died of unrelated causes.

A caution, based upon personal observation, is that newer radiation delivery modalities have the potential to be highly penetrative, and that the use of such therapy has the potential to cause injury to deeper structures. Since the localization of HS is largely dermal, such depth may not be needed for clinical response. In some patients, skin breakdown and delayed healing have been noted (PH personal observation). Currently, there is inadequate data to evaluate such therapy.

Peeling Agents

Resorcinol, a vitamin A derivative, is the only peeling agent reported in the literature as a treatment for HS. The suggestion that HS is a disease in which follicular occlusion plays a part suggests that topical keratolytic like resorcinol and retinoids could represent a logical treatment. Topical retinoids such as adapalene, tazarotene, and tretinoin have long been used for their keratolytic action in acne, but there are no studies of these medicines in HS, perhaps because they do not have enough peeling effect.[19]

Based on several case reports showing resorcinol to be of help in HS,[20,21] an open trial was created to evaluate resorcinol cream's ability to mitigate flares and reduce pain.[22] The study looked at 12 patients with Hurley stage I or II disease. All participants had significant flares and a high pain score. Resorcinol 15% cream was applied twice daily when flares began and could be used once daily as maintenance. Most reported significant pain reduction within 2 days of inception. Breakthrough flares were more easily controlled with the topical resorcinol. While the topical had little control on limiting the number of flares, they were more easily controlled when they did occur, and pain levels were significantly reduced.

In a more recent study, resorcinol 15% was again evaluated in an open trial of Hurley stage I and II patients, using both clinical and ultrasonographic measures.[23] A total of 32 patients were evaluated. Topical resorcinol was again shown to reduce pain and clinical size of the treated lesions. However, ultrasound showed persistence of inflammation after it was clinically resolved, suggesting incomplete response.

The mechanism of action for resorcinol is its putative keratolytic action. However, other factors may be at work. Resorcinol is a derivative of phenol, which is well-known for its topical anesthetic effects.[24] This may be the reason for its ability to ameliorate pain when used topically in HS, while its keratolytic action mitigated flares. Resorcinol cream appears to offer real effect regarding pain control and reduction of acute flares. However, resorcinol USP is no longer available in the United States, due to a lack of manufacturers, and there appears to be no change in these circumstances expected in the immediate future.

Cryoinsufflation

Although generally suggested for more chronic HS lesions, cryodestruction can also be used as an ablative therapy for acute lesions. The agent may be delivered by spray or through direct contact with a cotton-tipped applicator. It has generally been recommended for smaller lesions, and in the experience of the authors, may require multiple applications to achieve complete resolution.[25]

Cryoinsufflation was introduced to help those patients suffering from stage II or III HS and who could not use or tolerate systemic medical therapies, or who had chosen to defer or had failed other surgical techniques. Pagliarello et al. published the first paper in 2014, detailing two patients who desired definitive treatment but were not able to tolerate standard medical therapies.[26]

The technique is straightforward (Video 26.1). A hollow needle or catheter is placed within a tract and liquid nitrogen is introduced via a standard cryo-gun and a Luer-lock attachment. The gas expands to pass through and fill the existing tracts, and then advances through distant fistulous openings to the exterior. Treatments are repeated up to three times at monthly intervals to allow for the greatest healing. Both patients in the original paper[26] achieved clearance of the localized disease treated, with no additional scarring or color change. Local anesthesia was used and gave adequate pain control. Post-procedural pain was reported to be minimal and managed with paracetamol (acetaminophen).

In 2015, the same group presented some technical refinements to the original procedure. These changes were prompted by concerns for air embolus and necrosis at the entry points. The possibility that the needle could potentially be advanced into the subcutaneous space, and redirect gas flow from the tunnels into the subcutaneous space, was worrisome. The use of a 21–gauge olive–tipped catheter was proposed, which, with its blunted tip, would obviate the concern for placing the gas in the subcutaneous space. A chlorhexidine solution was sprayed onto the site to gauge gas outflow by the appearance of bubbles at points of exit.[27]

There was also concern that the use of metal needles might produce necrosis at the entry points as a result of ice-ball formation where the needle shaft meets the overlying skin. Short pulses of liquid nitrogen would seemingly serve to reduce the possibility of formation, while allowing enough gas to traverse the tunnels. The use of small plastic intravenous catheters was alternately proposed in an attempt to decrease the likelihood of formation of ice–balls at the entry points.

In 2019, Daveluy suggested that cryoinsufflation might be a valuable diagnostic tool in other surgical approaches such as unroofing and CO_2 staged marsupialization. Running liquid nitrogen through the affected skin would help delineate the area to be treated, and possibly reveal tracts not obvious to palpation.[28]

In an interesting modification to the standard technique of I&D, Molina-Leyva et al. reported a technique using liquid nitrogen for either acute or chronic abscesses of HS.[29] After the contents of an abscess were drained, liquid nitrogen was used to scar the pocket closed. A 4 to 5 mm disposable punch biopsy trocar was used to incise the abscess. The abscess contents were drained and the resultant pocket flushed with saline. The trocar was then reintroduced, and liquid nitrogen was introduced into the pocket by the simple expedient of placing the tip of the cryosurgical unit flush to the rear handle opening of the hollow trocar. They used 5 second applications, repeated twice. The area was then drained with the drain hole left open. Complete resolution, defined as no inflammatory signs observed, and no persistence of fluid collection noted by clinical and ultrasound examination, was achieved in 70% (7/10) of the treated lesions in one month. Post-procedural pain was minimal, and no adverse effects were noted in the treated population.

This technique is relatively straightforward and is not equipment intensive. One of us (BR) has used it for a number of patients since it was delineated, with variable results. Patients whose circumstances would make them good candidates for cryoinsufflation most often had so much involvement that it precluded use of the technique. Those who completed the course of treatment were uniformly pleased with the results. Although there is relatively little published data, the authors believe that it should be included in the procedural options for appropriate patients. A cautionary note reflects the observation that the contents of the abscess or scarred tract being treated will be expelled along with the gas. Placing a gauze over the treated area while injecting the gas will contain any expelled contents.

Neurotoxins

Neurotoxins such as onabotulinum toxin A and abobotulinum toxin A have shown some positive effect in the treatment of HS. The mechanism of action is proposed to be a downregulation of apocrine gland function, possibly reducing the potential for follicular occlusion.[30] Alternatively, reduction of sweating may change the environment by reducing humidification.

Neurotoxin was first used in 2005 to treat a young woman with HS (stage not noted).[30] Its use was prompted by symptoms of hyperhidrosis, although a diagnosis of focal hyperhidrosis had not been made. A total of 250 units of abobotulinum toxin A was used for both axillae and the patient experienced a cessation of symptoms beginning 2 weeks after injection, and lasting for 10 months.

In 2009, onabotulinum toxin A was used in a 7-year-old girl with stage I HS who had failed several topical and oral therapies.[31] A total of 40 units was injected in both inguinal folds in the standard 1 cm point model used in hyperhidrosis. She experienced 6 months of remission. A few lesions occurring towards the end of that period responded to a second treatment in the same way as the first.

Khoo and Burova reported on their results with botulinum toxin A in three patients.[32] Their most successful case involved a 46-year-old woman with stage II disease who had failed numerous topical and oral therapies. Noting the presence of hyperhidrosis in the axillae, onabotulinum toxin A 50 units was injected in each axilla. She showed some response and went into remission after the second treatment 3 months later, and remained in remission and was discharged from follow-up after her fourth treatment. They note that this degree of response was not mirrored in their other two patients, although each experienced disease-free intervals of 5 to 6 months after treatment.

Successful use of onabotulinum toxin A in a 41-year-old woman with stage III HS and obesity has also been reported.[33] The patient had failed all treatments and presented to the authors' physical medicine and rehabilitation clinic for chronic pain management. She was initially treated with 400 units into the bilateral axillary and inframammary folds (100 units in each site). She had good response on follow-up and reported 50% pain relief. Additional injections at a dosage of 50 units per site showed effect, but symptoms returned more quickly. With resumption of 100 units per site administration, treatment was more successful, and she remained "open-wound-free" with periodic injection sessions. This success was notable as most of the previously reported patients had been stage I and II. Its success in a Stage III patient is exciting.

Campanati et al. treated two patients with botulinum toxin A, both Hurley stage II.[34] The first, with disease limited to the axillae, had failed topical and oral therapies. A dose of 50 units per axilla was used. The second patient had disease involving the groin and thighs. Topical and oral therapies did not reduce the pain and drainage. A dose of 100 units per area was used. Both patients experienced close to 10 months of little to no pain and no evidence of active disease. Like the results experienced in hyperhidrosis treatment, both patients began to experience recurrence of their disease symptoms at this time.

Based on these reports, botulinum toxin A and B remain viable options for both pain and disease control. The treatment regimens differ wildly, as do the unit counts. Because the areas are those concomitantly involved in hyperhidrosis, a starting point for standardization would be dosing used in that disease, typically a 5cc dilution resulting in a 2 units per 0.1cc dosing scheme. The authors' experience and communications among US colleagues regarding the use and success of botulinum toxin A and B in the treatment of their HS patients reveals that it is rarely used. When it is used, it does not deliver the dramatic effects evident in the literature. Standardization of treatment regimens may help augment its success. However, significant financial barriers to the wide-spread use of neurotoxins exist in the United States and many other countries. This technique is off-label for HS and is usually denied by insurance companies and governmental health benefit payers. It is expensive if paid for privately, and patients may have unreasonable expectations if an expensive therapy requires multiple sessions to generate variable results.

Excision/Removal

Wide Local Excision

Wide local excision has been the most common surgical treatment in patients with chronic or extensive disease. It will be discussed in detail in Chapters 23 and 24.

Electrosurgical Stripping Excision

A procedure similar to scalpel excision, skin tissue-saving excision with electrosurgical peeling (STEEP) employs electrosurgical instrumentation to remove diseased tissue in a tangential, stepwise fashion. The goals are preservation of unaffected tissue and the production of improved healing.[35] This technique is also discussed in Chapter 24.

CO2 Laser Excision

In 1996, Finley and Ratz reported the use of CO_2 laser to excise lesions of HS in 7 patients and 12 sites. A single recurrence was reported in follow-up of 10 to 27 months.[36] Additionally, in 2008, Madan et al. reported similar results in 9 patients involving 27 sites treated with laser-excision.[37]

In contrast to carbon dioxide laser ablation, CO_2 laser excision uses the energy of the instrument in focused mode to excise individual lesion(s) of HS. It is primarily indicated for Hurley stage II to III lesions that are refractory to pharmacological management. After determining a pre-surgical margin, the laser is used as a cutting tool to carry out the removal process; it is similar in concept to that performed using scalpel excision or electrosurgical stripping.

The technique generally used is as follows. The margins of the individual lesion are defined, and local anesthesia administered. The CO_2 laser is then used in continuous, cutting mode as a scalpel to excise the delineated lesion. It is not used to address an entire physical unit, such as an axillary or groin plaque. It differs from CO_2 laser ablation in that the energy is delivered in focused mode, and that affected tissue is physically removed. Healing generally takes place by secondary intention. The procedure is associated with high patient satisfaction and good qualities of wound healing.

Staged CO2 Laser Marsupialization

En bloc excision with primary closure is the most common surgical procedure performed for patients with HS and is designed to remove the scarred skin in a large block, including a significant amount of subcutaneous tissue. The extent of surgery is driven by visual assessment, palpation and inspection for possible sinus tracts. The resulting defect is then primarily closed with sutures, staples, split-thickness skin graft, or a musculocutaneous flap. The healing process may be long and involved, with bed rest and wound vacs the norm. Postoperative complications including wound dehiscence, graft and flap failures, infections, and reduced range of motion are common. Recurrence rates after excision and primary closure are high, ranging from 20% to 70%, and the resulting scars can be quite disfiguring.[38–40]

In 2010, Hazen and Hazen reported success in managing a series of 61 patients with CO_2 laser using a technique they termed excision and marsupialization. Patient selection was based on physical findings as well as symptoms of pain, drainage, odor, itching, the frequency and severity of flares, and the degree of functional impairment as reflected by the Dermatologic Life Quality Index (DLQI) score. The procedure used the CO_2 laser as a cutting tool, followed by the intrasurgical evaluation and removal of occult areas of HS. The procedure resulted in a pocket-like (marsupial) defect. The technique had the advantages of office delivery, local anesthesia, minimal surgical complications, and low recurrence rates. Areas treated included the axilla, groin, vulva, perirectal skin, scrotum, abdomen, breast, neck, scalp, and face. Recurrence rates were less than 2%.[41]

Since the original description, the authors have had significant opportunity to perform and evaluate this technique. This highly regarded procedure is predicated on the observation that HS begins within the mid deep dermis and is concentrated within the skin. It is not a primary disease of the subcutaneum or muscle.

Medical therapy is intended to suppress as completely as possible the chronic inflammatory nature of the disease. However, the scarred, oozing disfiguring plaques will almost always be a source of pain. The ability to eliminate the plaques and nodules reduces the burden of HS in a patient. Frequently, all physical evidence of disease can be removed in patients who undergo the procedure. Many of these patients can stop all medicines, with the understanding that suppressive therapy may be reinstituted at the onset of a new inflammatory lesion.

Almost all patients with scarred plaques, nodules and sinus tracts are candidates for this surgical procedure. It is therefore usually reserved for Hurley stage II or III disease. Most patients are candidates for in-office surgery under local anesthesia. In our experience, lidocaine with epinephrine or tumescent anesthesia, which may be coupled with inhaled nitrous oxide or oral anxiolytics, make the procedure more comfortable for both patient and surgeon. General anesthesia may be needed for those patients with recurrence in an area of previous surgical treatment, as adequate anesthesia can be difficult to achieve in these areas due to scar tissue blocking diffusion into all targeted areas. Many patients will require general anesthesia for extensive disease, or extensive perianal, vaginal, and scrotal involvement. Patients with significant surgical anxiety or allergies to the components of local anesthesia may also desire general anesthesia.

Contraindications to treatment primarily relate to associated patient co-morbidities. Pre-surgical evaluation of clotting capabilities, as well as cardiovascular, endocrine, infectious, or wound and pain management issues should be performed. This is true especially if a general anesthesia is to be employed. The procedure is usually performed in an office setting using either intradermal or tumescent local anesthesia. If medically appropriate, anticoagulants may be withheld before and during surgery. It has always been the authors' practice to maintain all HS-suppressive medicines including biologics before, during, and after surgery. It has been observed that healing is more rapid with controlled disease. Both authors have a zero percent infection rate, which mitigates the prevailing and long-held fear that biologic medicines may precipitate infection in surgical wounds.

The extent and borders of HS lesions to be considered for surgery are determined by visual and palpatory evaluation. To improve the identification of occult disease, some investigators have suggested that injectable dye material be injected into prospective surgical lesions to further identify the extent and location of involved areas.[42] Recently, ultrasound of Hurley stage II to III lesions has confirmed the identification of dermal scars, abscesses, and interconnecting epithelial-lined sinus tracts.[43] Furthermore, evaluation of the ultrasound findings seems to be able to identify those patients, and occult areas, most likely to benefit from surgical intervention.[44] Whether the information gained with injectable dye or ultrasound will better guide the surgical process than the visual and palpatory examination is uncertain.

In contrast to pre-surgical dye or ultrasound evaluation of HS lesions, Staged CO_2 Laser Marsupialization uses an intrasurgical evaluation process to aid in the identification and treatment of affected areas. In concept, the technique is very similar to the standard of care for staged removal of cutaneous malignancies, Mohs micrographic surgery. Like Mohs, the concept is to intrasurgically identify occult areas of disease, thereby facilitating as complete a removal of HS tissue as possible, while preserving uninvolved tissue.

The surgery is performed as follows: The extent of the planned marsupialization is outlined with a skin marker. Local anesthesia is placed. Using the CO_2 laser in focused mode, a 2mm margin is used to excise the area of HS. Minimal bleeding and minimal tissue contraction allow for the preservation of the internal architecture of the wound. Additional areas of occult disease may be identified visually or with a probe or a 1mm ice-cream curette, which is used to "run the border," physically searching for additional missed tunnels (Video 26.2).

Four potential abnormalities may be noted on the underside of the plaque as it is carefully freed from the subcutaneous tissue:

1. A translucent, bubble-like outcropping or "bulge." This is usually seen to extend from the underside of the inflammatory mass.
2. Epithelial-lined sinus tracts. The extent and direction of such tracts may be identified by use of a 1mm ice-cream scoop curette placed within the lumen of the tract. Transit through the tract may identify a distant cutaneous exit point (Fig. 26.1).
3. A "Blind Loop": Marginal or deep extensions of epithelial-lined channels, without a distant exit point or overlying epidermal connection, may be identified (Figs. 26.2 and 26.3).
4. Marginal "pockets" may be identified (Figs. 26.4 and 26.5).

Using the laser in focused mode, these areas are then removed, focally enlarging the surgical defect by reflecting the flap and working "under" the extension until there is only fat at the base, creating a marsupialized (pocket) wound. Note that although the HS process is concentrated in the upper, mid, and lower dermis, there may be extensions that can be tracked

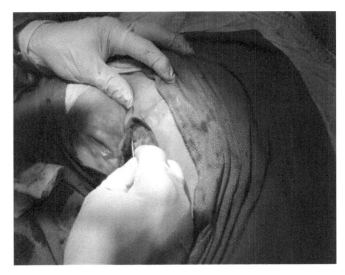
• **Fig. 26.2** Blind Loop Inner Thigh.

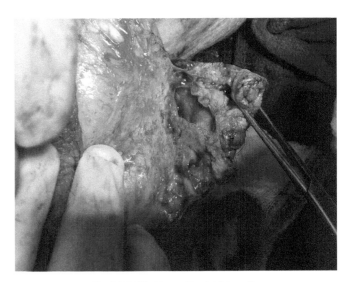
• **Fig. 26.3** Blind Loop Scrotal Dissection.

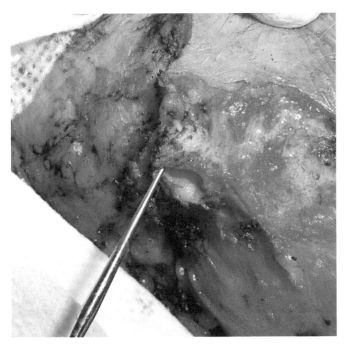
• **Fig. 26.1** Epithelial-lined Sinus Tract.

to the overlying follicular epithelium or more deeply into the subcutaneum. Involvement of the muscle is exceedingly rare. Elimination to the muscular fascia is generally necessary only in the axillary and scrotal areas. It is particularly important to be aware of the various tissue planes when working on the scrotum, as there is only skin, fascia, cremasteric muscle, and then scrotal fascia. It is important to frequently confirm that surgery is occurring in the proper plane, to both ensure removal of only diseased skin and confirm the integrity of the scrotal lining. (Video 26.3, Figs. 26.6–26.8) At completion of the marsupialization process, the laser is used in defocused mode to even the plane of the surgical base.

Because of the need for meticulous determination of occult disease, and because of the frequently large size and complexity of the areas needing treatment, such surgery is significantly more time-consuming than traditional dermatologic surgery. Additionally, prolonged patient healing time with large areas may make it impractical to remove the entirety of disease in a single surgical session. However, it is possible to return to the site to complete the

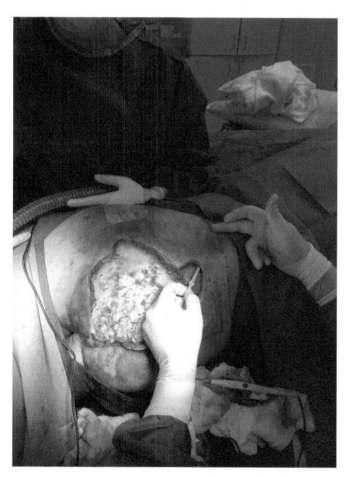

• **Fig. 26.4** Marginal Pocket Found Upon Second Evaluation.

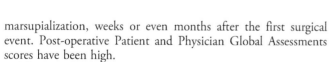

• **Fig. 26.5** Large Marginal Pocket Left Buttock.

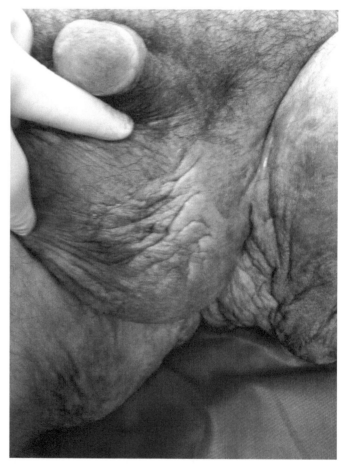

• **Fig. 26.6** Left Scrotal and Left Inguinal Fold/Inner Thigh Plaques Preoperative View.

marsupialization, weeks or even months after the first surgical event. Post-operative Patient and Physician Global Assessments scores have been high.

The post-operative wounds are dressed with petrolatum, non-stick pads, gauze and tape. Mesh tubing can be cut and worn across the chest and arm to support axillary dressings. Inguinal wounds benefit from disposable mesh underwear or compression boxer-briefs (both genders). Patients are urged to shower daily with the bandages in place, remove them while in the shower, and allow water to run over the areas. Microfiber towels are used to gently remove accumulated dressing. Extreme wound cleaning is not necessary and interrupts granulation. An impermeable barrier under the bedclothes will protect from incidental bleeding and leakage.

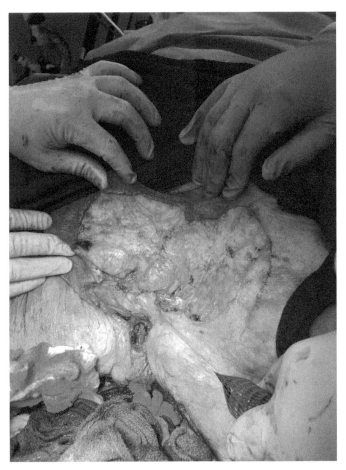

• **Fig. 26.7** Left Scrotal and Left Inguinal Fold/Inner Thigh Plaques Immediate Postoperative View.

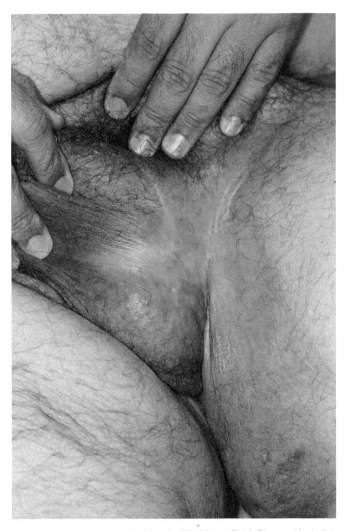

• **Fig. 26.8** Left Scrotal and Left Inguinal Fold/Inner Thigh Plaques Healed at 9 Months.

The more occluded the wound is kept, the less the wound will hurt. Granulation generally occurs in 2 weeks, and the dressing is changed from petrolatum to a barrier cream that is less greasy and just as occlusive.

Most patients are back to a reduced work schedule in 2 to 3 days. There are no movement restrictions; patients are urged to use common sense. Normal and natural movement will decrease the formation of adhesions in skin fold wounds and enhance range of motion when healed.

Post-operative complications are few and usually easily dealt with. Bleeding, if it occurs, is generally seen within the first 24 to 48 hours after the surgery. Prolonged healing time (9 to 16 weeks) is common with larger areas. Pain is generally most notable in the first 2 weeks. Hypertrophic granulation tissue may occur in 10% to 25% of patients and is usually managed with topical silver nitrate. Recurrence rates have generally been less than 2%, with follow-up of up to 17 years after surgery. A history of keloidal healing after previous surgery, or the presence of hypertrophic scars or keloids within sites of HS, has not been associated with post-treatment keloidal or hypertrophic scars. Wound contracture may occur, but in our experience has not been associated with compromised range of motion.

Post-operative infection has not been reported to date. Medications normally used to control the inflammatory lesions of HS, including the biologics, have not been associated with an increased incidence of postoperative infection or delayed healing. Rarely,

there may be a paradoxical flare of HS in non-contiguous areas post-operatively. Because the resulting scar has no follicles, the issue of new HS developing within the scar is moot. An occult blind pouch or tunnel, however, may develop and extend into the scar.

Prolonged healing can occur and last up to a year or more, but the sites are small and do not compromise the patient's ability to live life. Silver nitrate therapy, debridement with curettage, or primary excision with closure are all effective methods to treat this uncommon issue.

All patients are excited at the prospect of exchanging a leaking, oozing, ugly painful plaque of HS for a very cosmetically acceptable scar. Almost all of them note that the pain of healing after surgery is "one-tenth the pain of a flare."

Pearls for the Surgeon
• The intrasurgical findings of a "bulge" on the underside of involved areas of HS, or epithelial-lined sinus tracts, or the presence of "blind loops" of extended cavities, or the presence of small marginal pockets are all helpful guides in determining extent of HS needing removal.
• The use of tumescent anesthesia often ameliorates pain for up to 12 hours after surgery.

- Do not be daunted by overwhelming involvement that appears to be inoperable because of the size of the expected defect. Planning surgery in stages will allow treatment of even the largest areas.
- It is common for patients to want all areas removed at one time, secondary to financial burden and healing time requirements. It is wise to dissuade this approach and treat areas that experience dictates will be manageable for the patient.
- For patients with bilateral involvement of both axillae and groin, surgical treatment of the right axilla and right groin is easier to manage for the patient. Treating both underarms understandably makes it difficult if not impossible for the patient to manage alone. A dedicated spouse or significant other can make this work but is challenging for both patient and assistant when they are dealing with 24/7 care.
- Numbness of the skin of the upper inner arm or chest wall following treatment of axillary HS, or of the upper medial thigh after groin treatment, may occur. Such hypoesthesia may persist but usually improves over a period of 18 months.
- The surgical therapy of scrotal HS often requires treatment to the level of the cremasteric muscle but does not compromise scrotal contents. This area heals amazingly well, with excellent cosmesis and no functional impairment of the scrotal sac or its contents. HS can and does involve external labial skin. HS plaque can be removed up to the verge of the labia majora. However, HS seldom involves the vaginal mucosa. If sinus tracts should involve vaginal mucosa or extend deeply to the internal rectal sphincter, consider cutaneous Crohn's disease rather than HS.

Concomitant medical therapy, including biologic agents, should be continued without interruption before, during, and after surgery. The authors routinely work in "dirty" areas of the body, including perirectal, perineal, buttock, scrotal, and vaginal sites, and have never noted a post-operative infection. Maintaining disease suppression with biologics does not make it easier for infection to occur. Indeed, it appears to allow more rapid healing.

Summary

The selection of procedural care for the lesions of HS should be made based upon the acute versus chronic nature of the lesions, and the response of the patient to pharmacologic treatments. A summary of procedural treatments for HS is shown at the end of this chapter. While the stigmata of HS can look the same, its response to different treatments varies tremendously. Keeping all of these techniques on the palette of therapies allows us to give the best care to our patients. In our experience, staged CO_2 laser marsupialization has a 2% recurrence rate and a 0% infection rate. Healing is generally uncomplicated and does not require the patient to be immobile for any period of time. It will also dramatically reduce the burden of HS in patients. This burden is a very real weight on both the physical and mental well-being of people who suffer from HS. The ability to wear the clothes they desire, move freely without concern for bandages or stains on clothes, and be able to sit on furniture or a car seat without concern for staining is dramatically liberating. The simple act of raising one's arms to hug a loved one can now be a reality.

Summary of Procedural Options for Hidradenitis Suppurativa

These modalities should be used in conjunction with medical therapies and lifestyle modifications.

Acute Lesions

Goal of therapy is the relief of acute pain, drainage, or odor:
- Intralesional corticosteroids
- Peels with resorcinol: effective at pain reduction and some anti-inflammatory effect
- Incision and drainage: for painful, solitary abscess. Comment: There is a high risk of recurrence, but generally able to be performed quickly, and relieves acute pain.
- Unroofing/deroofing: Preferred over I&D for the painful, solitary abscess. Less effective in the setting of scarring, or multiple layers of sinus tract formation. It is more time-consuming, but more lastingly effective than I&D.
- Cryosurgical or electrosurgical destruction: Little data to determine effectiveness. Might be helpful in the small, thin inflammatory lesion.
- Nd:YAG laser: Appropriate for subacute, solitary or multiple lesions
- Double pulse each area to be treated. Treatment will depend on the availability of the laser. Management may require repeated sessions, at monthly intervals if lesions remain.
- CO_2 laser ablation: More likely to be helpful if the acute element is part of a larger chronic area of HS

Chronic Lesions

Goal of therapy is to give lasting resolution of inflammatory, scarred, draining areas:
- Intralesional corticosteroids
- Nd:YAG laser. Management may require repeated sessions, at monthly intervals
- Electrosurgical peeling
- Questionable effects: Cryosurgical or electrosurgical destruction: Little data to determine effectiveness. Might be helpful in the small, thin inflammatory lesion.
- Wide local excision
- CO_2 Laser ablation/destruction
- CO_2 Laser excision
- Staged CO_2 Laser marsupialization

References

1. Kohorst JJ, Baum CL, Otley CC, et al. Surgical Management of Hidradenitis Suppurativa: Outcomes of 590 Consecutive Patients. *Dermatol Surg.* 2016;42(9):1030–1040.
2. van der Zee HH, Prens EP, Boer J. Deroofing: a tissue-saving surgical technique for the treatment of mild to moderate hidradenitis suppurativa lesions. *J Am Acad Dermatol.* 2010;63(3):475–480.
3. Dalrymple JC, Monaghan JM. Treatment of hidradenitis suppurativa with the carbon dioxide laser. *Br J Surg.* 1987;74(5):420.
4. Sherman AI, Reid R. CO_2 laser for suppurative hidradenitis of the vulva. *J Reprod Med.* 1991;36(2):113–117.
5. Lapins J, Sartorius K, Emtestam L. Scanner-assisted carbon dioxide laser surgery: a retrospective follow-up study of patients with hidradenitis suppurativa. *J Am Acad Dermatol.* 2002;47(2):280–285.
6. Mikkelsen PR, Dufour DN, Zarchi K, Jemec GBE. Recurrence rate and patient satisfaction of CO2 laser evaporation of lesions in patients

with hidradenitis suppurativa: a retrospective study. *Dermatol Surg.* 2015;41(2):255–260.

7. McMullan FH, Zeligman I. Perifolliculitis capitis abscedens et suffodiens; its successful treatment with x-ray epilation. *AMA Arch Derm.* 1956;73(3):256–263.

8. MacKee GM, Cipollaro AC. *X-rays and Radium in the Treatment of Diseases of the Skin.* Philadelphia: Lea & Febriger; 1946.

9. Schenck SG. Hidradenitis suppurativa axillaris; an analysis of 54 cases treated with roentgen rays. *Radiology.* 1950;54(1):74–77. illust.

10. Zeligman I. Temporary x-ray epilation therapy of chronic axillary hidradenitis suppurativa. *Arch Dermatol.* 1965;92(6):690–694.

11. Lauge-Hansen N, Lyndrup S. Hidrosadenitis axillaris and its roentgen treatment; optimum total dose and intenseness. *Acta Radiol.* 1949; 31(2):129–144.

12. Myers JN, Mason AR, Gillespie LK, Salkey KS. Treatment of acne conglobata with modern external beam radiation. *J Am Acad Dermatol.* 2010;62(5):861–863.

13. Chinnaiyan P, Tena LB, Brenner MJ, Welsh JS. Modern external beam radiation therapy for refractory dissecting cellulitis of the scalp. *Br J Dermatol.* 2005;152(4):777–779.

14. Fröhlich D, Baaske D, Glatzel M. Radiotherapy of hidradenitis suppurativa—still valid today? *Strahlenther Onkol.* 2000;176(6):286–289.

15. Pape R, Golles D. Effect of roentgen microdosage in axillar hidrosadenitis. *Strahlentherapie.* 1950;81(4):565–576.

16. Trombetta M, Werts ED, Parda D. The role of radiotherapy in the treatment of hidradenitis suppurativa: case report and review of the literature. *Dermatol Online J.* 2010;16(2):16.

17. Patel SH, Robbins JR, Hamzavi I. Radiation Therapy for Chronic Hidradenitis Suppurativa. *J Nucl Med Radiat Ther.* 2013;4:146.

18. Maher M, Larsen L. A case of radiation-induced localized exacerbation of hidradenitis suppurativa. *JAAD Case Rep.* 2016;2(1):44–46.

19 Sartorius K, Boer J, Jemec GBE. Topical treatment. In: Jemec GBE, Revuz J, Leyden JJ, eds. *Hidradenitis Suppurativa.* Springer, Berlin, Heidelberg 2006.

20. Boer J, Bos BW, van der Meer JB. Hidradenitis suppurativa (acne inversa): behandeling met deroofing en resorcine [English abstract]. *Ned Tijdschr Derm Venereol.* 2004;14:274–278.

21. Boer J, Dijkstra AT, Baar TJM, van der Meer JB. Hidradenitis suppurativa (acne inversa): Lokale behandeling met resorcine. *Ned Tijdschr Derm Venereol.* 2001;11:348–349.

22. Boer J, Jemec GB. Resorcinol peels as a possible self-treatment of painful nodules in hidradenitis suppurativa. *Clin Exp Dermatol.* 2010;35(1):36–40.

23. Pascual JC, Encabo B, de Apodaca RFR, et al. Topical 15% resorcinol for hidradenitis suppurativa: An uncontrolled prospective trial with clinical and ultrasonographic follow-up. *J Am Acad Dermatol.* 2017;77(6):1175–1178.

24. Bensimon R. Phenol-Croton oil peels. In: Obagi S, ed. *Chemical Peels.* 3rd ed. *Procedures of Cosmetic Dermatology Series.* Philadelphia, PA: Elsevier; 2020:81–99.

25. Bong JL, Shalders K, Saihan E. Treatment of persistent painful nodules of hidradenitis suppurativa with cryotherapy. *Clin Exp Dermatol.* 2003;28(3):241–244.

26. Pagliarello C, Fabrizi G, Feliciani C, Di Nuzzo S. Cryoinsufflation for Hurley stage II hidradenitis suppurativa: a useful treatment option

27. Pagliarello C, Fabrizi G, di Nuzzo S. Cryoinsufflation for Hidradenitis Suppurativa: Technical Refinement to Prevent Complications. *Dermatol Surg.* 2016;42(1):130–132.

28. Daveluy S. Cryoinsufflation in the presurgical assessment of hidradenitis suppurativa. *J Am Acad Dermatol.* 2020;82(4), e127.

29. Molina-Leyva A, Salvador-Rodriguez L, Martinez-Lopez A, Cuenca-Barrales C. Effectiveness, safety and tolerability of drainage and punch-trocar-assisted cryoinsufflation (cryopunch) in the treatment of inflammatory acute fluid collections in hidradenitis suppurativa patients. *J Eur Acad Dermatol Venereol.* 2019;33(5):e221–e223.

30. O'Reilly DJ, Pleat JM, Richards AM. Treatment of hidradenitis suppurativa with botulinum toxin A. *Plast Reconstr Surg.* 2005; 116(5):1575–1576.

31. Feito-Rodriguez M, Sendagorta-Cudós E, Herranz-Pinto P, de Lucas-Laguna R. Prepubertal hidradenitis suppurativa successfully treated with botulinum toxin A. *Dermatol Surg.* 2009;35(8):1300–1302.

32. Khoo AB, Burova EP. Hidradenitis suppurativa treated with Clostridium botulinum toxin A. *Clin Exp Dermatol.* 2014;39(6):749–750.

33. Shi W, Schultz S, Strouse A, Gater DR. Successful treatment of stage III hidradenitis suppurativa with botulinum toxin A. *BMJ Case Rep.* 2019;12(1), e226064.

34. Campanati A, Martina E, Giuliodori K, et al. Two cases of Hidradenitis suppurativa and botulinum toxin type a therapy: a novel approach for a pathology that is still difficult to manage. *Dermatol Ther.* 2019;32(3), e12841.

35. Janse IC, Hellinga J, Blok JL, et al. Skin-Tissue-sparing Excision with Electrosurgical Peeling: A Case Series in Hidradenitis Suppurativa. *Acta Derm Venereol.* 2016;96(3):390–391.

36. Finley EM, Ratz JL. Treatment of hidradenitis suppurativa with carbon dioxide laser excision and second-intention healing. *J Am Acad Dermatol.* 1996;34(3):465–469.

37. Madan V, Hindle E, Hussain W, August PJ. Outcomes of treatment of nine cases of recalcitrant severe hidradenitis suppurativa with carbon dioxide laser. *Br J Dermatol.* 2008;159(6):1309–1314.

38. Knaysi Jr GA, Cosman B, Crikelair GF. Hidradenitis suppurativa. *JAMA.* 1968;203(1):19–22.

39. Rompel R, Petres J. Long-term results of wide surgical excision in 106 patients with hidradenitis suppurativa. *Dermatol Surg.* 2000;26 (7):638–643.

40. Watson JD. Hidradenitis suppurativa—a clinical review. *Br J Plast Surg.* 1985;38(4):567–569.

41. Hazen PG, Hazen BP. Hidradenitis suppurativa: successful treatment using carbon dioxide laser excision and marsupialization. *Dermatol Surg.* 2010;36(2):208–213.

42. Grimstad O, Ingvarsson G. Carbon Dioxide Laser Treatment Using Methylene Blue-Assisted Sinus Tract Identification in Hidradenitis Suppurativa. *Dermatol Surg.* 2016;42(11):1303–1304.

43. Martorell A, Wortsman X, Alfageme F, et al. Ultrasound Evaluation as a Complementary Test in Hidradenitis Suppurativa: Proposal of a Standardized Report. *Dermatol Surg.* 2017;43(8):1065–1073.

44. Martorell A, Giovanardi G, Gomez-Palencia P, Sanz-Motilva V. Defining Fistular Patterns in Hidradenitis Suppurativa: Impact on the Management. *Dermatol Surg.* 2019;45(10):1237–1244.

when systemic therapies should be avoided. *JAMA Dermatol.* 2014;150(7):765–766.

27

Lifestyle Modifications

JENNIFER M. FERNANDEZ, LYDIA JOHNSON, AND JOI LENCZOWSKI

CHAPTER OUTLINE

Introduction

Hidradenitis suppurativa (HS) is a chronic inflammatory disorder with a profoundly negative impact on quality of life in patients with active disease. Many lifestyle factors are associated with disease incidence, severity, and exacerbation. This chapter addresses potentially modifiable lifestyle factors that may affect disease activity, including diet, obesity, tobacco use, and psychological stress.

Diet

Emerging evidence indicates that dietary modifications may be a viable adjunctive therapy for HS.[1,2] More than 75% to 90% of HS patients have made dietary changes in an attempt to manage HS symptoms, altering at least one food item from their diet (gluten, dairy, and refined carbohydrates were the most common).[1,2]

Half to two-thirds of HS patients perceive improvement from dietary changes, while less than 5% reported worsening of HS.[1,2]

Though dietary changes are very common in HS, evidence supporting dietary recommendations in HS is weak to moderate at best.[3] There is a dearth of literature evaluating the impact of dietary choices on HS severity, and no randomized controlled studies. The little that is known about diet in HS comes from several small studies,[1,4–6] and support for dietary recommendations in HS is frequently extrapolated from the literature on acne, due to its pathologic similarities to HS.[4,7]

Mechanism of Diet in Follicular Occlusion

The proposed initiating event in the pathogenesis of HS involves occlusion of the folliculopilosebaceous unit.[8] Keratotic debris accumulates in the occluded follicle, eventually leading to follicular rupture and triggering an inflammatory cascade.[7] Diet, particularly dairy products and simple carbohydrates, may contribute to follicular occlusion through hormonal or other cellular signaling pathways (Fig. 27.1).[9–11]

Dairy products increase insulin and insulin-like growth factor 1 (IGF-1) levels, and refined carbohydrates increase insulin levels, leading to hyperinsulinemia.[9] Normally, forkhead box transcription factor O1 (FoxO1), the gatekeeper in the pathogenesis of acne, suppresses androgen receptor activation in the nucleus.[10] Hyperinsulinemia and elevated levels of IGF-1 lead to phosphorylation and subsequent expulsion of FoxO1 from the nucleus to the cytoplasm, where it no longer suppresses androgen receptors.[10] Without nuclear FoxO1, androgen receptors are exposed and susceptible to binding circulating androgens.[9,11] In addition to suppressing androgenic signaling, FoxO1 regulates immune responses, modulates regulatory proteins that control sebaceous lipogenesis, opposes oxidative damage, and regulates mTORC1 (the kinase mammalian target of rapamycin complex 1).[10] mTORC1 regulates cellular metabolic activity, growth, and proliferation.[9] Cytoplasmic FoxO1 indirectly activates the mTORC1 signaling pathway, which acts on sterol regulatory binding protein (SREBP-1), inducing lipogenesis in sebaceous (oil-producing glands) in acne.[10,12] Because dairy and refined carbohydrates can contribute to the dysregulation of FoxO1 and mTORC1, limiting consumption of these items may be beneficial in treating acne. Elevated levels of IGF-1 and increased cytoplasmic expression of FoxO1 have been observed in acne,[13] and given the pathologic similarities between acne and HS, these dietary interventions may also be beneficial in HS.

Additionally, cow's milk often contains androgenic hormones.[4] The increased propensity to have open androgen receptors along

• **Fig. 27.1** Hypothesized Mechanism of Dietary Exacerbation of Hidradenitis Suppurativa.

1. Ingestion of carbohydrates increases insulin. Dairy increases insulin, IGF-1, and circulating androgens.
2. FoxO1 is normally bound to the androgen receptor to suppress androgenic signaling. Increased insulin and IGF-1 levels lead to phosphorylation of nuclear FoxO1, which causes subsequent expulsion of FoxO1 from the nucleus to the cytoplasm.
3. In the cytoplasm, FoxO1 stimulates mTORC, which acts on STEBP to increase lipogenesis.
4. Circulating endogenous and exogenous androgens bind to androgen receptors, leading to hyperkeratinization of the hair follicle which eventually ruptures.

FoxO1, Forkhead box transcription factor O1; IGF-1, insulin-like growth factor-1; mTORC1, mammalian target of rapamycin complex 1; P, phosphorylation; SREBP-1, sterol regulatory binding protein 1 (From Danby FW. Turning acne on/off via mTORC1. *Exp Dermatol.* 2013;22(7):505–506. https://doi.org/10.1111/exd.12180; Melnik BC, Zouboulis CC. Potential role of FoxO1 and mTORC1 in the pathogenesis of Western diet-induced acne. *Exp Dermatol.* 2013;22(5):311–315. https://doi.org/10.1111/exd.12142; Melnik BC, Schmitz G. Role of insulin, insulin-like growth factor-1, hyperglycaemic food and milk consumption in the pathogenesis of acne vulgaris. *Exp Dermatol.* 2009;18(10):833–841. https://doi.org/10.1111/j.1600-0625.2009. 00924.x; Melnik B. Diet in acne: further evidence for the role of nutrient signalling in acne pathogenesis—a commentary. *Acta Derm Venerol.* 2012;92 (3):228–231. https://doi.org/10.2340/00015555-1358)

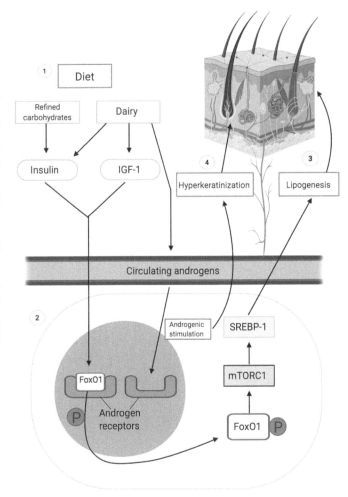

with the addition of exogenous androgens from dairy products can lead to excessive androgenic activation and subsequent follicular hyperproliferation seen in acne.[9,11] Due to androgenic stimulation, the hair follicle becomes occluded with poorly differentiated keratinocytes in HS, contents accumulate in the hair follicle, and it eventually ruptures.[4] Androgens such as progesterone, estrogen, and testosterone have been hypothesized to affect HS disease activity, although the effects of each hormone have yet to be elucidated.[14] While the exact role of androgens in HS is poorly understood, it appears that ingestion of dairy and refined carbohydrates may contribute to an overactive androgenic response, which exacerbates follicular occlusion and perpetuates the inflammatory cascade triggered by follicular rupture.

Mechanism of Diet in Inflammation

Inflammation is key to the development of active disease in HS. The majority of our current medical interventions for HS target inflammation to attenuate disease activity. Patients with HS often have co-morbidities, such as metabolic syndrome and obesity, which produce states of chronic non-specific inflammation. Diet is a potentially important source of pro- and anti-inflammatory nutrients (Table 27.1). The specific type of macronutrients and their relative amounts play a role in regulating inflammation. This section reviews scientific data on impact of carbohydrates, fats, and

sodium on inflammation. While there are case reports of worsening acne after consumption of supplemental whey protein, its effect on HS is unknown.[15]

Carbohydrates

Consumption of refined and excessive carbohydrates can lead to chronically elevated glucose levels. Hyperglycemia increases circulating cytokines such as interleukin (IL) 6, IL-18, and tumor necrosis factor alpha (TNF-alpha).[16] Chronic hyperglycemia leads to chronic hyperinsulinemia, which prompts increased metabolism of omega-6 fatty acid in production of arachidonic acid and its downstream inflammatory components.[17] In addition, hyperglycemia can increase nuclear factor κB (NF-κB) activation in monocytes, increasing levels of pro-inflammatory TNF-alpha.[18] Elevated glucose levels after eating induce macrophages to secrete IL-1 beta, which in turn promotes postprandial inflammation.[19]

Carbohydrate ingestion results in production of advanced glycation end products (AGEs), which are formed by the non-enzymatic reaction between reducing sugars and proteins, lipids, and DNA. AGEs can be increased by either endogenous or exogenous sources. Endogenous sources of AGEs are secondary to chronic hyperglycemia, while exogenous sources are found in foods processed at high temperatures, including commercially processed carbohydrates. AGEs trigger increases in NF-κB and as such are pro-inflammatory.[20] In addition, AGEs have hormonal effects leading to elevations in testosterone,

TABLE 27.1	Nutrients and Impact on Inflammation
Nutrient	**Response**
Carbohydrates	
Hyperglycemia: PRO-inflammatory	Increases non-specific inflammation by triggering pro-inflammatory NF-κB activation in monocytes
	Postprandial elevated glucose levels trigger macrophage production of IL-1β and insulin. Insulin then enhances macrophage production of IL-1β, in a positive inflammatory feedback loop of insulin and IL-1β, resulting in chronic inflammatory cycle
Hyperinsulinemia: PRO-inflammatory	Increased non-specific inflammation, promotes omega-6 metabolism, increasing inflammatory eicosanoids
Increases levels of advanced glycation end-products (AGEs) with hyperglycemia: PRO-inflammatory	Increased non-specific inflammation via multiple signaling pathways, increase TNF-α and IL-1 Promote increased levels of androgens and insulin in women with PCOS
Fiber: ANTI-inflammatory	Reduces glycemic index of carbohydrates thus decreases level of hyperglycemia
	Improves gut microbiome diversity with decreases in inflammation Healthy gut microbiome modulates systemic Treg/Th17 balance with decrease in non-specific inflammation
Whole vegetables: ANTI-inflammatory	Antioxidants, block reactive oxygen species and thus decrease inflammation triggered by ROS
	Dampen inflammatory response by increasing threshold for activation of NF-κB and reducing pro-inflammatory cytokines
Lipids	
Saturated fats: PRO-inflammatory	Activates inflammasome, increases production of IL-1β Decreases microbiome diversity
Omega 6 fatty acids: PRO-inflammatory	Metabolism leads to Arachidonic acid and pro-inflammatory eicosanoids
Omega 3 fatty acids: ANTI-inflammatory	Metabolism leads to DHA/EPA and production of anti-inflammatory eicosanoids Production of resolvins and protectins with resolution of inflammatory cascade
Proteins	
Mammalian meats: PRO-inflammatory	Contain Arachidonic acid If cooked at high temperatures (grilling) lead to production of AGEs
Dairy/eggs: PRO-inflammatory	Contain Arachidonic acid
Fish, fatty cold temperature: ANTI-inflammatory	Contain anti-inflammatory omega-3 Fatty acids
Electrolytes	
Sodium chloride: PRO-inflammatory	Reduce activation of IL-4 and IL-13 stimulated macrophages
	Alters gut microbiome Induces Th17 differentiation

AGE, advanced glycation end-products; *DHA*, docosahexaenoic acid; *EPA*, eicosapentaenoic acid; *IL*, Interleukin; *NF-κB*, nuclear factor κB; *PCOS*, polycystic ovary syndrome; *ROS*, reactive oxygen species; *Th17*, T-helper 17 cells (Th17); *TNF-α*, tumor necrosis factor alpha; *T regs*, regulatory T cells (Tregs).

insulin, and reactive oxygen species in women with polycystic ovary syndrome.[21] These pro-inflammatory effects of hyperglycemia can be detrimental to health and immunity.

Fat

While omega-3 and omega-6 fatty acids are both essential nutrients, omega-3 fats are anti-inflammatory and omega-6 fats are pro-inflammatory. Through the arachidonic acid pathway, omega-6 fats act as precursors for the production of pro-inflammatory eicosanoids.[17] While the ideal ratio of omega-6 fats to omega-3 fats is unknown, it is hypothesized that a ratio greater than 10:1 promotes inflammation.[17] It is thought that humans evolved consuming a 1:1 ratio of omega-6:omega-3 fats.[22] Our current typical pro-inflammatory Western diet (high in refined sugars, meats, processed foods, and fat) has an elevated pro-inflammatory omega-6 to omega-3 ratio of approximately 15:1.[22] Saturated fats, often present in animal products and baked goods, also exert pro-inflammatory effects.[23]

Sodium

Processed foods are frequently high in saturated fats, refined carbohydrates, and sodium. Not only does excessive sodium intake contribute to hypertension, but high salt intake may inhibit proper immune cell function. Excessive salt intake alters the intestinal microbiome (depleting beneficial bacterial species important for gut health and immunity) and promotes a pro-inflammatory T helper (Th) 17 phenotype.[24] High dietary salt intake also suppresses anti-inflammatory macrophage activity in mouse models, reducing noninflammatory innate immune cell activation, which may lead to an overall imbalance in immune homeostasis.[25]

Dietary Considerations in Hidradenitis Suppurativa

Multiple reports on restrictions of specific dietary components are present in HS literature. Most notable are reports on limiting dairy and brewer's yeast. Nightshades have been addressed as a potential dietary trigger for HS, and intermittent fasting as an intervention has also been reported. Potential benefits of the Mediterranean diet in HS have also been described.

Dairy

Dairy products include milk as well as products made from milk, such as cheese, yogurt, and cottage cheese. Eggs are typically not considered to be dairy products as they are not milk-based. Dairy is hypothesized to contribute to follicular occlusion in HS by way of exogenous hormones and hyperinsulinemia. Danby et al. reported that of 47 patients who followed a dairy-free diet, 83% improved while none reported worsening symptoms.[4] Another study revealed that patients who eliminated dairy were twice as likely to report HS improvement as those who did not.[1] Of the limited available evidence, it appears the reduction or elimination of dairy may be one of the more effective dietary recommendations in HS. However, because dairy is an important dietary source of calcium, patients following a dairy-free diet may require supplemental calcium and vitamin D.

Brewer's Yeast

Brewer's yeast (also called baker's yeast) has been implicated as a dietary trigger in HS.[5] Brewer's yeast contains *Saccharomyces cerevisiae*, a fungus that ferments alcohol and allows bread products to rise. A small study was conducted in 12 HS patients who followed a wheat and brewer's yeast-free diet for 12 months postoperatively after surgical excision of HS lesions.[5] Patients were instructed to eliminate all baked products, vinegar, soy sauce, beer, wine, fermented cheeses, and mushrooms. All patients experienced regression of HS lesions post-operatively while on the brewer's yeast-free diet, and all reported recurrence of skin lesions with reintroduction of wheat or yeast, and subsequent regression after removing these products from the diet again.[5] Study participants also reported improved quality of life after surgical and dietary intervention.[5] While elimination of brewer's yeast shows disease-attenuating potential, this study was done in conjunction with surgical excision, making it difficult to distinguish between the benefit of surgery and elimination of brewer's yeast.

Glycemic Load

Low-glycemic-load diets have not been studied in HS, but they have been investigated in acne. Glycemic load refers to the amount of carbohydrate consumed multiplied by the rate at which the carbohydrate is metabolized and enters the bloodstream (glycemic index).[17] A study conducted in male acne patients comparing a low-glycemic-load diet to a carbohydrate-dense diet showed a greater decrease in total number of acne lesions in the low-glycemic-load group compared to the control group.[26] In addition to improvement in acne, the low-glycemic-load diet resulted in greater weight reduction and improvement in insulin sensitivity than the control diet.[18] While acne and HS have a similar pathogenesis, HS primarily affects women, and this study was conducted using only male subjects, so results are not necessarily generalizable to HS patients. Still, there may be some theoretical benefit to a low-glycemic-load diet in HS, as high carbohydrate intake can lead to hyper-insulinemia, which may exacerbate follicular occlusion and inflammation.[9,27]

Nightshades

Nightshades, plants from the Solanaceae family, typically contain high amounts of alkaloids, which have the potential to be toxic.[28] Tomatoes, potatoes, eggplants, peppers (both bell and hot), and tobacco are included in this group.[1,28] While discussions on HS internet platforms reveal that some HS patients feel nightshades exacerbate HS, evidence is lacking. Current literature indicates that HS symptom improvement is not significant after elimination of peppers or eggplants. Those who eat tomatoes are more likely to experience HS improvement than those who do not.[1] While the elimination of nightshades may be a common practice among HS patients, it is not well-supported by evidence.

Fasting

The impact of intermittent fasting has been evaluated in a study of 55 patients with HS who fasted (abstained from food and beverages from sunrise to sunset) for one month during Ramadan.[6] Mean International Hidradenitis Suppurativa Severity Score System (IHS4) scores from before and after Ramadan decreased significantly. The greatest changes in IHS4 score were observed in those receiving topical antibiotics followed by systemic antibiotics, and the smallest changes were in those receiving biologics. Mean weight change during Ramadan was 0 kg, indicating that score changes were not related to weight loss. By the end of Ramadan, abscesses and draining fistulas decreased for 69% and 37.5%, respectively. However, of those that improved, the improvement only persisted in one-fourth of those patients at one month post completion of fasting. As the disease recurred with reinstitution of normal dietary patterns, all changes were likely dependent on persistent intermittent fasting, which may be impractical for most patients. The authors hypothesized that study results could be due to a fasting-induced downregulation of Th1, Th17, and antigen-presenting cells, as intermittent fasting has been shown to affect the composition of T cells in the gut with a reduction of IL-17-producing T cells and increased numbers of regulatory T cells. Additionally, intermittent fasting has been shown to increase gut microbiome diversity and activate microbial metabolic pathways that modulate systemic immune responses.[29]

Mediterranean Diet

In a cross-sectional study, Barrea et al. evaluated how closely dietary intake from 7-day food records resembled the Mediterranean diet in 41 HS patients and 41 healthy controls.[30] This study revealed that, despite comparable total caloric consumption, HS patients consumed lower amounts of complex carbohydrates, monounsaturated fat, and omega-3 polyunsaturated fats, and higher amounts of saturated and omega-6 fats than healthy controls. Those consuming diets with poor resemblance to the Mediterranean diet tended to have more severe HS than those consuming a more Mediterranean-style diet.[30] HS severity was also positively correlated with both total and simple carbohydrate intake, and negatively correlated with omega-3 fat intake.[30] Authors surmised that these observations could be due to anti-inflammatory properties of the Mediterranean diet, such as antioxidants and polyphenols found in plant foods. Given that consumption patterns reflective of the Mediterranean diet were associated with decreased HS severity, the Mediterranean diet may be a valuable dietary intervention in HS. However, cost may preclude some patients from adhering to this dietary pattern.

Anti-Inflammatory Diet

Certain dietary patterns have been described as anti-inflammatory due to an increase in components that can decrease inflammation while minimizing foods that increase inflammation. The most well-studied diet that is considered anti-inflammatory is the Mediterranean diet; studies have shown that it can reduce mortality, cardiovascular disease, cancer, neurodegenerative diseases, and diabetes.[31] This plant-based diet is high in fruits, vegetables, fiber, beans, lentils, nuts, and omega-3 fats, and low in animal protein and saturated fats. Fruits and vegetables are high in vitamins, minerals, fiber, and phytonutrients that counteract inflammation. Fish is an important source of protein in an anti-inflammatory diet as it is high in omega-3 fats, while meat and dairy products can have high levels of omega-6 fats that promote inflammation via generation of arachidonic acid.[32] Refined, commercially processed carbohydrates are often stripped of nutrients and result in rapid increases in serum glucose and hyperinsulinemia, which contribute to systemic inflammation. Whole-grain carbohydrates retain nutrients and fiber, moderating blood sugar fluctuation and promoting a healthy diverse gut microbiome. When recommending a healthy and potentially anti-inflammatory diet, it is important to recognize that dietary components work synergistically to combat the effects of inflammation. Culinary recommendations for a healthful diet are summarized in Box 27.1.

Summary of Diet in Hidradenitis Suppurativa

As HS is an inflammatory follicular disorder, pro-inflammatory foods may exacerbate this condition. However, studies that evaluate food as triggers for HS flares are lacking. Conducting clinical trials to evaluate dietary interventions in complex disease states is difficult and complicated by the potential impact of weight loss, which independently improves HS disease activity. To date, data is minimal and low quality. The improvement in HS reported by interventions in diet may be due to decreased promotion of follicular hyperkeratosis and occlusion, decreased induction of pro-inflammatory biomolecules, or by impact on gut microbiome. The gut microbiome is impacted by numerous external factors, including diet, smoking, and antibiotic uses. A healthy, diverse gut microbiome prevents non-specific systemic inflammation, which can translate into improved mental health and well-being. Dietary changes can greatly and rapidly alter the gut microbiota.[33]

• BOX 27.1 **Recommendations for Preparing Healthful Anti-inflammatory Meals**

- Incorporate fresh fruits and vegetables into each meal, ideally 50% of plate
- Add whole grains to diet
- Aim to eat fish two times per week
- Eat healthy sources of protein and fiber, including beans, lentils, and nuts
- Use healthy fats, including olive oil, canola oil, and vegetable oil
- To limit sodium, use spices and herbs for flavoring rather than salt
- Limit added fat when cooking; bake, steam, or boil foods
- Avoid highly processed, commercially prepared foods

- Limit consumption of red meat to two-three times per week
- Avoid frying and deep frying due to added fats
- Avoid using shortening, butter, and coconut oil due to high levels of saturated fat
- Chose produce that is in season, as it will often taste better and be less expensive than produce that is out-of-season
- When fresh produce is not available, consider using frozen rather than canned foods to avoid added sodium

---

Given that disease worsening from supervised dietary intervention is rare, and preliminary evidence indicates that dietary modifications may lead to improvement,[1,4] dietary interventions may have increasing relevance as an adjunctive therapy for HS. Avoiding foods such as dairy and refined carbohydrates that promote follicular occlusion and incorporating anti-inflammatory foods may be beneficial for attenuating HS disease activity. Key recommendations for HS patients are to consume appropriate portions of healthy food and beverages and to maintain a healthy weight. Some patients may benefit from keeping a food and HS symptom diary to identify triggers.

Key Points (for "Diet" Section)

Evidence to support dietary recommendations in HS is limited with a level of 3 to 5.

Limiting dairy and refined carbohydrates may provide some symptom relief in HS.

The Mediterranean diet may be beneficial for HS patients through improvement in HS as well as associated comorbidities.

Current evidence does not support removal of nightshades from the diet in HS patients.

Weight and Hidradenitis Suppurativa

Higher rates of obesity and metabolic syndrome are reported in patients with HS, and obesity prevalence in HS ranges from 22% to 61%.[34,35] A meta-analysis of case-controlled studies across Asia, Europe, and the United States concluded that HS patients are four times more likely to be obese compared to the general population.[36] There appears to be an association of disease severity with increased body mass index and decreased remission in obese compared to non-obese patients.[37–40] Obesity can contribute to follicular occlusion due to physical follicular obstruction as well as follicular hyperkeratosis secondary to effects of hyperandrogenism triggered by hyper-insulinemia. Mechanical stress can cause hyperkeratinization at the upper region of the hair follicle, which leads to follicular dilation and occlusion.

Obesity may contribute to disease activity by induction of inflammation, direct frictional exacerbation, and mechanical obstruction. Adipose tissue contributes to inflammation due to pro-inflammatory signaling from adipocytes and resident immune cells. In particular, adipose tissue contains distinct populations of M1 and M2 macrophages. M1 macrophages are increased in number in the adipose tissue of obese patients and produce pro-inflammatory cytokines, including IL-1beta and TNF-alpha. M2 macrophages dominate the adipose tissue of lean patients and produce anti-inflammatory cytokines such as IL-10. Thus, in the obese patient, resident macrophages of adipose tissue are a primary source of inflammation. Additionally, the adipokine balance is shifted in patients with hidradenitis, with increased expression of pro-inflammatory resistin and leptin as well as decreased anti-inflammatory adiponectin. This shift is the result of obesity-related increased production of leptin by adipocytes.[41] Leptin is pro-inflammatory and up-regulates the secretion of multiple inflammatory cytokines including TNF-alpha, IL-6, and IL-12. TNF-alpha and IL-1 positively regulate leptin and promote further increases in leptin level, thus promoting increased inflammation.[42,43] Additionally, leptin has been shown to promote a shift in T cell populations to pro-inflammatory Th17 cells.[44,45] Unfortunately, leptin resistance develops with increased levels and this prevents recognition of satiety, with subsequent increased caloric intake and further increased adiposity.[41] Adipose tissue also functions as an endocrine organ and expresses enzymes that produce androgens. Androgens likely play a role in HS pathogenesis as they stimulate epidermal hyperplasia and modulate epidermal differentiation. Testosterone can enhance sebum production and clog pores. Additionally, insulin, growth hormone, and insulin-like growth factors are elevated in obese patients and have been demonstrated to activate sebaceous glands and influence acne severity and likely contribute, as noted above, to hidradenitis HS activity.[11]

Effect of Weight Loss on Hidradenitis Suppurativa

Weight loss has been reported as a treatment for HS. The largest study, by Kromann et al., of 383 patients who underwent bariatric surgery reported stable to resolved disease in 89% of patients (resolution in 49%, decreased disease in 20%, stable disease in 20%, and worsening in 11%).[46] Intervention with bariatric surgery showed that weight reduction greater than 15% was associated with a significant reduction in HS disease severity.[46] Several other case reports also show remission following bariatric surgery.[47,48] There is a potential for worsening of disease following bariatric surgery due to micronutrient deficiencies or increase in skin folds; these issues can be corrected by intervention with nutritional support or surgical removal of excess skin, respectively.[49,50]

Cigarette Smoking and Hidradenitis Suppurativa

In addition to specific medical and surgical therapies, behavioral components may influence the severity of disease and response to therapy. Cigarette smoking is considered a risk factor for the disease. The proposed mechanism involves nicotine, a major toxin in cigarette smoke, which may act on the nicotinic acetylcholine receptors (nAChR) on immune cells present in HS lesions and thereby promote infundibular epithelial hyperplasia and follicular plugging.[51,52]

There is a high prevalence of smoking among HS patients, with estimates ranging from 40% to 89%.[53,54] In addition, the incidence of HS appears to be doubled among tobacco smokers,[55] and disease severity is worse in smokers compared to non-smokers.[53] There may be a link between duration of smoking and development of HS, as a longer duration of smoking is seen in patients with sporadic forms compared to those with familial forms.[54]

The association between smoking and HS may involve inflammatory abnormalities both from HS and from smoking. As such, active smokers may not respond to therapeutic anti-inflammatory agents.[54] A single retrospective cohort study of patients with HS over the course of 22 years found that non-smokers and former smokers were more likely to respond to first-line therapy with antibiotics or intralesional corticosteroids than current smokers.[39]

Smoking Cessation

While there are no studies showing that cessation of smoking leads to resolution of HS, remission has been noted more frequently in non-smokers compared to current smokers with HS.[39] Additionally, many patients with HS suffer from chronic medical comorbidities and increased cardiovascular risk, making smoking cessation an excellent intervention for their overall health; it may also improve their response to treatment. There are more former smokers than current smokers, indicating that people are able to quit smoking. However, this is an extremely challenging endeavor that may require several attempts. People who stop smoking often restart because of withdrawal symptoms, which can increase anxiety and stress. Weight gain due to increased hunger adds another layer of complexity.

Comprehensive, evidence-based treatment should be offered to all patients with HS who want to quit smoking. Interventions include the United States Food and Drug Administration-approved medications, such as varenicline, bupropion, and nicotine replacement therapy. Behavioral counseling can be very effective and often includes brief physician guidance, individual, group and telephone counseling, and social support. In general, counseling and medication are more effective together than using either one alone.[52]

Physical Irritants and Hidradenitis Suppurativa

Patients with HS are often advised to wear loose-fitting clothes, a recommendation based on expert opinion. The goal is to decrease mechanical occlusion and to inhibit accumulation and persistence of moisture in affected areas. Mechanical occlusion promotes keratinocyte differentiation and proliferation, contributing to epidermal thickening and retention of hair follicle debris. Friction also increases keratinocyte-derived matrix metalloproteinase 9 (MMP-9), which promotes inflammation and fibrosis. Several genes related to wound healing are down-regulated following mechanical stress.[56] Additionally, HS most commonly affects intertriginous areas and prolonged exposure to sweat and humidity in these regions increases inflammation and exacerbates disease.[57]

Specific clothing may help minimize frictional triggers as well as control sweat, moisture, and increased humidity in affected areas. Undergarment choices are particularly important, as undergarments are designed to fit closely to affected skin, particularly inframammary skin, the groin, and the perineum. To minimize friction from tight bra bands or straps, recommend sports bras or camisole tanks with built-in bras; avoid bras with thin straps, tight elastic, and metal wires. Underwear for women should be loose-fitting without seams or tight bands along the inguinal creases or across the abdomen. Men should be encouraged to wear loose-fitting boxers rather than tight briefs. These choices can minimize shearing forces from clothing rubbing on skin. Additionally, fabric selection is important, as some fabrics can assist in moisture wicking, including rayon cellulose fabric, polyproylene/nylon, bamboo fiber cloth, silver-impregnated fabric, and cotton. These fabrics decrease humidity, heat, and microbial colonization, thus improving the local skin environment and potentially decreasing HS exacerbations.

Many patients report exacerbation of their disease due to shaving and the use of antiperspirants. Recommend avoid shaving affected skin and consider laser hair removal for patients who prefer smooth skin. Avoid wearing perfume or scented deodorants in the affected areas. Topical clindamycin will decrease bacterial burden in these areas, thus decreasing "sweat odor."

Exercise

Exercise is recommended for patients with HS to assist in weight management and glucose and insulin regulation while also promoting overall good physical and mental health. Unfortunately, exercise can lead to disease exacerbation due to sweating and friction. Overheating and sweat induced by exercise can cause additional irritation in areas already affected by HS.

Swimming is the ideal exercise for patients with HS. Swimming keeps the body in motion while staying cool in the water and wicking away sweat. Aqua fitness options for patients with access to pools include treading water, water aerobics, aqua jogging, and traditional lap swimming.

Other forms of minimal sweating exercise options exist, including yoga, tai chi, pilates, slow walking, and low weight slow weightlifting. Recommend calming varieties of yoga, such as restorative, deep stretch, and yin yoga, which will provide multiple benefits for patients with HS, including a muscle workout, increasing flexibility, and reducing stress and anxiety. Tai chi, through a series of slow, flowing movements, keeps the body active without sweating and provides significant stress reduction.[58] If patients do not have significant active disease in their groin, slow walking in an indoor air-conditioned setting is a low-intensity cardiovascular workout that burns calories. Alternatively, if the lower body is affected but the upper body is mostly spared, upper body low-weight weightlifting can help burn calories and increase muscle mass, which is more metabolically active than adipose tissue.

As with day-to-day life while dealing with HS, clothing choices are important when exercising. Patients should choose loose, ventilated clothing that reduces friction and sweating. They should wear sweat-wicking materials that do not rub along affected areas.

Work and Hidradenitis Suppurativa

A key part of life satisfaction is derived from pursuing a worthwhile occupation. This can be a challenge for individuals with HS, as they have pain and associated loss of mobility, malodorous drainage, embarrassment, and low self-esteem. Patients often report that, due to flares and pain, they are unable to go to work and may even lose their jobs due to numerous sick days. Just over 58% of patients with HS miss work, and patients missed an average of 33.6 days from work.[59] However, another study showed that patients with HS missed less work days than controls.[60] The unemployment rate of adult HS patients eligible for a job was 25.1%, compared with 6.2% for the general population in Denmark.[61] Unemployed patients more commonly suffer from extensive axillary and mammary involvement and score higher on the Dermatology Life Quality Index (DLQI).[62] No data are available on the reason for unemployment; this may be due to pain and psychological impacts or the burden of disease, which may prevent patients from undertaking education, thus diminishing employment options.

Individuals with HS should consider career options carefully, with an understanding of common triggers and the potential need for accommodations in the workplace. Hot, humid work environments should be avoided, as heat and sweat are common HS triggers. Additionally, pressure and occlusion as experienced in many jobs from sitting may be modified with a standing desk/work setting. Appropriate consultation with a career counseling professional is recommended.

Stress Management

Patients with HS experience a great deal of daily stress due to the impact of their disease on overall quality of life, financial burdens, impairment of sex life, increased loneliness, and stigmatization; this

can lead to a significantly increased risk of suicide. Patients commonly report stress as a trigger for HS flares. A study of coping mechanisms showed that avoidant coping skills correlate with lower health-related quality of life (HRQOL) and partially mediate the negative impact of depression on quality-of-life assessment by patients.[63] There are no controlled trials investigating the direct effect of psychological stress on HS disease activity. However, studies of psychological stress impact on epidermal barrier, inflammation, and wound healing show that stress has a negative impact on skin integrity, and stress reduction techniques can mitigate the effects of stress.[64-66]

While initial evaluation of patients should include screening for psychiatric conditions such as depression and anxiety as well as appropriate referral to mental health professionals, it may be useful to recommend stress-reduction interventions for all patients. This can include relaxation techniques, mindfulness, increased attachment, and use of support networks (including support groups).[66,67] Additionally, physical exercise is associated with decreased stress and should be recommended due to positive impact on stress and mental health; it can also improve insulin resistance and enhance weight reduction. Given the detrimental effects of alcohol, drugs, and isolation, HS patients should not rely on these coping mechanisms to manage stress.

Conclusion

HS is a chronic, recurrent inflammatory disease. High-quality studies on diet are difficult to conduct, as patients have unique dietary needs and preferences. Dietary intake varies greatly from day to day, and foods are not eaten in isolation, making it challenging to identify the impact of specific foods or combinations of foods. Studies on lifestyle interventions (such as smoking cessation) may require long-term behavior changes, which may dissuade some patients from participating. Patients' treatment goals and their level of motivation should be considered during the creation of patient-specific treatment plans. Patients have individual, specific triggers and responses to interventions. As no single current treatment option is curative for all patients, it is essential to consider adjuvant interventions, including lifestyle modification, for each and every patient (Box 27.2). Lifestyle components as discussed in this chapter may exacerbate disease, and thus intervention to decrease lifestyle triggers may result in improvement in disease activity. Additionally, several interventions can be therapeutic, as evidenced by patients who have disease remission with dietary interventions and weight loss. It is important to consider lifestyle modification as part of a comprehensive treatment plan, along with medication and surgical interventions. Lifestyle modifications empower patients with tools for managing their disease.

• BOX 27.2 Summary Recommendations for Lifestyle Modifications

- Eat a healthful diet
- Avoid foods that trigger flares
- Decrease obesity
- Smoking cessation
- Wear loose-fitting clothing made of fabrics that wick moisture
- Exercise (recommend pool-based activities, yoga, walking)
- Avoid shaving affected skin
- Pursue a career that does not exacerbate disease, or request accommodations in work environments
- Manage stress (counseling, medication, support networks including support groups)

References

1. Dempsey A, Butt M, Kirby JS. Prevalence and Impact of Dietary Avoidance among Individuals with Hidradenitis Suppurativa. *Dermatology.* 2019;1–7. https://doi.org/10.1159/000503063. Published online November 1.
2. Price KN, Thompson AM, Rizvi O, et al. Complementary and Alternative Medicine Use in Patients With Hidradenitis Suppurativa. *JAMA Dermatol.* 2020. https://doi.org/10.1001/jamadermatol.2019.4595. Published online January 29.
3. Silfvast-Kaiser A, Youssef R, Paek SY. Diet in hidradenitis suppurativa: a review of published and lay literature. *Int J Dermatol.* 2019;58 (11):1225–1230. https://doi.org/10.1111/ijd.14465.
4. Danby FW. Diet in the prevention of hidradenitis suppurativa (acne inversa). *J Am Acad Dermatol.* 2015;73(5):S52–S54. https://doi.org/10.1016/j.jaad.2015.07.042.
5. Cannistrà C, Finocchi V, Trivisonno A, Tambasco D. New perspectives in the treatment of hidradenitis suppurativa: surgery and brewer's yeast–exclusion diet. *Surgery.* 2013;154(5):1126–1130. https://doi.org/10.1016/j.surg.2013.04.018.
6. Damiani G, Mahroum N, Pigatto PDM, et al. The Safety and Impact of a Model of Intermittent, Time-Restricted Circadian Fasting ("Ramadan Fasting") on Hidradenitis Suppurativa: Insights from a Multicenter, Observational, Cross-Over, Pilot, Exploratory Study. *Nutrients.* 2019;11(8):1781. https://doi.org/10.3390/nu11081781.
7. Yu CC, Cook MG. Hidradenitis suppurativa: a disease of follicular epithelium, rather than apocrine glands. *Br J Dermatol.* 1990;122(6):763–769. https://doi.org/10.1111/j.1365-2133.1990.tb06264.x.
8. Vossen ARJV, van der Zee HH, Prens EP. Hidradenitis Suppurativa: A Systematic Review Integrating Inflammatory Pathways Into a Cohesive Pathogenic Model. *Front Immunol.* 2018;9:2965. https://doi.org/10.3389/fimmu.2018.02965.
9. Danby FW. Turning acne on/off via mTORC1. *Exp Dermatol.* 2013;22(7):505–506. https://doi.org/10.1111/exd.12180.
10. Melnik BC, Zouboulis CC. Potential role of FoxO1 and mTORC1 in the pathogenesis of Western diet-induced acne. *Exp Dermatol.* 2013;22(5):311–315. https://doi.org/10.1111/exd.12142.
11. Melnik BC, Schmitz G. Role of insulin, insulin-like growth factor-1, hyperglycaemic food and milk consumption in the pathogenesis of acne vulgaris. *Exp Dermatol.* 2009;18(10):833–841. https://doi.org/10.1111/j.1600-0625.2009.00924.x.
12. Melnik B. Diet in acne: further evidence for the role of nutrient signalling in acne pathogenesis—a commentary. *Acta Derm Venerol.* 2012;92(3):228–231. https://doi.org/10.2340/00015555-1358.
13. Agamia NF, Abdallah DM, Sorour O, et al. Skin expression of mammalian target of rapamycin and forkhead box transcription factor O1, and serum insulin-like growth factor-1 in patients with acne vulgaris and their relationship with diet. *Br J Dermatol.* 2016;174(6):1299–1307. https://doi.org/10.1111/bjd.14409.
14. Perng P, Zampella JG, Okoye GA. Considering the impact of pregnancy on the natural history of hidradenitis suppurativa. *Br J Dermatol.* 2018;178(1). https://doi.org/10.1111/bjd.15735.
15. Simonart T. Acne and Whey Protein Supplementation among Bodybuilders. *Dermatology.* 2012;225(3):256–258. https://doi.org/10.1159/000345102.
16. Esposito K, Nappo F, Marfella R, et al. Inflammatory cytokine concentrations are acutely increased by hyperglycemia in humans: role of oxidative stress. *Circulation.* 2002;106(16):2067–2072. https://doi.org/10.1161/01.CIR.0000034509.14906.AE.
17. Ricker MA, Haas WC. Anti-Inflammatory Diet in Clinical Practice: A Review. *Nutr Clin Pract.* 2017;32(3):318–325. https://doi.org/10.1177/0884533617700353.
18. Aljada A, Friedman J, Ghanim H, et al. Glucose ingestion induces an increase in intranuclear nuclear factor κB, a fall in cellular inhibitor κB, and an increase in tumor necrosis factor α messenger RNA by mononuclear cells in healthy human subjects. *Metabolism.* 2006;55 (9):1177–1185. https://doi.org/10.1016/j.metabol.2006.04.016.
19. Dror E, Dalmas E, Meier DT, et al. Postprandial macrophage-derived IL-1β stimulates insulin, and both synergistically promote glucose disposal and inflammation. *Nat Immunol.* 2017;18(3):283–292. https://doi.org/10.1038/ni.3659.
20. Semba RD, Nicklett EJ, Ferrucci L. Does accumulation of advanced glycation end products contribute to the aging phenotype? *J Gerontol A Biol Sci Med Sci.* 2010;65A(9):963–975. https://doi.org/10.1093/gerona/glq074.
21. Tantalaki E, Piperi C, Livadas S, et al. Impact of dietary modification of advanced glycation end products (AGEs) on the hormonal and metabolic profile of women with polycystic ovary syndrome (PCOS). *Hormones.* 2014;13(1):65–73. https://doi.org/10.1007/BF03401321.
22. Simopoulos AP. Omega-6/omega-3 essential fatty acid ratio and chronic diseases. *Food Rev Int.* 2004;20(1):77–90. https://doi.org/10.1081/FRI-120028831.
23. Ralston JC, Lyons CL, Kennedy EB, et al. Fatty Acids and NLRP3 Inflammasome–Mediated Inflammation in Metabolic Tissues. *Annu Rev Nutr.* 2017;37(1):77–102. https://doi.org/10.1146/annurev-nutr-071816-064836.
24. Binger KJ, Gebhardt M, Heinig M, et al. High salt reduces the activation of IL-4– and IL-13–stimulated macrophages. *J Clin Invest.* 2015;125(11):4223–4238. https://doi.org/10.1172/JCI80919.
25. Wilck N, Matus MG, Kearney SM, et al. Salt-responsive gut commensal modulates TH17 axis and disease. *Nature.* 2017;551 (7682):585–589. https://doi.org/10.1038/nature24628.
26. Smith RN, Mann NJ, Braue A, et al. A low-glycemic-load diet improves symptoms in acne vulgaris patients: a randomized controlled trial. *Am J Clin Nutr.* 2007;86(1):107–115. https://doi.org/10.1093/ajcn.86.1.107.
27. Margesson LJ, Danby FW. Hidradenitis suppurativa. *Best Pract Res Clin Obstet Gynaecol.* 2014;28(7):1013–1027. https://doi.org/10.1016/j.bpobgyn.2014.07.012.
28. Cárdenas PD, Sonawane PD, Heinig U, et al. The bitter side of the nightshades: genomics drives discovery in Solanaceae steroidal alkaloid metabolism. *Phytochemistry.* 2015;113:24–32. https://doi.org/10.1016/j.phytochem.2014.12.010.
29. Cignarella F, Cantoni C, Ghezzi L, et al. Intermittent Fasting Confers Protection in CNS Autoimmunity by Altering the Gut Microbiota. *Cell Metab.* 2018;27(6):1222–1235. e6 https://doi.org/10.1016/j.cmet.2018.05.006.
30. Barrea L, Fabbrocini G, Annunziata G, et al. Role of Nutrition and Adherence to the Mediterranean Diet in the Multidisciplinary Approach of Hidradenitis Suppurativa: Evaluation of Nutritional Status and Its Association with Severity of Disease. *Nutrients.* 2019;11 (1):57. https://doi.org/10.3390/nu11010057.
31. Dinu M, Pagliai G, Casini A, Sofi F. Mediterranean diet and multiple health outcomes: an umbrella review of meta-analyses of observational studies and randomised trials. *Eur J Clin Nutr.* 2018;72 (1):30–43. https://doi.org/10.1038/ejcn.2017.58.
32. Li D, Ng A, Mann NJ, Sinclair AJ. Contribution of meat fat to dietary arachidonic acid. *Lipids.* 1998;33(4):437–440.
33. Serino M, Luche E, Gres S, et al. Metabolic adaptation to a high-fat diet is associated with a change in the gut microbiota. *Gut.* 2012;61 (4):543–553. https://doi.org/10.1136/gutjnl-2011-301012.
34. Vazquez BG, Alikhan A, Weaver AL, et al. Incidence of hidradenitis suppurativa and associated factors: a population-based study of Olmsted County, Minnesota. *J Invest Dermatol.* 2013;133(1):97–103. https://doi.org/10.1038/jid.2012.255.
35. Prens EP, Lugo-Somolinos AM, Paller AS, et al. Baseline Characteristics from UNITE: An Observational, International, Multicentre Registry to Evaluate Hidradenitis Suppurativa (Acne Inversa) in Clinical Practice. *Am J Clin Dermatol.* 2020. https://doi.org/10.1007/s40257-020-00504-4. Published online February 19.
36. Choi F, Lehmer L, Ekelem C, Mesinkovska NA. Dietary and metabolic factors in the pathogenesis of hidradenitis suppurativa: a systematic review. *Int J Dermatol.* 2019. https://doi.org/10.1111/ijd.14691. Published online October 25. ijd.14691.

37. Crowley JJ, Mekkes JR, Zouboulis CC, et al. Association of hidradenitis suppurativa disease severity with increased risk for systemic comorbidities. *Br J Dermatol.* 2014;171(6):1561–1565. https://doi.org/10.1111/bjd.13122.

38. Schrader AMR, Deckers IE, Van Der Zee HH, et al. Hidradenitis suppurativa: a retrospective study of 846 Dutch patients to identify factors associated with disease severity. *J Am Acad Dermatol.* 2014;71(3):460–467. https://doi.org/10.1016/j.jaad.2014.04.001.

39. Kromann CB, Deckers IE, Esmann S, et al. Risk factors, clinical course and long-term prognosis in hidradenitis suppurativa: a cross-sectional study. *Br J Dermatol.* 2014;171(4):819–824. https://doi.org/10.1111/bjd.13090.

40. Kromann C, Ibler K, Kristiansen V, Jemec G. The influence of body weight on the prevalence and severity of hidradenitis suppurativa. *Acta Derm Venereol.* 2014;94(5):553–557. https://doi.org/10.2340/00015555-1800.

41. Malara A, Hughes R, Jennings L, et al. Adipokines are dysregulated in patients with hidradenitis suppurativa. *Br J Dermatol.* 2018;178(3):792–793. https://doi.org/10.1111/bjd.15904.

42. Lumeng CN, Bodzin JL, Saltiel AR. Obesity induces a phenotypic switch in adipose tissue macrophage polarization. *J Clin Invest.* 2007;117(1):175–184. https://doi.org/10.1172/JCI29881.

43. Rosen ED, Spiegelman BM. What we talk about when we talk about fat. *Cell.* 2014;156(1–2):20–44. https://doi.org/10.1016/j.cell.2013.12.012.

44. Cava AL, Matarese G. The weight of leptin in immunity. *Nat Rev Immunol.* 2004;4(5):371–379. https://doi.org/10.1038/nri1350.

45. Naylor C, Petri WA. Leptin Regulation of Immune Responses. *Trends Mol Med.* 2016;22(2):88–98. https://doi.org/10.1016/j.molmed.2015.12.001.

46. Kromann C, Ibler K, Kristiansen V, Jemec G. The influence of body weight on the prevalence and severity of hidradenitis suppurativa. *Acta Derm Venereol.* 2014;94(5):553–557. https://doi.org/10.2340/00015555-1800.

47. Boer J. Resolution of hidradenitis suppurativa after weight loss by dietary measures, especially on frictional locations. *J Eur Acad Dermatol Venereol.* 2016;30(5):895–896. https://doi.org/10.1111/jdv.13059.

48. Thomas CL, Gordon KD, Mortimer PS. Rapid resolution of hidradenitis suppurativa after bariatric surgical intervention. *Clin Exp Dermatol.* 2014;39(3):315–318. https://doi.org/10.1111/ced.12269.

49. Garcovich S, De Simone C, Giovanardi G, et al. Post-bariatric surgery hidradenitis suppurativa: a new patient subset associated with malabsorption and micronutritional deficiencies. *Clin Exp Dermatol.* 2019;44(3):283–289. https://doi.org/10.1111/ced.13732.

50. Golbari NM, Lee Porter M, Kimball AB. Response to: remission of hidradenitis suppurativa after bariatric surgery. *JAAD Case Rep.* 2018;4(3):278–279. https://doi.org/10.1016/j.jdcr.2017.11.024.

51. Hana A, Booken D, Henrich C, et al. Functional significance of non-neuronal acetylcholine in skin epithelia. *Life Sci.* 2007;80(24–25):2214–2220. https://doi.org/10.1016/j.lfs.2007.02.007.

52. Shiels MS, Katki HA, Freedman ND, et al. Cigarette smoking and variations in systemic immune and inflammation markers. *J Natl Cancer Inst.* 2014;106(11). https://doi.org/10.1093/jnci/dju294.

53. Prens EP, Lugo-Somolinos AM, Paller AS, et al. Baseline Characteristics from UNITE: An Observational, International, Multicentre Registry to Evaluate Hidradenitis Suppurativa (Acne Inversa) in Clinical Practice. *Am J Clin Dermatol.* 2020. https://doi.org/10.1007/s40257-020-00504-4. Published online February 19.

54. Konig A, Lehmann C, Rompel R, Happle R. Cigarette smoking as a triggering factor of hidradenitis suppurativa. *Dermatology.* 1999;198(3):261–264. https://doi.org/10.1159/000018126.

55. Garg A, Papagermanos V, Midura M, Strunk A. Incidence of hidradenitis suppurativa among tobacco smokers: a population-based retrospective analysis in the U.S.A. *Br J Dermatol.* 2018;178(3):709–714. https://doi.org/10.1111/bjd.15939.

56. Cherbuin T, Movahednia MM, Toh WS, Cao T. Investigation of human embryonic stem cell-derived keratinocytes as an in vitro research model for mechanical stress dynamic response. *Stem Cell Rev and Rep.* 2015;11(3):460–473. https://doi.org/10.1007/s12015-014-9565-5.

57. Boer J, Nazary M, Riis PT. The Role of Mechanical Stress in Hidradenitis Suppurativa. *Dermatol Clin.* 2016;34(1):37–43. https://doi.org/10.1016/j.det.2015.08.011.

58. Zou L, Sasaki J, Wei G-X, et al. Effects of Mind–Body Exercises (Tai Chi/Yoga) on Heart Rate Variability Parameters and Perceived Stress: A Systematic Review with Meta-Analysis of Randomized Controlled Trials. *J Clin Med.* 2018;7(11):404. https://doi.org/10.3390/jcm7110404.

59. Matusiak Ł, Bieniek A, Szepietowski JC. Hidradenitis suppurativa markedly decreases quality of life and professional activity. *J Am Acad Dermatol.* 2010;62(4):706–708. e1 https://doi.org/10.1016/j.jaad.2009.09.021.

60. Onderdijk AJ, van der Zee HH, Esmann S, et al. Depression in patients with hidradenitis suppurativa: Depression in HS patients. *J Eur Acad Dermatol Venereol.* 2013;27(4):473–478. https://doi.org/10.1111/j.1468-3083.2012.04468.x.

61. Theut Riis P, Thorlacius L, Knudsen List E, Jemec GBE. A pilot study of unemployment in patients with hidradenitis suppurativa in Denmark. *Br J Dermatol.* 2017;176(4):1083–1085. https://doi.org/10.1111/bjd.14922.

62. Riis P, Vinding G, Ring H, Jemec G. Disutility in Patients with Hidradenitis Suppurativa: A Cross-sectional Study Using EuroQoL-5D. *Acta Derm Venereol.* 2016;96(2):222–226. https://doi.org/10.2340/00015555-2129.

63. Butt M, Sisic M, Silva C, et al. The associations of depression and coping methods on health-related quality of life for those with hidradenitis suppurativa. *J Am Acad Dermatol.* 2019;80(4):1137–1139. https://doi.org/10.1016/j.jaad.2018.09.045.

64. Maarouf M, Maarouf CL, Yosipovitch G, Shi VY. The impact of stress on epidermal barrier function: an evidence-based review. *Br J Dermatol.* 2019;181(6):1129–1137. https://doi.org/10.1111/bjd.17605.

65. Garg A, Chren M-M, Sands LP, et al. Psychological stress perturbs epidermal permeability barrier homeostasis: implications for the pathogenesis of stress-associated skin disorders. *Arch Dermatol.* 2001;137(1). https://doi.org/10.1001/archderm.137.1.53.

66. Kabat-Zinn J, Wheeler E, Light T, et al. Influence of a mindfulness meditation-based stress reduction intervention on rates of skin clearing in patients with moderate to severe psoriasis undergoing phototherapy (UVB) and photochemotherapy (PUVA). *Psychosom Med.* 1998;60(5):625–632. https://doi.org/10.1097/00006842-199809000-00020.

67. Robinson H, Jarrett P, Broadbent E. The Effects of Relaxation Before or After Skin Damage on Skin Barrier Recovery: A Preliminary Study. *Psychosom Med.* 2015;77(8):844–852. https://doi.org/10.1097/PSY.0000000000000222.

28

Complementary and Alternative Medicine

KYLA N. PRICE, ALYSSA M. THOMPSON, AND VIVIAN Y. SHI

Introduction

Hidradenitis suppurativa (HS) poses many challenges to patients, including delays in diagnosis, recurring pain, discomfort, and inadequate symptom coverage with conventional therapies. A survey study of 303 HS patients reported that half of HS patients using conventional therapies reported these methods as "not very successful."[1] As a result, many patients resort to complementary and alternative medicine (CAM) methods to treat and optimize their symptoms. The same survey study reported that 86% of HS patients used CAM for their HS and 65% of those that used CAM reported it at least "mildly successful." The most commonly reported reasons for using CAM included frustration with conventional treatment and a desire to try something "new" and more "natural." The majority (72%) of CAM users would recommend it to others. Many CAM modalities have not been specifically studied for HS, so data has been extrapolated from other inflammatory diseases with overlapping pathogenesis and symptoms.

The National Center for Complementary and Integrative Health (NCCIH) defines CAM as medical and health practices that are not currently considered to be part of conventional medicine.[2] CAM can be divided into two categories: natural products and mind and body practices. Natural products include herbs, vitamins, minerals, and probiotics. Mind and body practices include procedures or techniques such as yoga,

meditation, acupuncture, and hypnotherapy. Complementary health approaches outside of these two groups include cultural practices, such as Ayurvedic medicine, traditional Chinese medicine, homeopathy, and naturopathy. In this chapter, we will highlight the current knowledge and impact of CAM modalities on HS.

Complementary and Alternative Medicine Methods

A summary of CAM methods examined in this chapter, including their proposed mechanism of action, side effects, and special considerations are included in Table 28.1.

Vitamin D

There is evidence to suggest a relationship between vitamin D and the pathogenesis of HS. While the exact role vitamin D plays in HS is unknown, it appears to modulate immune function systemically within the folliculo-pilosebaceous subunit. Vitamin D supplementation increases the synthesis of antimicrobial peptides, which subsequently may reduce secondary infections and skin inflammation.

Pro-inflammatory cytokines, including tumor necrosis factor-alpha (TNF-α), interleukin (IL)-1β, IL-10, IL-17, and IL-18 are elevated in lesional and non-lesional skin of HS patients.[3,4] Vitamin D and its metabolites can promote anti-inflammatory activity through inhibition of IL-1, IL-17, TNF-α, or other proinflammatory pathways, such as the nuclear factor-κB (NF-κB) pathway.[5,6] In-vitro studies have shown that vitamin D can reduce cytokine production and downregulate antigen presentation.[7,8] Additionally, vitamin D has demonstrated some potential benefit in wound healing for patients with diabetic foot ulcers.[9]

HS patients have abnormal hair growth cycles as well as keratinocyte proliferation and differentiation. Vitamin D receptors play a significant role in epidermal homeostasis;[10,11] activation of vitamin D receptors regulates keratinocyte proliferation and differentiation.[12] In HS, supplementation with vitamin D may help control and normalize keratinocyte proliferation and differentiation to reduce follicular obstruction.[13]

Two previous studies have established a potential relationship between vitamin D deficiency and patients with HS. Serum levels of 25-hydroxyvitamin D were tested in patients with HS; the majority had insufficient (<50 nmol/L) levels, while over a third

TABLE 28.1 Overview of Complementary and Alternative Medicine Treatments

CAM Treatments	Hypothesized Mechanism of Action	Adverse Side Effects	Studied in HS?
Vitamin D	• Anti-inflammatory: Modulates the immune system by increasing the synthesis of antimicrobial peptides while also controlling keratinocyte proliferation and differentiation. Inhibition of pro-inflammatory cytokines found in HS lesions including IL-1β, IL-10 IL-17, IL-18, and TNF-α. • Inhibits keratinocyte proliferation and differentiation	• Hypercalcemia, hypercalciuria	Yes
Vitamin B12 (Cobalamin)	• Anti-inflammatory: overcomes impaired methionine synthetase and reduces TNF-α	• None	Yes
Zinc	• Anti-inflammatory: Inhibits NK cell activity, chemotaxis of granulocytes, keratinocyte activation, the production of damaging free radicals, and proinflammatory cytokines	• Nausea, vomiting, epigastric pain, loss of appetite, abdominal cramps, diarrhea, and headaches. Recommend combining with copper, especially when taking higher doses, to avoid copper deficiency.	Yes
Cannabinoids	• Analgesic and anti-pruritic: regulates nociceptive signals to the peripheral nervous system through interactions with vanilloid receptors. Inhibits the release of calcitonin gene-related peptide involved in the transmission of pain • Inhibits keratinocyte proliferation • Anti-inflammatory: inhibits the NF-κB pathway	• Systemic: Tachycardia (acute), bradycardia (chronic), decreased systemic vascular resistance, nystagmus, conjunctival injection, decreased intraocular pressure, lethargy, decreased concentration, and generalized psychomotor impairment	Yes

	Mechanism	Side effects	
Curcumin (Turmeric)	• Anti-inflammatory: Inhibits the production of IL-6, IL-8, MIP-1α, IL-1β, and TNF-α • Microbiome modulation: inhibits *Cutibacterium acne* growth	• Diarrhea, nausea, headache, yellow stool, and rash	No
Magnesium	• Anti-inflammatory: Reduces markers of systemic inflammation demonstrated by reduced C-reactive protein, IL-6, and TNF-α receptor 2 • Anti-nociceptive: noncompetitive inhibitor of N-methyl-D-aspartate preventing influx of calcium into cells	• Weakness, nausea, dizziness, confusion, cardiovascular complication, neurological disorder	No
Niacinamide (Nicotinamide)	• Anti-inflammatory: Decreases production of IL-8	• Oral: Insulin resistance, Parkinson's disease, liver toxicity • Topical: burning, pruritus, erythema	No
Balneotherapy, Magnesium sulfate bath	• Anti-inflammatory: decreases the production of inflammatory markers such as human beta-defensin-2, skin-derived antileukoproteinase, TNF-α, IL-6, and IL-1α	• Skin irritation, itching	No
Acupuncture/Acupressure	• Anti-inflammatory: Downregulation of pro-inflammatory cytokines, pro-inflammatory neuropeptides, and neurotrophins • Analgesic: Hypothesized to be due to stimulation of inhibitory nerve fibers, neurotransmitter modulation, and/or endorphin release	• Acupuncture: fever, pain, dizziness • Acupressure: bruising, soreness, and itch	No

CAM, Complementary and alternative medicine; *IL*, interleukin; *MIP*, macrophage inflammatory protein; *NF*, nuclear factor; *NK*, natural killer; *TNF*, tumor necrosis factor.

of HS patients in one study were severely deficient (<10 nmol/L).[13,14] Serum vitamin D deficiency correlated with disease severity based on Hurley stage. Patients with insufficient vitamin D levels who received supplementation according to their level of deficit had a significant decrease in the number of HS nodules at six months. These findings suggest that vitamin D may have a role in immune modulation and inhibiting keratinocyte proliferation.

The North American HS clinical management guidelines report that there is insufficient evidence to support routine use of vitamin D, so the inclusion of vitamin D supplementation is a grade C recommendation, which indicates recommendation based on opinion, consensus, case series, or disease-oriented evidence.[15,16] Supplementation should be done with caution as excess vitamin D can lead to hypercalcemia and hypercalciuria.

Vitamin B$_{12}$ (Cobalamin)

Vitamin B$_{12}$, also known as cobalamin, is generally safe, inexpensive, accessible, and has been shown to contribute to improvement in other dermatologic conditions.[17,18] Some patients are thought to have reduced S-adenosyl-L-methionine due to impairment of the vitamin B$_{12}$-dependent enzyme, methionine synthetase.[19] S-adenosyl-L-methionine has been shown to reduce serum TNF-α levels in mouse models.[20] Therefore, patients with reduced S-adenosyl-L-methionine may have higher TNF-α levels contributing to HS pathogenesis. Cobalamin deficiency has also been associated with increased TNF-α expression.[21] Supplementation with vitamin B$_{12}$ therefore may help to overcome impaired methionine synthetase activity and to reduce TNF-α levels.

Three patients with HS and concomitant inflammatory bowel disease who were given high dose vitamin B$_{12}$ (1000 micrograms for six weeks and then monthly thereafter) experienced reduction in the eruption of new lesions.[19] Vitamin B$_{12}$ has a low potential for toxicity but has been implicated in the development of acne in certain individuals.[22,23] Future investigations are warranted to better understand the role of vitamin B$_{12}$ as a potential adjuvant therapy for HS.

Zinc

Zinc is essential for cellular processes such as cell proliferation, differentiation, and apoptosis.[24] As a result, zinc plays a role in the modulation of both the innate and adaptive immune functions. There is evidence to suggest that zinc deficiency can decrease natural killer (NK) cell activity, including cell signaling and recognition.[25,26] Zinc also inhibits granulocyte chemotaxis, keratinocyte activation, and production of damaging free radicals and proinflammatory cytokines.[27–30] Both IL-17 producing cells and neutrophils are implicated in the pathogenesis of HS; zinc suppresses the development of IL-17 producing cells, which consequentially reduces the neutrophil count [31,32].

Toll-like receptors (TLRs) lead to inflammatory cytokines production. Enhanced TLR2 expression by infiltrating macrophages and dendritic cells in HS lesions is thought to contribute to the disease pathogenesis.[33] Zinc exhibits anti-inflammatory effects by downregulating TLR response and inhibiting keratinocyte expression of TLRs.[34,35]

A potential relationship between HS and zinc deficiency has been demonstrated by patients who developed new-onset HS or had worsening HS following bariatric surgery and weight loss.[36] After bariatric surgery, these patients were found to exhibit several nutritional deficiencies, including zinc deficiency. Patients who

developed HS or had worsening HS following bariatric surgery had significantly lower serum zinc levels than typical HS patients.

The efficacy of zinc supplementation in HS patients has been evaluated in open label studies. The most commonly studied zinc formulation is zinc gluconate; zinc picolinate has better absorption but is more expensive.[37] HS patients with Hurley stage I and II who were treated with 90mg of zinc gluconate daily in conjunction with topical triclosan experienced improvement in their HS disease and quality of life, as measured by the modified HS score and Dermatology Life Quality Index (DLQI), respectively.[38,39] Patients who initially achieved remission experienced exacerbation when their zinc dosage was reduced to 30 to 60 mg/day, indicating the potential suppressive rather than curative nature of zinc treatment. Oral zinc gluconate in combination with nicotinamide for maintenance therapy has also demonstrated a significant reduction in the number and duration of acute flares as well as extended disease-free survival.[40] Based on insufficient evidence to support routine use, the North American clinical management guidelines for HS lists zinc with a grade C recommendation, indicating support of use based on opinion, consensus, case series, or disease-oriented evidence.[15,16]

Common side effects of zinc supplementation include nausea, vomiting, and loss of appetite; these can be mitigated by adhering to the recommended dose.[41] Zinc can also affect the intestinal absorption of copper at the mucosal level by stimulating the production of metallothionein, a metal-binding protein which sequesters copper. Therefore, it is recommended that patients who chronically receive high dose zinc supplementation also take copper to avoid copper deficiency.[42] The typical ratio for co-administration of zinc:copper is 10:1. Even with copper co-supplementation, patients should be monitored for signs and symptoms of copper deficiency, which include hair loss, diarrhea, eye and skin sores, loss of appetite,[41] hypochromic microcytic anemia, and neutropenia.[43–45]

Cannabinoids

Cannabinoids have drawn increasing public attention with expanding legalization and accessibility. Cannabinoids are a group of compounds that are biologically and structurally similar to the chemical compounds of *Cannabis sativa*.[46] There are three classes of cannabinoids: plant-derived cannabinoids (phytocannabinoids), endogenous cannabinoids (endocannabinoids), and synthetic cannabinoids. Phytocannabinoids are plant-derived cannabinoids that are historically derived from *cannabis sativa*.[47] The most notable phytocannabinoids are Δ^9-tetrahydrocannabinol (THC), which can have psychotropic effects, and cannabidiols (CBD), which are mostly non-psychotropic. Endocannabinoids are endogenous lipids that function as ligands for cannabinoid receptors.[46] Synthetic cannabinoids are developed in laboratories and mimic phytocannabinoids and endocannabinoids.

The effects of cannabinoids are mediated by cannabinoid receptors CB1 and CB2. CB1 is responsible for the psychoactive effects through the release of various neurotransmitters,[48] while CB2 is presumed to mediate immunomodulation and the anti-inflammatory effects of cannabinoids.[49] Generally, oral cannabinoids have been shown to target systemic symptoms such as anorexia, nausea, and pain, whereas topically applied cannabinoids often target localized pain and inflammation.[50–54]

The pathogenesis of HS includes a complex relationship between pilosebaceous unit occlusion due to keratinocyte proliferation, sebaceous gland disruption, and an overlapping, autoinflammatory response.[3,4,55,56] Cannabinoids have been shown to inhibit keratinocyte proliferation in vitro CBD, and other phytocannabinoids have also been shown to inhibit a number of inflammatory pathways, including the NF-κB pathway.[57]

Anandamide is a CB1 agonist that interacts with vanilloid receptors to transduce and regulate nociceptive signals (including pain and itch) to the peripheral nervous system.[58,59] Phytocannabinoids and cannabinoid agonists have demonstrated clinical improvements for patients with pain associated with chronic medical conditions.[60–62] CB1 and CB2 agonists have been shown to reduce itch for patients with lichen simplex chronicus, uremic pruritus, atopic dermatitis (AD), and prurigo nodularis.[63,64] In a study of acne patients, application of topical cannabis seed extract cream resulted in significant decreases in skin sebum and erythema.[65] Cannabinoids may have an analgesic effect in HS due to inhibition of the release of calcitonin gene-related peptide, which is stored in sensory neurons and involved in the transmission of pain.[66]

Despite the growing interest in the therapeutic applications of cannabinoids, there remains a lack of high quality randomized controlled trials that evaluate their effects in dermatology. In a recent HS CAM survey, marijuana and topical CBD oil were both among the more commonly used CAM methods by respondents. Most users reported them as helpful, with 57% reporting marijuana as helpful and 45% reporting topical CBD oil as helpful. Systemic toxicity can occur as a result of overstimulation of the endocannabinoid system from exogenous cannabinoid use through ingestion or inhalation.[67] Notable side effects of cannabinoid systemic toxicity include tachycardia (acute), bradycardia (chronic), decreased systemic vascular resistance, nystagmus, conjunctival injection, decreased intraocular pressure, lethargy, decreased concentration, and generalized psychomotor impairment.

Curcumin/Turmeric

Curcumin (diferuloylmethane) is a naturally occurring, active polyphenol derived from the plant *Curcuma longa* (turmeric) of the ginger family.[68,69] There has been a growing interest in the potential therapeutic applications of curcumin because of its low cost and good safety profile. To date, there have been no studies examining the efficacy of curcumin in the treatment of patients with HS. However, there have been some promising findings with topical and oral curcumin in other inflammatory skin conditions (such as psoriasis and AD).[70–73] Curcumin is known for its anti-inflammatory properties and is thought to inhibit the production of cytokines that have been implicated in HS, such as IL-6, IL-8, macrophage inflammatory protein-1α, IL-1β, and TNF-α.[74–78] Inhibition of proinflammatory cytokine production may help restore skin homeostasis by hindering the cyclical immune activation. Curcumin also appears to play a role in microbiome modulation, such as inhibiting the growth of *Cutibacterium acnes*.[79]

Concomitant use of both oral curcumin and curcumin topical cream had more improvement compared to placebo, oral curcumin alone, and oral curcumin combined with a curcumin topical gel in a phase II clinical trial of patients with acne vulgaris.[80] In dermatology clinical trials, oral curcumin has been administered with benefit at doses ranging from 2000 to 6000 mg/day.[81–83] Oral curcumin has poor bioavailability due to rapid elimination, fast metabolism, and poor absorption.[84,85] As a result, it is recommended to consume piperine (black pepper) with curcumin, at a curcumin to piperine ratio of 100 to 1 to increase its bioavailability.[85]

Diarrhea, headache, yellow stool, rash, and nausea have been reported with curcumin use, often at higher doses.[86,87] In some cases, the symptoms resolved with continued use or improved with reduction in the curcumin dose. Gastrointestinal side effects may be reduced by taking curcumin with food and yogurt concurrently. For bothersome symptoms despite dose reduction, cessation of use may be recommended. Curcumin use may inhibit platelet aggregation and should be avoided in patients taking anticoagulants or antiplatelet medications.[88,89] Future investigations are warranted to further understand the relationship of curcumin in HS, especially since 60% of respondents in a recent survey stated that they use curcumin for their HS, although the route of administration was unknown.[1]

Magnesium

Magnesium is a noncompetitive inhibitor of N-methyl-D-aspartate and inhibits the entry of calcium ions into cells, leading to an antinociceptive effect.[90] Magnesium therapy has been shown effective in reducing pain for a number of conditions, including primary dysmenorrhea, headaches, and perioperative pain.[91–93] Elevations in C-reactive protein have been seen in magnesium depletion and may be a predisposing factor to chronic inflammatory stress.[94,95] Magnesium intake has also been inversely associated with other markers of systemic inflammation including high-sensitivity C-reactive protein, IL-6, and TNF-α receptor 2.[96–98] Supplementation with magnesium may be beneficial in alleviating pain associated with HS lesions as well as minimizing inflammatory stress. Hypermagnesemia is relatively uncommon but can occur in patients with renal disease or increased magnesium intake.[99] Patients who receive magnesium supplementation should be monitored for symptoms of hypermagnesemia which range from weakness, nausea, dizziness, and confusion in mild cases, to serious systemic symptoms including cardiovascular complications, flaccid paralysis, lethargy, and coma.

Niacinamide (Nicotinamide)

Niacinamide has demonstrated some clinical benefit in acne and may be beneficial for patients with HS, though more research is needed. In patients with acne vulgaris, *C. acnes* interacts with TLR2, leading to activation of IL-8.[100] Through the NF-κB and mitogen-activated protein kinase pathway, nicotinamide decreases the production of IL-8 and subsequently reduces inflammation. Combined supplementation of nicotinamide 750 mg, zinc 25 mg, copper 1.5 mg, and folic acid 500 µg has been shown to improve acne.[101] Another study found that topical 4% niacinamide exhibited comparable clinical efficacy for acne as topical clindamycin, particularly in patients with oily skin types.[102] Oral niacinamide in combination with zinc gluconate as maintenance therapy has been shown to extend disease-free survival and significantly reduce the rate and duration of flares.[40] Burning, pruritus, and erythema have been reported with topical niacinamide.[103,104]

Bathing Regimens

For HS patients with multiple widely separated areas of involvement, bathing treatments can be useful, as they treat a wide body surface area. Sodium hypochlorite (bleach) baths are discussed in Chapter 15. In addition to bleach baths, HS patients may consider using magnesium sulfate (Epsom salt) baths. A magnesium sulfate bath was among the most common CAM methods (60%) used by survey respondents, and 48% of users found magnesium sulfate baths helpful for their HS.[1] A discussion about magnesium sulfate baths can be found in Chapter 15.

Balneotherapy is a method of bathing or immersing in mineral water. Often, studies examining balneotherapy are conducted using mineral water with elevated levels of magnesium along with other Dead Sea minerals such as sodium, potassium, calcium, chloride, sulfate, and carbonate.[105] In patients with AD, balneotherapy has been shown to control flare symptoms in refractory cases, clear lesions, reduce itch, and reduce the amount of *Staphylococcus aureus* on the skin surface.[106,107] Balneotherapy has also demonstrated benefits for patients with psoriasis and acne.[108,109] Dead sea water and selenium-rich thermal spring water have been shown to decrease levels of psoriasis-associated inflammatory markers such as human β-defensin-2, skin-derived antileukoproteinase, TNF-α, IL-6, and IL-1α.[110–112] Side effects of balneotherapy are rare and include itch and skin irritation.[113]

In addition to the anti-inflammatory and anti-itch benefits of different bathing techniques, the act of bathing has been shown to reduce stress, pain, and fatigue.[114] The heat from thermal baths stimulates the release of β-endorphin and enkephalin, endogenous opioid peptides which can influence pain reception.[115,116] It should be noted that not every patient has access to a bathtub for the purpose of implementing bathing techniques.

Acupuncture and Acupressure

Acupuncture is a practice of traditional Chinese medicine in which the body's meridian lines are stimulated via insertion of thin needles through the skin.[117–119] The meridian lines are thought to host channels in which energy known as Qi flows, and may influence the autonomic system. Acupuncture helps to reduce inflammation, pain, and itch. The anti-inflammatory effects of acupuncture are thought to be mediated by downregulation of pro-inflammatory cytokines, pro-inflammatory neuropeptides, and neurotrophins while altering the Th1/Th2 cytokine balance.[120–122] The precise mechanism of acupuncture pain reduction is not completely understood but may be due to stimulation of inhibitory nerve fibers to reduce pain signals to the brain, endorphin release, and/or neurotransmitter modulation.[123–128].

Battlefield acupuncture involves five sequentially placed acupoints on the ear: intertragic notch, antitragus, helix, helix crus, and antihelix crura.[129] The use of battlefield and ear acupuncture among veterans has consistently resulted in immediate pain reduction.[130–133] The immediate pain reduction associated with acupuncture may be beneficial for patients with HS, especially during acute flares where pain is often a predominant symptom. Battlefield acupuncture has also demonstrated some success and benefit in opioid weaning for patients with chronic pain.[134] An alternative to acupuncture for patients that have a fear of needles is acupressure, which consists of applying external pressure without puncturing the skin to similarly designated acupoints. Both acupuncture and acupressure have resulted in improvements to psoriasis and AD symptoms, such as pruritus as well as improvement in disease severity measures including the Eczema and Psoriasis Area and Severity Indexes.[135,136] Research is needed to investigate whether the notable improvements in pain and pruritus seen in other chronic cutaneous diseases may be achieved in HS. Adverse effects reported with acupuncture-related techniques include fever,

pain, and dizziness.[137] Potential side effects of acupressure include bruising, soreness, and itch at the pressure sites.[138,139]

Conclusion

HS patients often express frustration with conventional therapies in treating their disease, so many resort to CAM completely or concurrently with their conventional treatment regimens. However, there is limited level one evidence supporting the use of various CAM methods, and many have not been studied in HS. As a result, several CAM modalities have been anecdotally tried by patients in hopes of achieving the potential clinical benefits seen in other diseases. Especially for more severe disease, CAM may be more beneficial when used in conjunction with other conventional therapies. In most countries, CAM is not covered by insurance and can result in additional out-of-pocket expenses for patients. Future investigations are warranted to understand the potential benefits of various CAM methods in HS and how they can safely and effectively be incorporated into the conventional HS treatment paradigm. Increases in governmental regulations and standardized safety testing for CAM treatment modalities is needed.

References

1. Price KN, Thompson AM, Rizvi O, et al. Complementary and Alternative Medicine Use in Patients With Hidradenitis Suppurativa. *JAMA Dermatol.* 2020;156(3):345–348. https://doi.org/10.1001/jamadermatol.2019.4595.
2. National Library of Medicine. *Complementary and Alternative Medicine*; 2020. Retrieved from https://www.ncbi.nlm.nih.gov/books/NBK518811/.
3. Kelly G, Hughes R, McGarry T, et al. Dysregulated cytokine expression in lesional and nonlesional skin in hidradenitis suppurativa. *Br J Dermatol.* 2015;173(6):1431–1439. https://doi.org/10.1111/bjd.14075.
4. Van Der Zee HH, De Ruiter L, Van Den Broecke DG, et al. Elevated levels of tumour necrosis factor (TNF)-α, interleukin (IL)-1β and IL-10 in hidradenitis suppurativa skin: a rationale for targeting TNF-α and IL-1β. *Br J Dermatol.* 2011;164(6):1292–1298. https://doi.org/10.1111/j.1365-2133.2011.10254.x.
5. Janjetovic Z, Zmijewski MA, Tuckey RC, et al. 20-Hydroxycholecalciferol, product of vitamin D3 hydroxylation by P450scc, decreases NF-κB activity by increasing IκBα levels in human keratinocytes. *PLoS One.* 2009;4(6). https://doi.org/10.1371/journal.pone.0005988, e5988.
6. Janjetovic Z, Tuckey RC, Nguyen MN, Thorpe EM, Slominski AT. 20,23-dihydroxyvitamin D3, novel P450scc product, stimulates differentiation and inhibits proliferation and NF-κB activity in human keratinocytes. *J Cell Physiol.* 2009. https://doi.org/10.1002/jcp.21992. n/a-n/a.
7. van Etten E, Decallonne B, Bouillon R, Mathieu C. NOD bone marrow-derived dendritic cells are modulated by analogs of 1,25-dihydroxyvitamin D3. *J Steroid Biochem Mol Biol.* 2008;89–90 (1–5):457–459. https://doi.org/10.1016/j.jsbmb.2004.03.017.
8. Van Halteren AGS, Van Etten E, De Jong EC, et al. Redirection of human autoreactive T-cells upon Interaction with dendritic cells modulated by TX527, an analog of 1,25 dihydroxyvitamin D(3). *Diabetes.* 2002;51(7):2119–2125. https://doi.org/10.2337/diabetes.51.7.2119.
9. Razzaghi R, Pourbagheri H, Momen-Heravi M, et al. (2017). The effects of vitamin D supplementation on wound healing and metabolic status in patients with diabetic foot ulcer: A randomized, double-blind, placebo-controlled trial. *J Diabetes Complications.*

2017;31(4):766–772. https://doi.org/10.1016/j.jdiacomp.2016.06.017.

10. Li YC, Pirro AE, Amling M, et al. Targeted ablation of the vitamin D receptor: an animal model of vitamin D-dependent rickets type II with alopecia. *Proc Natl Acad Sci.* 1997;94(18):9831–9835. https://doi.org/10.1073/pnas.94.18.9831.

11. Erben RG, Soegiarto DW, Weber K, et al. Deletion of deoxyribonucleic acid binding domain of the vitamin D receptor abrogates genomic and nongenomic functions of vitamin D. *Mol Endocrinol.* 2002;16(7):1524–1537. https://doi.org/10.1210/mend.16.7.0866.

12. Xie Z, Komuves L, Yu QC, et al. Lack of the vitamin D receptor is associated with reduced epidermal differentiation and hair follicle growth. *J Investig Dermatol.* 2002;118(1):11–16. https://doi.org/10.1046/j.1523-1747.2002.01644.x.

13. Guillet A, Brocard A, Bach Ngohou K, et al. Verneuil's disease, innate immunity and vitamin D: a pilot study. *J Eur Acad Dermatol Venereol.* 2015;29(7):1347–1353. https://doi.org/10.1111/jdv.12857.

14. Kelly G, Sweeney CM, Fitzgerald R, et al. Vitamin D status in hidradenitis suppurativa. *Br J Dermatol.* 2014;170(6):1379–1380. https://doi.org/10.1111/bjd.12900.

15. Alikhan A, Sayed C, Alavi A, et al. North American clinical management guidelines for hidradenitis suppurativa: a publication from the United States and Canadian Hidradenitis Suppurativa Foundations. *J Am Acad Dermatol.* 2019;81(1):76–90. https://doi.org/10.1016/j.jaad.2019.02.067.

16. Ebell MH, Siwek J, Weiss BD, et al. Strength of recommendation taxonomy (SORT): a patient-centered approach to grading evidence in the medical literature. *J Am Board Fam Med.* 2004;17(1):59–67. https://doi.org/10.3122/jabfm.17.1.59.

17. Stucker M, Pieck C, Stoerb C, et al. Topical vitamin B12-a new therapeutic approach in atopic dermatitis-evaluation of efficacy and tolerability in a randomized placebo-controlled multicentre clinical trial. *Br J Dermatol.* 2004;150(5):977–983. https://doi.org/10.1111/j.1365-2133.2004.05866.x.

18. Simon SW. Vitamin B12 therapy in allergy and chronic dermatoses. *J Allergy.* 1951;22(2):183–185. https://doi.org/10.1016/0021-8707(51)90059-7.

19. Mortimore M, Florin THJ. A role for B12 in inflammatory bowel disease patients with suppurative dermatoses? An experience with high dose vitamin B12 therapy. *J Crohn's Colitis.* 2010;4(4):466–470. https://doi.org/10.1016/j.crohns.2010.02.007.

20. Watson WH, Zhao Y, Chawla RK. S-adenosylmethionine attenuates the lipopolysaccharide-induced expression of the gene for tumour necrosis factor alpha. *Biochem J.* 1999;342(Pt 1):21–25.

21. Scalabrino G, Peracchi M. New insights into the pathophysiology of cobalamin deficiency. *Trends Mol Med.* 2006;12(6):247–254. https://doi.org/10.1016/j.molmed.2006.04.008.

22. Institute of Medicine. *Dietary Reference Intakes for Thiamin, Riboflavin, Niacin, Vitamin B6, Folate, Vitamin B12, Pantothenic Acid, Biotin, and Choline.* Washington, DC: The National Academies Press; 1988.

23. Kang D, Shi B, Erfe MC, et al. Vitamin B12 modulates the transcriptome of the skin microbiota in acne pathogenesis. *Sci Transl Med.* 2015;7(293). https://doi.org/10.1126/scitranslmed.aab2009.293ra103-293ra103.

24. Brocard A, Dréno B. Innate immunity: a crucial target for zinc in the treatment of inflammatory dermatosis. *J Eur Acad Dermatol Venereol.* 2011;25(10):1146–1152. https://doi.org/10.1111/j.1468-3083.2010.03934.x.

25. Mocchegiani E, Santarelli L, Muzzioli M, Fabris N. Reversibility of the thymic involution and of age-related peripheral immune dysfunctions by zinc supplementation in old mice. *Int J Immunopharmacol.* 1995;17(9):703–718. doi:https://doi.org/10.1016/0192-0561(95)00059-B (web archive link).

26. Rajagopalan S, Winter CC, Wagtmann N, Long EO. The Ig-related killer cell inhibitory receptor binds zinc and requires zinc for recognition of HLA-C on target cells. *J Immunol.* 1995;155(9):4143–4146. Retrieved from https://www.jimmunol.org/content/jimmunol/155/9/4143.full.pdf.

27. Frank S, Kämpfer H, Podda M, et al. Identification of copper/zinc superoxide dismutase as a nitric oxide-regulated gene in human (HaCaT) keratinocytes: implications for keratinocyte proliferation. *Biochem J.* 2000;346(Pt 3):719–728.

28. Dreno B, Trossaert M, Boiteau HL, Litoux P. Zinc salts effects on granulocyte zinc concentration and chemotaxis in acne patients. *Acta Derm Venereol.* 1992;72(4):250–252.

29. Yamaoka J, Kume T, Akaike A, Miyachi Y. Suppressive effect of zinc ion on iNOS expression induced by interferon-gamma or tumor necrosis factor-alpha in murine keratinocytes. *J Dermatol Sci.* 2000;23(1):27–35. https://doi.org/10.1016/s0923-1811(99)00062-6.

30. Driessen C, Hirv K, Rink L, Kirchner H. Induction of cytokines by zinc ions in human peripheral blood mononuclear cells and separated monocytes. *Lymphokine Cytokine Res.* 1994;13(1):15–20.

31. Kitabayashi C, Fukada T, Kanamoto M, et al. Zinc suppresses Th17 development via inhibition of STAT3 activation. *Int Immunol.* 2010;22(5):375–386. https://doi.org/10.1093/intimm/dxq017.

32. Lima AL, Karl I, Giner T, et al. Keratinocytes and neutrophils are important sources of proinflammatory molecules in hidradenitis suppurativa. *Br J Dermatol.* 2016;174(3):514–521. https://doi.org/10.1111/bjd.14214.

33. Hunger RE, Surovy AM, Hassan AS, et al. Toll-like receptor 2 is highly expressed in lesions of acne inversa and colocalizes with C-type lectin receptor. *Br J Dermatol.* 2008;158(4):691–697. https://doi.org/10.1111/j.1365-2133.2007.08425.x.

34. Jarrousse V, Castex-Rizzi N, Khammari A, et al. Zinc salts inhibit in vitro Toll-like receptor 2 surface expression by keratinocytes. *Eur J Dermatol.* 2007;17(6):492–496. https://doi.org/10.1684/ejd.2007.0263.

35. Gon Y, Asai Y, Hashimoto S, et al. A20 inhibits toll-like receptor 2– and 4–mediated interleukin-8 synthesis in airway epithelial cells. *Am J Respir Cell Mol Biol.* 2004;31(3):330–336. https://doi.org/10.1165/rcmb.2003-0438oc.

36. Garcovich S, De Simone C, Giovanardi G, et al. Post-bariatric surgery hidradenitis suppurativa: a new patient subset associated with malabsorption and micronutritional deficiencies. *Clin Exp Dermatol.* 2019;44(3):283–289. https://doi.org/10.1111/ced.13732.

37. Barrie SA, Wright JV, Pizzorno JE, et al. Comparative absorption of zinc picolinate, zinc citrate and zinc gluconate in humans. *Agents Actions.* 1987;21(1–2):223–228. https://doi.org/10.1007/bf01974946.

38. Hessam S, Sand M, Meier NM, et al. Combination of oral zinc gluconate and topical triclosan: an anti-inflammatory treatment modality for initial hidradenitis suppurativa. *J Dermatol Sci.* 2016;84(2):197–202. https://doi.org/10.1016/j.jdermsci.2016.08.010.

39. Brocard A, Knol AC, Khammari A, Dréno B. Hidradenitis suppurativa and zinc: a new therapeutic approach. A pilot study. *Dermatology.* 2007;214(4):325–327. https://doi.org/10.1159/000100883.

40. Molinelli E, Brisigotti V, Campanati A, et al. Efficacy of oral zinc and nicotinamide as maintenance therapy for mild/moderate hidradenitis suppurativa: a controlled retrospective clinical study. *J Am Acad Dermatol.* 2020;83(2):665–667. https://doi.org/10.1016/j.jaad.2020.04.092.

41. Zinc Fact Sheet for Health Professionals. National Institutes of Health Office of Dietary Supplements. Published 2019. Accessed August 2020.

42. Fischer PW, Giroux A, L'Abbe MR. Effects of zinc on mucosal copper binding and on the kinetics of copper absorption. *J Nutr.* 1983;113(2):462–469. https://doi.org/10.1093/jn/113.2.462.

43. Roeser HP, Lee GR, Nacht S, Cartwright GE. The role of ceruloplasmin in iron metabolism. *J Clin Investig.* 1970;49(12):2408–2417. https://doi.org/10.1172/jci106460.

44. Cartwright GE. The relationship of copper, cobalt, and other trace elements to hemopoiesis. *Am J Clin Nutr.* 1955;3(1):11–19. https://doi.org/10.1093/ajcn/3.1.11.

45. Zidar BL, Shadduck RK, Zeigler Z, Winkelstein A. Observations on the anemia and neutropenia of human copper deficiency. *Am J Hematol.* 1977;3:177–185. https://doi.org/10.1002/ajh.2830030209.

46. Lu HC, Mackie K. An Introduction to the Endogenous Cannabinoid System. *Biol Psychiatry.* 2016;79(7):516–525. https://doi.org/10.1016/j.biopsych.2015.07.028.

47. Gülck T, Møller BL. Phytocannabinoids: Origins and Biosynthesis. *Trends Plant Sci.* 2020. https://doi.org/10.1016/j.tplants.2020.05.005.

48. Nikan M, Nabavi SM, Manayi A. Ligands for cannabinoid receptors, promising anticancer agents. *Life Sci.* 2016;146:124–130. https://doi.org/10.1016/j.lfs.2015.12.053.

49. Eagleston LRM, Kalani NK, Patel RR, et al. Cannabinoids in dermatology: a scoping review. *Dermatol Online J.* 2018;24(6). Retrieved from https://www.ncbi.nlm.nih.gov/pubmed/30142706.

50. Meiri E, Jhangiani H, Vredenburgh JJ, et al. Efficacy of dronabinol alone and in combination with ondansetron versus ondansetron alone for delayed chemotherapy-induced nausea and vomiting. *Curr Med Res Opin.* 2007;23(3):533–543. https://doi.org/10.1185/030079907X167525.

51. Costiniuk CT, Mills E, Cooper CL. Evaluation of oral cannabinoid-containing medications for the management of interferon and ribavirin-induced anorexia, nausea and weight loss in patients treated for chronic hepatitis C virus. *Can J Gastroenterol.* 2008;22(4):376–380. https://doi.org/10.1155/2008/725702.

52. Rog DJ, Nurmikko TJ, Friede T, Young CA. Randomized, controlled trial of cannabis-based medicine in central pain in multiple sclerosis. *Neurology.* 2005;65(6):812–819. https://doi.org/10.1212/01.wnl.0000176753.45410.8b.

53. Chelliah MP, Zinn Z, Khuu P, Teng JMC. Self-initiated use of topical cannabidiol oil for epidermolysis bullosa. *Pediatr Dermatol.* 2018;35(4):e224–e227. https://doi.org/10.1111/pde.13545.

54. Hammell DC, Zhang LP, Ma F, et al. Transdermal cannabidiol reduces inflammation and pain-related behaviours in a rat model of arthritis. *Eur J Pain.* 2016;20(6):936–948. https://doi.org/10.1002/ejp.818.

55. Xiao X, He Y, Li C, et al. Nicastrin mutations in familial acne inversa impact keratinocyte proliferation and differentiation through the Notch and phosphoinositide 3-kinase/AKT signalling pathways. *Br J Dermatol.* 2016;174(3):522–532. https://doi.org/10.1111/bjd.14223.

56. Yu CC, Cook MG. Hidradenitis suppurativa: a disease of follicular epithelium, rather than apocrine glands. *Br J Dermatol.* 1990;122(6):763–769. https://doi.org/10.1111/j.1365-2133.1990.tb06264.x.

57. Oláh A, Tóth BI, Borbíró I, et al. Cannabidiol exerts sebostatic and antiinflammatory effects on human sebocytes. *J Clin Invest.* 2014;124(9):3713–3724. https://doi.org/10.1172/jci64628.

58. Clapper JR, Moreno-Sanz G, Russo R, et al. Anandamide suppresses pain initiation through a peripheral endocannabinoid mechanism. *Nat Neurosci.* 2010;13(10):1265–1270. https://doi.org/10.1038/nn.2632.

59. Boillat A, Alijevic O, Kellenberger S. Calcium entry via TRPV1 but not ASICs induces neuropeptide release from sensory neurons. *Mol Cell Neurosci.* 2014;61:13–22. https://doi.org/10.1016/j.mcn.2014.04.007.

60. Blake DR, Robson P, Ho M, et al. Preliminary assessment of the efficacy, tolerability and safety of a cannabis-based medicine (Sativex) in the treatment of pain caused by rheumatoid arthritis. *Rheumatology.* 2006;45(1):50–52. https://doi.org/10.1093/rheumatology/kei183.

61. Capano A, Weaver R, Burkman E. Evaluation of the effects of CBD hemp extract on opioid use and quality of life indicators in chronic pain patients: a prospective cohort study. *Postgrad Med.* 2020;132(1):56–61. https://doi.org/10.1080/00325481.2019.1685298.

62. Hoggart B, Ratcliffe S, Ehler E, et al. A multicentre, open-label, follow-on study to assess the long-term maintenance of effect, tolerance and safety of THC/CBD oromucosal spray in the management of neuropathic pain. *J Neurol.* 2015;262(1):27–40. https://doi.org/10.1007/s00415-014-7502-9.

63. Dvorak M, Watkinson A, McGlone F, Rukwied R. Histamine induced responses are attenuated by a cannabinoid receptor agonist in human skin. *Inflamm Res.* 2003;52(6):238–245. https://doi.org/10.1007/s00011-003-1162-z.

64. Ständer S, Reinhardt HW, Luger TA. Topische Cannabinoidagonisten. *Hautarzt.* 2006;57(9):801–807. https://doi.org/10.1007/s00105-006-1180-1.

65. Ali A, Akhtar N. The safety and efficacy of 3% Cannabis seeds extract cream for reduction of human cheek skin sebum and erythema content. *Pak J Pharm Sci.* 2015;28(4):1389–1395.

66. Ellington HC, Cotter MA, Cameron NE, Ross RA. The effect of cannabinoids on capsaicin-evoked calcitonin gene-related peptide (CGRP) release from the isolated paw skin of diabetic and non-diabetic rats. *Neuropharmacology.* 2002;42(7):966–975. https://doi.org/10.1016/S0028-3908(02)00040-0.

67. Kelly BF, Nappe TM. Cannabinoid Toxicity. In: *StatPearls.* Treasure Island (FL): StatPearls Publishing; 2020.

68. Gupta SC, Kismali G, Aggarwal BB. Curcumin, a component of turmeric: from farm to pharmacy. *Biofactors.* 2013;39(1):2–13. https://doi.org/10.1002/biof.1079.

69. Gupta SC, Patchva S, Koh W, Aggarwal BB. Discovery of curcumin, a component of golden spice, and its miraculous biological activities. *Clin Exp Pharmacol Physiol.* 2012;39(3):283–299. https://doi.org/10.1111/j.1440-1681.2011.05648.x.

70. Rawal RC, Shah BJ, Jayaraaman AM, Jaiswal V. Clinical evaluation of an Indian polyherbal topical formulation in the management of eczema. *J Altern Complement Med.* 2009;15(6):669–672. https://doi.org/10.1089/acm.2008.0508.

71. Bilia AR, Bergonzi MC, Isacchi B, et al. Curcumin nanoparticles potentiate therapeutic effectiveness of acitrein in moderate-to-severe psoriasis patients and control serum cholesterol levels. *J Pharm Pharmacol.* 2018;70(7):919–928. https://doi.org/10.1111/jphp.12910.

72. Bahraini P, Rajabi M, Mansouri P, et al. Turmeric tonic as a treatment in scalp psoriasis: a randomized placebo-control clinical trial. *J Cosmet Dermatol.* 2018;17(3):461–466. https://doi.org/10.1111/jocd.12513.

73. Antiga E, Bonciolini V, Volpi W, et al. Oral Curcumin (Meriva) Is Effective as an Adjuvant Treatment and Is Able to Reduce IL-22 Serum Levels in Patients with Psoriasis Vulgaris. *Biomed Res Int.* 2015;2015:283634. https://doi.org/10.1155/2015/283634.

74. Abe Y, Hashimoto S, Horie T. Curcumin inhibition of inflammatory cytokine production by human peripheral blood monocytes and alveolar macrophages. *Pharmacol Res.* 1999;39(1):41–47. https://doi.org/10.1006/phrs.1998.0404.

75. Jain SK, Rains J, Croad J, et al. Curcumin supplementation lowers TNF-α, IL-6, IL-8, and MCP-1 secretion in high glucose-treated cultured monocytes and blood levels of TNF-α, IL-6, MCP-1, glucose, and glycosylated hemoglobin in diabetic rats. *Antioxid Redox Signal.* 2009;11(2):241–249. https://doi.org/10.1089/ars.2008.2140.

76. Aggarwal BB, Gupta SC, Sung B. Curcumin: an orally bioavailable blocker of TNF and other pro-inflammatory biomarkers. *Br J Pharmacol.* 2013;169(8):1672–1692. https://doi.org/10.1111/bph.12131.

77. Zhang Z, Li K. Curcumin attenuates high glucose-induced inflammatory injury through the reactive oxygen species-phosphoinositide 3-kinase/protein kinase B-nuclear factor-κB signaling pathway in rat thoracic aorta endothelial cells. *J Diabetes Investig.* 2018;9(4):731–740. https://doi.org/10.1111/jdi.12767.

78. Yu S, Wang M, Guo X, Qin R. Curcumin Attenuates Inflammation in a Severe Acute Pancreatitis Animal Model by Regulating TRAF1/ASK1 Signaling. *Med Sci Monit.* 2018;24:2280–2286. Retrieved from https://europepmc.org/articles/PMC5921955. (Accession No. 29657313).

79. Liu CH, Huang HY. in vitro anti-propionibacterium activity by curcumin containing vesicle system. *Chem Pharm Bull.* 2013;61(4):419–425. https://doi.org/10.1248/cpb.c12-01043.

80. Lalla JK, Nandedkar SY, Paranjape MH, Talreja NB. Clinical trials of ayurvedic formulations in the treatment of acne vulgaris. *J Ethnopharmacol.* 2001;78(1):99–102. https://doi.org/10.1016/s0378-8741(01)00323-3.

81. Chainani-Wu N, Collins K, Silverman S. Use of curcuminoids in a cohort of patients with oral lichen planus, an autoimmune disease. *Phytomedicine.* 2012;19(5):418–423. https://doi.org/10.1016/j.phymed.2011.11.005.

82. Chainani-Wu N, Madden E, Lozada-Nur F, Silverman S. High-dose curcuminoids are efficacious in the reduction in symptoms and signs of oral lichen planus. *J Am Acad Dermatol.* 2012;66 (5):752–760. https://doi.org/10.1016/j.jaad.2011.04.022.

83. Chainani-Wu N, Silverman S, Reingold A, et al. A randomized, placebo-controlled, double-blind clinical trial of curcuminoids in oral lichen planus. *Phytomedicine.* 2007;14(7–8):437–446. https://doi.org/10.1016/j.phymed.2007.05.003.

84. Wahlström B, Blennow G. A study on the fate of curcumin in the rat. *Acta Pharmacol Toxicol (Copenh).* 1978;43(2):86–92. https://doi.org/10.1111/j.1600-0773.1978.tb02240.x.

85. Shoba G, Joy D, Joseph T, et al. Influence of piperine on the pharmacokinetics of curcumin in animals and human volunteers. *Planta Med.* 1998;64(4):353–356. https://doi.org/10.1055/s-2006-957450.

86. Lao CD, Ruffin MT, Normolle D, et al. Dose escalation of a curcuminoid formulation. *BMC Complement Altern Med.* 2006;6:10. https://doi.org/10.1186/1472-6882-6-10.

87. Sharma RA, Euden SA, Platton SL, et al. Phase I clinical trial of oral curcumin: biomarkers of systemic activity and compliance. *Clin Cancer Res.* 2004;10(20):6847–6854. https://doi.org/10.1158/1078-0432.Ccr-04-0744.

88. Srivastava KC, Bordia A, Verma SK. Curcumin, a major component of food spice turmeric (Curcuma longa) inhibits aggregation and alters eicosanoid metabolism in human blood platelets. *Prostaglandins, Leukot Essent Fatty Acids.* 1995;52(4):223–227. https://doi.org/10.1016/0952-3278(95)90040-3.

89. Shah BH, Nawaz Z, Pertani SA, et al. Inhibitory effect of curcumin, a food spice from turmeric, on platelet-activating factor- and arachidonic acid-mediated platelet aggregation through inhibition of thromboxane formation and Ca2+ signaling. *Biochem Pharmacol.* 1999;58(7):1167–1172. https://doi.org/10.1016/s0006-2952(99)00206-3.

90. Na HS, Ryu JH, Do SH. The role of magnesium in pain. In: Vink R, Nechifor M, eds. *Magnesium in the Central Nervous System.* Adelaide (AU): University of Adelaide Press; 2011.

91. Mauskop A, Altura BT, Cracco RQ, Altura BM. Intravenous magnesium sulfate rapidly alleviates headaches of various types. *Headache.* 1996;36(3):154–160. https://doi.org/10.1046/j.1526-4610.1996.3603154.x.

92. Benassi L, Barletta FP, Baroncini L, et al. Effectiveness of magnesium pidolate in the prophylactic treatment of primary dysmenorrhea. *Clin Exp Obstet Gynecol.* 1992;19(3):176–179.

93. Tramer MR, Schneider J, Marti RA, Rifat K. (1996). Role of magnesium sulfate in postoperative analgesia. *Anesthesiology.* 1996;84 (2):340–347.

94. Markaki A, Kyriazis J, Stylianou K, et al. The role of serum magnesium and calcium on the association between adiponectin levels and all-cause mortality in end-stage renal disease patients. *PLoS One.* 2012;7(12). https://doi.org/10.1371/journal.pone.0052350, e52350.

95. Hata A, Doi Y, Ninomiya T, et al. Magnesium intake decreases Type 2 diabetes risk through the improvement of insulin resistance and inflammation: the Hisayama Study. *Diabetic Med.* 2013;30 (12):1487–1494. https://doi.org/10.1111/dme.12250.

96. Chacko SA, Song Y, Nathan L, et al. Relations of dietary magnesium intake to biomarkers of inflammation and endothelial dysfunction in an ethnically diverse cohort of postmenopausal women. *Diabetes Care.* 2010;33(2):304–310. https://doi.org/10.2337/dc09-1402.

97. Guerrero-Romero F, Rodríguez-Morán M. Relationship between serum magnesium levels and C-reactive protein concentration, in non-diabetic, non-hypertensive obese subjects. *Int J Obes Relat Metab Disord.* 2002;26(4):469–474. https://doi.org/10.1038/sj.ijo.0801954.

98. Rodríguez-Morán M, Guerrero-Romero F. Serum magnesium and C-reactive protein levels. *Arch Dis Child.* 2008;93(8):676–680. https://doi.org/10.1136/adc.2006.109371.

99. Cascella M, Vaqar S. Hypermagnesemia. In *StatPearls.* Treasure Island (FL): StatPearls Publishing; 2020. Copyright © 2020, StatPearls Publishing LLC.

100. Grange PA, Raingeaud J, Calvez V, Dupin N. Nicotinamide inhibits Propionibacterium acnes-induced IL-8 production in keratinocytes through the NF-κB and MAPK pathways. *J Dermatol Sci.* 2009;56 (2):106–112. https://doi.org/10.1016/j.jdermsci.2009.08.001.

101. Niren NM, Torok HM. The Nicomide Improvement in Clinical Outcomes Study (NICOS): results of an 8-week trial. *Cutis.* 2006;77(1 Suppl):17–28.

102. Khodaeiani E, Fouladi RF, Amirnia M, et al. Topical 4% nicotinamide vs. 1% clindamycin in moderate inflammatory acne vulgaris. *Int J Dermatol.* 2013;52(8):999–1004. https://doi.org/10.1111/ijd.12002.

103. Navarrete-Solís J, Castanedo-Cázares JP, Torres-Álvarez B, et al. A Double-Blind, Randomized Clinical Trial of Niacinamide 4% versus Hydroquinone 4% in the Treatment of Melasma. *Dermatol Res Pract.* 2011;2011:379173. https://doi.org/10.1155/2011/379173.

104. Kaymak Y, Önder M. An Investigation of Efficacy of Topical Niacinamide for the Treatment of Mild and Moderate Acne Vulgaris. *J Turk Acad Dermatol.* 2008;2(4).

105. Nasermoaddeli A, Kagamimori S. Balneotherapy in medicine: a review. *Environ Health Prev Med.* 2005;10(4):171–179. https://doi.org/10.1007/bf02897707.

106. Inoue T, Inoue S, Kubota K. Bactericidal activity of manganese and iodide ions against Staphylococcus aureus: a possible treatment for acute atopic dermatitis. *Acta Derm Venereol.* 1999;79(5):360–362. https://doi.org/10.1080/000155599750010265.

107. Kubota K, Machida I, Tamura K, et al. Treatment of refractory cases of atopic dermatitis with acidic hot-spring bathing. *Acta Derm Venereol.* 1997;77(6):452–454. https://doi.org/10.2340/0001555577452454.

108. Abels DJ, Rose T, Bearman JE. Treatment of psoriasis at a Dead Sea dermatology clinic. *Int J Dermatol.* 1995;34(2):134–137. https://doi.org/10.1111/j.1365-4362.1995.tb03599.x.

109. Shani J, Seidl V, Hristakieva E, et al. Indications, contraindications and possible side-effects of climatotherapy at the Dead-Sea. *Int J Dermatol.* 1997;36(7):481–492. https://doi.org/10.1046/j.1365-4362.1997.00286.x.

110. Gambichler T, Skrygan M. Expression of human β-defensin-2 in psoriatic epidermis models treated with balneophototherapy. *J Eur Acad Dermatol Venereol.* 2015;29(1):169–173. https://doi.org/10.1111/jdv.12325.

111. Gambichler T, Demetriou C, Terras S, et al. The impact of salt water soaks on biophysical and molecular parameters in psoriatic epidermis equivalents. *Dermatology.* 2011;223(3):230–238. https://doi.org/10.1159/000332983.

112. Celerier P, Litoux P, Dreno B, Richard A. Modulatory effects of selenium and strontium salts on keratinocyte-derived inflammatory cytokines. *Arch Dermatol Res.* 1995;287(7):680–682. https://doi.org/10.1007/bf00371742.

113. Huang A, Seité S, Adar T. The use of balneotherapy in dermatology. *Clin Dermatol.* 2018;36(3):363–368. https://doi.org/10.1016/j.clindermatol.2018.03.010.

114. Goto Y, Hayasaka S, Kurihara S, Nakamura Y. Physical and Mental Effects of Bathing: A Randomized Intervention Study. *Evid Based Complement Alternat Med.* 2018;2018:9521086. https://doi.org/10.1155/2018/9521086.

115. Nissen JB, Avrach WW, Hansen ES, et al. Increased levels of enkephalin following natural sunlight (combined with salt water bathing at the Dead Sea) and ultraviolet A irradiation. *Br J Dermatol.* 1998;139(6):1012–1019. https://doi.org/10.1046/j.1365-2133.1998.02557.x.

116. Kubota K, Kurabayashi H, Tamura K, et al. A transient rise in plasma beta-endorphin after a traditional 47 degrees C hot-spring

bath in Kusatsu-spa. *Japan Life Sci.* 1992;51(24):1877–1880. https://doi.org/10.1016/0024-3205(92)90039-r.

117. Chon TY, Lee MC. Acupuncture. *Mayo Clin Proc.* 2013;88 (10):1141–1146. https://doi.org/10.1016/j.mayocp.2013.06.009.

118. Andersson S, Lundeberg T. Acupuncture—from empiricism to science: functional background to acupuncture effects in pain and disease. *Med Hypotheses.* 1995;45(3):271–281. https://doi.org/10.1016/0306-9877(95)90117-5.

119. Becker RO, Reichmanis M, Marino AA, Spadaro JA. Electrophysiological correlates of acupuncture points and meridians. *Psychoenergetic Systems.* 1976;1(106):195–212.

120. McDonald JL, Cripps AW, Smith PK, et al. The Anti-Inflammatory Effects of Acupuncture and Their Relevance to Allergic Rhinitis: A Narrative Review and Proposed Model. *Evid Based Complement Alternat Med.* 2013;2013:591796. https://doi.org/10.1155/2013/591796.

121. McDonald JL, Cripps AW, Smith PK. Mediators, Receptors, and Signalling Pathways in the Anti-Inflammatory and Antihyperalgesic Effects of Acupuncture. *Evid Based Complement Alternat Med.* 2015;2015:975632. https://doi.org/10.1155/2015/975632.

122. Zijlstra FJ, Van Den Berg-De Lange I, Huygen FJPM, Klein J. Anti-inflammatory actions of acupuncture. *Mediators Inflamm.* 2003;12 (2):59–69. https://doi.org/10.1080/09629350310001114943.

123. Melzack R, Wall PD. Pain mechanisms: a new theory. *Science.* 1965;150(3699):971–979. Retrieved from www.jstor.org/stable/1717891.

124. Clement-Jones V, Tomlin S, Rees L, et al. (1980). Increased beta-endorphin but not met-enkephalin levels in human cerebrospinal fluid after acupuncture for recurrent pain. *Lancet.* 1980;316 (8201):946–949. https://doi.org/10.1016/s0140-6736(80)92106-6.

125. Eriksson SV, Lundeberg T, Lundeberg S. Interaction of diazepam and naloxone on acupuncture induced pain relief. *Am J Chin Med.* 1991;19(1):1–7. https://doi.org/10.1142/s0192415x91000028.

126. Harris RE, Zubieta JK, Scott DJ, et al. Traditional Chinese acupuncture and placebo (sham) acupuncture are differentiated by their effects on mu-opioid receptors (MORs). *NeuroImage.* 2009;47(3):1077–1085. https://doi.org/10.1016/j.neuroimage.2009.05.083.

127. Yoshimoto K, Fukuda F, Hori M, et al. Acupuncture stimulates the release of serotonin, but not dopamine, in the rat nucleus accumbens. *Tohoku J Exp Med.* 2006;208(4):321–326. https://doi.org/10.1620/tjem.208.321.

128. Clement-Jones V, McLoughlin L, Tomlin S, et al. Increased beta-endorphin but not met-enkephalin levels in human cerebrospinal fluid after acupuncture for recurrent pain. *Lancet.* 1980;2(8201):946–949. https://doi.org/10.1016/s0140-6736(80)92106-6.

129. Niemtzow RC. Battlefield acupuncture. *Med Acupunct.* 2007;19 (4):225–228. https://doi.org/10.1089/acu.2007.0603.

130. Federman DG, Zeliadt SB, Thomas ER, et al. Battlefield Acupuncture in the Veterans Health Administration: Effectiveness in Individual and Group Settings for Pain and Pain Comorbidities. *Med Acupunct.* 2018;30(5):273–278. https://doi.org/10.1089/acu.2018.1296.

131. Jan AL, Aldridge ES, Rogers IR, et al. Does Ear Acupuncture Have a Role for Pain Relief in the Emergency Setting? A Systematic Review and Meta-Analysis. *Med Acupunct.* 2017;29(5):276–289. https://doi.org/10.1089/acu.2017.1237.

132. Goertz CM, Niemtzow R, Burns SM, et al. Auricular acupuncture in the treatment of acute pain syndromes: a pilot study. *Mil Med.* 2006;171(10):1010–1014. https://doi.org/10.7205/milmed.171.10.1010.

133. Allais G, Romoli M, Rolando S, et al. Ear acupuncture in the treatment of migraine attacks: a randomized trial on the efficacy of appropriate versus inappropriate acupoints. *Neurol Sci.* 2011;32 (Suppl 1):S173–S175. https://doi.org/10.1007/s10072-011-0525-4.

134. Tillmann HL, Nelson WR, Freedman M. Opioid weaning made possible by pain control with Battlefield Acupuncture. *Acupunct Med.* 2020. https://doi.org/10.1177/0964528420929342.964528420929342.

135. Lee KC, Keyes A, Hensley JR, et al. Effectiveness of acupressure on pruritus and lichenification associated with atopic dermatitis: a pilot trial. *Acupunct Med.* 2012;30(1):8–11. https://doi.org/10.1136/acupmed-2011-010088.

136. Kang S, Kim YK, Yeom M, et al. Acupuncture improves symptoms in patients with mild-to-moderate atopic dermatitis: a randomized, sham-controlled preliminary trial. *Complement Ther Med.* 2018;41:90–98. https://doi.org/10.1016/j.ctim.2018.08.013.

137. Yeh ML, Ko SH, Wang MH, et al. Acupuncture-Related Techniques for Psoriasis: A Systematic Review with Pairwise and Network Meta-Analyses of Randomized Controlled Trials. *J Altern Complement Med.* 2017;23(12):930–940. https://doi.org/10.1089/acm.2016.0158.

138. Zick SM, Sen A, Wyatt GK, et al. Investigation of 2 Types of Self-administered Acupressure for Persistent Cancer-Related Fatigue in Breast Cancer Survivors: A Randomized Clinical Trial. *JAMA Oncol.* 2016;2(11):1470–1476. https://doi.org/10.1001/jamaoncol.2016.1867.

139. Xue CC, Zhang CS, Yang AW, et al. (2011). Semi-self-administered ear acupressure for persistent allergic rhinitis: a randomised sham-controlled trial. *Ann Allergy Asthma Immunol.* 2011;106(2):168–170. https://doi.org/10.1016/j.anai.2010.11.006.

29

Pediatric Hidradenitis Suppurativa

ARISTEIDIS G. VAIOPOULOS, GEORGIOS NIKOLAKIS, AND CHRISTOS C. ZOUBOULIS

Introduction

Hidradenitis suppurativa/acne inversa (HS) is a chronic, inflammatory, recurrent, debilitating skin disease of the hair follicle which affects apocrine gland-rich areas of the body. The disease usually presents after puberty, but it can, although uncommonly, also affect adolescents (onset after initiation of puberty, older than 10 to 12 years) and children. Typical clinical symptoms include painful, deep-seated, inflamed lesions (nodules, abscesses), tunnels, and scarring.[1] In this chapter, we present the main aspects of the disease in pediatric populations. The major features of HS in children and adolescents are summarized in Table 29.1.

Pathogenesis

Pathogenetic mechanisms of HS are not yet fully elucidated. In general, genetic susceptibility, obesity/metabolic syndrome, and smoking have been implicated. A positive family history is often observed in patients with early onset of the disease. Familial occurrence varies from 20% to 55% among different studies, whereas a small Danish cohort of obese children reported a positive family history in 80% (4/5) of the patients.[2–9] Moreover, genetic predisposition may also lead to pediatric HS. Mutations in the γ-secretase genes complex as well as aberrations in the Notch signaling cascade are implicated in the inflammatory process.[4–6] Data from case reports or small case series show that early-onset HS is also associated with underlying hormonal disorders, such as precocious

puberty, premature adrenarche, or adrenal hyperplasia. These conditions are more commonly seen in children than in adults with HS. In the pathogenetic pathway of pediatric HS, the elevated sensitivity of the pilosebaceous unit to circulating sex hormones has also been postulated.[4,10–14] Moreover, apocrine glands may also be secondarily involved. Apocrine glands become active during puberty. They empty their content into the follicular canal and not into the skin surface in contrast to eccrine glands. Keratinocytes of the pilosebaceous unit contain androgen receptors, which may promote follicular plugging due to hyperkeratinization, resulting in inflammation, rupture of follicles, abscess, and tunnel (sinus tract) formation.[6,15]

Another factor propagating HS in adult and pediatric patients is obesity.[16] Recent data suggest that the majority of patients are overweight or obese, with a reported rate varying from about 50% to 80%. Additionally, obesity is likely associated with a more serious disease course as well as precocious puberty. In a recent multicenter study, patients' body mass index (BMI) were correlated with the average parent BMI, showing that our therapeutic approach and weight counseling strategies should also include the patient's family.[2,4,8,9,17–20]

Despite being a pivotal player in adult HS cases, smoking habits do not seem to play a key role in cases of early-onset HS. According to recent studies, only a small proportion of pediatric HS patients were active smokers. However, bear in mind that children may be subject to passive tobacco exposure.[2,8,9,17]

Epidemiology

Overall, HS has a prevalence of 0.03% (Europe) to 0.053% (USA) and a calculated prevalence of 0.4%.[21,22,23] Pediatric HS seems to represent a rather small cluster of the disease.[21–25] However, the data regarding disease onset shows a wide age range. Although older reports documented an early onset in 2% of HS patients, a recent study from the Netherlands reported that 8% of patients show a disease onset before the age of 13.5 years, whereas according to an Italian study, 90 out of 235 patients (38%) recalled that the first symptoms occurred before the age of 16.[6–8] On the other hand, a recent US cohort study presented an overall standardized prevalence of 0.02% for pediatric HS patients (0 to 17) and demonstrated that the pediatric age group only represents 1020 of 47620 documented HS cases in the USA (2.2%), affecting pediatric patients of African American or biracial descent significantly more often.[25] A very young disease onset in prepubertal patients (age 10 years or younger), with or without precocious puberty or premature adrenarche, has only been presented in case reports or small case series.[4,10–14]

TABLE 29.1	**Summary of the Major Features of Hidradenitis Suppurativa in Pediatric Patients**
Epidemiology	2%–8% of HS patients Rare in children (≤10 years), uncommon in adolescents (after initiation of puberty >10–12 years)
Predisposing factors	Obesity (50%–70% overweight or obese) Tobacco exposure • Active small proportion • Passive smoking Familial occurrence Genetic predisposition
Clinical features	Axillary and inguinal regions most commonly involved Mostly mild or moderate severity Similar clinical course as adults Female predominance
Severe complications (rare)	Infections Fistulas to surrounding organs (e.g., urinary bladder, rectum, etc.) Anemia Lymphedema
Comorbid disorders	Obesity/metabolic syndrome Dermatologic conditions Hormonal disorders Down's syndrome Hypothyroidism Pyoderma gangrenosum Psychiatric disorders
Therapy	*Topical* • Clindamycin 1% gel • Azelaic acid • Chlorhexidine or zinc pyrithione washes *Systemic* • Clindamycin/rifampicin • Tetracyclines (should not be administered to patients younger than 8 years old due to risk of discoloration of permanent teeth) • Anti-Tumor Necrosis Factor-alpha (adalimumab, infliximab) *Other* • Anakinra, dapsone, finasteride, zinc gluconate, oral contraceptives • Photodynamic therapy • Intralesional injection of corticosteroids or botulinum toxin A *Surgical* • Deroofing • Total excision • Endoscopic treatment of tunnels • CO_2-laser (scarring) • Nd:YAG-laser and intense pulsed light (hair removal) *Adjuvant* • Weight reduction, nutrition counseling • Pain management • Treatment of complications and comorbidities • Psychological support

Note: These therapies have been used to treat HS in adults, but few studies have been conducted for their use in pediatric patients with HS.

HS, Hidradenitis Suppurativa; *Nd:YAG*, neodymium-doped yttrium aluminum garnet.

Clinical Features

HS in pediatric patients is also characterized by the presence of inflammatory nodules, abscesses, tunnels, and scarring in the apocrine gland-rich areas of the body. According to recent data, it seems that most subjects suffer from a mild or moderate disease and show a similar clinical course when compared with adult patients. However, it has been suggested that pediatric patients may not have reached their peak severity. Ethnicity may also affect the clinical course and areas of involvement in HS patients. Cases with excessive scarring and numerous abscesses and sinus tracts have been documented. In most patients, the axillary and inguinal regions are involved, although with varying frequency among different studies. Other affected anatomic areas include the buttocks, the submammary area, and the mons pubis. Additionally, most recent studies have demonstrated a female predominance in cases of early-onset HS.[1–3,7–9,26]

Complications

The clinical course of HS in children and adults may be complicated by a wide variety of sometimes serious clinical conditions, such as anemia, lymphoedema, and fistulae to the surrounding organs (urinary bladder, rectum, etc.). Additionally, various, occasionally life-threatening cutaneous, extracutaneous, and systemic infections may also complicate the course of HS patients.[1,4,5,27,28] Theoretically, HS patients represent a high-risk group for potential infections due to the dysfunction of the epidermal barrier, treatment with immunomodulators/immunosuppressants, and associated comorbidities, such as diabetes mellitus. However, infections in HS patients are rarely documented.

Scoring Systems

The most commonly used classification system is Hurley's classification.[29] Dynamic scoring systems used to assess disease severity in adults are also applied in pediatric patients and include the International Hidradenitis Suppurativa Severity Score System (IHS4), the Sartorius score, and the HS Physician Global Assessment (HS-PGA), whereas Children's Dermatology Life Quality Index (CDLQI) is used to evaluate the influence of HS on patients' quality of life.[1,18]

Comorbid Disorders

Various studies, case series, and case reports have tried to identify the most common comorbid disorders associated with HS. In most cases, a statistically significant difference between early and adult onset could not be documented. The most commonly reported comorbid disorder is acne vulgaris. Furthermore, pediatric HS patients display a wide variety of other dermatological conditions such as atopic dermatitis, hirsutism, pilonidal sinus, seborrheic dermatitis, and acanthosis nigricans. As mentioned before, in some early onset cases, hormonal dysregulation, such as premature adrenarche, precocious puberty, congenital adrenal hyperplasia, and polycystic ovary syndrome, may play a pivotal role in the pathogenetic mechanism and/or propagation of HS. Recently, the association of pediatric HS with metabolic disorders/syndrome, including obesity, diabetes mellitus, hyperlipidemia, and hypertension, has also been highlighted. Additionally, autoimmune/autoinflammatory conditions, such as rheumatoid arthritis, inflammatory bowel disease, and various inflammatory disorders, may also associate with HS. Other conditions, including hypothyroidism, pyoderma gangrenosum, and HIV infection, have also been reported. A small proportion of early-onset HS, about 2% to 5%, coexists with Down syndrome, while a prevalence of 38% was reported in a study from Saudi Arabia.[a] Finally, it must be noted that affected individuals often suffer from psychiatric conditions due to a significant life quality alteration and fear of stigmatization, which further perplex the clinical course and management of HS patients.[1,2,3,9,32]

---

[a]References 2, 4–6, 8, 9, 17, 26, 30, 31.

Treatment

Therapeutic strategies in pediatric HS patients are based on the guidelines for adult patients and depend on the disease severity. Despite being relatively widely used, they are based on extrapolations that highlight the need for specific pediatric HS guidelines. In general, mild cases are treated with topical agents, whereas more severe cases are treated with antibiotics or biologics. Extended or resistant disease may sometimes require a surgical approach. Pain management, weight counseling, and psychological consulting should also be included in the therapeutic arsenal. In the treatment of early-onset HS, the management of comorbid disorders as well as complications such as severe infections are also essential.[9,27,33]

Topical

Clindamycin 1% gel applied twice daily for 3 months seems to be the treatment of choice for most mild cases. A recent study suggested the topical use of resorcinol; however, its use should probably be avoided due to lethal cases of resorcinol poisoning in infants and young children.[33,34] Azelaic acid and chlorhexidine or zinc pyrithione washes have also been used.[4,9,33]

Systemic

Systemic therapeutic approaches may be needed for patients who do not respond to first-line topical agents, or in more severe cases. In such cases, antibiotic treatment with tetracyclines or clindamycin alone or in combination with rifampicin, in adapted dosing for children and adolescents, is preferred. Tetracyclines should not be used before the age of 8 years, as they can cause an irreversible discoloration of the permanent teeth. Doxycycline displays the lowest affinity for calcium binding and has the lowest risk of teeth or bone discoloration. Additionally, the use of azithromycin has been proposed to control the flares. However, in severe cases, biologics combined with surgery may be needed. Adalimumab is the only approved biological treatment for HS in adults and children older than 12 years with moderate or severe HS. Infliximab has been administered off-label in non-responders as a second-line therapy, while treatment with Anakinra has been mentioned in small case series. Dapsone, finasteride, oral contraceptives, oral zinc supplementation, photodynamic therapy, and intralesional injection of corticosteroids or botulinum toxin A are also regarded as alternative treatment options. Isotretinoin did not prove to be effective in adults with HS, and its use is not recommended when treating children for HS.[4,9,33,35]

Surgery

Pediatric patients may also need surgical treatment in cases of severe and extensive HS. Surgical management seems to be relatively safe and effective, although there is a risk of recurrence. Deroofing or total excision (local or wide) of the affected area has been used. A simple incisions has been proven ineffective in most cases, although they are sometimes used to manage an acute painful abscess. Recently, an endoscopic approach for the treatment of tunnels has been proposed, following a procedure similar to the treatment of pediatric endoscopic pilonidal sinus. Laser therapy with a fractionated CO_2 laser is another effective treatment option with a relatively good safety profile, especially for the management of scarring. Neodymium-doped yttrium aluminum garnet (Nd:YAG) lasers, as well as intense pulsed light, can be used for hair removal.[4,9,20,33,36]

Adjuvant Therapeutic Strategies

Apart from the standard treatment of HS, the diagnosis and management of complications such as anemia and infections are of crucial importance. It is also important to notice that endocrine and metabolic disorders should be diagnosed early and treated properly. Weight reduction strategies and nutrition counseling, as well as pain management and psychological support, should also be included in the therapeutic arsenal.[9,19,32,33]

Conclusion

HS in children is rare and uncommon in adolescents with varying prevalence among different studies. The disease shows a similar clinical course to adult patients, with most subjects exhibiting a mild or moderate severity. The majority of pediatric patients are overweight or obese and non-smokers, with a female predominance. Acne vulgaris, accompanying infections, and endocrine, metabolic, or psychological disorders may complicate the clinical course. Treatment is based on guidelines for adult patients and depends on disease severity. Management of mild cases includes topical measures such as clindamycin gel, whereas antibiotic treatment or biologics should be used for more advanced cases. Surgical management should also be considered for more severe or refractory cases. Therapeutic algorithms should also include pain management, treatment of superinfections, weight counseling, and psychological consulting.

References

1. Zouboulis CC, Desai N, Emtestam L, et al. European S1 guideline for the treatment of hidradenitis suppurativa/acne inversa. *J Eur Acad Dermatology Venereol.* 2015;29:619–644.
2. Vaiopoulos AG, Nikolakis G, Zouboulis CC. Hidradenitis suppurativa in paediatric patients: a retrospective monocentric study in Germany and review of the literature. *J Eur Acad Dermatol Venereol.* 2020;34:2140–2146.
3. Lindsø Andersen P, Kromann C, Fonvig CE, et al. Hidradenitis suppurativa in a cohort of overweight and obese children and adolescents. *Int J Dermatol.* 2019;20:47–51.
4. Offidani A, Molinelli E, Sechi A, et al. Hidradenitis suppurativa in a prepubertal case series: a call for specific guidelines. *J Eur Acad Dermatology Venereol.* 2019;33(S6):28–31.
5. Liy-Wong C, Pope E, Lara-Corrales I. Hidradenitis suppurativa in the pediatric population. *J Am Acad Dermatol.* 2015;73:S36–S41.
6. Palmer RA, Keefe M. Early-onset hidradenitis suppurativa. *Clin Exp Dermatol.* 2001;26:501–503.
7. Bettoli V, Ricci M, Zauli S, et al. Hidradenitis suppurativa-acne inversa: a relevant dermatosis in paediatric patients. *Br J Dermatol.* 2015;173:1328–1330.
8. Deckers IE, Van Der Zee HH, Boer J, et al. Correlation of early-onset hidradenitis suppurativa with stronger genetic susceptibility and more widespread involvement. *J Am Acad Dermatol.* 2015;72:485–488.
9. Riis PT, Saunte DM, Sigsgaard V, et al. Clinical characteristics of pediatric hidradenitis suppurativa: a cross-sectional multicenter study of 140 patients. *Arch Dermatol Res.* 2020;312:715–724.
10. Mengesha YM, Holcombe TC, Hansen RC. Prepubertal hidradenitis suppurativa: two case reports and review of the literature. *Pediatr Dermatol.* 1999;16:292–296.
11. Stojkovic-Filipovic JM, Gajic-Veljic MD, Nikolic M. Prepubertal onset of hidradenitis suppurativa in a girl: a case report and literature review. *Indian J Dermatol Venereol Leprol.* 2015;81:294–298.
12. Jourdain JC, Le Lorier B, Mourier C, et al. Virilisation par déficit en 21-hydroxylase et hyperplasie sudorale axillaire. *Ann Dermatol Venereol.* 1988;115:1136–1138.
13. Lewis F, Messenger AG, Wales JKH. Hidradenitis suppurativa as a presenting feature of premature adrenarche. *Br J Dermatol.* 1993;129:447–448.
14. Lopes S, Gomes N, Trindade E, et al. Hidradenitis suppurativa in a prepubertal girl. *Acta Dermatovenerol Alp Pannonica Adriat.* 2019;28:139–141.
15. Karagiannidis I, Nikolakis G, Sabat R, et al. Hidradenitis suppurativa/Acne inversa: an endocrine skin disorder? *Rev Endocr Metab Disord.* 2016;17:335–341.
16. Kaleta KP, Nikolakis G, Hossini AM, et al. Metabolic disorders/obesity is a primary risk factor in hidradenitis suppurativa: an immunohistochemical real-world approach. *Dermatology.* 2021; [online ahead of print].
17. Choi E, Cook AR, Chandran NS. Hidradenitis suppurativa: an Asian perspective from a Singaporean institute. *Skin Appendage Disord.* 2018;4:281–285.
18. Zouboulis CC, Tzellos T, Kyrgidis A, et al. Development and validation of the International Hidradenitis Suppurativa Severity Score System (IHS4), a novel dynamic scoring system to assess HS severity. *Br J Dermatol.* 2017;177:1401–1409.
19. Reichert B, Fernandez Faith E, Harfmann K. Weight counseling in pediatric hidradenitis suppurativa patients. *Pediatr Dermatol.* 2020;37:480–483.
20. Ge S, Ngaage LM, Orbay H, et al. Surgical Management of Pediatric Hidradenitis Suppurativa. *Ann Plast Surg.* 2020;84:570–574.
21. Kirsten N, Petersen J, Hagenström K, et al. Epidemiology of hidradenitis suppurativa in Germany—an observational cohort study based on a multisource approach. *J Eur Acad Dermatology Venereol.* 2020;34:174–179.
22. Cosmatos I, Matcho A, Weinstein R, et al. Analysis of patient claims data to determine the prevalence of hidradenitis suppurativa in the United States. *J Am Acad Dermatol.* 2013;68:412–419.
23. Jfri A, Nassim D, O'Brien E, et al. Prevalence of hidradenitis suppurativa: A systematic review and meta-regression study. *JAMA Dermatol.* 2021;137:924–931.
24. Vazquez BG, Alikhan A, Weaver AL, et al. Incidence of hidradenitis suppurativa and associated factors: a population-based study of Olmsted County, Minnesota. *J Invest Dermatol.* 2013;133:97–103.
25. Garg A, Kirby JS, Lavian J, et al. Sex- and age-adjusted population analysis of prevalence estimates for hidradenitis suppurativa in the United States. *JAMA Dermatol.* 2017;153:760–764.
26. Braunberger TL, Nicholson CL, Gold L, et al. Hidradenitis suppurativa in children: The Henry Ford experience. *Pediatr Dermatol.* 2018;35:370–373.
27. Scheinfeld N. Hidradenitis suppurativa in prepubescent and pubescent children. *Clin Dermatol.* 2015;33:316–319.
28. Lee HH, Patel KR, Singam V, et al. Associations of cutaneous and extracutaneous infections with hidradenitis suppurativa in U.S. children and adults. *Br J Dermatol.* 2020;182:327–334.
29. Hurley HJ. Hidradenitis suppurativa. In: Roenigk RK, Roenigk Jr HH, eds. *Roenigk & Roenigk's Dermatologic Surgery: Principles and Practice.* 2nd ed. New York: Marcel Dekker, Inc.; 1996:623–645.
30. Firsowicz M, Boyd M, Jacks SK. Follicular occlusion disorders in Down syndrome patients. *Pediatr Dermatol.* 2020;37:219–221.
31. Veraldi S, Guanziroli E, Benzecry V, et al. Hidradenitis suppurativa in patients with Down syndrome. *J Eur Acad Dermatology Venereol.* 2019;33(S6):34–35.

32. Tiri H, Jokelainen J, Timonen M, et al. Somatic and psychiatric comorbidities of hidradenitis suppurativa in children and adolescents. *J Am Acad Dermatol.* 2018;79:514–519.

33. Mikkelsen PR, Jemec GBE. Hidradenitis suppurativa in children and adolescents: a review of treatment options. *Paediatr Drugs.* 2014;16:483–489.

34. Cunnigham AA. Resorcin poisoning. *Arch Dis Child.* 1956;31:173–176.

35. Fougerousse A-C, Reguiai Z, Roussel A, et al. Hidradenitis suppurativa management using TNF inhibitors in patients under the age of 18: a series of 12 cases. *J Am Acad Dermatol.* 2020;83:199–201.

36. Esposito C, Del Conte F, Cerulo M, et al. Pediatric endoscopic hidradenitis treatment: a new minimally invasive treatment for pediatric patients with hidradenitis suppurativa. *J Laparoendosc Adv Surg Tech A.* 2020;30:464–470.

30

Skin of Color

SHANTHI NARLA, MARSHA HENDERSON, AND ILTEFAT H. HAMZAVI

ABBREVIATIONS USED

HS hidradenitis suppurativa
IL interleukin
Nd:YAG neodymium-doped yttrium-aluminum-garnet laser
MetS metabolic syndrome
IBD inflammatory bowel disease
OR odds ratio
SIR standardized incidence ratios
QOL quality of life
SD standard deviation
SES socioeconomic status
NAMCS National Ambulatory Medical Care
NHAMCS National Hospital Ambulatory Medical Care Survey
IPV intimate partner violence
CD Crohn's disease
UC ulcerative colitis
SCC squamous cell carcinoma
US United States

Prevalence of Hidradenitis Suppurativa in Skin of Color Individuals

While the overall US prevalence of hidradenitis suppurativa (HS), obtained through US claims data, has been reported to be 0.10% or 98 per 100,000 persons, HS disproportionally affects women (137 per 100,000), African Americans (296 per 100,000), and biracial (African American/Caucasian) (218 per 100,000) patient groups. In comparison, the rates of HS among white patients are closer to the overall reported US prevalence at 95 per 100,000 persons. Conversely, HS affects Asians, Pacific Islanders, Native Americans, Latin Americans, and Native Hawaiians at much lower rates, with a standard prevalence of 0.04%.[1] However, these prevalence rates may be underestimations due to underdiagnosis and the inability to capture those who did not seek care in the healthcare systems included in the databases analyzed.[1] Further, adult patients with HS may have symptoms for up to 7 years before diagnosis. Consequently, if the same is true among children with HS, then prevalence in younger age groups may also be underestimated.[1,2]

Classical teachings have supported this claim that people of African descent have a higher incidence than those of European descent.[3] However, the majority of previously published studies on HS report prevalence and incidence in a largely Caucasian cohort.[4] Recently, additional retrospective studies have emerged supporting the classical teachings, demonstrating that African

Americans appear to be more commonly affected and with higher severity of HS.[5,6] The true prevalence of HS in the general US population may likely be higher due to limitations in diagnosis, underdiagnosis, misdiagnosis, and patient reluctance to seek treatment.[7] This may be especially true in skin of color populations due to limited access to medical care, implicit biases, anatomical differences, genetics, and increased prevalence of lower socioeconomic status (SES) among these groups.[8,9]

HS presents with painful, erythematous, and often malodorous abscesses, nodules, dermal tunnels, double- and multi-ended comedones, along with scar formation followed by hyperpigmentation in apocrine gland-bearing skin such as the axillae, inguinal, perianal, and perineal regions. Further, HS lesions in skin of color patients may be purplish in color, more hyperpigmented, and the erythema and tunnels may be more difficult to identify in comparison to Caucasian patients. Gentle palpation can be used to help identify them(Fig. 30.1).[8,10,11]

Skin of Color Representation in Hidradenitis Suppurativa Clinical Trials

This discrepancy in reporting HS prevalence amongst skin of color patients also appears to extend to clinical trials. Using Clinicaltrials.gov and PubMed, Price et al. examined the race

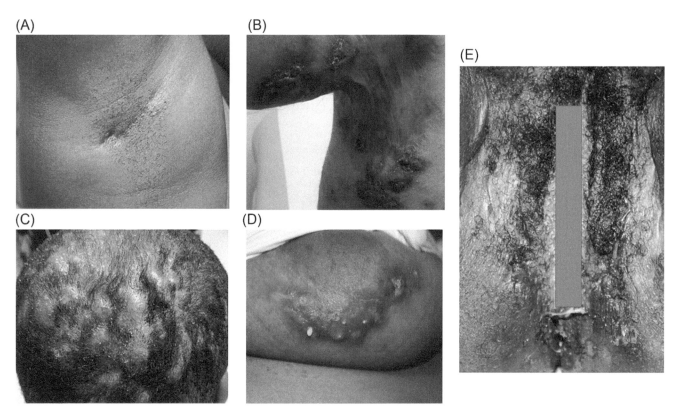

• **Fig. 30.1** Clinical Presentation of Hidradenitis Suppurativa in Skin of Color. (A) Axilla. (B) Axilla. (C) Dissecting cellulitis of the scalp. (D) Breast. (E) Vulva. Hidradenitis suppurativa (HS) presents with painful, erythematous, and often malodorous abscesses, nodules, dermal tunnels, and scar formation followed by hyperpigmentation in apocrine gland-bearing skin, such as the axillae, inguinal, perianal, and perineal regions. HS lesions in skin of color patients may be purplish in color, more hyperpigmented, and the erythema and tunnels may be more difficult to identify in comparison to Caucasian patients. Gentle palpation can be used to help identify them.

and ethnicity demographics in phase II and phase III HS treatment trials published from 2000 to August 2019. Fifteen trials were included in the analysis. Among these trials, 669 (68.0%) of the participants were Caucasian and 138 (14.0%) were of African descent. Asians, American Indian or Alaskan Natives, and Native Hawaiian or other Pacific Islanders comprised 29 (2.9%), 3 (0.3%), and 1 (0.1%) participants, respectively. Only 15 participants were reported as Hispanic, as only three trials reported ethnicity data. While these percentages may reflect the breakdown of the US population in terms of race/ethnicity,[12] they do not reflect the disproportionate rates of HS in African Americans. The remaining 144 (14.6%) participants were recorded as "other/unspecified" (36 self-identified, 108 lacked race reporting). None of the trials included a sub-analysis of treatment efficacy based on race or ethnicity.[9]

Adalimumab is the only currently approved systemic medication for the treatment of HS. However, clinical trials for adalimumab did not sufficiently examine the treatment response in patients with skin of color.[13–16] One study was conducted solely in Caucasian and Romany individuals,[13] while another study consisted of 80% to 85% Caucasians.[15] Further, none of the trials reported the percentage of patients that were Hispanic/Latino or stratified the responses to adalimumab by race.[9] The other systemic biologic agent trials for HS (e.g., etanercept, infliximab, anakinra, and ustekinumab) either did not report race or largely had a Caucasian population.[17–20] Reduced enrollment in clinical trials by skin of color populations may be due to distance from clinical trial sites, lack of education regarding clinical trials, lack of awareness that clinical trials are available for the particular disorder, language barriers, and mistrust of researchers from historical experiences such as the Tuskegee Syphilis Study.[21] Moreover, these results suggest that populations represented in clinical trials may not truly reflect the diverse patient populations affected by HS, and that these medications may only work in a subset of HS patients.

Light/Laser and Other Treatment Considerations

In HS treatment, there are differences in dosing for standard phototherapeutic options in patients with skin of color. In randomized controlled trials, typical settings used for the neodymium-doped yttrium-aluminum-garnet laser (Nd:YAG) were generally a 10-mm spot size with a 20-ms pulse duration and 40 to 50 J/cm^2 in patients with Fitzpatrick skin type I to III and a 35-ms pulse duration and 25 to 35 J/cm^2 in patients with skin types IV to VI.[22] This treatment is discussed further in Chapter 25. Carbon dioxide laser excision and marsupialization has also been shown to be an effective therapy for the management of Hurley Stage II or III disease.[23] Notably, it has been our experience in clinical practice that the risk of keloid formation following the excision of HS lesions has rarely been seen. Due to this observation, the authors strongly suggest that this modality be offered to skin of color patients. Additional light-based treatment options for HS include photodynamic therapy (PDT) and intense pulsed light.[24] However, these treatment modalities are not well-studied in skin of color HS patients and their general efficacy appears to be very limited.

Genetics and Anatomy

In a Dutch cohort of 846 HS patients, 283 (35.5%) were identified as having a family history of HS. Further, patients with a family history of HS were more often female, had a lower mean age of disease onset, and had longer disease duration.[25] Familial HS proves to be autosomal dominant with mutations in genes (*NCSTN, PSENEN, PSEN1*) that code for parts of γ-secretase, an enzyme that normally cleaves the Notch receptor involved in epidermal and follicular development and differentiation. Of note, these studies were conducted primarily in Chinese populations.[26–28] Only one case report has been published identifying a mutation in the *NCSTN* gene in an African American family with HS.[29] Further, a retrospective chart review of patients who underwent surgical treatment for HS was performed at the University of Illinois Medical Center. The results showed that 81.6% of patients who had surgery were African American, and African American women with axillary HS were more likely to have a recalcitrant disease with progressive symptomology over approximately nine years before surgical intervention.[30]

Older studies (pre-1965) found that patients of African American descent had larger, more numerous, and more productive apocrine glands than Caucasians.[31] The scalp hair of African Americans has been examined, and cross-sections have shown that the hair shaft tends to be elliptical or flattened and spiraled or tightly curled in its tertiary structure. Moreover, the curled hair does not emanate from a straight follicle. Instead, the follicle where the hair is formed is just as curved as the hair itself.[32] The hair shaft structure in Asian patients tends to be round in cross-section and relatively large in diameter. In comparison, Caucasian patients' hair shaft structure appears to fall somewhere between those of Asian and African American patients.[32] These results suggest that skin of color populations may have an anatomical predisposition for both HS and more severe forms of HS warranting further studies into genetic and anatomical variations and epigenetics in skin of color HS patients. Thus far, no ultrasound differences of hair follicles in skin of color patients versus Caucasian patients have been published.

Keloids

Individuals of African, Latino, or Asian descent appear to be at increased risk for keloids.[33] In individuals prone to keloid formation, the chronic inflammatory lesions of HS may lead to keloid formation. It has been hypothesized that the same pathway underlying tissue destruction and scar formation in HS subsequently triggers keloid formation in these patients. HS has been associated with the upregulation of cytokines such as interleukin (IL)-1, similar to general keloids.[34]

Previously, one case report existed of HS keloids being successfully treated with adalimumab.[35] However, in 2019, a North American case series was performed consisting of 10 patients with keloid formation in HS wounds. Patient ethnicities were African, Asian, Middle Eastern, and White. The most frequently affected sites were the chest (6 out of 10 cases) followed by axillae, and the severity of HS ranged from mild to severe disease. Some of the patients' keloids were either treated with intralesional injections of triamcinolone or received no specific treatment. Three of the 10 patients received adalimumab for the treatment of HS with subsequent reduction in both keloidal size and pruritis.[34]

Treating a patient with both HS and keloids within the same area can be complex. In the setting of no residual HS inflammation, the keloids formed from HS scars may respond to traditional therapies such as intralesional corticosteroid injections. However, keloids that occur in chronically inflamed HS lesions first require treating the underlying HS inflammation.[34] Intralesional corticosteroid injections have been used for the management of localized flares in HS. In 3 of the 10 patients mentioned above, patients who received adalimumab for their HS also saw a subsequent reduction in both keloidal size and pruritis. However, it cannot be said for certain whether the effects of the biologics were due to directly acting on keloids or whether it was due to early control of inflammation.[34] Optimal treatment of patients with HS and keloids in HS scars requires further investigation, and currently, prevalence rates of keloids in HS scars are unknown. However, our anecdotal experience is that the keloidal-type lesions in areas affected by HS are amenable to surgery.

Comorbidities

There are a number of comorbidities associated with HS. A higher cardiovascular risk is associated with HS due to several factors, including metabolic syndrome (MetS), diabetes mellitus type II, and smoking. Endocrine comorbidities include diabetes mellitus and polycystic ovarian syndrome. HS has also been linked to inflammatory bowel disease (IBD) and spondyloarthropathy.[11] A recent population-based study of 22,468 patients with HS in the Republic of Korea demonstrated an increased risk of HS patients having cancer overall, specifically higher rates of Hodgkin lymphoma, oral cavity and pharyngeal cancer, central nervous system cancer, nonmelanoma skin cancer, prostate cancer, and colorectal cancer.[36] Moreover, HS patients experience significant mental health disease burden, have an increased risk of completed suicide, and are vulnerable to substance use disorders.[11]

Metabolic Syndrome

HS is known to be associated with MetS and shares several major risk factors, including non-Caucasian race (African Americans and Hispanics) and female gender.[37] African Americans and Hispanics are less likely to engage in regular exercise compared to Caucasians.[38] Further, HS disease severity has been correlated with morbid obesity more commonly in patients with high versus medium disease burden (37% vs. 22%). Non-obese HS patients report more frequent HS remission in comparison to obese patients (45 vs. 23%), and in younger patients, HS onset occurs earlier in patients with comorbid MetS.[8] Taken together, these findings suggest that African American and Hispanic HS patients are at greater risk for MetS, chronic HS, and more severe forms.

Inflammatory Bowel Disease

In a retrospective study of a single US tertiary medical care center, the prevalence of HS in patients with IBD was 0.7%, while the prevalence of IBD in patients with HS was 3.6%. Among the 93 patients with both IBD and HS (IBD-HS), 75 (80%) had Crohn's disease (CD). When compared to controls with only IBD, the IBD-HS population had more women, African Americans, and higher rates of smoking.[39] Further, in another retrospective cohort study using the National Inpatient Sample (NIS) 2004 to 2014, a total of 3,079,332 admissions with IBD were recorded, of which 4,369 had a concurrent diagnosis of HS. From this IBD cohort, 1,962,733 (64%) patients had a diagnosis of CD, while 1,116,599 (36%) of patients were diagnosed with ulcerative colitis

(UC). IBD-HS patients were associated with 3732 cases (85%) of CD and 637 cases (15%) of UC. Compared to IBD-only patients, IBD-HS patients were significantly younger (mean age 39 [IQR: 28 to 49] vs. 51 [IQR: 34 to 66]; $P < .001$), more likely to be female (61.6% vs. 57.2%; $P = .008$), and African American (46.8% vs. 10.0%; $P < .001$); they were also more likely to be smokers, obese, and have diabetes mellitus, depression, and anemia.[40] Overall, these two studies show that patients with IBD and HS are more likely to be African American than IBD patients without HS.

Squamous Cell Carcinoma

Lapins et al. found that statistically significant risk elevations were observed for nonmelanoma skin cancer in HS patients (5 cases; SIR, 4.6; 95% confidence interval, 1.5 to 10.7).[41] As mentioned previously, a Korean cohort demonstrated an increased risk of HS patients having nonmelanoma skin cancer.[36] The transformation of chronic HS to squamous cell carcinoma (SCC) is considered the most severe complication of HS but is an extremely rare phenomenon.[42] The most important risk factor for the development of SCC in African Americans is chronic scarring processes and areas of chronic inflammation. Moreover, chronic scarring processes including ulcers, discoid lupus erythematosus, lupus vulgaris, granuloma annulare, osteomyelitis, and HS have been noted in 20% to 40% of cases of SCC in African American people.[43] Therefore, any nonhealing ulcers or nodules adjacent to an area of chronic scarring or inflammation should be biopsied to exclude malignancy.[43] In general, African Americans with SCC have a higher mortality rate than Caucasians.[44] Currently, there are no studies that examine whether there are higher rates of SCC in African American patients vs Caucasian patients with HS.

Psychiatric Comorbidity

HS patients have higher quality-of-life (QOL) impairment than patients with psoriasis, acne, neoplasms, strokes, and heart transplant candidates,[8] and HS has been shown to be associated with increased odds of depression, antidepressant use, anxiety, anxiolytic use, and suicidality.[45] Further, depression was found to be more prevalent in those with higher disease burden than those with medium disease burden (52% vs. 35%).[46] This has serious implications for African Americans and Latinos compared to Caucasians because they are already at risk for a wide range of psychosocial stressors.[47] A study that oversampled African Americans and Hispanics/Latinos in relation to Caucasians found that major depression was most prevalent amongst Latinos (11%), followed by African Americans (8%), and then Caucasians (8%). The differences in depression rates are thought to be due to functional limitations, lack of health insurance, and lifestyle factors such as smoking and exercise, which varied amongst the racial groups.[48] Rates of chronic major depressive disorder are higher in African Americans than Caucasians (57% vs. 39%), and African Americans were more likely to rate their depression as severe/very severe and more disabling.[49] Given these findings, African American and Latino patients with HS may be at higher risk for developing depression and more severe forms of depression in comparison to the overall HS population.

In addition, there is increased mental health stigma in African American and Latino communities.[50] Thus, if there is an underlying medical condition that is causing or exacerbating an individual's mental health, treatment of that underlying medical condition is imperative since the patient may not seek treatment for their mental health. Further, in a study conducted to determine the incidence of long-term opioid use in previously opioid-naïve patients with HS, there was a 53% higher risk of long-term opioid use among patients with HS (OR 1.53, 95% CI 1.20 to 1.95; $P < .001$). Among patients with HS, a history of depression (OR, 1.97; 95% CI, 1.21 to 3.19, $P = .006$) was associated with higher odds of long-term opioid use. However, no association was found between race/ethnicity and increased risk of long-term opioid use among the HS patients.[51] These finding should still be seriously considered in skin of color HS patients as well as other racial and ethnic groups who also suffer from depression.

Access to Adequate and Empathetic Care

Studies have shown that HS is associated with low SES, potentially because low SES is also associated with lifestyle factors such as smoking and obesity.[52] Moreover, low SES is more prevalent in African and Latino populations, especially in the US.[53] A recent retrospective analysis examined HS patients presenting to Montefiore Medical Center HS Treatment Center between January 2015 and November 2017. Patient SES was based on factor analysis from census block groups and a z-score reflecting SES deviation from the New York State mean. Demographics of 375 HS patients were analyzed. Females with low SES (z-score $\leq$ -1.00) were more likely to present with Hurley stage II/III disease (OR, 1.72; $P = .049$), and there were more African American patients in stage III than non-African Americans (50% vs. 28%, $P < .001$). African American patients were more likely to have stage II/III than others (OR 2.46, $P = .0003$). The median SES of HS patients was -2.3 standard deviations (SD). African American patients with HS demonstrated a median SES of -2.3 SD, while non-African American patients had a median SES of -1.6 SD ($P = .001$).[54] In summary, approximately one-third of HS patients were African American and had more severe disease and significantly lower SES.

Patients with low SES may have HS and more severe HS due to healthcare barriers. Conversely, patients with HS may have low SES due to pain, drainage, and medical comorbidities leading to lost employment and educational opportunities.[54] Low SES makes it difficult for families to buy fresh produce, and their neighborhoods may prevent them from exercising outside for safety reasons, thereby contributing to obesity and metabolic syndrome. In addition, an important barrier to optimal HS treatment is proper wound care management. The cost of the dressings can be mitigated by insurance coverage, but some insurance plans do not cover the expense of wound dressings.[55]

In 2016, data from the 2005 to 2011 National Ambulatory Medical Care Survey (NAMCS) and the National Hospital Ambulatory Medical Care Survey (NHAMCS) were analyzed to assess factors that were predictive of outpatient visits for HS. Non-Hispanic, non-Latino patients were more likely to experience clinic visits for HS than Hispanic/Latino patients (OR 5.49, $P = .002$). The difference in patient visits for HS observed in Latinos and Hispanics may not represent a true difference in disease burden within this population but may reflect decreased access to healthcare resources.[56]

A recent study examined the demographic patterns and geographic patterns of inpatient hospitalizations for HS in the United States. African American patients accounted for almost half (47%) of HS patients discharged. Patients from zip codes with the lowest quartile for income accounted for 41% of HS hospitalizations. Nearly one-third (29%) of HS discharges from 2012 through

2014 were from the South Atlantic census division (Delaware, Maryland, Virginia, West Virginia, North Carolina, South Carolina, Georgia, Florida, and the District of Columbia). In contrast, the New England division and the Mountain division each accounted for only 3% of HS discharges. The study suggested there may be a significant link between the geographic distribution of HS discharges, the racial distribution of African Americans, and the prevalence of adult obesity across the US.[57] Further, a recent study demonstrated that urban zip codes with higher percentages of African Americans tended to have fewer dermatologists, while urban zip codes with lower percentages of African Americans tended to have more dermatologists. In the areas with a higher representation of African Americans, dermatologists were responsible for more people per provider than recommended (>25,000 people/dermatologist).[58] Hence, limited access to care and a higher number of comorbidities may contribute to more severe disease, necessitating higher hospitalization rates amongst African Americans.

Sisic et al. found that individuals with HS were significantly more likely to report being victimized by intimate partner violence (IPV).[59] Moreover, ethnic minority women (i.e., Black/African American, Hispanic/Latina, Native American/Alaska Native, Asian American) are disproportionately affected by IPV. According to the 2010 National Intimate Partner and Sexual Violence Survey, non-Hispanic Black and Native American/Alaska Native women reported higher prevalence rates of lifetime IPV (43.7% and 46%, respectively) compared to non-Hispanic White women (34.6%); the rate for Hispanic women was slightly higher (37.1%). These disproportionate rates have also been consistently documented in multiple US studies.[60] Screening for IPV should be incorporated into the care of HS patients, especially those with skin of color.

Conclusion

Despite a growing database of literature demonstrating a higher prevalence of HS in skin of color patients, especially in African Americans, few large-scale studies exist focusing on HS in skin of color. Significant differences may exist in treatment response for different racial/ethnic groups; however, clinical studies have primarily been performed in the Caucasian population. Greater representation of skin of color patients is needed in HS clinical trials. Skin of color populations may have forms of HS that are more severe and less responsive to treatment due to genetic variations, warranting further studies into genetic and anatomic variations and epigenetics in skin of color patients. Further, African American and Latino patients are at greater risk for MetS and more chronic and severe forms of HS. They may also be at higher risk for other comorbidities of HS, including IBD, SCC, and depression exacerbated by lower SES and higher rates of IPV. There is a crucial need for improved access to effective and culturally appropriate care for skin of color patients with HS and future research focusing on skin of color patients is needed to fully elucidate HS and its burden in these patient populations.

Note: In writing this chapter, we used the terminology presented by the National Institutes of Health regarding racial and ethnic categories.[61] However, we would like to bring awareness that these terms, while acceptable in scientific literature, may not always be the preferred terms of these communities. For example, Latino and Latina are gender specific, so Latinx may actually be the preferred term to include individuals of the LGBTQIA (Lesbian, Gay, Bisexual, Transsexual, Queer, Intersex, Asexual)

community. In all permissible instances, we have tried to be respectful and thoughtful of these considerations.

References

1. Garg A, Kirby JS, Lavian J, et al. Sex- and Age-Adjusted Population Analysis of Prevalence Estimates for Hidradenitis Suppurativa in the United States. *JAMA Dermatol.* 2017;153(8):760–764.
2. Ingram JR, Jenkins-Jones S, Knipe DW, et al. Population-based Clinical Practice Research Datalink study using algorithm modelling to identify the true burden of hidradenitis suppurativa. *Br J Dermatol.* 2018;178(4):917–924.
3. Browning J. Dermatology, Edited by Jean L. Bolognia, Julie V. Schaffer, Lorenzo Cerroni Fourth edition, China: Elsevier, 2018, ISBN 978-0-7020-6275-9. *Pediatr Dermatol.* 35:289–289. https://doi.org/10.1111/pde.13439.
4. Vazquez BG, Alikhan A, Weaver AL, et al. Incidence of hidradenitis suppurativa and associated factors: a population-based study of Olmsted County. *Minnesota J Invest Dermatol.* 2013;133(1):97–103.
5. Vlassova N, Kuhn D, Okoye GA. Hidradenitis suppurativa disproportionately affects African Americans: a single-center retrospective analysis. *Acta Derm Venereol.* 2015;95(8):990–991.
6. Reeder VJ, Mahan MG, Hamzavi IH. Ethnicity and hidradenitis suppurativa. *J Invest Dermatol.* 2014;134(11):2842–2843.
7. Garg A, Wertenteil S, Baltz R, et al. Prevalence Estimates for Hidradenitis Suppurativa among Children and Adolescents in the United States: A Gender- and Age-Adjusted Population Analysis. *J Invest Dermatol.* 2018;138(10):2152–2156.
8. Lee DE, Clark AK, Shi VY. Hidradenitis Suppurativa: Disease Burden and Etiology in Skin of Color. *Dermatology.* 2017;233(6):456–461.
9. Price KN, Hsiao JL, Shi VY. Race and Ethnicity Gaps in Global Hidradenitis Suppurativa Clinical Trials. *Dermatology.* 2019;1–6.
10. Ben-Gashir MA, Seed PT, Hay RJ. Reliance on erythema scores may mask severe atopic dermatitis in black children compared with their white counterparts. *Br J Dermatol.* 2002;147(5):920–925.
11. Nguyen TV, Damiani G, Orenstein LAV, Hamzavi I, Jemec GB. Hidradenitis suppurativa: an update on epidemiology, phenotypes, diagnosis, pathogenesis, comorbidities and quality of life. *J Eur Acad Dermatol Venereol.* 2021;35(1):50–61. https://doi.org/10.1111/jdv.16677.
12. Bureau USC. *Quick Facts United States*; 2019. https://www.census.gov/quickfacts/fact/table/US/HSG010218#HSG010218.
13. Arenbergerova M, Gkalpakiotis S, Arenberger P. Effective long-term control of refractory hidradenitis suppurativa with adalimumab after failure of conventional therapy. *Int J Dermatol.* 2010;49(12):1445–1449.
14. Kimball AB, Kerdel F, Adams D, et al. Adalimumab for the treatment of moderate to severe Hidradenitis suppurativa: a parallel randomized trial. *Ann Intern Med.* 2012;157(12):846–855.
15. Kimball AB, Okun MM, Williams DA, et al. Two Phase 3 Trials of Adalimumab for Hidradenitis Suppurativa. *N Engl J Med.* 2016;375(5):422–434.
16. Miller I, Lynggaard CD, Lophaven S, et al. A double-blind placebo-controlled randomized trial of adalimumab in the treatment of hidradenitis suppurativa. *Br J Dermatol.* 2011;165(2):391–398.
17. Blok JL, Li K, Brodmerkel C, et al. Ustekinumab in hidradenitis suppurativa: clinical results and a search for potential biomarkers in serum. *Br J Dermatol.* 2016;174(4):839–846.
18. Pelekanou A, Kanni T, Savva A, et al. Long-term efficacy of etanercept in hidradenitis suppurativa: results from an open-label phase II prospective trial. *Exp Dermatol.* 2010;19(6):538–540.
19. Grant A, Gonzalez T, Montgomery MO, et al. Infliximab therapy for patients with moderate to severe hidradenitis suppurativa: a randomized, double-blind, placebo-controlled crossover trial. *J Am Acad Dermatol.* 2010;62(2):205–217.

20. Tzanetakou V, Kanni T, Giatrakou S, et al. Safety and Efficacy of Anakinra in Severe Hidradenitis Suppurativa: A Randomized Clinical Trial. *JAMA Dermatol.* 2016;152(1):52–59.
21. Kailas A, Dawkins M, Taylor SC. Suggestions for Increasing Diversity in Clinical Trials. *JAMA Dermatol.* 2017;153(7):727.
22. Xu LY, Wright DR, Mahmoud BH, et al. Histopathologic study of hidradenitis suppurativa following long-pulsed 1064-nm Nd:YAG laser treatment. *Arch Dermatol.* 2011;147(1):21–28.
23. Alikhan A, Sayed C, Alavi A, et al. North American clinical management guidelines for hidradenitis suppurativa: a publication from the United States and Canadian Hidradenitis Suppurativa Foundations: Part I: Diagnosis, evaluation, and the use of complementary and procedural management. *J Am Acad Dermatol.* 2019;81(1):76–90.
24. Panduru M, Salavastru CM, Panduru NM, Tiplica GS. Birth weight and atopic dermatitis: systematic review and meta-analyis. *Acta Dermatovenerol Croat.* 2014;22(2):91–96.
25. Schrader AM, Deckers IE, van der Zee HH, et al. Hidradenitis suppurativa: a retrospective study of 846 Dutch patients to identify factors associated with disease severity. *J Am Acad Dermatol.* 2014; 71(3):460–467.
26. Xu H, Xiao X, Hui Y, et al. Phenotype of 53 Chinese individuals with nicastrin gene mutations in association with familial hidradenitis suppurativa (acne inversa). *Br J Dermatol.* 2016;174(4):927–929.
27. Yang JQ, Wu XJ, Dou TT, et al. Haploinsufficiency caused by a nonsense mutation in NCSTN underlying hidradenitis suppurativa in a Chinese family. *Clin Exp Dermatol.* 2015;40(8):916–919.
28. Jiao T, Dong H, Jin L, et al. A novel nicastrin mutation in a large Chinese family with hidradenitis suppurativa. *Br J Dermatol.* 2013; 168(5):1141–1143.
29. Chen S, Mattei P, You J, et al. γ-Secretase Mutation in an African American Family With Hidradenitis Suppurativa. *JAMA Dermatol.* 2015;151(6):668–670.
30. Thomas C, Rodby KA, Thomas J, et al. Recalcitrant Hidradenitis Suppurativa: An Investigation of Demographics, Surgical Management, Bacterial Isolates, Pharmacologic Intervention, and Patient-reported Health Outcomes. *Am Surg.* 2016;82(4):362–368.
31. Shelley WB, Hurley HJ. The physiology of the human axillary apocrine sweat gland. *J Invest Dermatol.* 1953;20:285–297. https://doi.org/10.1038/jid.1953.35.
32. McMichael AJ. Hair and scalp disorders in ethnic populations. *Dermatol Clin.* 2003;21(4):629–644.
33. Bayat A, McGrouther DA, Ferguson MW. Skin scarring. *BMJ.* 2003;326(7380):88–92.
34. Jfri A, O'Brien E, Alavi A, Goldberg SR. Association of hidradenitis suppurativa and keloid formation: a therapeutic challenge. *JAAD Case Rep.* 2019;5(8):675–678.
35. Singer E, Kundu R. Hidradenitis suppurativa with extensive secondary keloid formation. *JAMA Dermatol.* 2017;76(6)(suppl. 1), AB153.
36. Jung JM, Lee KH, Kim YJ, et al. Assessment of Overall and Specific Cancer Risks in Patients With Hidradenitis Suppurativa. *JAMA Dermatol.* 2020;156(8):844–853.
37. Moore JX, Chaudhary N, Akinyemiju T. Metabolic Syndrome Prevalence by Race/Ethnicity and Sex in the United States, National Health and Nutrition Examination Survey, 1988-2012. *Prev Chronic Dis.* 2017;14, E24.
38. Saffer H, Dave D, Grossman M, Leung LA. Racial, Ethnic, and Gender Differences in Physical Activity. *J Hum Cap.* 2013;7 (4):378–410.
39. Campbell P, Sayed C, Long MD. Clinical Characteristics of Patients With Hidradenitis Suppurativa and Inflammatory Bowel Diseases. *Am J Gastroenterol.* 2017;112:S411–S412.
40. Ramos-Rodriguez AJ, Timerman D, Khan A, et al. The in-hospital burden of hidradenitis suppurativa in patients with inflammatory bowel disease: a decade nationwide analysis from 2004 to 2014. *Int J Dermatol.* 2018;57(5):547–552.
41. Lapins J, Ye W, Nyrén O, Emtestam L. Incidence of cancer among patients with hidradenitis suppurativa. *Arch Dermatol.* 2001; 137(6):730–734.
42. Chapman S, Delgadillo III D, Barber C, Khachemoune A. Cutaneous squamous cell carcinoma complicating hidradenitis suppurativa: a review of the prevalence, pathogenesis, and treatment of this dreaded complication. *Acta Dermatovenerol Alp Pannonica Adriat.* 2018; 27(1):25–28.
43. Gloster Jr HM, Neal K. Skin cancer in skin of color. *J Am Acad Dermatol.* 2006;55(5):741–760, quiz 761–744.
44. Halder RM, Bridgeman-Shah S. Skin cancer in African Americans. *Cancer.* 1995;75(2 Suppl):667–673.
45. Patel KR, Lee HH, Rastogi S, Vakharia PP, Hua T, Chhiba K, Singam V, Silverberg JI. Association between hidradenitis suppurativa, depression, anxiety, and suicidality: a systematic review and meta-analysis. *JAMA Dermatol.* 2020;83(3):737–744.
46. Crowley JJ, Mekkes JR, Zouboulis CC, et al. Association of hidradenitis suppurativa disease severity with increased risk for systemic comorbidities. *Br J Dermatol.* 2014;171(6):1561–1565.
47. Williams DR, Priest N, Anderson NB. Understanding associations among race, socioeconomic status, and health: Patterns and prospects. *Health Psychol.* 2016;35(4):407–411.
48. Dunlop DD, Song J, Lyons JS, et al. Racial/ethnic differences in rates of depression among preretirement adults. *Am J Public Health.* 2003;93(11):1945–1952.
49. Williams DR, Gonzalez HM, Neighbors H, et al. Prevalence and distribution of major depressive disorder in African Americans, Caribbean blacks, and non-Hispanic whites: results from the National Survey of American Life. *Arch Gen Psychiatry.* 2007; 64(3):305–315.
50. DeFreitas SC, Crone T, DeLeon M, Ajayi A. Perceived and Personal Mental Health Stigma in Latino and African American College Students. *Front Public Health.* 2018;6:49.
51. Reddy S, Orenstein LAV, Strunk A, Garg A. Incidence of Long-term Opioid Use Among Opioid-Naive Patients With Hidradenitis Suppurativa in the United States. *JAMA Dermatol.* 2019;155(11): 1284–1290.
52. Deckers IE, Janse IC, van der Zee HH, et al. Hidradenitis suppurativa (HS) is associated with low socioeconomic status (SES): a cross-sectional reference study. *J Am Acad Dermatol.* 2016;75(4): 755–759.e751.
53. Williams DR, Priest N, Anderson NB. Understanding associations among race, socioeconomic status, and health: patterns and prospects. *Health Psychol.* 2016;35(4):407–411.
54. Soliman YS, Hoffman LK, Guzman AK, et al. African American Patients With Hidradenitis Suppurativa Have Significant Health Care Disparities: A Retrospective Study. *J Cutan Med Surg.* 2019; 23(3):334–336.
55. Kazemi A, Carnaggio K, Clark M, et al. Optimal wound care management in hidradenitis suppurativa. *J Dermatol Treat.* 2018;29 (2):165–167.
56. Udechukwu NS, Fleischer Jr AB. Higher Risk of Care for Hidradenitis Suppurativa in African American and Non-Hispanic Patients in the United States. *J Natl Med Assoc.* 2017;109(1):44–48.
57. Anzaldi L, Perkins JA, Byrd AS, Khazzari H, Okoye GA. Characterizing inpatient hospitalizations for hidradenitis suppurativa in the United States. *JAMA Dermatol.* 2020 Feb;82(2):510–513.
58. Vengalil N, Nakamura M, Helfrich Y. *Analyzing the Distribution of Dermatologists in the Urban Setting: Comparing Zip Codes with High and Low Representation of African Americans.* American Academy of Dermatology Annual Meeting (virtual), June 12–14, 2020.
59. Sisic M, Tan J, Lafreniere KD. Hidradenitis Suppurativa, Intimate Partner Violence, and Sexual Assault. *J Cutan Med Surg.* 2017; 21(5):383–387.
60. Stockman JK, Hayashi H, Campbell JC. Intimate Partner Violence and its Health Impact on Ethnic Minority Women [corrected]. *J Womens Health (Larchmt).* 2015;24(1):62–79.
61. National Institutes of Health, 2015. Racial and Ethnic Categories and Definitions for NIH Diversity Programs and for Other Reporting Purposes. [online] Available at: https://grants.nih.gov/grants/guide/notice-files/NOT-OD-15-089.html.

31

Hidradenitis Suppurativa in Women

ERIN K. COLLIER, VIVIAN Y. SHI, AND JENNIFER L. HSIAO

Introduction

In many epidemiologic studies, hidradenitis suppurativa (HS) has been found to disproportionately affect women of childbearing age. Nearly three-quarters of new diagnoses are in women, with the highest incidence in female patients aged 30 to 39. Furthermore, the reported average annual incidence in the United States is 12.1 per 100,000 for women, which is more than twice that of men (5.1 per 100,000).[1] Women may also have an earlier onset of disease coincident with the earlier onset of puberty in girls.[2] In women, HS can be found in the inframammary folds, breasts, and vulva, in addition to the axilla, inguinal, and buttock regions, as well as other anatomic sites.[3] A hormonal influence on HS in women is strongly suggested given changes observed in HS disease status peri-menstruation and during pregnancy.[4] Female sex hormones present in high levels, such as estrogen and progesterone, have been thought to play a role in the sexual dichotomy of HS prevalence.[5] Women face unique challenges in managing their HS related to menses, pregnancy, lactation, and menopause. Special consideration should be taken to provide comprehensive care to women with HS and improve their quality of life.

Menses

The range of peri-menstrual HS flares has been reported to be between 44% and 63%.[6] The ovarian cycle enters the luteal phase after ovulation, where the remaining granulosa cells undergo luteinization and combine with theca-lutein cells to form the corpus luteum.[7] The corpus luteum functions as an endocrine organ and primarily secretes progesterone to prepare the endometrium for possible embryo implantation.[7] Typically, eight or nine days after ovulation, during the mid-luteal phase, serum levels of progesterone and estradiol peak.[7] If human chorionic gonadotropin (hCG) is not produced as a result of pregnancy, the corpus luteum will undergo luteolysis, leading to a decline in progesterone production and resulting in the menstrual period.[7] Estradiol also decreases during the luteal phase of the ovarian cycle, though to a lesser degree. Premenstrual HS flares are hypothesized to be caused by the change in steroid sex hormone levels immediately preceding the onset of menstruation (Fig. 31.1),[6] which leads to immunologic changes; however, the definitive relationship between progesterone, estrogen, and HS disease status has yet to be established.

Hormonally Mediated Immune Alterations That Impact Hidradenitis Suppurativa

Immune dysregulation has been implicated in HS pathogenesis, with studies reporting elevation in several pro-inflammatory (and some anti-inflammatory) cytokines, including TNF-α, interleukin (IL)-1β, IL-10, IL-17, IL-12, IL-23, IL-22, and IL-20 in lesional HS skin compared to healthy control skin.[8]

Estrogen and progesterone have been shown to differentially modulate immune tolerance through varying physiological mechanisms (Fig. 31.2). Estrogen stimulates the production of interferon alpha (IFN-α) by plasmacytoid dendritic cells. In mice, this has been shown to occur via estrogen receptor alpha (ER-α)-mediated upregulation of the transcription of type 1 interferon (IFN) producing genes.[9] Type 1 IFNs (including IFN-α, β, ε, τ, and δ) then further increase estrogen signaling within immune cells by inducing expression of more ER-α, resulting in a "feed-forward" loop.[9] Estrogen can

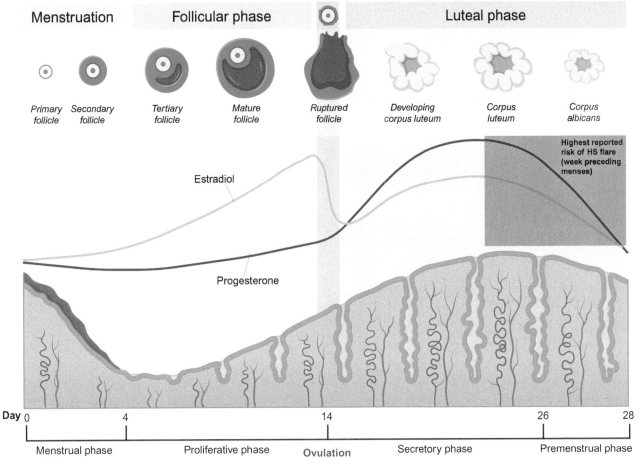

• **Fig. 31.1** Phases of the Menstrual Cycle.

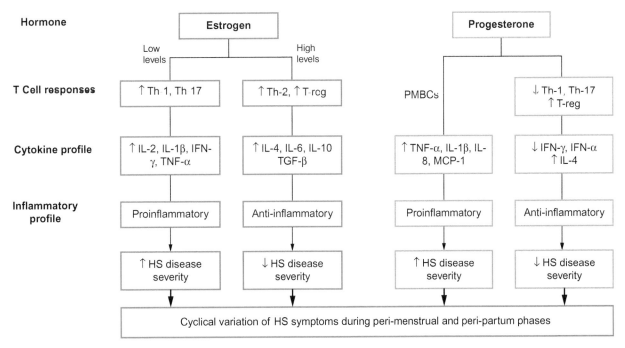

• **Fig. 31.2** Theoretical impact of how estrogen and progesterone may influence hidradenitis suppurativa disease course. *HS*, Hidradenitis suppurativa; *IFN*, interferon; *IL*, interleukin; *MCP*, monocyte chemoattractant protein; *PMBCs*, peripheral blood mononuclear cells; *TGF-β*, transforming growth factor beta; *Th*, T helper cell; *TNF-α*, tumor necrosis factor alpha; *Treg*, regulatory T cell.

also enhance the release of inflammatory cytokines including IL-1 and TNF-α from human monocytes and macrophages and pro- and anti-inflammatory cytokine IL-6.[10] In addition, in vivo mouse studies suggest that estrogen induces ER-α mediated differentiation of naïve CD4+ T cells into T helper (Th) 1 cells, which secrete pro-inflammatory IFN-γ.[11]

Though these results suggest that estrogen plays a predominantly pro-inflammatory role, discordant mouse studies have demonstrated inhibition of CD4+ T cell differentiation into Th1 and Th17 cells via ER-α signaling in T lymphocytes.[12] Other in vivo mice studies have suggested that the effects of estrogen on cell-mediated immunity vary according to dose, with low doses of estrogen promoting enhanced pro-inflammatory Th1 responses and high doses leading to anti-inflammatory Th2 responses.[10,13,14] Estrogens have also been shown to have a biphasic effect on TNF-α in human T cell clones, with enhancement at low concentrations and inhibition at high concentrations.[10,15]

The anti-inflammatory effects of progesterone have been well-documented. Progesterone has been found to suppress type 1 IFN production as well as production of IFN-γ from Th1 cells in mouse studies.[9] Studies have shown that medroxyprogesterone acetate at doses sufficient for contraceptive efficacy can suppress IFN-α production by plasmacytoid dendritic cells in mice in vivo[16] and human plasmacytoid dendritic cells in vitro.[9,17] Moreover, progesterone suppresses proliferation of CD4+ T cells and Th17 cells, which are involved with chronic inflammation seen in HS.[11] Evidence from mouse models also supports the role of progesterone in facilitating regulatory T cells (Treg) differentiation involved in preventing autoimmunity and mitigating the damaging inflammation from naïve CD4+ T cells via progesterone receptor signaling.[9]

Few studies suggest that progesterone may also have pro-inflammatory effects. Yuan et al. (2008) studied the effects of progesterone on the spontaneous production of TNF-α, IL-1β, IL-8, and macrophage chemotactic protein by unstimulated peripheral blood mononuclear cells (PMBCs) from patients with chronic hepatitis C. They discovered that the levels of each cytokine increased significantly in PBMCs treated with progesterone.[18]

Premenstrual HS exacerbation has been suggested to result from a reduction in anti-inflammatory mediators due to lower progesterone levels prior to menses.[11] However, the timing of HS symptom onset needs further elucidation; it is unclear if HS symptoms are triggered by high levels of progesterone and estrogen in the mid-luteal phase, or by the declining levels of progesterone and estrogen right before menses. One study found that, compared to patients with premenstrual HS flares, women without premenstrual flare had lower progesterone levels and higher testosterone and androstenedione levels.[19] Additional research is needed to fully elucidate the role of steroid sex hormone in HS immunology.

Medical Therapy

Oral Contraceptive Pills

Evidence is mixed regarding the use of oral contraceptive pills (OCPs) in the management of HS flares. Early cases have suggested a temporal relationship between HS onset and initiation of OCPs, with complete resolution occurring with either discontinuation of OCPs or switching to a formulation with a higher estrogen:progestogen ratio.[20] Other studies have shown no differences in HS symptoms between OCP and non-OCP groups,[21] or have shown substantial disease improvement with either ethinyloestradiol 50 μg/cyproterone acetate (CPA) 50 mg EKC or ethinyloestradiol 50 μg/norgestrel 500 μg.[22] The literature also contains anecdotal

reports of OCPs with high estrogen to progesterone ratio and low androgenic progestogens leading to HS disease amelioration.[23] Current evidence does not allow for concrete recommendations on which specific OCP to use for the management of HS. However, if OCPs are being considered, choosing one with a less androgenic progestogen, such as norgestimate, desogestrel, gestodene, or drospirenone, may be beneficial.[24] Though further investigation is needed, some studies suggest that progesterone-only pills, progesterone implants, or depot progesterone can cause HS exacerbation.[24]

Spironolactone

Spironolactone, a potassium-sparing diuretic with anti-androgenic properties, has demonstrated varying efficacy in HS management. Studies have shown HS clinical improvement with spironolactone at 3 months follow-up.[25] One study found no differences in improvement between patients who received less than 75 EKC mg of spironolactone daily and those who received over 100 mg daily EKC.[26] The 2019 North American HS management guidelines recommend the use of hormonal therapies, such as spironolactone and OCPs, in female patients with mild-to-moderate HS or as adjunctive agents in severe disease, and suggest that those with perimenstrual flares may be most likely to benefit.[27]

Wound Care During Menstruation

Mechanical friction has been suggested as a pathogenic mechanism in the development of HS, supported by cases of HS lesions arising in areas of amputated limbs with prostheses-related friction and the development of new HS lesions at sites exposed to excess friction.[28] Women may potentially experience discomfort and exacerbation of vulvar or perineal lesions during menstruation due to mechanical friction imposed by sanitary napkins. Therefore, the use of tampons[29] in lieu of menstrual pads can help reduce friction and moisture in the area. For women who prefer menstrual pads, choosing non-fragranced pads made from gentle materials such as cotton or bamboo may be beneficial. For painful or heavily draining wounds in the groin region, women may benefit from the use of a hydro-fiber dressing with silver, calcium alginates, or foams. Appropriately fitting biker shorts can be worn to help hold dressings in place.[30]

Fertility

Limited evidence from prospective studies suggests that approximately 12% to 18% of women in the U.S. are not pregnant within 12 months of attempting conception.[31] There is a paucity of data in the literature regarding the impact of HS on female fertility. However, it is well known that HS is associated with several somatic and psychiatric comorbidities associated with fertility issues.

Somatic Diseases and Infertility

The pathophysiology of infertility in women often involves anatomical dysfunctions, including history of tubal infections, endometriosis, and various uterine pathologies such as adhesions, polyps, fibroids, or asymptomatic tumors.[32] There is a higher prevalence of polycystic ovarian syndrome (PCOS) among HS patients than the general population (9.0% vs. 2.9%, respectively),[33] which could contribute to increased infertility.[34] Lifestyle and modifiable behavioral factors can also negatively impact fertility in female HS patients. The overall incidence rate of HS in tobacco smokers is nearly double the incidence rate among nonsmokers (0.20% vs. 0.11%, respectively);[35] chronic smoking can cause rapid depletion of ovarian follicles, conception delay, and increased risk of spontaneous abortion.[36] Obesity is also significantly associated with HS (pooled OR of 3.45 found in the systematic review);[37] obese women have a threefold higher risk of infertility compared to non-obese women. This risk is potentially due to derangements in gonadotrophin secretion as a result of peripheral aromatization of androgens to estrogens and hyperandrogenemia from insulin resistance and hyperinsulinemia.[32]

Psychologic Stress and Infertility

HS patients may suffer from stress related to their illness, financial hardship from disease burden, and psychiatric comorbidities.[3] Persistent psychological stress can alter oocyte maturation and lead to infertility.[32] Female HS patients struggling with infertility should be screened for comorbid conditions such as PCOS and psychiatric disorders if that has not already been done. Lifestyle modifications should be encouraged to achieve and maintain a healthy weight and join smoking cessation programs if applicable. Large population-based studies exploring infertility rates in HS patients compared to the general population are needed.

Pregnancy

The effects of pregnancy on HS disease course are mixed. Two European survey studies found that pregnancy is associated with HS symptom improvement in 20% and 30.2% of patients, worsening in 8% and 16.7%, with the majority reporting no change (72% and 53.1%).[38,39] However, a recent retrospective chart review study of patients at an academic referral center in the U.S. found that the majority (62%) of HS patients reported HS disease worsening during pregnancy.[40] There remains a lack of consensus in the literature regarding the impact of pregnancy on HS; thus, patients should be counseled to monitor their HS disease during pregnancy and contact their healthcare providers if symptoms are worsening.

Pregnancy-Related Protective Factors for Hidradenitis Suppurativa

Progesterone and estrogen levels rise throughout pregnancy, which has been implicated in the amelioration of HS symptoms reported by some pregnant women. Estrogens produced by the placenta are primarily derived from fetal dehydroepiandrosterone (DHEA) sulfate, which is then converted to androstenedione and testosterone through enzymatic pathways in steroid-producing tissues. The placenta then aromatizes these androgens to estrone and estradiol. 17α-hydroxysteroid dehydrogenase type II catalyzes the conversion of estradiol to estrone. A third type of estrogen, estriol, is formed as a metabolite from DHEA sulfate. Throughout pregnancy, serum estrone and estradiol concentrations increase to approximately 50-fold their maximal pre-pregnancy values, while estriol increases 1000-fold.[41]

This excess estrogen affects inflammatory pathways in various ways. Human in vitro and mouse in vivo studies show that estrogens can affect T helper cells in a biphasic way, with low doses of estrogen enhancing Th1 responses, and high levels augmenting Th2 responses (see Fig. 31.2). Therefore, as estrogens rise during

pregnancy, there is a shift in the Th cytokine profile from pro-inflammatory (IL-2, IFN-γ, TNF-α) to anti-inflammatory (IL-4, IL-6, IL-10, TGF-β).[10] During pregnancy, estrogen also activates regulatory T cells (Treg), promoting their proliferation via the PI3K/AKT signaling pathway and augmenting their immune-suppressive capabilities.[42] Improvement of other chronic inflammatory diseases during pregnancy, such as rheumatoid arthritis, has been correlated with elevated and sustained levels of Treg activity.[9] Thus, the high levels of estrogen during pregnancy may confer beneficial effects on patients' HS disease; however, the precise mechanisms for estrogen-induced immunomodulation during pregnancy and the impact on HS disease remain unclear.

Progesterone-mediated anti-inflammatory effects may also contribute to the amelioration of HS symptoms during pregnancy. Around the tenth week of pregnancy, the placenta takes over progesterone production and the corpus luteum involutes. The placental enzymes cleave maternal cholesterol sidechains to yield pregnenolone, which is later isomerized to progesterone. By the third trimester, 250 to 350 mg of progesterone are produced daily, with the majority entering the maternal circulation.[41] As mentioned, progesterone promotes an anti-inflammatory cytokine milieu. Progesterone also induces the release of IL-4, an important cytokine for the suppression of inflammation (mediates Th2 cell function and regulates Treg activity), and together, both act to inhibit Th1 responses during pregnancy.[43]

In addition to the immune-modulating activities of estrogen and progesterone during pregnancy, there are also immunological changes that are not directly hormonally influenced, which take place within the pregnant female body that may mitigate HS disease symptoms. For example, uterine natural killer cells (NK cells), monocytes, and Tregs within the decidua (the membrane lining the uterus during pregnancy) are key producers of IL-10, which inhibits excess inflammation. IL-10 production is increased during the first and second trimester, falls by the third trimester, and then increases again postpartum. Furthermore, IL-4 can be produced by immune cells of the placenta, maternal decidua, amniochorionic membranes, cytotrophoblasts, and maternal and fetal endothelial cells.[43]

Cytokine receptor antagonists, such as IL1Ra, can also act to inhibit pro-inflammatory mechanisms by blocking receptor binding.[44] A study by Østensen et al. found that levels of IL1Ra and soluble TNF receptor (TNFR) were elevated in healthy pregnant women and pregnant women with rheumatoid arthritis, when compared to non-pregnant controls, with a significant decrease in the post-partum phase.[44] Thus, increased levels of IL-10, IL-4, IL1Ra, and TNFR seen in pregnancy could contribute to the amelioration of HS disease experienced by some patients during pregnancy.

Pregnancy-Related Harmful Factors for Hidradenitis Suppurativa

Pregnancy begins with an inflammatory reaction triggered by implantation of the embryo within the uterine wall. During this reaction, inflammatory cytokines, such as IL-1, IL-6, and leukemic inhibitory factors are upregulated.[45] Various leukocytes migrate to the decidua and directly interact with the trophoblasts of the developing placenta, promoting their survival.[45] This initial pro-inflammatory state could be a contributing factor in those patients with HS disease worsening with the onset of pregnancy.

Weight gain during pregnancy may increase friction and maceration at intertriginous sites, which may contribute to HS flares.

Additionally, adipocytes may independently promote the secretion of pro-inflammatory cytokines, such as TNF-α.[11] One cross-sectional study of 186 patients did not demonstrate a correlation between body mass index and severity of HS symptoms during pregnancy; however, the impact of increased weight gain during pregnancy on the severity of HS symptoms was not evaluated.[39]

Medical Therapy During Pregnancy and Lactation

When deciding on a therapeutic agent for a pregnant HS patient, important considerations include: (1) expected efficacy of the intervention for HS and (2) safety profile of the intervention for both the mother and the fetus. The U.S. Food and Drug Administration (FDA) pregnancy categories have now been replaced by individual medication risk summaries[46]; however, these former pregnancy categories will still be included in this chapter for historical reference (Table 31.1). A list of commonly used HS medications and their associated pregnancy and lactation safety information is found in Table 31.2.

Hidradenitis Suppurativa Medications to Avoid During Pregnancy and Lactation

Medications with former FDA pregnancy categories D and X are contraindicated during pregnancy; select category C drugs, as described in this section, are also best avoided (Table 31.3).

Tetracyclines class (D) have been the mainstay of HS treatment for many decades and have traditionally been used for Hurley stage I or mild stage II disease.[27,83] Though not associated with congenital anomalies with first-trimester use, tetracyclines class antibiotics deposit within developing bones in the second and third trimester, leading to yellow dental staining and enamel hypoplasia. They have also been associated with acute fatty liver of pregnancy, a potentially fatal condition that occurs during the third trimester.[49] Therefore, oral tetracyclines are contraindicated during pregnancy, especially after the first trimester.[51,84] The American Academy of Pediatrics considers tetracyclines compatible with lactation;[85] however, administration for longer than three weeks at a time is contraindicated in order to prevent dental staining.[69] Overall, the use of tetracyclines during pregnancy and lactation should generally be avoided.

TABLE 31.1	Former Food and Drug Administration Pregnancy Categories[a]
Category	**Risk**
A	Well-controlled studies in pregnant women have failed to demonstrate fetal risk
B	Animal reproduction studies have failed to demonstrate fetal risk and no well-controlled studies exist for pregnant women; animal reproduction studies have demonstrated adverse effects, but well-controlled studies in pregnant women show no adverse fetal effects
C	Animal reproduction studies have shown adverse fetal effects; or no animal reproduction studies exist and no well-controlled studies in humans exist
D	Positive evidence of fetal risk; benefits may outweigh risks
X	Positive evidence of fetal risk; risks clearly outweigh possible benefits

[a]FDA pregnancy categories have been replaced by medication specific risk summaries (effective June 30, 2015); however, they are included here for historical reference.[46]

Systemic retinoids, such as acitretin (X) and isotretinoin (X) are strictly contraindicated during pregnancy and lactation.[79] Exposure to either medication, at any point during pregnancy, is associated with severe birth defects including craniofacial, cardiac, thymic, and central nervous system malformations.[51,86] Acitretin should be discontinued at least three years prior to conception,[78] and recommendations for isotretinoin suggest discontinuation at least one month before conception.[49] Finasteride (X) is contraindicated in pregnancy due to teratogenic effects and is not indicated for use during lactation.[80] Spironolactone (C) has been shown to affect sex differentiation and lead to feminization of male rat fetuses in animal studies and should be avoided during pregnancy. Long-term data in nursing mothers is lacking, though no evidence of adverse effects on infants has been noted with short-term exposure. Manufacturers suggest switching to an alternative form of infant feeding if spironolactone is deemed essential.[81]

Methotrexate (X) has also been used in the treatment of HS, though limited amounts of data support its use in the literature.[87] Methotrexate is a known teratogen, causing embryotoxicity, spontaneous abortion, and fetal defects (growth restriction, hypoplastic supraorbital ridges, micrognathia, limb abnormalities, low-set ears, and intellectual disability).[49] It is strictly contraindicated in pregnancy and lactation. Pregnancy should be avoided for at least one ovulatory cycle in female patients who were receiving methotrexate.[82]

Procedural Therapies for Pregnant Hidradenitis Suppurativa Patients

Certain procedural therapies may be considered compatible with pregnancy and lactation, especially for those with severe, recalcitrant disease. Office-based procedures that can be considered include intralesional triamcinolone for individual lesions that are flaring, incision and drainage for acute pain relief, de-roofing of sinus tracts, local excisional surgeries, and cryoinsufflation. Chapters 22 and 24 discuss office-based procedural therapies for HS. Table 31.4 presents safety comments on select procedural interventions in pregnant women.[51] Data are lacking in the literature regarding the use of lasers for HS treatment during pregnancy. A systematic review of 22 studies on laser therapy (CO_2 laser, pulsed-dye laser, Nd:YAG laser, and potassium titanyl phosphate laser) for cutaneous conditions during pregnancy found only one case of premature rupture of membranes in a woman who had CO_2 treatment of genital condyloma (unclear if there was a causal relationship). There were no reported cases of spontaneous abortion, preterm labor, or congenital malformation related to laser treatment.[88]

Pregnancy and Hidradenitis Suppurativa-Related Comorbidities

Several HS-associated comorbidities may exacerbate HS symptoms or impose maternal or fetal harm. Special care should be taken to adhere to prenatal screening guidelines in pregnant women with HS.[89]

Anemia occurs at higher rates among HS patients,[3] and pregnancy is also a risk factor for anemia[90]; therefore, the risk of anemia is compounded for pregnant HS patients. Iron-deficiency anemia increases the risk of preterm labor, intrauterine growth restriction, and perinatal depression.[91] Current guidelines recommend screening all pregnant women for anemia in early pregnancy,[91] and this is especially important in HS patients who may be anemic at baseline.

HS patients also have higher rates of obesity and metabolic syndrome, which may worsen during pregnancy due to weight

TABLE 31.2 Safety of Hidradenitis Suppurativa Medications During Pregnancy and Breastfeeding

Medication	Former FDA Pregnancy Category[a]	Safety Comments for Pregnancy	Safety Comments for Breastfeeding
Topical Antibiotics			
Clindamycin	B	Minimal systemic absorption; no evidence of teratogenicity with systemic exposure during 2nd and 3rd trimester[47]; remote cases of pseudomembranous colitis with topical use[48]	Not known if excreted in breast milk with topical application; considered compatible[49]
Erythromycin	B	Low levels of systemic absorption; no evidence of teratogenicity or any other adverse effects in animal studies[50]	Not known if excreted in human milk after topical application; considered compatible[51]
Metronidazole	B	Negligible systemic absorption; no evidence of embryotoxicity or teratogenicity[52]	May be present in low levels in breast milk; considered compatible[51]
Systemic Antibiotics			
Clindamycin	B	No evidence of congenital abnormalities when given in 2nd and 3rd trimester; lack of adequate studies during 1st trimester[47]	Can pass into breast milk; has the potential to cause adverse effects on infant's gastrointestinal flora[49]; considered compatible[47]
Dapsone	C	No evidence of fetal abnormalities with administration during any trimester[53]; has been shown to cause neonatal hyperbilirubinemia and hemolysis; G6PD screening recommended due to risk of hemolytic anemia[49]	Excreted in breast milk in substantial amounts; possible hemolysis in neonate[53]; caution advised with breastfeeding
Ertapenem	B	No adequate studies in pregnant women; no evidence of teratogenicity in animal studies; slight decrease in fetal weight and effects on vertebral ossification in mice[53]	Present in human milk; limited data regarding effects on breastfed infant; considered compatible[49]
Metronidazole	B	Crosses placental barrier and enters fetal circulation rapidly; no evidence of fetotoxicity in mice[54]; no well-controlled studies in pregnant women; evidence in observational studies suggest low risk[49]	Secreted in breast milk in concentrations similar to plasma levels; discontinue 12–24 h before breastfeeding[55]
Moxifloxacin	C	No human studies; animal studies show no teratogenicity but there may be other possible harmful effects to the fetus, such as decreased weight and delayed skeletal development[56]; safer alternatives are generally preferred	Unknown if excreted in human breast milk, but likely[49]; caution advised with breastfeeding
Rifampin	C	No adequate well-controlled studies in pregnant women; reported to cross the placental barrier and appear in cord blood; congenital malformations reported in animal studies[57]; postnatal hemorrhages in mothers and infants following exposure during last few weeks of pregnancy[57,58]; use only if benefits outweigh risks	Excreted in breast milk but no evidence of adverse effects in infants; considered compatible[55]
Immunosuppressants			
Corticosteroids	C	Animal studies have shown cleft palate, increased fetal lethality, and decreased body weights; observational studies in women report intrauterine growth retardation and fetal hypoadrenalism with high doses[59]; recommended to limit prolonged use to 7.5 mg/day (avoid doses at or above 20 mg daily)[60]	Minimal excretion in breast milk; wait 4 h prior to breastfeeding[51]
Cyclosporine	C	Embryo- and fetotoxic in animals at 2–5 times human dose; no well-controlled studies in pregnant women[61]; increased risk of premature birth and low birth weight shown in observational studies [62]	Present in breast milk; not recommended during breastfeeding due to concern that drug may interfere with cellular metabolism in infant[55]
Biologics			
Adalimumab	B	Studies do not reliably establish an association with birth defects; increased active transfer across placenta in 3rd trimester and may affect the immune response of infant; in animal studies, no fetal harm or malformations was observed[63]; consider discontinuing at end of 2nd trimester[64]	Data suggest systemic exposure to adalimumab in the breastfed infant is low because it is a large molecule and degraded in the gastrointestinal tract; no reports of adverse effects on the infant[63]; likely compatible

(Continued)

TABLE 31.2 Safety of Hidradenitis Suppurativa Medications During Pregnancy and Breastfeeding—cont'd

Medication	Former FDA Pregnancy Category[a]	Safety Comments for Pregnancy	Safety Comments for Breastfeeding
Anakinra	B	No evidence of fetal harm in animal studies; insufficient data in pregnant women to determine the risk of birth defects or maternal adverse events[65]; animal studies suggest low risk but may be best avoided until additional safety data is available[49]	Limited data precludes risk assessment; case reports on use during lactation have not shown adverse effects on breastfed infants[65]
Infliximab	B	Unknown if causes fetal harm; no evidence of maternal toxicity, embryotoxicity, or teratogenicity in mice; crosses the human placenta in late gestation and has been detected in infants up to 6 months after delivery[66]; congenital anomalies reported in observational studies though causation not established[67]; consider discontinuing at the end of the 2nd trimester[64]	Minimal transfer into breastmilk; case reports of exposure in nursing infants show no adverse effects[68]; likely compatible[69]
Ustekinumab	B	Insufficient data in pregnant women to inform risk assessment; animal studies show no adverse effects; additional safety data required[70]	Present in milk in animal studies; exposure to infant expected to be low[70]
Other Immunomodulators			
Apremilast	C	Animal studies reveal possible increased risk of fetal loss; data on pregnant women are extremely limited[71]	Detected in the milk of lactating mice; no data on presence in human milk or effects on the breastfed infant[71]; caution advised with breastfeeding
Colchicine	C	No adequate well-controlled studies in pregnant women; crosses the human placenta; animal studies demonstrate teratogenicity, embryofetal toxicity, and altered postnatal development[72]; human observational studies suggest risk to the fetus is low [49]	Excreted in human milk; may affect gastrointestinal cell renewal and permeability in infants[72]; caution advised with breastfeeding
Other Medications			
Acetaminophen	B	Analgesic of choice in pregnancy[51]; no known teratogenicity; possible increased risk of childhood attention-deficit/hyperactivity disorder and autism spectrum disorder after in-utero exposure[73]	Low excretion in breast milk; one case report of rash in newborn following exposure; compatible[49]
Ibuprofen	B/D[b]	Avoid during late pregnancy to prevent premature closing of the ductus arteriosus[74]	Low levels in breast milk; compatible[55]
Metformin	B	Not teratogenic in animal studies; crosses human placenta[75]	Excreted into breast milk; potential risk of hypoglycemia in the infant; benefits and risks should be weighed[75]; considered compatible
Zinc gluconate	Not assigned	No adverse effects on maternal or neonatal outcomes in review studies with the use of up to 50 mg daily; excess zinc consumption may lead to copper deficiency[51]	Does not appear to be transferred into breast milk[51]; considered compatible

[a]The United States Food and Drug Administration (FDA) pregnancy categories have been replaced by medications specific risk summaries (effective June 30, 2015); however, they are included here for historical reference
[b]Ibuprofen is former FDA pregnancy category B in the 1st and 2nd trimester, and pregnancy category D in the 3rd trimester

gain. At-risk patients with HS should be counseled on appropriate weight gain and glucose control during pregnancy or pre-pregnancy planning. Mechanical stress on intertriginous sites from excess weight can further deteriorate HS symptoms.[3] HS patients also have a higher prevalence of diabetes compared to controls.[92] A retrospective cohort study of 202 pregnancies in 127 HS patients found higher rates of gestational diabetes (9.3% vs. 6% to 8%, though not statistically significant) and gestational hypertension (14.9% vs. 10%, $P = .022$) compared to the general U.S. population.[93] In accordance with published clinical recommendations, pregnant women should undergo a glucose tolerance test between 24 and 28 weeks gestation to screen for gestational diabetes.[91]

Increased risk of psychiatric comorbidities, such as depression, among HS patients[94] may result in significant morbidity to a mother and infant. Complications associated with maternal perinatal depression include prematurity, low birth weight, neurodevelopmental delays, and decreased maternal-infant bonding.[95] As many as 15% of healthy mothers suffer from postpartum depression, which can have short- and long-term effects on child development.[96] Thus, women

TABLE 31.3 Hidradenitis Suppurativa Medications to Avoid During Pregnancy

Medication	Former FDA Pregnancy Category*	Safety Comments for Pregnancy	Safety Comments for Breastfeeding
Antibiotics			
Tetracyclines	D	No adequate well-controlled studies of use in short-term, 1st-trimester exposure; no human data on long-term therapy; therapeutic doses unlikely to pose substantial teratogenic risk[76]; positive association was seen with total malformations and use of doxycycline during pregnancy in a case-control study[77]	Tetracyclines are excreted in breast milk but the extent of absorption by the infant is unknown; short-term use by lactating women not necessarily contraindicated; however, prolonged exposure is best avoided to prevent dental staining[69]
Retinoids			
Acitretin	X	Causes major human fetal anomalies; embryotoxic and teratogenic in animal studies; avoid pregnancy for at least 3 years after discontinuing acitretin[78]	Contraindicated; rat studies show etretinate excretion in milk; one case report of acitretin excretion in human milk[78]
Isotretinoin	X	High risk of severe birth defects with any amount, for even short lengths of time;[79] discontinue one month prior to conception[49]	Unknown excretion in human breast milk; should be avoided given the potential for adverse effects[79]
Hormonal Therapy			
Finasteride	X	Causes abnormal development of genitalia in male fetuses[80]	Not indicated; unknown if excreted in human milk[80]
Spironolactone	C	Animal studies show effect on sex differentiation and feminization of male fetuses during embryogenesis, and endocrine dysfunction in females[81]	Not present in breast milk though limited human data on the presence of active metabolite (canrenone) in low amounts; no evidence of adverse effects with short-term exposure; no data on long-term exposure. Manufacturers suggest an alternate form of feeding infant if the drug is deemed essential[81]; caution advised with breastfeeding
Immunosuppressant			
Methotrexate	X	Can cause fetal death and congenital anomalies[82]	Potential for serious adverse events in infant; contraindicated[82]

TABLE 31.4 Safety of Select Procedural Interventions in Pregnancy

Procedure	Safety Comments for Pregnancy
Cryoinsufflation	Safety uncertain
De-roofing of sinus tracts	Lidocaine (+/- epinephrine) is the preferred local anesthetic for procedures during pregnancy
Incision and drainage	Lidocaine (+/- epinephrine) is the preferred local anesthetic for procedures during pregnancy
Intralesional corticosteroids	Compatible with use during pregnancy and lactation
Laser therapy[88]	
CO₂ Laser	One case of possible association with premature rupture of membranes (CO_2 laser was used to treat genital condyloma); risk of complications is considered low
Nd:YAG laser	No fetal or maternal complications reported to date with the treatment of genital condyloma.
Local excisional surgery	Lidocaine (+/- epinephrine) is the preferred local anesthetic; procedures requiring general anesthesia should be avoided

Adapted from Perng P, Zampella JG, Okoye GA. Management of hidradenitis suppurativa in pregnancy. *J Am Acad Dermatol.* 2017;76(5):979–989. https://doi.org/10.1016/j.jaad.2016.10.032

with HS who become pregnant should be adequately screened for mental illness both during and after pregnancy.[91]

Pregnancy Outcomes

A retrospective single-center cohort study of 202 pregnancies found that pregnant women with HS did not have higher rates of miscarriage, cesarean section, stillbirths, prematurity, or perinatal mortality compared to that of the general U.S. population.[93] Larger prospective pregnancy registries are needed to collect data on the influence of HS and HS treatments on maternal and neonatal outcomes.

Lactation

Breastfeeding is highly encouraged among new mothers and is the feeding method for most infants.[91] However, women with HS may experience difficulty with breastfeeding. One retrospective study found that about a quarter of infants born to mothers with HS were bottle-fed, and having HS lesions on the breast was associated with not breastfeeding.[93] Pregnant HS patients should have anticipatory counseling regarding the feasibility of breastfeeding and be referred to lactation specialists if needed. For patients with breast lesions who are planning on nursing, early treatment with intralesional corticosteroids or other medications may make breastfeeding more feasible.[97]

Menopause

Menopause is the final hormonal transition in women. It is characterized by loss of ovarian follicular activity and a subsequent drop in estradiol levels by approximately 50% by the time of their final menstrual period; estradiol levels continue to fall as menopause progresses.[98] Much like the other events that occur throughout a woman's life course, menopause may also lead to variable changes in HS disease severity. One survey study found that 48% of women with HS reported improvement of symptoms, 38% reported no changes, and 15% reported the deterioration of HS following menopause.[38] Further studies are needed to clarify the impact of menopause on HS and if there are any predictors of which individuals are at increased risk of disease worsening during menopause to help providers counsel patients.

Women's General Preventive Health Care and Lifestyle Considerations

Comprehensive care of women with HS includes general preventive care and lifestyle modifications. Weight loss via exercise and dietary modifications should be encouraged for overweight women. Physical activities with minimal friction to anatomic regions with active lesions can be helpful for women struggling with exercise.[97] Individuals with HS have also been found to be more likely to experience intimate partner violence.[99] It is important to elicit and address these challenges and refer for psychosocial support as needed.

Appropriate clothing selection can minimize excess mechanical friction and irritation on HS lesions and improve quality of life for some patients. Patients should be encouraged to wear soft fabrics made with 100% cotton, cellulose-derived rayon, or bamboo fibers that are loose-fitting and breathable.[100] Patients should also be counseled to avoid shaving in regions of active flare and to instead consider clipping their hairs short or pursuing laser hair removal if they desire hairless skin. Recommendations for wound care may include hygiene pads, postpartum mesh underwear, and adult diapers for draining vulvar, perineal, and gluteal lesions.

Conclusion

HS is a debilitating disease that disproportionately affects women of childbearing age and can significantly impact patients' health-related quality of life. Comprehensive care for women with HS involves optimization of management during menstruation, pregnancy, lactation, and menopause. Further research is needed to improve the understanding of hormone-mediated mechanisms in HS. Large prospective studies on infertility, medication safety during pregnancy, and maternal and neonatal outcomes in HS are warranted.

References

1. Garg A, Lavian J, Lin G, et al. Incidence of hidradenitis suppurativa in the United States: a sex- and age-adjusted population analysis. *J Am Acad Dermatol.* 2017. https://doi.org/10.1016/j.jaad.2017.02.005. Published online.
2. Naik HB, Paul M, Cohen SR, et al. Distribution of Self-reported Hidradenitis Suppurativa Age at Onset. *JAMA Dermatol.* 2019; 155(8):971–973. https://doi.org/10.1001/jamadermatol.2019.0478.
3. Alikhan A, Lynch P, Eisen D. Hidradenitis suppurativa: a comprehensive review. *J Am Acad Dermatol.* 2009;60(4):539–561. https://doi.org/10.1016/j.jaad.2008.11.911.
4. Jemec GB. The symptomatology of hidradenitis suppurativa in women. *Br J Dermatol.* 1988;119(3):345–350. https://doi.org/10.1111/j.1365-2133.1988.tb03227.x.
5. Karagiannidis I, Nikolakis G, Zouboulis CC. Endocrinologic Aspects of Hidradenitis Suppurativa. *Dermatol Clin.* 2016;34(1):45–49. https://doi.org/10.1016/j.det.2015.08.005.
6. Riis PT, Ring HC, Themstrup L, Jemec GB. The role of androgens and estrogens in hidradenitis suppurativa—a systematic review. *Acta Dermatovenerologica Croat.* 2016;24(4):239–249.
7. Reed B, Carr B. The normal menstrual cycle and the control of ovulation. In: Feingold K, Anawalt B, Boyce A, Al E, eds. *Endotext [Internet].* South Dartmouth, MA: MDText.com, Inc.; 2000. https://www.ncbi.nlm.nih.gov/books/NBK279054/.
8. Kelly G, Sweeney CM, Tobin AM, Kirby B. Hidradenitis suppurativa: the role of immune dysregulation. *Int J Dermatol.* 2014; 53(10):1186–1196. https://doi.org/10.1111/ijd.12550.
9. Hughes GC, Choubey D. Modulation of autoimmune rheumatic diseases by oestrogen and progesterone. *Nat Rev Rheumatol.* 2014; 10(12):740–751. https://doi.org/10.1038/nrrheum.2014.144.
10. Kassi E, Moutsatsou P. Estrogen receptor signaling and its relationship to cytokines in systemic lupus erythematosus. *J Biomed Biotechnol.* 2010;2010. https://doi.org/10.1155/2010/317452.
11. Perng P, Zampella JG, Okoye GA. Considering the impact of pregnancy on the natural history of hidradenitis suppurativa. *Br J Dermatol.* 2018;178(1):e13–e14. https://doi.org/10.1111/bjd.15735.
12. Lélu K, Laffont S, Delpy L, et al. Estrogen receptor α signaling in T lymphocytes is required for estradiol-mediated inhibition of Th1 and Th17 cell differentiation and protection against experimental autoimmune encephalomyelitis. *J Immunol.* 2011;187(5):2386–2393. https://doi.org/10.4049/jimmunol.1101578.
13. Bao M, Yang Y, Jun HS, Yoon JW. Molecular mechanisms for gender differences in susceptibility to T cell-mediated autoimmune diabetes in nonobese diabetic mice. *J Immunol.* 2002;168(10):5369–5375. https://doi.org/10.4049/jimmunol.168.10.5369.
14. Maret A, Coudert JD, Garidou L, et al. Estradiol enhances primary antigen-specific CD4 T cell responses and Th1 development in vivo. Essential role of estrogen receptor α expression in hematopoietic cells. *Eur J Immunol.* 2003;33(2):512–521. https://doi.org/10.1002/immu.200310027.
15. Gilmore W, Weiner LP, Correale J. Effect of estradiol on cytokine secretion by proteolipid protein-specific T cell clones isolated from multiple sclerosis patients and normal control subjects. *J Immunol.* 1997;158(1):446–451.
16. Hughes GC, Thomas S, Li C, et al. Cutting edge: progesterone regulates IFN-α production by plasmacytoid dendritic cells. *J Immunol.* 2008;180(4). https://doi.org/10.4049/jimmunol.180.4.2029. 2029 LP–2033.
17. Huijbregts RPH, Helton ES, Michel KG, et al. Hormonal contraception and HIV-1 infection: medroxyprogesterone acetate suppresses innate and adaptive immune mechanisms. *Endocrinology.* 2013;154(3):1282–1295. https://doi.org/10.1210/en.2012-1850.
18. Yuan Y, Shimizu I, Shen M, et al. Effects of estradiol and progesterone on the proinflammatory cytokine production by mononuclear cells from patients with chronic hepatitis C. *World J Gastroenterol.* 2008;14(14):2200–2207. https://doi.org/10.3748/wjg.14.2200.
19. Harrison BJ, Read GF, Hughes LE. Endocrine basis for the clinical presentation of hidradenitis suppurativa. *Br J Surg.* 1988;75(10):972–975. https://doi.org/10.1002/bjs.1800751011.
20. Stellon AJ, Wakeling M. Hidradenitis suppuritiva associated with use of oral contraceptives. *Br Med J.* 1989;298(6665):28–29. https://doi.org/10.1136/bmj.298.6665.28.
21. Jemec GBE, Heidenheim M, Nielsen NH. Hidradenitis suppurativa—characteristics and consequences. *Clin Exp Dermatol.* 1996; 21(6):419–423. https://doi.org/10.1111/j.1365-2230.1996.tb00145.x.

22. Mortimer P, Dawber R, Gales M, Moore R. A double-blind controlled cross-over trial of cyproterone acetate in females with hidradenitis suppurativa. *Br J Dermatol.* 1986;115(3):263–268.

23. Clark AK, Quinonez RL, Saric S, Sivamani RK. Hormonal therapies for hidradenitis suppurativa: review. *Dermatol Online J.* 2017;23(10):0–6.

24. Collier F, Smith RC, Morton CA. Diagnosis and management of hidradenitis suppurativa. *BMJ.* 2013;346(7905):f2121. https://doi.org/10.1136/bmj.f2121.

25. Lee A, Fischer G. A case series of 20 women with hidradenitis suppurativa treated with spironolactone. *Australas J Dermatol.* 2015;56(3):192–196. https://doi.org/10.1111/ajd.12362.

26. Golbari N, Porter M, Kimball A. Antiandrogen therapy with spironolactone for the treatment of hidradenitis suppurativa. *J Am Acad Dermatol.* 2019;80(1):114. https://doi.org/10.1016/j.jaad.2018.06.063.

27. Alikhan A, Sayed C, Alavi A, et al. North American clinical management guidelines for hidradenitis suppurativa: a publication from the United States and Canadian Hidradenitis Suppurativa Foundations: Part II: topical, intralesional, and systemic medical management. *J Am Acad Dermatol.* 2019;81(1):91–101. https://doi.org/10.1016/j.jaad.2019.02.068.

28. De Winter K, Van Der Zee HH, Prens EP. Is mechanical stress an important pathogenic factor in hidradenitis suppurativa? *Exp Dermatol.* 2012;21(3):176–177. https://doi.org/10.1111/j.1600-0625.2012.01443.x.

29. Margesson LJ, Danby FW. Hidradenitis suppurativa. *Best Pract Res Clin Obstet Gynaecol.* 2014;28(7):1013–1027. https://doi.org/10.1016/j.bpobgyn.2014.07.012.

30. Kazemi A, Carnaggio K, Clark M, et al. Optimal wound care management in hidradenitis suppurativa. *J Dermatolog Treat.* 2018;29(2):165–167. https://doi.org/10.1080/09546634.2017.1342759.

31. Thoma ME, McLain AC, Louis JF, et al. Prevalence of infertility in the United States as estimated by the current duration approach and a traditional constructed approach. *Fertil Steril.* 2013;99(5). https://doi.org/10.1016/j.fertnstert.2012.11.037. 1324–1331.e1.

32. Silvestris E, de Pergola G, Rosania R, Loverro G. Obesity as disruptor of the female fertility. *Reprod Biol Endocrinol.* 2018;16(1):1–13. https://doi.org/10.1186/s12958-018-0336-z.

33. Garg A, Neuren E, Strunk A. Hidradenitis Suppurativa Is Associated with Polycystic Ovary Syndrome: A Population-Based Analysis in the United States. *J Invest Dermatol.* 2018;138(6):1288–1292. https://doi.org/10.1016/j.jid.2018.01.009.

34. Hanson B, Johnstone E, Dorais J, et al. Female infertility, infertility-associated diagnoses, and comorbidities: a review. *J Assist Reprod Genet.* 2017;34(2):167–177. https://doi.org/10.1007/s10815-016-0836-8.

35. Garg A, Papagermanos V, Midura M, Strunk A. Incidence of hidradenitis suppurativa among tobacco smokers: a population-based retrospective analysis in the U.S.A. *Br J Dermatol.* 2018;178(3):709–714. https://doi.org/10.1111/bjd.15939.

36. Dorfman SF. Tobacco and fertility: our responsibilities. *Fertil Steril.* 2008;89(3):502–504. https://doi.org/10.1016/j.fertnstert.2008.01.011.

37. Tzellos T, Zouboulis CC, Gulliver W, et al. Cardiovascular disease risk factors in patients with hidradenitis suppurativa: a systematic review and meta-analysis of observational studies. *Br J Dermatol.* 2015;173(5):1142–1155. https://doi.org/10.1111/bjd.14024.

38. Kromann CB, Deckers IE, Esmann S, et al. Risk factors, clinical course and long-term prognosis in hidradenitis suppurativa: a cross-sectional study. *Br J Dermatol.* 2014;171(4):819–824. https://doi.org/10.1111/bjd.13090.

39. Vossen ARJV, van Straalen KR, Prens EP, van der Zee HH. Menses and pregnancy affect symptoms in hidradenitis suppurativa: a cross-sectional study. *J Am Acad Dermatol.* 2017;76(1):155–156. https://doi.org/10.1016/j.jaad.2016.07.024.

40. Lyons AB, Peacock A, McKenzie SA, et al. Evaluation of Hidradenitis Suppurativa Disease Course during Pregnancy and Postpartum. *JAMA Dermatol.* 2020;90404:1–5. https://doi.org/10.1001/jamadermatol.2020.0777.

41. Patel B, Nitsche JF, Taylor RN. The endocrinology of pregnancy. In: Gardner DG, Shoback D, eds. *Greenspan's Basic & Clinical Endocrinology.* 10th ed. New York, NY: McGraw-Hill Education; 2017. http://accessmedicine.mhmedical.com/content.aspx?aid=1144818385.

42. Nadkarni S, McArthur S. Oestrogen and immunomodulation: new mechanisms that impact on peripheral and central immunity. *Curr Opin Pharmacol.* 2013;13(4):576–581. https://doi.org/10.1016/j.coph.2013.05.007.

43. Chatterjee P, Chiasson VL, Bounds KR, Mitchell BM. Regulation of the anti-inflammatory cytokines interleukin-4 and interleukin-10 during pregnancy. *Front Immunol.* 2014;1. https://doi.org/10.3389/fimmu.2014.00253. 5(MAY).

44. Østensen M, Förger F, Nelson JL, et al. Pregnancy in patients with rheumatic disease: anti-inflammatory cytokines increase in pregnancy and decrease post partum. *Ann Rheum Dis.* 2005;64(6):839–844. https://doi.org/10.1136/ard.2004.029538.

45. Yockey LJ, Iwasaki A. Interferons and Proinflammatory Cytokines in Pregnancy and Fetal Development. *Immunity.* 2018;49(3):397–412. https://doi.org/10.1016/j.immuni.2018.07.017.

46. Pernia S, DeMaagd G. The New Pregnancy and Lactation Labeling Rule. *P T.* 2016;41(11):713–715.

47. Cleocin T [package insert]. Pfizer. Published online 2020. https://www.accessdata.fda.gov/drugsatfda_docs/label/2014/050537s035,050600s013,050615s012lbl.pdf.

48. Parry MF, Rha CK. Pseudomembranous colitis caused by topical clindamycin phosphate. *Arch Dermatol.* 1986;122(5):583–584. https://doi.org/10.1001/archderm.1986.01660170113031.

49. Briggs G, Freeman R, Yaffe S, eds. *Drugs in Pregnancy and Lactation.* 10th ed. Philadelphia, PA: Wolters Kluwer Health; 2015.

50. Erythromycin topical gel [package insert]. Perrigo New York Inc. Arbor Pharmaceuticals, Inc. Published online 2020. https://dailymed.nlm.nih.gov/dailymed/fda/fdaDrugXsl.cfm?setid=dd64459e-c88f-4ca8-b63b-fb96377a3921&type=display.

51. Perng P, Zampella JG, Okoye GA. Management of hidradenitis suppurativa in pregnancy. *J Am Acad Dermatol.* 2017;76(5):979–989. https://doi.org/10.1016/j.jaad.2016.10.032.

52. Metronidazole 0.75% gel [package insert]. Fougera Pharmaceuticals Inc. Published online 2020. https://dailymed.nlm.nih.gov/dailymed/drugInfo.cfm?setid=43ed872b-63ac-4a22-9c9e-cc0e05bcc41e.

53. Dapsone [package insert]. Jacobus Pharmaceutical Company, Inc. Published online 2011. https://dailymed.nlm.nih.gov/dailymed/lookup.cfm?setid=0792169d-c6f9-4af0-93ae-b75d710c47a9.

54. Flagyl [package insert]. Pfizer. Published online 2013. 2021. http://labeling.pfizer.com/showlabeling.aspx?id=570.

55. Committee on Drugs, American Academy of Pediatrics. The Transfer of drugs and other chemicals into human milk. *Pediatrics.* 2001;108:776–789.

56. Avelox [package insert]. Merck & Co., Inc. Published online 2012. https://www.merck.com/product/usa/pi_circulars/a/avelox/avelox_pi.pdf.

57. Rifampin [package insert]. Sanofi-aventis. Published online 2010. https://www.accessdata.fda.gov/drugsatfda_docs/label/2010/050420s073,050627s012lbl.pdf.

58. Eggermont E, Logghe N, Van De Casseye W, et al. Haemorrhagic disease of the newborn in the offspring of rifampicin and isoniazid treated mothers. *Acta Paediatr Belg.* 1976;29:87–90.

59. RAYOS (prednisone) [package insert]. Horizon Pharma USA, Inc. Published online 2012. https://www.accessdata.fda.gov/drugsatfda_docs/label/2012/202020s000lbl.pdf.

60. Murase JE, Heller MM, Butler DC. Safety of dermatologic medications in pregnancy and lactation: Part I. Pregnancy. *J Am Acad Dermatol.* 2014;70(3):401.e1–401.e14. https://doi.org/10.1016/j.jaad.2013.09.010.

61. Cyclosporine [package insert]. Apotex Corp. Published online 2020. https://www1.apotex.com/products/us/downloads/pre/cycl_imcp_ins.pdf.

62. Neoral [package insert]. Novartis. Published online 2009. https://www.accessdata.fda.gov/drugsatfda_docs/label/2009/050715s027,050716s028lbl.pdf.

63. Humira [package insert]. AbbVie Inc. Published online 2008. https://www.rxabbvie.com/pdf/humira.pdf.

64. Puchner A, Gröchenig HP, Sautner J, et al. Immunosuppressives and biologics during pregnancy and lactation: a consensus report issued by the Austrian Societies of Gastroenterology and Hepatology and Rheumatology and Rehabilitation. *Wien Klin Wochenschr.* 2019;131(1–2):29–44. https://doi.org/10.1007/s00508-019-1448-y.

65. Kineret [package insert]. Swedish Orphan Biovitrum AB. Published online 2012. https://www.accessdata.fda.gov/drugsatfda_docs/label/2012/103950s5136lbl.pdf.

66. Remicade [package insert]. Janssen Biotech, Inc. Published online 2013. https://www.accessdata.fda.gov/drugsatfda_docs/label/2013/103772s5359lbl.pdf.

67. Carter JD, Ladhani A, Ricca LR, et al. A safety assessment of tumor necrosis factor antagonists during pregnancy: a review of the food and drug administration database. *J Rheumatol.* 2009;36(3):635–641. https://doi.org/10.3899/jrheum.080545.

68. Fritzsche J, Pilch A, Mury D, et al. Infliximab and adalimumab use during breastfeeding. *J Clin Gastroenterol.* 2012;46(8):718–719. https://doi.org/10.1097/MCG.0b013e31825f2807.

69. Butler DC, Heller MM, Murase JE. Safety of dermatologic medications in pregnancy and lactation Part II. Lactation. *J Am Acad Dermatol.* 2014;70(3):417.e1–417.e10. https://doi.org/10.1016/j.jaad.2013.09.009.

70. Stelara [package insert]. Published online 2012.

71. Otezla [package insert]. Published online 2020.

72. Colcrys [package insert]. Published online 2012.

73. Ji Y, Azuine RE, Zhang Y, et al. Association of Cord Plasma Biomarkers of in Utero Acetaminophen Exposure with Risk of Attention-Deficit/Hyperactivity Disorder and Autism Spectrum Disorder in Childhood. *JAMA Psychiatry.* 2020;77(2):180–189. https://doi.org/10.1001/jamapsychiatry.2019.3259.

74. Motrin [package insert]. Published online 2007.

75. Glucophage XR [package insert]. Published online 2017.

76. Doryx [package insert]. Published online 2008.

77. Czeizel AE, Rockenbauer M. Teratogenic study of doxycycline. *Obstet Gynecol.* 1997;89(4):524–528. https://doi.org/10.1016/S0029-7844(97)00005-7.

78. Acitretin [package insert]. Stiefel Laboratories, Inc. Published online 2019. https://www.accessdata.fda.gov/drugsatfda_docs/label/2017/019821s028lbl.pdf.

79. Accutane [package insert]. Roche Laboratories Inc. Published online 2008. https://www.accessdata.fda.gov/drugsatfda_docs/label/2008/018662s059lbl.pdf.

80. Propecia [package insert]. Merck & Co., Inc. Published online 2012. https://www.accessdata.fda.gov/drugsatfda_docs/label/2011/020788s018lbl.pdf.

81. Aldactone [package insert]. Pfizer. Published online 2008. https://www.accessdata.fda.gov/drugsatfda_docs/label/2008/012151s062lbl.pdf.

82. Methotrexate [package insert]. Dava Pharmaceuticals, Inc. Published online 2011. https://www.accessdata.fda.gov/drugsatfda_docs/label/2016/008085s066lbl.pdf.

83. Zouboulis CC, Desai N, Emtestam L, et al. European S1 guideline for the treatment of hidradenitis suppurativa/acne inversa. *J Eur Acad Dermatology Venereol.* 2015;29(4):619–644. https://doi.org/10.1111/jdv.12966.

84. Tyler KH, Zirwas MJ. Pregnancy and dermatologic therapy. *J Am Acad Dermatol.* 2013;68(4):663–671. https://doi.org/10.1016/j.jaad.2012.09.034.

85. Committee on Drugs, American Academy of Pediatrics. The transfer of drugs and other chemicals into human milk. *Pediatrics.* 1994;93(1):137–150.

86. Koh YP, Tian EA, Oon HH. New changes in pregnancy and lactation labelling: review of dermatologic drugs. *Int J Women's Dermatology.* 2019;5(4):216–226. https://doi.org/10.1016/j.ijwd.2019.05.002.

87. Savage KT, Brant EG, Rosales Santillan M, et al. Methotrexate shows benefit in a subset of patients with severe hidradenitis suppurativa. *Int J Women's Dermatology.* 2020;6(3):159–163. https://doi.org/10.1016/j.ijwd.2020.02.007.

88. Wilkerson EC, Van Acker MM, Bloom BS, Goldberg DJ. Utilization of laser therapy during pregnancy: a systematic review of the maternal and fetal effects reported from 1960 to 2017. *Dermatologic Surg.* 2019;45(6):818–828. https://doi.org/10.1097/DSS.0000000000001912.

89. Brouillette RT. Guidelines for Perinatal Care. *JAMA.* 1989;261(12):1809. https://doi.org/10.1001/jama.1989.03420120151044.

90. Suryanarayana R, Chandrappa M, Santhuram AN, et al. Prospective study on prevalence of anemia of pregnant women and its outcome: a community based study. *J Fam Med Prim Care.* 2017;6(4):739–743. https://doi.org/10.4103/jfmpc.jfmpc_33_17.

91. Zolotor AJ, Carlough MC. Update on prenatal care. *Am Fam Physician.* 2014;89(3):199–208.

92. Phan K, Charlton O, Smith SD. Hidradenitis suppurativa and diabetes mellitus: updated systematic review and adjusted meta-analysis. *Clin Exp Dermatol.* 2019;44(4):e126–e132. https://doi.org/10.1111/ced.13922.

93. Lyons AB, Peacock A, McKenzie SA, et al. Retrospective cohort study of pregnancy outcomes in hidradenitis suppurativa. *Br J Dermatol.* 2002;183(5):945–947. Published online 2020:0–3 https://doi.org/10.1111/bjd.19155.

94. Machado MO, Stergiopoulos V, Maes M, et al. Depression and Anxiety in Adults With Hidradenitis Suppurativa: A Systematic Review and Meta-analysis. *JAMA dermatology.* 2019;155(8):939–945. https://doi.org/10.1001/jamadermatol.2019.0759.

95. Bonari L, Pinto N, Ahn E, et al. Perinatal risks of untreated depression during pregnancy. *Can J Psychiatry.* 2004;49(11):726–735.

96. Pearlstein T, Howard M, Salisbury A, Zlotnick C. Postpartum depression. *Am J Obstet Gynecol.* 2009;200(4):357–364. https://doi.org/10.1016/j.ajog.2008.11.033.

97. Collier E, Shi VY, Parvataneni RK, et al. Special considerations for women with hidradenitis suppurativa. *Int J Women's Dermatology.* 2020;6(2):85–88. https://doi.org/10.1016/j.ijwd.2020.02.005.

98. Burger HG, Hale GE, Robertson DM, Dennerstein L. A review of hormonal changes during the menopausal transition: focus on findings from the Melbourne Women's Midlife Health Project. *Hum Reprod Update.* 2007;13(6):559–565. https://doi.org/10.1093/humupd/dmm020.

99. Sisic M, Tan J, Lafreniere KD. Hidradenitis suppurativa, intimate partner violence, and sexual assault. *J Cutan Med Surg.* 2017;21(5):383–387. https://doi.org/10.1177/1203475417708167.

100. Loh TY, Hendricks AJ, Hsiao JL, Shi VY. Undergarment and Fabric Selection in the Management of Hidradenitis Suppurativa. *Dermatology.* 2019;85718. https://doi.org/10.1159/000501611.

Combined Approach

32

Building a Multidisciplinary Hidradenitis Suppurativa Clinic

ALEXIS B. LYONS AND ILTEFAT H. HAMZAVI

Introduction

Successful treatment of a patient with hidradenitis suppurativa (HS) requires a multidisciplinary approach. As such, establishing a multidisciplinary HS clinic is crucial to address this multifaceted disease. Having a basic treatment algorithm, expertise in the field, access to other specialties for referral, knowledge and access to the latest research,[1] and quality improvement initiatives are all important in establishing a successful HS clinic.

Treatment Algorithm

Every patient with HS presents differently, and accordingly, every patient should have an individualized treatment approach. Having a multidisciplinary HS care plan has been associated with high levels of patient satisfaction.[2] Implementing a standard treatment algorithm can be a valuable implementation tool and starting point for residents, physicians, and other practitioners, particularly those who are new to treating patients with HS. Establishing an institutional treatment algorithm can allow for the inclusion of institution-specific information regarding local specialized pharmacies, collaboration with non-dermatology colleagues, and important institutional contact information. Various

international groups have provided information on region-specific guidelines that can be referenced as a starting point[3-6] and are discussed further in Chapter 14. Disease severity classification methods such as Hurley staging and stability questions should guide this initial treatment approach and algorithm. An example of an institution-specific algorithm from Henry Ford Hospital, Detroit, MI, has been published,[7] and a skeleton structure is shown in Fig. 32.1. The goal of medical treatment is to stabilize and maintain low HS activity, while the goal of surgical treatment is to debulk affected tissue with the possibility of potential remission. A multimodal, individualized, and multidisciplinary approach should be applied, and institutional and clinic resources will guide the creation of the algorithm with site-specific components.

Domains of Expertise

To establish a successful multidisciplinary HS clinic, the clinic should be customized to the needs of the patient. Billing and insurance coverage for HS medications are important considerations. Since adalimumab is the only FDA-approved medication for the treatment of HS, prior authorizations are often needed to obtain coverage for many medications including biologics as well as for procedural treatments and lasers (e.g., neodymium-doped yttrium aluminum garnet [Nd:YAG]). Having friendly and knowledgeable clinic staff who can help handle these issues and communicate effectively with the patient and insurance company is crucial. A staff member(s) dedicated to these tasks can help to reduce the administrative burden.

Having expertise in wound care is also fundamental in establishing a successful HS clinic. HS patients often require multiple dressing changes per day due to chronic wounds and persistent drainage. Wound care supplies can consequently result in an extremely costly burden for patients. Determining the optimal wound dressing regimen and having helpful and affordable wound care recommendation options for patients is therefore essential (see Chapter 20 for comprehensive wound care management). If the HS clinic performs more invasive surgical procedures, including traditional surgical excisions or carbon dioxide (CO_2) laser excisions, having nursing staff with expertise in wound care is necessary to manage patients postoperatively and at follow-up visits. Access to a specialized wound care clinic can also aid in caring for patients who have chronic or post-operative, slow-healing wounds.

"Institution Name" HS Treatment Algorithm

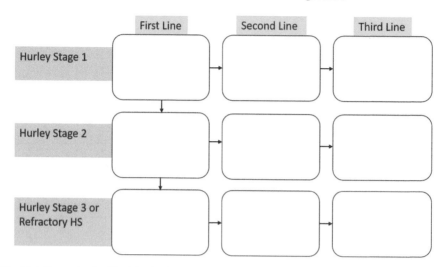

• **Fig. 32.1** Example of a Blank Institution-specific Hidradenitis Suppurativa *(HS)* Algorithm Structure.

Knowledge regarding cutting-edge HS research is important to be able to convey this information to patients with HS as well as answer questions that arise from patients regarding new treatments. Staying up to date with current treatments and guidelines is also paramount.[1] Having a research unit that conducts clinical trials or performs basic science research within your HS clinic offers a significant advantage, particularly with subject recruitment and the establishment of HS biobanks. Basic science HS research leads to a better understanding of the disease and leads to new treatment options with the goal being an eventual cure. Working closely, collaborating, and understanding the needs of basic scientists helps dramatically to advance the field of knowledge. If basic scientists researching HS require tissue or serum from patients with HS, where better to collaborate than with an HS specialty clinic? Having a dedicated and knowledgeable clinical research team can help facilitate the collaboration between clinical and basic science research. Understanding and working with institutional review boards is often an arduous process that can be managed effectively by a clinical research team.

Quality Improvement

Given the widespread prevalence of HS with an estimated 0.1% to 2% of the population affected[8–10] and the relatively small number of physicians with an expertise in HS, specialty HS clinics can quickly become saturated. Thus, quality improvement initiatives to continuously improve the clinic as it grows are important. Videos on the various HS procedures can be created to be viewed by patients so they can be aware of what to expect pre-, intra-, and postoperatively. This also cuts down on lengthy physician explanations in a clinic.

In addition, implementing a shared HS clinic with multiple providers can help to decrease patient wait times. Educating other physicians in the department about the institution-specific HS treatment algorithm can help facilitate bringing others on board to participate in the HS specialty clinic. Implementing sub-clinics within the HS specialty clinic can also be beneficial. Establishing a nursing wound care clinic and educating nursing staff to care for chronic and post-operative HS wounds can help with clinic flow. Establishing an urgent HS referral sub-clinic to triage complex

patients can also help with some of the more serious acute problems that patients with HS can experience, including flares, pain, and infection. Establishing a dedicated medical laser clinic can allow for patients to come in for scheduled laser treatments to be performed by nursing staff or residents to free up physician visit appointments for others with more acute needs. Additionally, given the ever-increasing research into HS, new treatments continue to emerge. Treatments including ertapenem and infliximab are administered intravenously; thus, establishing an infusion center within the clinic or having easy access and a partnership with a nearby infusion center can be of valuable assistance to patients.

Core Specialties for Referrals and Collaboration

As previously stated, the management of patients with HS is often a multidisciplinary effort. HS is associated with numerous comorbidities and often requires input from multiple specialties (Fig. 32.2). Given this fact, close collaboration is often required with colleagues within other specialties. Establishing these relationships for referrals and collaboration is essential. Compiling a handout for local physicians, medical staff, and patients with relevant contact information can be an invaluable tool. Comorbidities and systemic associations are discussed further in Chapter 8.

Surgery

One of the most common specialties to help manage patients with HS is surgery. While dermatologists and surgeons are capable of performing many deroofing office procedures for HS, general and plastic surgeons are often tasked with performing large excisions of affected HS areas that require utilization of general anesthesia. In HS clinics, dermatologists and surgeons are a complementary combination to evaluate patients together in the clinic, if possible. Colorectal surgeons are often needed in cases with extensive buttock and rectal involvement. Urologic or gynecologic evaluation is sometimes needed for those with penile, scrotal, urethral, or vaginal involvement, or for those who have HS involvement near these areas.

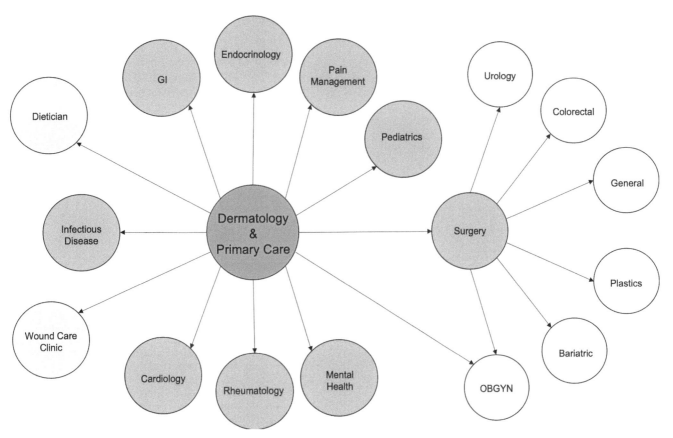

• **Fig. 32.2** Specialties Involved in Caring for Patients With Hidradenitis Suppurativa. *GI*, Gastrointestinal; *OBGYN*, obstetrics and gynecology.

Endocrinology, Weight Loss and Diet

Due to the fact that HS is associated with an increased risk for diabetes mellitus,[11,12] metabolic syndrome,[13] and polycystic ovarian syndrome (PCOS),[14] consultation and referral to endocrinology for management of these comorbid conditions are often necessary. In addition, dietary modifications can help in the management of some of these disease states. Accordingly, referral to a dietician can be helpful. Some patients report that the avoidance of dairy and brewer's yeast improves disease severity.[15,16] Dieticians can make helpful recommendations regarding avoidance of these patient-specific dietary triggers. The prevalence of overweight or obesity in patients with HS may be greater than 75%,[9,10,17] and as such, evaluation for bariatric surgery is sometimes warranted. Bariatric surgery can be beneficial for some patients with HS as improvement in the severity of the disease in one retrospective review was seen in 35% of patients after bariatric surgery.[18]

Cardiovascular Disease

HS has also been linked to major cardiovascular events including myocardial infarction (MI) and stroke with a 23% increased risk compared to those without HS.[19] As such, close collaboration between family practice, internal medicine, and cardiology is needed to evaluate and assess for the presence of modifiable risk factors and to screen for these comorbidities. In addition, the prevalence of smoking in patients with HS is between 70% and 75%.[8,20,21] Thus, taking a thorough smoking history is recommended, and smoking cessation counseling by providers is encouraged.

Comorbid Autoimmune and Inflammatory Conditions

Rheumatology can be brought on board to help manage patients with HS who also have fibromyalgia, polymyositis, and ankylosing spondylitis, among others.[22,23] Gastroenterology is often needed for the management of patients with HS who also have concomitant inflammatory bowel disease.[24] Often, some of these diseases can be treated using the same immunosuppressive or biologic medications. Close contact and collaboration between specialties to come up with individualized treatment regimens are key to optimizing patient outcomes.

Antibiotic Management

Infectious disease is also an important referral specialty for those with HS. Oral antibiotics are an important component of the HS treatment armamentarium. Administration of some intravenous antibiotics, including ertapenem,[25] require consultation with infectious disease colleagues to develop a collaborative management plan as well as to coordinate placement of vascular access lines for prolonged use. Concern for antibiotic resistance means that this treatment is typically reserved for more severe cases that have failed first-line treatments.

Obstetrics and Gynecology

Hormones affect HS; thus, many pregnant women with HS can experience improvement, no change, or worsening of the disease during pregnancy or in the post-partum period.[26,27] A recent single-institution study of 202 pregnancies revealed that 34.7% of pregnancies ($n = 70$) had worsened the severity of HS during pregnancy, 16.8% ($n = 34$) had no change, 4.5% ($n = 9$) had improvement, and 42.6% ($n = 86$) were unknown.[28] In addition, post-partum HS exacerbation was reported in 40.1% ($n = 81$) pregnancies. Treatment of HS during pregnancy also requires special attention to avoid the negative effects of some medications on the fetus that could cause birth defects. For instance, tetracyclines and retinoids are contraindicated during pregnancy due to the risk for teeth discoloration and fetal anomalies, respectively.[29–31] Thus, close collaboration between dermatology and obstetrics and gynecology (OB-GYN) is needed throughout pregnancy and in the post-partum period. In addition, OB-GYN physicians can aid in the early diagnosis of HS as well as the management of comorbid PCOS.

Pediatrics

HS can also be present in the pediatric population, and it has been suggested that HS in the pediatric population may be more severe than in the adult population.[32–34] Thus, early intervention and close collaboration between dermatology and pediatrics to avoid progression and scarring are warranted.

Pain Management

Pain is a major factor that negatively affects patient quality of life in those with HS. Management of acute and chronic pain are both important considerations, and collaboration with pain specialists is often necessary. One or a combination of topical and/or oral analgesics, anti-inflammatories, opiates, and anticonvulsants can be used. There are no HS-specific pain studies or recommendations, and treatment is based on pain guidelines, expert opinion, and patient preference.[35] Pain management is discussed further in Chapter 19.

Mental Health

Lastly, and perhaps most importantly, mental health in patients with HS should always be evaluated. HS is a chronic, painful, and often debilitating and disfiguring disease, and as such has a huge effect on patient quality of life and mental health. HS is associated with depression and anxiety,[36] and patients with HS also have a higher chance of committing suicide than those without HS.[37] Patients should be screened and be referred for psychology/psychiatry services to treat any depression, anxiety, and suicidal thoughts/behaviors. Psychosexual health should also be considered as those with HS are at a higher risk for sexual dysfunction when compared to those without HS.[38] Referral to a sex therapist who has experience treating patients with HS could be extremely helpful in select patients. Access to HS support groups such as Hope for HS (https://hopeforhs.org) or other chronic disease support groups also allows for a sense of community and the opportunity to express shared experiences and promote mental health. In fact, those participating in support groups have been reported to have lower levels of depression and anxiety as well as increased quality of life.[39,40] These support groups can also provide resources and recommendations for therapists and mental health experts for patients.

Conclusion

In conclusion, establishing a successful multidisciplinary clinic for the treatment of patients with HS is a multifaceted endeavor. A basic treatment algorithm can guide an initial treatment approach. Customizing the clinic to meet the needs of the patient is central. Quality improvement projects to help enhance the clinic should always be considered. And finally, close collaboration with colleagues in other specialties is crucial.

References

1. Collier EK, Hsiao JL, Shi VY, Naik HB. Comprehensive approach to managing hidradenitis suppurativa patients. *Inter J Dermatol.* 2020;59(6):744–747.
2. Timila Touhouche A, Chaput B, Marie Rouquet R, et al. Integrated multidisciplinary approach to Hidradenitis Suppurativa in clinical practice. *Inter J Women's Dermatol.* 2020;6(3):164–168.
3. Hendricks AJ, Hsiao JL, Lowes MA, Shi VY. A Comparison of International Management Guidelines for Hidradenitis Suppurativa. *Dermatol (Basel, Switzerland).* 2019;1–16.
4. Alikhan A, Sayed C, Alavi A, et al. North American clinical management guidelines for hidradenitis suppurativa: a publication from the United States and Canadian Hidradenitis Suppurativa Foundations: Part I: Diagnosis, evaluation, and the use of complementary and procedural management. *J Am Acad Dermatol.* 2019;81(1):76–90.
5. Gulliver W, Zouboulis CC, Prens E, et al. Evidence-based approach to the treatment of hidradenitis suppurativa/acne inversa, based on the European guidelines for hidradenitis suppurativa. *Rev Endocr Metab Disord.* 2016;17(3):343–351.
6. Hunger RE, Laffitte E, Läuchli S, et al. Swiss Practice Recommendations for the Management of Hidradenitis Suppurativa/Acne Inversa. *Dermatol (Basel, Switzerland).* 2017;233(2-3):113–119.
7. Smith MK, Nicholson CL, Parks-Miller A, Hamzavi IH. Hidradenitis suppurativa: an update on connecting the tracts. *F1000Research.* 2017;6:1272.
8. Vazquez BG, Alikhan A, Weaver AL, et al. Incidence of hidradenitis suppurativa and associated factors: a population-based study of Olmsted County, Minnesota. *J Invest Dermatol.* 2013;133(1):97–103.
9. Revuz JE, Canoui-Poitrine F, Wolkenstein P, et al. Prevalence and factors associated with hidradenitis suppurativa: results from two case-control studies. *J Am Acad Dermatol.* 2008;59(4):596–601.
10. Jemec GB, Kimball AB. Hidradenitis suppurativa: epidemiology and scope of the problem. *J Am Acad Dermatol.* 2015;73(5 Suppl 1):S4–S7.
11. Bui TL, Silva-Hirschberg C, Torres J, Armstrong AW. Hidradenitis suppurativa and diabetes mellitus: a systematic review and meta-analysis. *J Am Acad Dermatol.* 2018;78(2):395–402.
12. Garg A, Birabaharan M, Strunk A. Prevalence of type 2 diabetes mellitus among patients with hidradenitis suppurativa in the United States. *J Am Acad Dermatol.* 2018;79(1):71–76.
13. Shalom G, Freud T, Harman-Boehm I, et al. Hidradenitis suppurativa and metabolic syndrome: a comparative cross-sectional study of 3207 patients. *Br J Dermatol.* 2015;173(2):464–470.
14. Garg A, Neuren E, Strunk A. Hidradenitis Suppurativa Is Associated with Polycystic Ovary Syndrome: A Population-Based Analysis in the United States. *J Invest Dermatol.* 2018;138(6):1288–1292.
15. Danby FW. Diet in the prevention of hidradenitis suppurativa (acne inversa). *J Am Acad Dermatol.* 2015;73(5 Suppl 1):S52–S54.
16. Cannistra C, Finocchi V, Trivisonno A, Tambasco D. New perspectives in the treatment of hidradenitis suppurativa: surgery and brewer's yeast-exclusion diet. *Surgery.* 2013;154(5):1126–1130.
17. Canoui-Poitrine F, Revuz JE, Wolkenstein P, et al. Clinical characteristics of a series of 302 French patients with hidradenitis

suppurativa, with an analysis of factors associated with disease severity. *J Am Acad Dermatol.* 2009;61(1):51–57.

18. Kromann CB, Ibler KS, Kristiansen VB, Jemec GB. The influence of body weight on the prevalence and severity of hidradenitis suppurativa. *Acta Derm Venereol.* 2014;94(5):553–557.
19. Reddy S, Strunk A, Jemec GBE, Garg A. Incidence of Myocardial Infarction and Cerebrovascular Accident in Patients With Hidradenitis Suppurativa. *JAMA Dermatol.* 2019;1–7.
20. Sartorius K, Emtestam L, Jemec GB, Lapins J. Objective scoring of hidradenitis suppurativa reflecting the role of tobacco smoking and obesity. *Br J Dermatol.* 2009;161(4):831–839.
21. Schrader AM, Deckers IE, van der Zee HH, et al. Hidradenitis suppurativa: a retrospective study of 846 Dutch patients to identify factors associated with disease severity. *J Am Acad Dermatol.* 2014;71(3):460–467.
22. Fauconier M, Reguiai Z, Barbe C, et al. Association between hidradenitis suppurativa and spondyloarthritis. *Joint Bone Spine.* 2018;85(5):593–597.
23. Rondags A, Arends S, Wink FR, et al. High prevalence of hidradenitis suppurativa symptoms in axial spondyloarthritis patients: a possible new extra-articular manifestation. *Semin Arthritis Rheum.* 2019;48(4):611–617.
24. Chen WT, Chi CC. Association of Hidradenitis Suppurativa With Inflammatory Bowel Disease: A Systematic Review and Meta-analysis. *JAMA Dermatol.* 2019;155(9):1022–1027.
25. Join-Lambert O, Coignard-Biehler H, Jais JP, et al. Efficacy of ertapenem in severe hidradenitis suppurativa: a pilot study in a cohort of 30 consecutive patients. *J Antimicrob Chemother.* 2016;71(2):513–520.
26. Vossen AR, van Straalen KR, Prens EP, van der Zee HH. Menses and pregnancy affect symptoms in hidradenitis suppurativa: a cross-sectional study. *J Am Acad Dermatol.* 2017;76(1):155–156.
27. Kromann CB, Deckers IE, Esmann S, et al. Risk factors, clinical course and long-term prognosis in hidradenitis suppurativa: a cross-sectional study. *Br J Dermatol.* 2014;171(4):819–824.
28. Lyons AB, Peacock A, McKenzie SA, et al. Hidradenitis Suppurativa and Pregnancy: A Retrospective Review. In: *4th Annual Symposium on Hidradenitis Suppurativa Advances, Detroit, MI*; 2019.
29. Vennila V, Madhu V, Rajesh R, et al. Tetracycline-induced discoloration of deciduous teeth: case series. *J Int Oral Health.* 2014;6(3):115–119.
30. Lipson AH, Collins F, Webster WS. Multiple congenital defects associated with maternal use of topical tretinoin. *Lancet (London, England).* 1993;341(8856):1352–1353.
31. Centers for Disease Control and Prevention (CDC). Accutane-exposed pregnancies—California, 1999. *MMWR Morb Mortal Wkly Rep.* 2000;49(2):28–31.
32. Liy-Wong C, Pope E, Lara-Corrales I. Hidradenitis suppurativa in the pediatric population. *J Am Acad Dermatol.* 2015;73(5 Suppl 1):S36–S41.
33. Deckers IE, van der Zee HH, Boer J, Prens EP. Correlation of early-onset hidradenitis suppurativa with stronger genetic susceptibility and more widespread involvement. *J Am Acad Dermatol.* 2015;72(3):485–488.
34. Palmer RA, Keefe M. Early-onset hidradenitis suppurativa. *Clin Exp Dermatol.* 2001;26(6):501–503.
35. Smith HS, Chao JD, Teitelbaum J. Painful hidradenitis suppurativa. *Clin J Pain.* 2010;26(5):435–444.
36. Shavit E, Dreiher J, Freud T, et al. Psychiatric comorbidities in 3207 patients with hidradenitis suppurativa. *J Eur Acad Dermatol Venereol.* 2015;29(2):371–376.
37. Patel KR, Lee HH, Rastogi S, et al. Association between hidradenitis suppurativa, depression, anxiety, and suicidality: a systematic review and meta-analysis. *J Am Acad Dermatol.* 2019.
38. Slyper M, Strunk A, Garg A. Incidence of sexual dysfunction among patients with hidradenitis suppurativa: a population-based retrospective analysis. *Br J Dermatol.* 2018;179(2):502–503.
39. Wakefield JR, Bickley S, Sani F. The effects of identification with a support group on the mental health of people with multiple sclerosis. *J Psychosom Res.* 2013;74(5):420–426.
40. Geramita EM, Herbeck Belnap B, Abebe KZ, et al. The Association Between Increased Levels of Patient Engagement With an Internet Support Group and Improved Mental Health Outcomes at 6-Month Follow-Up: Post-Hoc Analyses From a Randomized Controlled Trial. *J Med Inter Res.* 2018;20(7): e10402.

33

Support Groups in Hidradenitis Suppurativa—Building a Community

SANDRA GUILBAULT, ALEXIS B. LYONS, AND ANGIE PARKS-MILLER

Introduction

Support groups are an invaluable tool to help individuals cope with a multitude of diseases, conditions, and phases in life. They are beneficial to patients as well as to family members and caregivers. Support groups can be in-person with scheduled meeting times for members to attend or online in the form of social media without time or geographic constraints. For a disease like hidradenitis suppurativa (HS) that impacts so many facets of an individual's life such as physical functioning, mental health, sexual health, and ability to work, support groups can offer individuals community support for what is otherwise an often isolating disease.

In this chapter, we offer guidance on setting up a support group from the perspective and experiences of Hope for HS (hopeforhs. org), a grassroots, 501c3 non-profit patient advocacy and support organization for the HS community. At face value, an HS support group requires only a time, a place, and a little effort to spread the word. The support group founder can reserve a suitable conference room and inform the surrounding patient community of the event via mail, online health system messages, posters, or flyers placed in a clinic exam or waiting rooms. The creation of a support group to meet the needs of the HS community is also an opportunity to repair trust in a patient population that has historically had their needs go unrecognized and been offered few treatment options. Thus, ensuring adequate time, resources, and level of commitment should be given due consideration before one decides to create a support group.

How to Get Started

The experience of creating a support group can be both rewarding and challenging at times. Support groups offer those who suffer from HS the empowerment to work on and solve problems in a constructive and validating way. They enrich the community of people undergoing the same issues. The Hope for HS support group platform encourages partnership with the medical community. This important partnership allows for honest and productive exchanges between patients and medical providers outside the context of a clinical visit without the same time constraints. The following are suggested steps to building a good foundation for your support group from the start (Fig. 33.1).

1. Select your core team members.

    A representative from the medical and from the patient communities is recommended.

- **Chapter Director**: Patient or Medical Community Member
- **Chapter Medical Director**: Attending Physician
- **Medical Lead:** Resident/Fellow/Medical Student
- **Patient Lead(s):** Trusted, dependable, motivated patient or caregiver

    You may also wish to enlist the help of support staff.

    When selecting any of the pillars of your support group team, there are a few questions you may want to pose before acceptance of the role:

- Do you have the time necessary to plan and publicize the meetings, coordinate special events, and talk with individual members who contact the support group with issues?
- Are you committed to attending the meetings, even if you are having a bad day?
- Do you feel comfortable in front of a group?
- Are you able to be assertive enough (in a kind way) to keep the meeting on track?
- Do you maintain a positive, encouraging, and hopeful attitude?
- Are you a good listener?

Initial Steps

Hope for HS

MEDICAL DIRECTOR/LEAD
- knowledgable & compassionate
- has HS patients - does not need to be dermatologist
- can provide meeting space

CHAPTER DIRECTOR
- handles logistics - secure meeting space, confirm speaker, collect RSVPs
- communicate with Hope for HS organization

SELECT DATE AND LOCATION
- 3-6 months lead time to receive materials and generate interest
- conference room or lobby is fine
- familiar spaces enjoy a better turn out

• **Fig. 33.1** Suggested Initial Steps to Form a Support Group.

2. Select a meeting location.
3. Select meeting frequency. Every other month meetings during the evening are recommended.
4. Select a target date. It is recommended to give 3 to 6 months lead time.
5. Find interested persons. You can start by targeting patients in the chapter Medical Director's clinic, but remember that only a percentage will attend. Casting a wide net will reach more potential participants.
6. Select meeting topic(s). Examples of initial meeting topics include Current HS Treatments, Knowledge Gaps, Addressing Mental Health.
7. Advertise. Create a support group information flyer that can be disseminated to patients via mail or email, passed out in clinics, and posted in the chapter Medical Director's clinic.
8. Create an intake questionnaire. This questionnaire can help you understand the needs of your respective HS community, which may vary geographically, and may be given to any newly attending support group member. Questions may be directed at seeking feedback on topics of interest, ideas for advocacy and awareness, and suggestions for support group organization growth.

Participant Interactions

Physician to Patient

Physician presence at each support group meeting allows patients to learn accurate information about their condition. Trust in the medical community that may have been eroded over years of disease progression and lack of treatment options can begin to be rebuilt by sharing optimistic news of research opportunities and the development of new treatment options. General questions may be answered for a group, away from the time constraints of individual appointments in a clinical setting (Fig. 33.2).

Meeting Format

Hope for HS

90 minute format

Welcome - 15 minutes
Presentation/Discussion topic – 15-30 mins
Question & Answer and open discussion
Flexibility is important
Meetings tend to naturally evolve
Medical lead always present

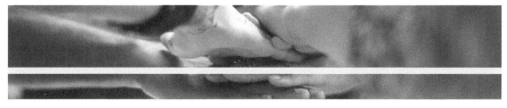

• **Fig. 33.2** Suggested Meeting Format.

TABLE 33.1 Topics of Concern in the Hidradenitis Suppurativa Community Can Be Utilized as Ice Breaker Questions

Topics	Questions
Pain Management	• How do you feel the medical community views HS pain? • How would you improve pain management for HS? • What tips could you offer to someone struggling with pain management?
Wound Care	• What information on wound care would you like to see from a medical provider? • What have you found to be most and/or least helpful to you in caring for your HS wounds? • How would you improve wound care for HS?
Access to Care	• Are you able to obtain coverage for your HS treatments? • Do you find it difficult to get an appointment for HS care when needed? • How would you improve reimbursement and insurance issues for HS?

HS, Hidradenitis suppurativa.

Patient to Physician

Patients provide insight into their daily lives with this condition to the participating medical professionals. Discussing negative experiences and unmet needs may illuminate opportunities to improve patient care. Personal observations, improvement or worsening from exposure to specific products, or lifestyle management may be considered for clinical use or future research.

Patient to Patient

Through connections with other HS patients, individuals are empowered to share stories, discuss first-hand treatment experiences, provide peer-to-peer support, and reduce the tremendous isolation that often accompanies a diagnosis of HS. Treatment success stories are especially meaningful to individuals with HS, caregivers, and the community support system.

Ice Breakers

Preparation of ice breaker questions may help facilitate group discussions. Even seasoned attendees of support groups may find it difficult to communicate at times (Table 33.1).

Use of Social Media in Support Groups

Clinicians may consider using social media to provide support for their patients, either on its own or as a supplement to in-person or virtual meetings. Social media allows for patients and caregivers to connect to peers at any time of day, regardless of location. This presents a potential opportunity for support group facilitators to reach HS patients outside of their own practices and institutions to provide accurate disease information, spread the word about their support group meetings, or recruit for ongoing research efforts. Managing a social media-based support requires time and effort

as well. Even after the initial effort of support group creation, a substantial time commitment must be made to screen or recruit members, maintain patient privacy, answer questions, and moderate discussions.

Informal peer support for HS can be found on numerous social media platforms, from hashtags on Twitter and Instagram to subreddits on Reddit and public pages and private groups on Facebook. Thus, these platforms are already being used to successfully raise awareness and provide peer support. Social media may be the first place that some patients feel comfortable discussing the devastating impacts of living with HS given the relative anonymity of the virtual setting. Clinicians may also consider recommending established social media groups to provide peer support for their patients rather than creating their own. However, these groups should not be recommended without thorough vetting.

Many of these online support groups have thousands of members; however, there are some potential limitations to be discussed. These groups may not be representative of the general HS population; for example, social media groups may attract more severe cases because patients that are well-controlled may not seek out support. Failed medical interventions for recalcitrant cases and poor experiences with individual doctors can create an unintended breeding ground for anti-medicine perspectives to flourish. Difficulty finding trustworthy disease information online could lead to sharing of misinformation. Desperation for relief may lead to discussions about potentially dangerous self-experimentation and self-management.

Despite this, the sheer number of members in these existing support groups, and the supportive peer connections that have formed within them, has led to many patients feeling empowered to be open about their diagnosis with their family, friends, and wider social media network. The HS community owes a tremendous debt to the people affected by HS who are using social media to raise awareness and support their peers.

Finally, although online support is a valuable resource, there is still no substitute for human interaction, especially in the case of a disease that requires vulnerability, trust, and respect for privacy from all group members. Therefore, it is recommended to carefully weigh options in consideration of creating or recommending an in-person or a social media-based support system and make a decision that best suits you and those you aim to serve.

Attendance

The physical and emotional toll of HS can certainly affect the ability of community members to attend in-person support groups. The inclusion of a remote access option can be helpful, along with choosing an optimal meeting frequency and promoting support system involvement.

Hope for HS encourages meetings to be an open forum. A loose agenda is recommended to keep the meeting on track, but diversions should be expected and prepared for, particularly as new members experience their first session. Many new attendees are encountering others with HS for the first time. Some become emotional, some are reserved, and some are elated to be at a support group designated for HS. Frequently, new attendees will want to share their experiences at length. The Medical Lead and Patient Lead should provide gentle direction to prevent a member from monopolizing meeting time; however, it is encouraged to allow new members to share, vent, and discuss their struggles.

Mental Health

Due to the deep emotional and quality of life-impacting nature of HS, occasionally, one may encounter a very depressed support group member. Such a person may make active or passive comments or threats about suicidal ideation that must be taken seriously. Before conducting a support group, it is crucial to have a plan in place for these situations. Resources, such as names for mental health referrals and a suicide hotline, should be readily available. One should familiarize oneself with institutional guidelines on suicidal ideation and follow them.

HS has been reported to have the worst quality of life scores when compared to other skin diseases. A study comparing HS to psoriasis found that the quality of life measured by the Skindex-17 questionnaire found that the mean symptom scores were 69.4 versus 53.7, respectively.[1] The same study found the mean psychosocial scores were 56.1 for HS versus 32.7 for psoriasis. Other studies have reported similar results with worse quality of life for patients with HS compared to other debilitating skin conditions including psoriasis, atopic dermatitis, chronic urticaria, and neurofibromatosis.[2] In addition, there is a high incidence of depression and anxiety in patients with HS.[3] This underscores the importance of having a good support system for HS patients, and support groups can help in this role. A more detailed discussion about the impact of HS on the quality of life can be found in Chapter 21.

The health and emotional benefits on the quality of life of both in-person and online support groups for chronic diseases have previously been reported.[4-6] In a recent survey study of 165 patients with HS, 77% reported participating in a support group, and of those who participated, 89% were in the form of online support groups. Those who participated in a support group had increases in resilience scores at 6 months.[7]

Community Perception and Transparency

Patient Advocacy Organizations (PAO) are critical partners for industry and other stakeholders. Partnerships with industry can provide much-needed funding to improve disease awareness, access to additional resources, and provide a seat at the table for key discussions surrounding research, drug development, and other important community interests and concerns.

Hope for HS is a grassroots organization that is run by volunteers and supported by voluntary donations. This organizational structure has allowed for growth of the organization while monitoring for any HS community concerns regarding bias. However, the lack of industry funding or sponsors is also a hindrance at times when resources are needed to accomplish organizational goals. Thus, it is important for organizations to be in touch with their members and the HS community to move forward with increasing diversity of funding sources or incorporating sponsorships when it is the right time to do so. Balance and transparency are key to maintaining trust.

A recent systematic review and meta-analysis of patient and health organizations[8] revealed that 20% to 83% of organizational funding is derived from industry, with most lacking policies on disclosures of conflicts of interest. Additionally, this review reported industry-funded groups generally supported sponsor interests. Thus, ensuring a PAO has a solid conflict of interest and disclosure policy and considering diversity in sponsorships are important.

Participant Perspectives

Hidradenitis Suppurativa Provider Perspective

Attending support group meetings as a provider is an invaluable experience. It allows for the opportunity to hear the patient perspective of the disease without the time constraints of a clinic visit. It also provides the opportunity to build and strengthen bonds between providers and patients and to disseminate new clinical and research updates regarding the disease. Providers are afforded the opportunity to gain a deeper insight into the disease than what would otherwise be possible.

Teaching physicians and other providers to effectively empathize with patients is critical during their training. Studies have shown that medical students and residents who have attended support group meetings develop improved attitudes and empathy toward patients.[9,10] Trainees report that attending support group meetings are educationally valuable experiences.[9] They also have had more confidence in referring patients to support groups after having attended a meeting themselves.[10]

Hidradenitis Suppurativa Community Perspectives

Being a part of the HS community means having a safe place to express and address the unique challenges that this disease presents. Because HS still carries misconception and stigma, patients like me really need safe places to discuss our needs without judgment or shame. The in-person support groups are my absolute favorite. At first, I had no idea that meeting other patients would be so empowering but now I understand why. The support groups help eliminate the isolation factor and teach patients how to vocalize their needs. In these meetings, we acknowledge, validate, and support each other in ways that really no one else can. Being an advocate in this community has empowered me so much. Contributing to a dialogue that spreads awareness helps other patients and teaches medical professionals about this disease is work that feeds my soul and helps me to overcome the trauma I have endured. As this work has done so much for me, it is my hope that other patients find the same comfort and strength in this community. There is much to be done and we need every single story and every single voice to accomplish our goal of effective, stigma free treatment.

ATHENA GIERBOLINI

As an HS patient, caregiver, speaker, advocate, and supporter, I have seen HS from many different angles. I have also seen the effects it has on not only the patient but on the patient's family and caregivers, work and social life, and on one's physical, mental and emotional health. For me, the importance of my involvement means that I can push for better care, information, and access for HS sufferers. It also means that I can call for an increase in research, development, and knowledge, all the while passing on hope to thousands of HS patients, standing up and presenting a face of HS to the medical and research community as a whole. The road is not easy, but the opportunity to make such a difference for HS sufferers, for myself, and ever so importantly, for my daughter, make every step forward, and even those sideways and sometimes backward, an unparalleled privilege. While my dream is for a cure, my hope is for better days, less pain and more dignity.

CHRISTINE YANNUZZI

Conclusion

The value of having a support group as a tool for the management of patients with HS cannot be overstated. Support groups provide a sense of community and camaraderie for patients, promote mental health, and allow providers the opportunity to connect with their patients on a deeper level which is not always possible in a busy clinical setting. They allow for the dissemination of information as well as provide a forum for open discussion. Whether in-person or online, support groups provide the opportunity for collaboration and advocacy between individuals with HS, the medical community, pharmaceutical companies, and government agencies. Participating in support groups can benefit patients, family members, and caregivers as well as providers and should be recommended to HS patients to help expand their support network and decrease the isolation of this oftentimes debilitating illness.

References

1. Sampogna F, Fania L, Mazzanti C, et al. The Broad-Spectrum Impact of Hidradenitis Suppurativa on Quality of Life: A Comparison with Psoriasis. *Dermatology (Basel, Switzerland).* 2019;235(4):308–314.
2. Wolkenstein P, Loundou A, Barrau K, et al. Quality of life impairment in hidradenitis suppurativa: a study of 61 cases. *J Am Acad Dermatol.* 2007;56(4):621–623.
3. Patel KR, Lee HH, Rastogi S, et al. Association between hidradenitis suppurativa, depression, anxiety, and suicidality: a systematic review and meta-analysis. *J Am Acad Dermatol.* 2020;83(3):737–744.
4. Han JY, Shah DV, Kim E, et al. Empathic exchanges in online cancer support groups: distinguishing message expression and reception effects. *Health Commun.* 2011;26(2):185–197.
5. Kim E, Han JY, Moon TJ, et al. The process and effect of supportive message expression and reception in online breast cancer support groups. *Psychooncology.* 2012;21(5):531–540.
6. Yoo W, Namkoong K, Choi M, et al. Giving and Receiving Emotional Support Online: Communication Competence as a Moderator of Psychosocial Benefits for Women with Breast Cancer. *Comput Human Behav.* 2014;30:13–22.
7. Butt M, Cotton C, Kirby JS. Support group utilization and impact for patients with hidradenitis suppurativa. *J Am Acad Dermatol.* 2020;83(1):216–219.
8. Alice F, Lisa P, Cinzia C, et al. Industry funding of patient and health consumer organisations: systematic review with meta-analysis. *BMJ.* 2020;368:l6925.
9. Kastenholz KJ, Agarwal G. A Qualitative Analysis of Medical Students' Reflection on Attending an Alcoholics Anonymous Meeting: Insights for Future Addiction Curricula. *Acad Psychiatry.* 2016;40(3):468–474.
10. Kennedy AJ, McNeil M, Hamm M, et al. Internal Medicine Resident Perceptions of Patients with Substance Use Disorder After Attending a Mutual Support Group Meeting. *J Gen Intern Med.* 2020;35(3):918–921.

34

Pipeline Therapeutics

ROB LELAND SHAVER, MICHELLE A. LOWES, AND NOAH GOLDFARB

CHAPTER OUTLINE

Introduction

Since early 2000, there has been a dramatic increase in the number of publications and clinical trials devoted to moderate to severe hidradenitis suppurativa (HS).[1] HS is a complex disease process in which a complete mechanism is still unknown. Recent data on pathogenesis are presented in earlier chapters, and a currently proposed model is presented in Fig. 34.1. Drugs currently in the therapeutic pipeline target a broad range of inflammatory pathways that may be important in the pathogenesis of HS.

This chapter summarizes the drugs, procedures, and complementary and alternative medicine (CAM) modalities currently in clinical trials for HS. Outcome measures for HS clinical trials have been presented in Chapter 13. Table 34.1 lists drug trials for HS registered at www.clinicaltrials.gov as of January 1, 2020, which are active, recruiting, not yet recruiting, or recently completed but results are unpublished. Potential therapeutic targets currently being studied in drug clinical trials include neutrophils, the complement pathway, inflammatory cytokine signaling pathways such as interleukin (IL)-17, IL-23, and IL-1α/β, as well as the Janus kinase (JAK)-signal transducer and activator of transcription (STAT) signaling pathway. Fig. 34.1 illustrates where these agents may act in the pathogenic pathway of HS. Surgical, procedural, CAM treatments, and wound care approaches currently under investigation and registered as of the same date are listed in Table 34.2.

Neutrophils and Complement

Hair follicle content exposed to the dermis, due to follicular occlusion and subsequent rupture, provokes a robust neutrophilic infiltration via inflammatory cytokines (e.g., IL-8), lipid signaling (e.g., leukotriene B4 [LTB4]), and complement activation (e.g., C3a, C5a).[2] These chemoattractants, as well as others, bind to over 30 chemokine, selectin, and integrin receptors on the neutrophil's surface. Neutrophils have been implicated in the pathogenesis of

HS due to the large number of neutrophils seen in early lesions and several case reports and series suggesting efficacy for anti-neutrophil agents, such as dapsone and colchicine, in HS.[3-5]

Primed neutrophils produce reactive oxygen species (ROS); secrete granules containing antimicrobial peptides (AMPs), alarmins, and proteases; and release neutrophil extracellular traps (NETs).[6] These result in tissue damage as well as recruitment and activation of macrophages, that produce pro-inflammatory cytokines, such as IL-1α/β, TNF-α, and granulocyte-colony stimulating factor (G-CSF), recruiting more neutrophils.[6] In vitro, stimulated neutrophils from HS patients secrete higher levels of ROS compared to healthy controls and produce NETs, even without stimulation.[7,8] In HS lesional tissue, NETs have been detected that correlate with disease activity.[8]

Currently, researchers are investigating two novel drugs that target neutrophil recruitment in HS. CSL324 is a fully human G-CSF receptor monoclonal antibody.[9] The G-CSF receptor signals via the JAK1/STAT3 signaling pathway. It regulates mobilization of neutrophils from the bone marrow into the peripheral circulation as well as neutrophil recruitment to tissues via changes to cellular adhesion and chemokine receptors on the neutrophil surface.[6] In animal models, G-CSF receptor inhibition reduces neutrophilic inflammation without causing neutropenia or reducing neutrophil function.[10] CSL324 is currently in its first-in-human study, a phase I, open-label, two-dose regimen trial in patients with HS and palmoplantar pustulosis.

LYS006, an inhibitor of LTA4 hydrolase,[9] is currently being studied for acne, Crohn's disease, and non-alcoholic fatty liver disease (NAFLD), in addition to HS. LTA4 hydrolase catalyzes the rate-limiting step in converting LTA4 into LTB4, a potent neutrophil chemotactic agent.[11] LTB4 has been shown to be critical for the recruitment and clustering of neutrophils into localized collections (abscess).[12] LTB4 and LTB4-induced pathways in HS have been found to be increased in lesional skin, suggesting that this lipid pathway could be an important target for HS

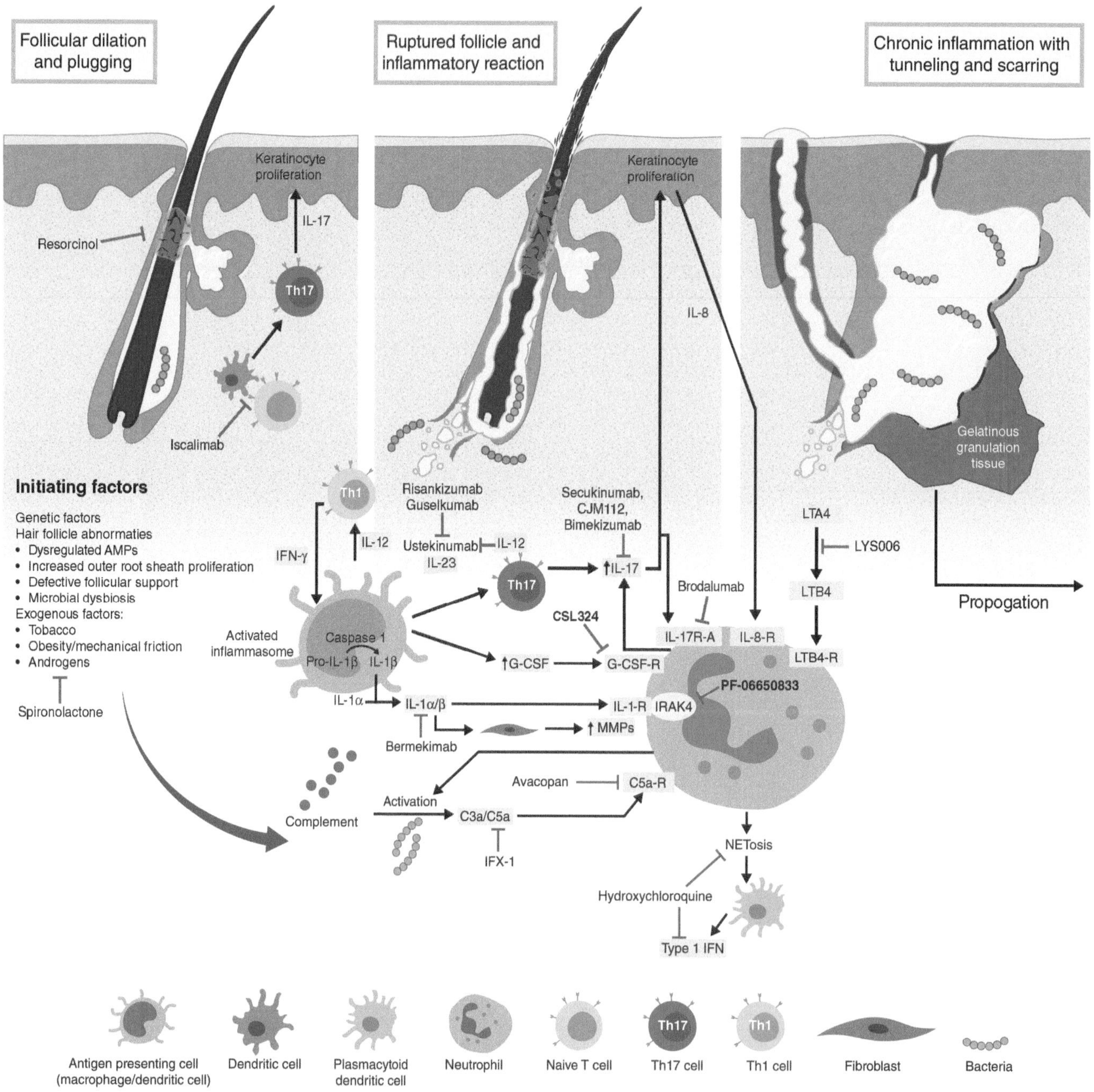

• **Fig. 34.1** Proposed Model of Hidradenitis Suppurativa (HS) Pathogenesis With Therapeutic Targets Currently in Clinical Trials. HS pathogenic pathway based on Vossen et al.[92] Drugs currently in the therapeutic pipeline target a broad range of inflammatory pathways that may be important in the pathogenesis of HS. Red bars indicate where these agents may act in the HS pathogenic pathway. *AMP,* Antimicrobial peptide; *G-CSF,* granulocyte-colony stimulating factor; *HBD,* human beta defensin; *IFN,* interferon; *IL,* interleukin; *LT,* leukotriene; *R,* receptor.

treatment.[13] A three-arm randomized controlled trial studying LYS006 vs. iscalimab (CFZ533, anti-CD40) vs. placebo is presently recruiting.

Activated neutrophils are able to initiate the complement alternative pathway on their cell surfaces. Anaerobic bacteria, such as *Porphyromonas* spp. can also cleave and activate complement.[14,15] The resulting complement fragments, including C3a and C5a, are strong chemoattractants for both neutrophils and macrophages. C5a has also been shown to induce NET release in activated

neutrophils and prime monocytes to produce TNF-α and IL-6.[16] In HS, the complement pathway may be an important contributor to the heightened neutrophilic inflammatory response. With increased levels of C5a found in both tissue and plasma of HS patients, C5a and its receptor have become therapeutic targets for HS treatment.[17]

IFX-1 is a monoclonal IgG4 kappa antibody against human C5a. Selective C5a inhibition leaves the membrane attack complex (MAC) intact, minimizing immunosuppression, especially for

TABLE 34.1 Drugs currently in clinical trials for Hidradenitis Suppurativa

Sections	Drug name	Target(s)	Structure	Sponsor	Trial number	Phase	Status
Complement/Neutrophils	CSL324	G-CSF receptor	Monoclonal antibody	CSL Behring	NCT03972280	I	Recruiting
	LYS006	LTA4 hydrolase	Small molecule	Novaritis Pharmaceuticals	NCT03827798	II	Recruiting
	IFX-1	C5a	Monoclonal antibody	InflaRx GmbH	NCT03487276	II	Completed
	Avacopan	C5a receptor	Small molecule	ChemoCentryx	NCT03852472	II	Recruiting
TNF-α	Adalimumab	TNF-α	Monoclonal antibody	Wake Forest University Health Sciences	NCT04132388	IV	Not yet recruiting
IL-17	Secukinumab	IL-17A	Monoclonal antibody	Novartis Pharmaceuticals	NCT03713632 / NCT03713619 / NCT04179175	III / III / III	Recruiting / Recruiting / Recruiting
	CJM112	IL-17A/F	Monoclonal antibody	Novartis Pharmaceuticals	NCT02421172	II	Completed
	Bimekizumab (vs adalimumab/placebo)	IL-17A/F	Monoclonal antibody	UCB Biopharma	NCT03248531	II	Completed
	Brodalumab	IL-17 receptor A	Monoclonal antibody	Florida Academic Dermatology Centers	NCT03910803	II	Not yet recruiting
IL-23	Risankizumab	IL-23p19	Monoclonal antibody	AbbVie	NCT03926169	II	Recruiting
	Guselkumab	IL-23p19	Monoclonal antibody	Rockefeller University University Medical Center Groningen	NCT04084665	I	Not yet recruiting
					NCT04061395	II	Not yet recruiting
				Janssen Research & Development	NCT03628924	II	Active, not recruiting
IL-1	Bermekimab (MABp1)	IL-1α	Monoclonal antibody	XBiotech, Inc.	NCT04019041	II	Recruiting
	PF-06650833	IRAK4	Small molecule	Pfizer	NCT04092452	II	Recruiting
JAK/STAT	PF-06700841	JAK1/TYK2	Small molecule	Pfizer	NCT04092452	II	Recruiting
	PF-06826647	TYK2	Small molecule	Pfizer	NCT04092452	II	Recruiting
	INCB054707	JAK1	Small molecule	Incyte Corporation	NCT03569371 / NCT03607487	II / II	Completed / Recruiting
Other Medications	Hydroxychloroquine	Multiple	Quinolone	University of Pittsburgh	NCT03275870	I/II	Completed
	Spironolactone	Androgens	Steroid	Medical University of South Carolina	NCT04100083	IV	Not yet recruiting
	Iscalimab (CFZ533)	CD40	Monoclonal antibody	Novartis Pharmaceuticals	NCT03827798	II	Recruiting
	15% Topical Resorcinol	Keratin	Benzenediol FIZEVI	FIZEVI, Fundación Pública Andaluza para la gestión de la Investigación en Sevilla;	NCT04099212	II	Recruiting

Clinical studies registered with clinicaltrials.gov as of January 1, 2020.

CD, Cluster of differentiation; *G-CSF*, granulocyte-colony stimulating factor; *IL*, interleukin; *JAK*, Janus kinase; *LTA*, leukotriene A; *IRAK*, interleukin-1 receptor-associated kinase; *TLR*, toll-like receptor; *TYK*, tyrosine kinase.

TABLE 34.2 Surgical, procedural, complementary, and alternative medicine (CAM) treatments currently under investigation for Hidradenitis Suppurativa

Sections	Drug name	Sponsor	Trial number	Status
Surgery/Procedures	Sclerotherapy	Beth Israel Deaconess Medical Center	NCT02805595	Recruiting
	Alexandrite Laser	Wayne State University	NCT03054155	Recruiting
	Radiotherapy	Montefiore Medical Center	NCT03040804	Recruiting
	Adalimumab Peri-surgically (SHARPS)	Abbvie	NCT02808975	Completed
	Adalimumab vs. Adalimumab/Surgery	Erasmus Medical Center	NCT03221621	Recruiting
	Axillary Perforator Flap vs. Secondary Intention Wound Healing	Assistance Publique - Hôpitaux de Paris	NCT03784313	Not yet recruiting
	Negative pressure therapy	Royal Free Hospital NHS Foundation Trust	NCT04325607	Recruiting
Wound Care	Methylene blue, gentian violet, and bovine forestomach	Wake Forest University Health Sciences	NCT04354012	Not yet recruiting
	Multiple Cutimed® dressings	University of Miami	NCT04194541	Recruiting
CAM	Cannabis oil	TO Pharmaceuticals	NCT03929835	Not yet recruiting
	Battlefield Acupuncture	Wayne State University	NCT04218422	Recruiting

Clinical studies registered with clinicaltrials.gov as of January 1, 2020.

encapsulated organisms.[18,19] An early open-label study of IFX-1 indicated an 83% treatment response rate after three months in patients with severe HS.[19] A phase IIb clinical trial for IFX-1 in HS patients was recently completed and the results were released in two press releases.[20,21] Unfortunately, IFX-1 failed to meet its primary end point (a statistically significant dose-dependent improvement in HS Clinical Response [HiSCR] over placebo), although there was a significant improvement in the DLQI. Secondary endpoint and post-hoc analysis demonstrated significant reductions in draining fistulas and IHS4 score in the high-dose IFX-1 group compared to controls.[20] The company has indicated that it plans to continue to develop IFX-1 as a treatment for HS, and an open-label extension study is continuing. Avacopan, an orally available small-molecule C5a receptor antagonist with demonstrated efficacy in ANCA-associated vasculitis, is now undergoing a Phase II clinical trial in moderate to severe HS patients.[22]

Cytokines

There are numerous cytokines that have been implicated in the pathogenesis of HS. To date, the inhibition of TNF-α has been the mainstay of medical treatment. Currently, the only United States Federal Drug Administration (FDA) approved medication for HS is adalimumab, a fully human, IgG1 monoclonal antibody targeting TNF-α. Unfortunately, only 40% to 60% of patients achieve HiSCR, and of those that achieve HiSCR, some lose their response over time.[23] Data from studies on inflammatory bowel disease suggest that secondary loss of response is either due to mechanistic failure or low drug concentrations, with or without the development of anti-drug antibodies.[24] Poor adherence to therapy has been associated with secondary loss of response due to low drug concentrations and increased immunogenicity.[25,26] A phase IV randomized trial is planning to evaluate the practical administration

of adalimumab for HS, specifically whether a novel electronic medication monitoring device compared with usual care can improve clinical outcomes and adherence compared with usual care. In addition to issues related to adherence and loss of response to TNF-α inhibitors, many patients are not able to tolerate or never respond to TNF-α inhibition initially. Thus, researchers have started investigating new cytokine targets, such as interleukin (IL)-17, IL-23, and IL-1α/β. The following section highlights each cytokine, its association with HS, and preliminary results from clinical studies. Clinical trials data of adalimumab are further discussed in Chapter 18.

IL-17

The family of interleukin-17 (IL-17) cytokines (IL-17A-F) signal through multiple IL-17 receptors formed from six unique IL-17 receptor subunits that exist as homodimers or heterodimers. While not critical for differentiation, IL-23 plays an important role in sustaining T_H17 differentiation and promoting IL-17 and IL-22 production.[27] In addition, IL-17A and IL-17F act synergistically with IL-1 and TNF-α to augment and perpetuate the inflammatory cascade triggered by these pro-inflammatory cytokines.[28] IL-17A activates keratinocyte proliferation and produces AMPs and numerous neutrophil-attracting chemokines, including IL-8 (also referred to as CXCL8).[27] IL-17F has similar functions biologically as IL-17A, signaling through the same receptor and forming a heterodimeric complex with IL-17A.[28] Multiple studies have demonstrated significantly increased IL-17 levels in HS lesions and perilesional tissue, compared to control skin.[29] The elevated levels of IL-17 in perilesional tissue may suggest an early role in HS pathogenesis.[29] In addition, IL-17 has also been found to be elevated in the serum of HS patients, which correlates with disease activity.[30]

Secukinumab is a human IgG1 monoclonal antibody that binds IL-17A, preventing its interaction with the IL-17 receptor.

Initially, several case reports were published demonstrating benefit to HS patients.[31] However, an in vitro study using HS skin lesions showed that secukinumab did not significantly lower overall cytokine (TNF-α, IFN-γ, IL-1β, IL-6, and IL-17A) levels compared with prednisolone, TNF-α inhibitors, or ustekinumab.[32] More recently, there has been increased enthusiasm for this approach after three open-label 16- to 24-week prospective studies for moderate to severe HS demonstrated benefit, with 67% to 75% achieving HiSCR.[33-35] Two core phase III multicenter, randomized, double-blinded placebo-controlled studies with two secukinumab dose regimens (300 mg every 2 or 4 weeks) are currently underway for moderate to severe HS. A randomized withdrawal extension study for the two core trials is already recruiting. The goal of the study is to assess the long-term maintenance of HiSCR out to week 104. Those participants that achieve HiSCR by week 52 of the two core studies will be randomized (2:1) to continue their regimen or placebo until week 104 to evaluate the loss of response. Those participants that either did not achieve HiSCR by week 52 in the core studies or lose response in the extension trial or complete the 104-week extension trial maintaining HiSCR will be offered to enroll in the open-label treatment study to week 260.

CJM112 is a fully human IgG1 monoclonal dual anti-IL-17A and anti-IL-17F antibody. It has higher potency compared with secukinumab, achieving similar results for psoriasis, but at significantly lower doses.[36] In addition, in vitro studies have demonstrated that dual IL-17A/F inhibition significantly lowers inflammatory mediators more than either IL-17A or IL-17-F alone.[28] Recently, a phase II randomized placebo-controlled trial for HS showed 32% (10/32) participants had a two-point drop in HS physician global assessment (HS-PGA) score, compared to only 12.5% (4/32) in the placebo group.[36]

Bimekizumab is also a human IgG1 monoclonal dual anti-IL-17A/F antibody. Phase II proof-of-concept and dose-ranging studies have already shown significant improvements in both plaque psoriasis and psoriatic arthritis at higher doses compared to controls.[37] A phase II randomized, double blind trial comparing two different doses of bimekizumab against adalimumab and placebo was recently completed. Results from this study have not been released, but two phase III randomized, placebo-controlled trials are currently being planned.

Brodalumab is a human monoclonal IgG2 antibody that binds with high affinity to the IL-17 receptor A, competitively inhibiting IL-17A, C, E, and F.[38] As the responses to direct IL-17A inhibition with secukinumab can take up to 12 to 24 weeks for HS,[33-35] the faster response rates seen for brodalumab in psoriasis makes it an attractive potential treatment for HS. Initially, a case report of brodalumab for HS showed rapid improvement in draining tunnels, global assessment, and quality of life over 12 weeks.[39] More recently, results from an open-label early Phase I study of 10 participants with moderate to severe HS showed that using the FDA-approved dose for psoriasis resulted in all 10 participants achieving HiSCR by 12 weeks.[40] Although there is a black box warning for suicidal ideation and behavior for brodalumab, no episodes of self-harm or suicidality were experienced by HS patients in this small study.[40]

IL-12/23

Interleukin-12 (IL-12) and interleukin-23 (IL-23) are cytokines secreted by macrophages and dendritic cells in response to wound healing and infection.[41] While IL-12 promotes T_H1 cell differentiation of naïve CD4 T cells, IL-23 contributes to the IL-17

producing T helper (T_H17) cell response. Both cytokines are highly expressed by infiltrating macrophages in lesional HS skin, and share a p40 subunit.[42] IL-12 is a heterodimer composed of the IL-12p40 and IL-12p35 subunits which signal through the IL-12 receptor.[41] IL-23 is a heterodimer composed of the IL-12p40 and IL-23p19 subunits that bind to the IL-23 receptor and signal through the JAK/STAT pathway.[41] IL-23 has become a therapeutic target for both HS, psoriasis, and Crohn's disease, three conditions with mechanistic as well as clinical overlap.[43,44] Ustekinumab, an IL-12/23 inhibitor, has been FDA approved for the treatment of Crohn's disease, while the data supporting its use in HS are less substantial.[4] Ustekinumab has been shown to inhibit HS-related cytokine production in vitro.[32] In addition to several case reports and case series suggesting benefit, moderate-to-marked improvements of the modified Sartorius score were seen in 82% of patients in a small open-label study of ustekinumab in 17 HS patients.[4,45] More recent case series have suggested more frequent and higher doses of ustekinumab, with an initial intravenous infusion, may be of added benefit.[46,47]

Recently, rizankizumab, a high-affinity monoclonal antibody to the p19 subunit of IL-23, demonstrated significantly increased rates of clinical remission of Crohn's disease compared to placebo.[48] They used doses of 600 mg intravenous infusion monthly, much higher than the FDA-approved dosing for psoriasis. Now there is increased interest in IL-23 specific antibodies for the treatment of HS. Currently, a phase II multicenter randomized double blinded placebo-controlled study is underway, evaluating the efficacy of rizankizumab at two dose levels for moderate to severe HS.

A similarly designed trial for HS is also starting for another IL23 p19 monoclonal antibody, guselkumab, at doses of 200 mg subcutaneously every 4 weeks, more than double the FDA-approved psoriasis dosing. One case report and a small case series of eight patients receiving guselkumab suggested benefit, with ~60% of patients demonstrating improvement over 2–4 months with typical psoriasis doses.[49,50]

IL-1α/β

IL-1α and IL-1β contribute to the initiation of an immune response through a shared IL-1 receptor (IL-1R).[51] IL-1R-associated kinase 4 (IRAK4) gets recruited to the internal domain of the IL1-R, resulting in downstream activation of pro-inflammatory transcription factors such as nuclear factor-kappa B (NF-κB). This results in the production of inflammatory mediators (i.e., IL-6), potent neutrophil chemoattractants (including G-CSF and IL-8), and MMPs.[29,52] In addition, IL-1 receptor signaling results in increased production of both IL-1α and IL-1β, resulting in a positive feedback loop.[51] IL-1α is constitutively expressed and actively secreted by many cells, most notably, myeloid cells, endothelial cells, and keratinocytes.[51] Moreover, IL-1α can activate its receptor while membrane-bound or through apoptotic bodies released after cell damage or death. Release of IL-1β from macrophages and dendritic cells; on the other hand, is mediated by caspase-1, which, in its inactive form, is a component of the NOD-, LRR-, and pyrin domain-containing protein 3 (NLRP3) inflammasome.[51] In order to be activated, the IL-1β precursor must be cleaved by caspase-1. The IL-1 receptor signaling cross-talks with various inflammation pathways, including interactions with Th17 and type I interferon signaling.[51,53] IL-1α and IL-1β act synergistically with IL-23 on T cells to produce IL-17.[51] Type I interferons antagonize IL-1 signaling via suppression of

IL-1α and IL-1β transcription, as well as several indirect mechanisms.[53]

The role of IL-1—especially IL-1α—has become of increasing interest recently in the pathogenesis of HS. While some conflicting data exist, several studies have demonstrated overexpression of IL-1β in lesional and perilesional HS skin compared to controls.[29] Similarly, elevated levels of IL-1α and IL-1β have been seen in pus from HS lesions.[54] Increased serum levels of IL-1β in HS patients have also been reported.[54]

Anakinra, a competitive antagonist of the shared IL-1 receptor, has demonstrated efficacy in case reports, case series, and a small randomized, placebo-controlled trial of 20 patients with severe HS.[31,55] Retrospective analysis of this trial revealed 78% of anakinra patients versus 30% of placebo patients achieved HiSCR at 12 weeks. Currently, anakinra is recommended as third-line treatment consideration after failed response to TNF-α inhibitors.[4] While anakinra has demonstrated some benefit in HS, canakinumab, a monoclonal antibody specifically targeting IL-1β, has had much more conflicting data.[31]

Current clinical trials targeting IL-1 include bermekimab (previously known as MABp1), an anti-IL-1α monoclonal antibody which has shown promising results for HS. In a randomized placebo-controlled small study of 20 patients with moderate HS refractory to TNF-α inhibition, 60% of HS patients achieved HiSCR compared to only 10% in the placebo group.[56] Similar responses were seen in a larger, multicenter, phase II open-label study of 42 patients with HS, with ~60 achieving HiSCR, with no difference between those that had failed TNF-α and those that were TNF-α inhibitor naïve.[57] It has been proposed that its efficacy may be linked to its roles in both angiogenesis, as well as upregulation of human beta-defensin 2.[56] A phase II clinical trial with bermekimab is currently ongoing.

PF-06650833, a small molecule inhibiting IL-1 receptor-associated kinase 4 (IRAK4), is also currently being investigated as a target for HS. Presently, a phase II, double-blind, randomized, placebo-controlled clinical trial is examining the efficacy and safety of PF-06650833 in moderate to severe HS alongside two other JAK family inhibitors.

JAK-STAT Signaling Pathway

The JAK/STAT signaling pathway is activated by numerous ligands, including cytokines and hormones, that are responsible for a large number of cellular functions in various cell types. In humans, there are four JAK family members identified (JAK1-3 and Tyrosine Kinase 2 [TYK2]), which associate with several different receptors and are also found in many different cell types.[58] Each pathway can activate one or more STAT family members (STAT1-4, STAT5A, STAT5B, and STAT6). Disruption of the JAK/STAT signaling pathway interferes with $T_H1/2/17$ differentiation, T- and B-cell function, as well as granulopoiesis and neutrophil release and chemotaxis, depending on which of the specific JAK/STAT receptor complexes are inhibited.[58]

JAK inhibitors have become of interest for HS due to the role that type I and II cytokines are thought to play in HS, as well as their indirect inhibition of IL-1β production and TNF-α signaling.[59,60] Recently, two severe Hurley stage III patients that had failed multiple biologics treatments were reported to have responded to adjunct tofacitib (JAK 1/2/3 inhibitor) 5 mg twice a day in addition to antibiotics and various immunosuppressive agents.[61] Due to cytokine profiles important for the various JAK

TABLE 34.3 JAK Family and Their Associated Cytokines and Inhibitors

	JAK1	JAK2	JAK3	TYK2
PERTINENT CYTOKINES AFFECTED	IL-2, -4, -6, -21 IFNα, IFNβ, IFN-γ	IL-6, -12, -23 IFN-γ	IL-2, -4, -21	IL-12, -23 IFNα, IFNβ
INHIBITORS				
Tofacitinib	X	X	X	
Ruxolitinib	X	X		
PF-06700841	X			X
PF-06826647				X
INCB054707	X			

IFN, Interferon; *IL*, Interleukin.
Adapted from Gadina et al.[62]

family members (Table 34.3), JAK1 and TYK2 are the most intriguing due to the current proposed HS pathogenesis.[62]

Several JAK inhibitors are currently under clinical investigation for HS. PF-06700841 is a small molecule dual JAK1/TYK2 inhibitor that has already demonstrated a good safety profile and significant benefit over controls in a phase IIa randomized placebo-controlled trial for psoriasis.[63] Currently, it is being studied in a phase IIa multicenter randomized double-blind placebo-controlled trial for HS alongside the IRAK4 inhibitor (PF-06650833) and a small molecule selective TYK2 inhibitor (PF-06826647). Two separate phase II trials evaluating the safety and efficacy of a selective JAK1 inhibitor (INCB054707) for HS were recently completed. The first was an open-label study in ten patients with moderate to severe HS, primarily evaluating adverse effects and pharmacokinetics of INCB054707, with clinical response evaluated as a secondary outcome measure. Of the 10 participants, 7 completed the 8-week study and 3 achieved HiSCR by 8 weeks and no serious adverse events were noted.[64] The results of the placebo-controlled dose escalation dose escalation trial are still pending.

Other Medications

Other medications currently undergoing clinical investigation for HS include hydroxychloroquine, spironolactone, iscalimumab, and topical resorcinol. In addition to its use in malaria, hydroxychloroquine is also FDA approved for the treatment of lupus erythematosus and rheumatoid arthritis, as well as several other autoimmune conditions.[65] The mechanism underlying its immunomodulating effects is poorly understood. HCQ is a 4-aminoquinolone that has a basic side chain, which promotes its accumulation within inflamed tissues and acidic intracellular compartments, such as lysozymes.[65] HCQ and its analog, chloroquine (CQ), inhibit enzymatic lysosomal activity, theorized to impair lymphocyte antigen presentation, and disrupt autophagy and phagocytosis.[65] Autophagy, which translates to "self-eating," refers to the cellular removal of defective proteins and damaged organelles and is found to play a critical role in NETosis.[66] As NETosis and phagocytosis are important to the role of neutrophils in HS, prevention of these functions could conceptually be important to treating HS.[8] Antimalarials, including HCQ and CQ, have also been shown to disrupt TLR and type I signaling with reduced production of cytokines such as TNF-α, IL-1, IL-6, IFN-γ, and IFN-α/β in vitro.[65] While these mechanisms of action suggest HCQ could be beneficial for HS, the recently completed phase I/II study unfortunately had too high a drop-out rate to draw any conclusions. While there was a significant decrease in Sartorius score at 6 months compared to baseline, only three of 17 subjects enrolled completed the study.[67]

Spironolactone has clinical data supporting its benefit for HS. Hormones, specifically androgens, are thought to play a role in the pathogenesis of HS.[68] It has been theorized that androgens may increase follicular plugging via proliferation of follicular keratinocytes as well as increase inflammatory cytokine production, such as TGF-β and TNF-α.[69] Several anti-androgen approaches for HS have been studied, including oral contraceptives, finasteride, and spironolactone; however, due to the lack of randomized placebo-controlled trials, evidence-based recommendations are limited.[4,69] Spironolactone is the most commonly utilized hormonal treatment for HS.[70] It is known to decrease testosterone production and block the binding of dihydrotestosterone (DHT) to its receptor.[71] Three retrospective chart reviews have demonstrated significant improvement in HS disease activity with spironolactone, one showing an 86% response rate.[4,72] While data supporting spironolactone is reassuring, the efficacy of spironolactone has still not been established in randomized-controlled trials and the appropriate dosage is still unknown. Therefore, a clinical trial evaluating the three-dose regimen (50 mg, 100 mg, 200 mg) for spironolactone will be an important addition to the literature.

Iscalimab (CFZ533) is a fully human, anti-CD40 monoclonal antibody in phase II clinical trials for HS. CD40 is primarily located on B-cells and antigen-presenting cells (APCs), including macrophages, monocytes, and dendritic cells. Iscalimab blocks the co-stimulatory interaction between CD40 and its ligand, CD154, located on activated T cells. The CD40-CD154 interaction results in mitogen-activated protein kinases (MAPK) and NF-κβ signaling in APCs and B-cells, resulting in APC activation and multiple T cell-dependent B-cell functions such as B-cell differentiation/proliferation and antibody isotype switching. While this pathway has not been well-studied in relationship to HS, the cytokines produced by APCs (TNF-α, IL-1, IL-6, IL-8, IL-12, IL-23), such as macrophages and dendritic cells, are central to HS pathophysiology. Theoretically, inhibiting APC activation and cytokine production could prove beneficial for HS.[73]

Finally, resorcinol (m-dihydroxybenzene) is a chemical similar to phenol. It has been used as an ingredient in various topical acne medications at low concentrations (1–2%) and has been used at higher concentrations (10–50%) as a chemical peel.[74] It was initially an attractive option for HS due to its keratolytic and bactericidal properties. After three encouraging case reports were published, a case series of 12 patients were prescribed topical resorcinol 15% cream daily for flares.[75] Resorcinol peels were found to reduce the duration of painful abscesses to 3.7 days on average, down from 5 or more, and dramatically reduced the average pain score, typically within 2 days. Subsequently, a prospective open-label trial of resorcinol 15% cream daily for HS flares demonstrated a significant decrease in mean lesion size and pain score by 7 days.[76] The current trial underway is an observational cross-sectional study in Hurley stage I and II patients to evaluate change in severity and quality of life after 16 weeks of topical resorcinol 15%.

Surgical and Procedural Treatments

Injectables

Intralesional injectable medications are not new *to* the management of HS. Corticosteroids have long been a commonly used modality for acute HS lesions.[4] Intralesional photodynamic therapy (PDT) using a 630 to 635 nm laser diode to activate intralesionally infused 5-aminolevulinic acid (ALA) has also been studied,[68] as well as small case series with intralesional liquid nitrogen (cryoinsufflation) and intralesional radiofrequency ablation.[68] Sclerotherapy with hypertonic saline was described in two HS patients with a total of three tunnels. The tunnels were injected with 0.1 to 0.4 mL of 23.4% hypertonic saline. Both patients reported decreased drainage, and one tract had documented complete resolution.[77] Due to these positive results seen in a small number of patients, a double-blind placebo-controlled trial is currently underway to evaluate the efficacy of sclerotherapy with 23.4% hypertonic saline on HS tunnels.

Light-Based treatments

Light-based treatments including photodynamic therapy, intense pulsed light, and lasers such as Nd-YAG (neodymium-doped yttrium aluminum garnet), diode, alexandrite, and CO₂, have been used to treat HS (discussed in Chapters 25 and 26). Currently, the literature supporting the alexandrite and diode lasers for HS is limited to single case reports.[68] The proposed single-blinded, split-body, randomized trial evaluating the efficacy of the long-pulsed 755 nm Alexandrite laser for HS will help determine whether a more superficial wavelength could expand our light-based armamentarium for HS.

Radiation

The evidence for radiotherapy in HS is limited to several case reports and one large case series of 231 patients.[68] In the large retrospective series by Fröhlich and colleagues (2000),[78] recalcitrant cases of HS were treated with fractions of 0.5 to 1.5 Gy over multiple sessions, with total dosages ranging from 3.0 to 8.0 Gy. Complete response was seen in 38% of patients and another 40% demonstrated improvement of symptoms. While these findings are promising, radiation treatment is limited due to its risk of secondary malignancies, local side effects, and the restricted amount of radiation that can be given to any one region.[79] Specific concerns related to HS include previous reports of HS either induced or exacerbated by radiation exposure as well as the intrinsic risk of squamous cell carcinoma within chronic HS lesions.[68,80] Recent technological advances have made radiation therapy safer, allowing more directed radiation to affected tissues and requiring lower total doses of radiation.[79] A small open-label single intervention trial using a Simon-two stage design is currently recruiting patients for low-dose radiation therapy. Patients will receive five doses of 1.5 Gy (total 7.5 Gy) over one week. Changes in lesional histology and quality of life and adverse events will be evaluated.

Surgery

Complete remission is typically unattainable with medical management alone in severe patients. Surgical excision of recalcitrant structural disease plays an important role in the management of Hurley stage II and III disease, but diffuse disease and high rates of recurrence also limit surgical management alone.[81] While combination medical and surgical treatment is recommended, inadequate number and quality of studies limit the strength of this recommendation.[68]

Two surgical studies are currently underway that will help patients and clinicians determine how to escalate medical therapy in the context of excising recalcitrant tissue. The Safety and Efficacy of Humira (Adalimumab) for HS Peri-Surgically (SHARPS Study) was recently completed. The SHARPS study was a multicenter, prospective, randomized, placebo-controlled trial in 206 HS patients comparing adalimumab versus placebo, given 12 weeks prior to a planned wide local excision for HS and then 2 weeks perioperatively and 10 weeks post-operatively. Preliminary results show a significant difference in patients achieving HiSCR at week 12 and 24 when given adalimumab prior to surgery vs. placebo, but there was no significant difference in those requiring less extensive or no surgery between the treatment arms.[82] A second study is planned to measure the 2-year cost-effectiveness of adalimumab monotherapy compared with adalimumab in combination with up to three wide local excisions within the first year. Patients in the adalimumab monotherapy group will be allowed to cross-over to the surgery group and will be offered escalation to infliximab as determined by clinical practice.

Two other studies are currently investigating the ideal closure techniques after wide local excision (WLE). The optimal approach is currently unknown, and while reconstruction may provide faster healing, it may come at the expense of higher rates of recurrence.[68,83] A multicenter prospective randomized trial is planned to compare axillary perforator flaps with secondary intention wound healing after WLE. The primary outcome being evaluated is complete wound healing at 6 months. A second study will evaluate if negative pressure wound therapy (NPWT) with versus without instillation improves HS outcomes after delayed closure with split-thickness skin grafting. Instillation therapy entails infusing antimicrobial fluid retrograde through the wound during NPWT and is typically used to manage acute and chronic wound infections. Outcomes evaluated in this study include mean days to grafting, percentage of grafts taking, and recurrence rates. This approach has been reported in HS patients previously with success.[84] Procedural treatments are further discussed in Chapters 22–26.

Wound Care

Limited research has been conducted on optimal wound care for HS. Wound care dressing guides have been proposed, emphasizing the importance of absorbency for exudative wounds and tunnels, as well as antibacterial modalities to reduce bacterial colonization and odor.[85] Two clinical studies are currently planned for evaluating various wound care products on healing time and quality of life. A phase II trial will prospectively evaluate wound healing time over eight weeks in five HS participants using a combination of Hydrofera BLUE® and Endoform®. Hydrofera BLUE® is an antimicrobial foam dressing containing gentian violet and methylene blue, which has broad-spectrum antimicrobial activity, without cytotoxic effects on healing tissue.[86] Endoform® is an ovine forestomach-derived dressing, which retains the collagen I and III extracellular matrix, after removal of the antigenic cellular material.[87] This combination was evaluated in a retrospective case series of 53 patients with chronic wounds that demonstrated ~90% wound surface area reduction over 12 weeks.[88] No literature on its use in HS is currently available, but the results from various types of chronic wounds are encouraging.

The other study that is currently recruiting compares the effects of three different Cutimed® wound products on quality of life in HS patients, including Cutimed® Sorbact Hydroactive B antimicrobial wound dressing, Cutimed® Siltect superabsorbent square adhesive wound dressing, and Cutimed® Sorbion® Sana superabsorbent four-leaf clover-shaped non-adhesive wound dressing. The various types of bandages in these studies will help determine what components of wound care have the largest impact on quality of life for people living with HS. Wound care is further discussed in Chapter 20.

Complementary and Alternative Medicine

CAM use is widespread in the HS patient community.[89] Marijuana and cannabidiol (CBD) oil, both topical and oral, are commonly tried CAM modalities, with relatively high reported success rates, ranging from 45% for topical CBD to 57% for marijuana.[89] CBD is one of the major cannabinoids found in marijuana, also known as cannabis. These are also discussed further in Chapter 19.

Given the high reported success rates from HS patients, a randomized placebo-controlled trial evaluating the efficacy of cannabinoids in HS will be a meaningful addition to the literature. In a phase II clinical trial, 40 patients are planned to be randomly assigned to cannabis oil versus placebo, with the primary end point being a one-point reduction in the HS physician global assessment (HS-PGA) score at 8 weeks. Secondarily, HiSCR response and changes in quality of life and pain will be assessed.

HS pain is a major unmet need that significantly impairs quality of life.[70] As HS patients are at increased risk for long-term opioid use, effective, non-opioid, pain management options are desperately needed. In response to this need, researchers are investigating ear acupuncture (EA), also known as battlefield acupuncture, as a possible adjuvant treatment for HS-related pain. EA incorporates inserting semi-permanent needles into five points on the ear.[90] Compared to traditional acupuncture, which is effective for chronic musculoskeletal pain, EA is less time consuming and requires less training.[90] Multiple systematic reviews and meta-analyses have been completed that suggest EA may be a promising modality for pain reduction, but large scientifically rigorous studies are still needed for definitive evidence.[91] In the proposed study, 32 HS patients will be randomly assigned to two EA versus sham treatments one week apart. The primary endpoint will be a change in average daily pain score (0–10) over the two weeks of EA vs sham treatment compared to the two weeks prior to treatment. As a non-pharmacologic option for pain that is quick and easy to learn, EA has the capacity to be an important tool to improve quality of life and reduce chronic opioid use in HS patients. CAM is further discussed in Chapter 28.

Summary

Since adalimumab received FDA approval for HS in 2015, there has been a remarkable increase in published research and clinical trials for HS. While the pathogenesis of HS is still not fully understood, we now have a better understanding of the underlying mechanisms driving this condition. This has led to identification of many potential treatment targets currently being examined in clinical trials. The medical interventions currently under investigation in clinical trials are primarily targeting neutrophils, complement and cytokine dysregulation. While the majority of these drugs being studied are monoclonal antibodies targeting specific cytokines and receptors, trials are also evaluating novel small-molecule JAK inhibitors that are capable of inhibiting multiple pathways related to T_H1/T_H17 cytokines as well type I interferons. These targeted medications have been primarily created for other diseases, such as psoriasis and Crohn's disease, and secondarily investigated for HS. As our understanding of HS pathogenesis expands, targeted therapies will hopefully advance concurrently. In addition to medical therapies, laser treatments, sclerotherapy, wound care products, various surgical approaches as well as some CAM modalities, are also under clinical investigation for HS. Although we are still far away from fully understanding the mechanisms underlying HS, the future of HS management looks bright, with numerous medical, procedural, and surgical treatments in the pipeline.

References

1. Naik H, Lowes MA. Call to Accelerate Hidradenitis Suppurativa Research and Improve Care-Moving Beyond Burden. *JAMA Dermatol.* 2019;155(9):1005–1006.
2. McDonald B, Kubes P. Cellular and molecular choreography of neutrophil recruitment to sites of sterile inflammation. *J Mol Med.* 2011;89(11):1079–1088.
3. Van Der Zee HH, De Ruiter L, Boer J, et al. Alterations in leucocyte subsets and histomorphology in normal-appearing perilesional skin and early and chronic hidradenitis suppurativa lesions. *Br J Dermatol.* 2012;166(1):98–106.
4. Alikhan A, Sayed C, Alavi A, et al. North American clinical management guidelines for hidradenitis suppurativa: A publication from the United States and Canadian Hidradenitis Suppurativa Foundations: Part II: Topical, intralesional, and systemic medical management. *J Am Acad Dermatol.* 2019;81(1):91–101.
5. Lima AL, Karl I, Giner T, et al. Keratinocytes and neutrophils are important sources of proinflammatory molecules in hidradenitis suppurativa. *Br J Dermatol.* 2016;174(3):514–521.
6. Soehnlein O, Steffens S, Hidalgo A, Weber C. Neutrophils as protagonists and targets in chronic inflammation. *Nat Rev Immunol.* 2017;17(4):248–261.
7. Lapins J, Åsman B, Gustafsson A, Bergström K, Emtestam L. Neutrophil-related host response in hidradenitis suppurativa: A pilot study in patients with inactive disease. *Acta Derm Venereol.* 2001; 81(2):96–99.
8. Byrd AS, Carmona-Rivera C, O'Neil LJ, et al. Neutrophil extracellular traps, B cells, and type I interferons contribute to immune dysregulation in hidradenitis suppurativa. *Sci Transl Med.* 2019;11 (508):1–13.
9. Markert C, T Gebhard, Sriniva H, et al. Discovery of LYS006, a Potent and Highly Selective Inhibitor of Leukotriene A 4 Hydrolase. *J Med Chem.* 2021;64(4):1889–1903.
10. Scalzo-Inguanti K, Monaghan K, Edwards K, et al. A neutralizing anti–G-CSFR antibody blocks G-CSF–induced neutrophilia without inducing neutropenia in nonhuman primates. *J Leukoc Biol.* 2017; 102(2):537–549.
11. Haeggström JZ. Leukotriene biosynthetic enzymes as therapeutic targets. *J Clin Invest.* 2018;128(7):2680–2690.
12. Lämmermann T, Afonso PV, Angermann BR, et al. Neutrophil swarms require LTB4 and integrins at sites of cell death in vivo. *Nature.* 2013;498(7454):371–375.
13. Penno CA, Jäger P, Laguerre C, et al. Lipidomics Profiling of Hidradenitis Suppurativa Skin Lesions Reveals Lipoxygenase Pathway Dysregulation and Accumulation of Pro-Inflammatory Leukotriene B4. *J Invest Dermatol.* 2020 May.
14. Camous L, Roumenina L, Bigot S, et al. Complement alternative pathway acts as a positive feedback amplification of neutrophil activation. *Blood.* 2011;117(4):1340–1349.
15. Jagels MA, Ember JA, Travis J, Potempa J, Pike R, Hugli TE. Cleavage of the human C5A receptor by proteinases derived from Porphyromonas gingivalis: cleavage of leukocyte C5a receptor. *Adv Exp Med Biol.* 1996;389:155–164.
16. Seow V, Lim J, Iyer A, et al. Inflammatory Responses Induced by Lipopolysaccharide Are Amplified in Primary Human Monocytes but Suppressed in Macrophages by Complement Protein C5a. *J Immunol.* 2013;191(8):4308–4316.
17. Hoffman LK, Tomalin LE, Alavi A, et al. Integrating the skin and blood transcriptomes and serum proteome in hidradenitis suppurativa reveals complement dysregulation and a plasma cell signature. *PLoS One.* 2018;13(9): e0203672.
18. Guo R, Habel M, Zenker O, Giamarellos-bourboulis EJ, Riedemann N, Gmbh I. IFX-1 blocking the anaphylatoxin C5a – an anti-inflammatory effect in patients with hidradenitis suppurativa. InflaRx GmbH, Jena, Ger 2017 Retrieved from https://www.inflarx.de/dam/jcr:ec982d1e-f82b-4992-a1b0-ff6e69a04b6b/Guo_2017_poster.pdf. Accessed 12 May 2020.
19. Giamarellos-Bourboulis EJ, Argyropoulou M, Kanni T, et al. Clinical efficacy of complement C5a inhibition by IFX-1 in hidradenitis suppurativa: an open-label single-arm trial in patients not eligible for adalimumab. *Br J Dermatol.* 2020;(c):5–6.
20. InflaRx. *11-2019-InflaRx Reports Positive Results from the Open Label Extension Part of the SHINE Study for IFX-1 in Hidradenitis Suppurativa*; 2019. Retrieved from https://www.inflarx.de/Home/Investors/Press-Releases/11-2019-InflaRx-Reports-Positive-Results-from-the-Open-Label-Extension-Part-of-the-SHINE-Study-for-IFX-1-in-Hidradenitis-Suppurativa.html. Accessed 12 May 2020.
21. InflaRx. 2019. 07-2019-InflaRx Reports Additional Analysis of the SHINE Phase IIb Results for IFX-1 in Hidradenitis Suppurativa. Retrieved from https://www.inflarx.de/Home/Investors/Press-Releases/07-2019-InflaRx-Reports-Additional-Analysis-of-the-SHINE-Phase-IIb-Results-for-IFX-1-in-Hidradenitis-Suppurativa-.htmlAccessed. Accessed 12 May 2020.
22. Jayne DRW, Bruchfeld AN, Harper L, et al. Randomized trial of C5a receptor inhibitor avacopan in ANCA-associated vasculitis. *N Engl J Med.* 2004;350(9):2756–2767.
23. Kimball AB, Okun MM, Williams DA, et al. Two phase 3 trials of adalimumab for hidradenitis suppurativa. *N Engl J Med.* 2016; 375(5):422–434.
24. Fine S, Papamichael K, Cheifetz AS. Etiology and management of lack or loss of response to anti–tumor necrosis factor therapy in patients with inflammatory bowel disease. *Gastroenterol Hepatol.* 2019;15(12):656–665.
25. Maser EA, Villela R, Silverberg MS, Greenberg GR. Association of trough serum infliximab to clinical outcome after scheduled maintenance treatment for Crohn's disease. *Clin Gastroenterol Hepatol Off Clin Pract J Am Gastroenterol Assoc.* 2006 Oct;4(10):1248–1254.
26. van der Have M, Oldenburg B, Kaptein AA, et al. Non-adherence to anti-TNF therapy is associated with illness perceptions and clinical outcomes in outpatients with inflammatory bowel disease: Results from a prospective multicentre study. *J Crohn's Colitis.* 2016;10(5): 549–555.
27. Hawkes JE, Yan BY, Chan TC, Krueger JG. Discovery of the IL-23/IL-17 Signaling Pathway and the Treatment of Psoriasis. *J Immunol.* 2018;201(6):1605–1613.
28. Glatt S, Baeten D, Baker T, et al. Dual IL-17A and IL-17F neutralisation by bimekizumab in psoriatic arthritis: Evidence from preclinical experiments and a randomised placebo-controlled clinical trial that IL-17F contributes to human chronic tissue inflammation. *Ann Rheum Dis.* 2018;77(4):523–532.
29. Frew JW, Hawkes JE, Krueger JG. A systematic review and critical evaluation of inflammatory cytokine associations in hidradenitis suppurativa. *F1000Research.* 2018;7:1930.
30. Matusiak Ł, Szczęch J, Bieniek A, et al. Increased interleukin (IL)-17 serum levels in patients with hidradenitis suppurativa: Implications for treatment with anti-IL-17 agents. *J Am Acad Dermatol.* 2017;76(4):670–675.

31. Lim SYD, Oon HH. Systematic review of immunomodulatory therapies for hidradenitis suppurativa. *Biol Targets Ther.* 2019;13:53–78.

32. Vossen ARJV, Ardon CB, van der Zee HH, et al. The anti-inflammatory potency of biologics targeting tumour necrosis factor-α, interleukin (IL)-17A, IL-12/23 and CD20 in hidradenitis suppurativa: an ex vivo study. *Br J Dermatol.* 2019;181(2):314–323.

33. Casseres RG, Prussick L, Zancanaro P, et al. Secukinumab in the treatment of moderate to severe hidradenitis suppurativa: Results of an open-label trial. *J Am Acad Dermatol.* 2020;82(6):1524–1526.

34. Prussick L, Rothstein B, Joshipura D, et al. Open-label, investigator-initiated, single-site exploratory trial evaluating secukinumab, an anti-interleukin-17A monoclonal antibody, for patients with moderate-to-severe hidradenitis suppurativa. *Br J Dermatol.* 2019;181(3):609–611.

35. Reguiaï Z, Fougerousse A, Maccari F, Bécherel P. Effectiveness of secukinumab in Hidradenitis Suppurativa: an open study (20 cases). *J Eur Acad Dermatol Venereol.* 2020;34(11):e750–e751.

36. Clinicaltrials.gov. Bethesda (MD): National Library of Medicine (US). 2000 Feb 29. NCT02421172: Efficacy, Safety, and Pharmacokinetics Study of CJM112 in Hidradenitis Suppurativa Patients. Accessed 2020 Aug 18.

37. Ritchlin CT, Kavanaugh A, Merola JF, et al. Bimekizumab in patients with active psoriatic arthritis: results from a 48-week, randomised, double-blind, placebo-controlled, dose-ranging phase 2b trial. *Lancet.* 2020;395(10222):427–440.

38. Printer A, Bonnekoh B, Hadshiew IM, Zimmer S. Brodalumab for the treatment of moderate-to-severe psoriasis: case series and literature review. *Clin Cosmet Investig Dermatol.* 2019;12:509–517.

39. Arenbergerova M, Arenberger P, Marques E, Gkalpakiotis S. Successful treatment of recalcitrant gluteal hidradenitis suppurativa with brodalumab after anti-TNF failure. *Int J Dermatol.* 2020; 733–735.

40. Frew JW, Facd M, Navrazhina K, et al. The Effect of Subcutaneous Brodalumab upon Clinical Disease Activity in Hidradenitis Suppurativa: An Open Label Cohort Study. *J Am Acad Dermatol.* 2020.

41. Teng MWL, Bowman EP, McElwee JJ, et al. IL-12 and IL-23 cytokines: From discovery to targeted therapies for immune-mediated inflammatory diseases. *Nat Med.* 2015;21(7):719–729.

42. Schlapbach C, Hänni T, Yawalkar N, Hunger RE. Expression of the IL-23/Th17 pathway in lesions of hidradenitis suppurativa. *J Am Acad Dermatol.* 2011;65(4):790–798.

43. Maxwell JR, Zhang Y, Brown WA, et al. Differential Roles for Interleukin-23 and Interleukin-17 in Intestinal Immunoregulation. *Immunity.* 2015;43(4):739–750.

44. Chen WT, Chi CC. Association of Hidradenitis Suppurativa with Inflammatory Bowel Disease: A Systematic Review and Meta-analysis. *JAMA Dermatology.* 2019;155(9):1022–1027.

45. Blok JL, Li K, Brodmerkel C, et al. Ustekinumab in hidradenitis suppurativa: Clinical results and a search for potential biomarkers in serum. *Br J Dermatol.* 2016;174(4):839–846.

46. Romani J, Vilarrasa E, Martorell A, et al. Ustekinumab with Intravenous Infusion: Results in Hidradenitis Suppurativa. *Dermatology.* 2020;236(1):21–24.

47. Scholl L, Hessam S, Garcovich S, Bechara FG. High-dosage ustekinumab for the treatment of severe hidradenitis suppurativa. *Eur J Dermatol.* 2019 Dec;29(6):659–661.

48. Feagan BG, Sandborn WJ, D'Haens G, et al. Induction therapy with the selective interleukin-23 inhibitor risankizumab in patients with moderate-to-severe Crohn's disease: a randomised, double-blind, placebo-controlled phase 2 study. *Lancet.* 2017;389(10080): 1699–1709.

49. Berman HS, Villa NM, Shi VY, Hsiao JL. Guselkumab in the treatment of concomitant hidradenitis suppurativa, psoriasis, and Crohn's disease. *J Dermatolog Treat.* 2019;1–3.

50. Casseres RG, Kahn JS, Her MJ, Rosmarin D. Guselkumab in the treatment of hidradenitis suppurativa: A retrospective chart review. *J Am Acad Dermatol.* 2019;81(1):265–267.

51. Mantovani A, Dinarello CA, Molgora M, Garlanda C. Interleukin-1 and Related Cytokines in the Regulation of Inflammation and Immunity. *Immunity.* 2019;50(4):778–795.

52. Sanchez J, Le Jan S, Muller C, et al. Matrix remodelling and MMP expression/activation are associated with hidradenitis suppurativa skin inflammation. *Exp Dermatol.* 2019;28(5):593–600.

53. Mayer-Barber KD, Yan B. Clash of the Cytokine Titans: Counter-regulation of interleukin-1 and type i interferon-mediated inflammatory responses. *Cell Mol Immunol.* 2017;14(1):22–35.

54. Kanni T, Tzanetakou V, Savva A, et al. Compartmentalized cytokine responses in hidradenitis suppurativa. *PLoS One.* 2015;10(6):1–15.

55. Tzanetakou V, Kanni T, Giatrakou S, et al. Safety and efficacy of anakinra in severe hidradenitis suppurativa a randomized clinical trial. *JAMA Dermatology.* 2016;152(1):52–59.

56. Kanni T, Argyropoulou M, Spyridopoulos T, et al. MABp1 targeting IL-1α for moderate to severe hidradenitis suppurativa not eligible for adalimumab: A randomized study. *J Invest Dermatol.* 2018;138(4): 795–801.

57. Gottlieb A, Natsis NE, Kerdel F, et al. A phase II open-label study of bermekimab in patients with hidradenitis suppurativa shows resolution of inflammatory lesions and pain. *J Invest Dermatol.* 2020.

58. Bharadwaj U, Kasembeli MM, Robinson P, Tweardy DJ. Targeting Janus kinases and signal transducer and activator of transcription 3 to treat inflammation, fibrosis, and cancer: Rationale, progress, and caution. *Pharmacol Rev.* 2020;72(2):486–526.

59. Furuya MY, Asano T, Sumichika Y, et al. Tofacitinib inhibits granulocyte–macrophage colony-stimulating factor induced NLRP3 inflammasome activation in human neutrophils. *Arthritis Res Ther.* 2018;20(1):196.

60. Yarilina A, Xu K, Chan C, Ivashkiv LB. Regulation of inflammatory responses in tumor necrosis factor-activated and rheumatoid arthritis synovial macrophages by JAK inhibitors. *Arthritis Rheum.* 2012; 64(12):3856–3866.

61. Savage KT, Santillan MR, Flood KS, et al. Tofacitinib shows benefit in conjunction with other therapies in recalcitrant hidradenitis suppurativa patients. *JAAD Case Reports [Internet].* 2020;6(2):99–102.

62. Gadina M, Johnson C, Schwartz D, et al. Translational and clinical advances in JAK-STAT biology: The present and future of jakinibs. *J Leukoc Biol.* 2018;104(3):499–514.

63. Forman SB, Pariser DM, Poulin Y, et al. TYK2/JAK1 Inhibitor PF-06700841 in Patients with Plaque Psoriasis: Phase IIa, Randomized, Double-blind, Placebo-controlled Trial. In: Society for Investigative Dermatology; 2020. Journal of Investigative Dermatology;.

64. Clinicaltrials.gov. Bethesda (MD): National Library of Medicine (US). 2000 Feb 29. NCT03569371: A Study of the Safety of INCB054707 in Participants With Hidradenitis Suppurativa. Accessed Aug 18, 2020.

65. Schrezenmeier E, Dörner T. Mechanisms of action of hydroxychloroquine and chloroquine: implications for rheumatology. *Nat Rev Rheumatol.* 2020;16(3):155–166.

66. Migliario M, Tonello S, Rocchetti V, Rizzi M, Renò F. Near infrared laser irradiation induces NETosis via oxidative stress and autophagy. *Lasers Med Sci.* 2018;33(9):1919–1924.

67. Clinicaltrials.gov. Bethesda (MD): National Library of Medicine (US). 2000 Feb 29. NCT03275870: Hydroxychloroquine for the Treatment of Hidradenitis Suppurativa. Accessed Aug 18, 2020.

68. Alikhan A, Sayed C, Alavi A, et al. North American clinical management guidelines for hidradenitis suppurativa: A publication from the United States and Canadian Hidradenitis Suppurativa Foundations: Part I: Diagnosis, evaluation, and the use of complementary and procedural management. *J Am Acad Dermatol.* 2019;81(1):76–90.

69. Riis PT, Ring HC, Themstrup L, Jemec GB. The role of androgens and estrogens in hidradenitis suppurativa - a systematic review. *Acta Dermatovenerologica Croat.* 2016;24(4):239–249.

70. Garg A, Neuren E, Cha D, et al. Evaluating patients' unmet needs in hidradenitis suppurativa: Results from the Global Survey Of Impact and Healthcare Needs (VOICE) Project. *J Am Acad Dermatol.* 2020;82(2):366–376.

71. Loriaux DL, Menard R, Taylor A, Santen R. Spironolactone and endocrine dysfunction. *Ann Intern Med.* 1976;85(5):630–636.

72. Lee A, Fischer G. A case series of 20 women with hidradenitis suppurativa treated with spironolactone. *Australas J Dermatol.* 2015; 56(3):192–196.

73. Ristov J, Espie P, Ulrich P, et al. Characterization of the in vitro and in vivo properties of CFZ533, a blocking and non-depleting anti-CD40 monoclonal antibody. *Am J Transplant.* 2018;18(12):2895–2904.

74. Bontemps H, Mallaret M, Besson G, et al. Confusion after topical use of resorcinol. *Arch Dermatol.* 1995;131(1):112.

75. Boer J, Jemec GBE. Resorcinol peels as a possible self-treatment of painful nodules in hidradenitis suppurativa. *Clin Exp Dermatol.* 2010;35(1):36–40.

76. Pascual JC, Encabo B, Ruiz de Apodaca RF, et al. Topical 15% resorcinol for hidradenitis suppurativa: An uncontrolled prospective trial with clinical and ultrasonographic follow-up. *J Am Acad Dermatol.* 2017;77(6):1175–1178.

77. Porter M, Kimball A, Prens L. Sclerotherapy for fistula tracts in hidradenitis suppurativa: Two case reports of a novel treatment option. *J Am Acad Dermatol.* 2017;76(6). AB226.

78. Frohlich D, Baaske D, Glatzel M. Radiotherapy of hidradenitis suppurativa-still valid today? *Strahlenther Onkol.* 2000;176(6):286–289.

79. Berkey FJ. Managing the adverse effects of radiation therapy. *Am Fam Physician.* 2010;82(4):381–388.

80. Haber R, Gottlieb J, Zagdanski AM, Battistella M, Bachelez H. Radiation-induced hidradenitis suppurativa: A case report. *JAAD Case Reports.* 2017;3(3):182–184.

81. Melendez Gonzalez M, del M, Sayed CJ. Surgery is an essential aspect of managing patients with hidradenitis suppurativa. *J Am Acad Dermatol.* 2020;1–2.

82. Clinicaltrials.gov. Bethesda (MD): National Library of Medicine (US). 2000 Feb 29. NCT02808975: Safety and Efficacy of Adalimumab (Humira) for Hidradenitis Suppurativa (HS) Peri-Surgically (SHARPS). Accessed Aug 18, 2020 [Internet].

83. Bouazzi D, Chafranska L, Saunte DML, Jemec GBE. Systematic Review of Complications and Recurrences After Surgical Interventions in Hidradenitis Suppurativa. *Dermatol Surg.* 2020;Jul; 46(7):914–921.

84. Ge S, Orbay H, Silverman RP, Rasko YM. Negative Pressure Wound Therapy with Instillation and Dwell Time in the Surgical Management of Severe Hidradenitis Suppurativa. *Cureus.* 2018;10(9):e3319.

85. Alavi A, Sibbald RG, Kirsner RS. Optimal hidradenitis suppurativa topical treatment and wound care management: a revised algorithm. *J Dermatolog Treat.* 2018;29(4):383–384.

86. Woo KY, Heil J. A prospective evaluation of methylene blue and gentian violet dressing for management of chronic wounds with local infection. *Int Wound J.* 2017;14(6):1029–1035.

87. Liden BA, May BCH. Clinical outcomes following the use of ovine forestomach matrix (endoform dermal template) to treat chronic wounds. *Adv Ski Wound Care.* 2013;26(4):164–167.

88. Lullove EJ. Use of Ovine-based Collagen Extracellular Matrix and Gentian Violet/Methylene Blue Antibacterial Foam Dressings to Help Improve Clinical Outcomes in Lower Extremity Wounds: A Retrospective Cohort Study. *Wounds.* 2017;29(4):107–114.

89. Price KN, Thompson AM, Rizvi O, et al. Complementary and Alternative Medicine Use in Patients With Hidradenitis Suppurativa. *JAMA dermatol.* 2020;156(3):345–348.

90. Levy CE, Casler N, FitzGerald DB. Battlefield Acupuncture: An Emerging Method for Easing Pain. *Am J Phys Med Rehabil.* 2018; 97(3):e18–e19.

91. Murakami M, Fox L, Dijkers MP. Ear acupuncture for immediate pain relief—A systematic review and meta-analysis of randomized controlled trials. *Pain Med (United States).* 2017;18(3): 551–564.

92. Vossen ARJV, van der Zee HH, Prens EP. Hidradenitis Suppurativa: A Systematic Review Integrating Inflammatory Pathways Into a Cohesive Pathogenic Model. *Front Immunol.* 2018;Dec 14;9:2965.

35

The Future

HALEY B. NAIK AND MICHELLE A. LOWES

CHAPTER OUTLINE

Introduction

This chapter is our vision for the way forward from *gaps* to *goals*. We first summarize the major gaps that exist in order to provide optimal care for HS patients. We then outline the journey to address these gaps and the programs and initiatives required to do this (Fig. 35.1).

Major Gaps to Address Now for Optimal Care of HS Patients in the Future

1. Delayed diagnosis and treatment may lead to uninhibited disease progression

   It is unacceptable that there is a prolonged delay for most patients to be diagnosed with HS, on average, about a decade.[1] It is critical that patients are diagnosed promptly so they may be treated much earlier in their disease course. As inflammation progresses, it causes irreversible tissue destruction and scarring in the region of disease activity. Given the relapsing and remitting nature of HS, a dynamic treatment plan is often needed to care for HS both during flares and periods of remission. Treatment goals are to improve quality of life, prevent permanent disfigurement, and reduce the need for visits to acute care settings. Another major gap is that it has not yet been definitively demonstrated that preventing HS from advancing will avert progression and scar formation.[2] Early and proactive treatment has been shown in other destructive inflammatory diseases, including rheumatoid arthritis, to limit disease progression via the treat-to-target paradigm[3] wherein treatment modalities are aggressively and proactively managed to maximize long-term health-related quality of life.

2. Suboptimal access to care impedes HS management

   Patients deserve timely access to knowledgeable care and effective treatment that leads to disease remission.[4] HS patients describe insufficient access to healthcare providers who are educated about HS, as well as geographical restrictions to HS providers. In terms of treatment limitations, there is only one FDA-approved treatment for HS; adalimumab (Humira, AbbVie) based on the PIONEER I and II studies.[5] Patients in some states face challenges accessing this therapy. There are also issues with access to off-label and procedural therapies, as well as financial difficulties in obtaining wound care supplies. Disparities in access to care have been suggested in this disease that predominates in women and Blacks,[6] and it is already documented that Blacks with HS experience significant healthcare disparities.[7]

3. Limited understanding of HS clinical course, clinical phenotypes and disease burden prevents personalized medicine approaches

   The ultimate goal of providing personalized treatment requires comprehensive knowledge of clinical course, clinical phenotypes, and disease burden. These features may hold important clues to predict disease prognosis and treatment response. Patients progressing along a given clinical course, as well as patients with different phenotypes, may respond to specific treatment approaches more positively than others. In addition, it is now appreciated that there are significant systemic co-morbidities associated with HS.[8] Understanding these cardiometabolic, rheumatologic, oncologic, and psychological co-morbidities may also help tailor treatment for patients with HS.

4. Insufficient understanding of HS pathogenesis inhibits therapeutic development

   The unique HS pathogenic signature is still not known; this has hindered the development of novel targeted therapies. Accelerated basic and translational research is imperative to rationally target dysregulated pathways and guide therapeutic development.

5. Paucity of novel therapeutics currently limits finding a permanent remission or a cure

   There is a paucity of high-quality evidence for HS treatments.[9,10] To address this deficit, carefully designed randomized controlled trials (RCTs) of novel targeted therapies are needed. While developing these HS clinical

The future for hidradenitis suppurativa

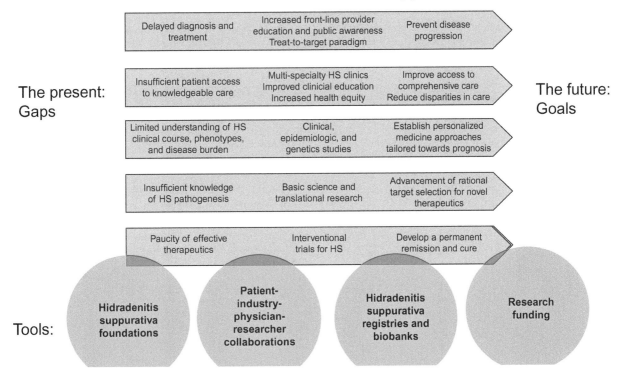

The present: Gaps

The future: Goals

Tools:

• **Fig. 35.1** The Future of Hidradenitis Suppurativa. Major current gaps in the management of hidradenitis suppurativa (HS) are listed (*left*), with steps to address these gaps (*middle*) to achieve future goals for optimal care for those living with HS (*right*). The tools to achieve these goals are identified (*circles*).

trial programs, special considerations include patient selection and recruitment, development of outcome measures, the role of placebo or active treatment comparators, and conduct of concomitant translational research for pathogenesis and biomarkers during the RCTs.

The Journey From Gaps to Goals

1. Clinician, patient, and public education

   To improve time to diagnosis and treatment, education of clinicians, patients, and the general public is paramount. Increasing awareness of HS diagnostic criteria across medical specialties will reduce under-diagnosis, misdiagnosis, and diagnostic delay. Education programs for front-line providers who first encounter patients with HS symptoms and signs could reduce the time to diagnosis and dermatology referral. Another major goal is to educate clinicians as treatment paradigms are developed to induce early disease remission and prevent progression, such as treat-to-target approaches. In addition, increased awareness of the clinical signs and symptoms of HS in the general public could decrease the stigma associated with HS. Physicians can work with patient organizations to improve patient education.

   Given the high disease burden and healthcare costs associated with HS,[11] efforts should be made to improve both pharmacologic and nonpharmacologic treatment plans. An individualized written home-management action plan has shown efficacy in other chronic inflammatory conditions, such as asthma and atopic dermatitis.[12,13] Patients are provided with written instructions on flare recognition and corresponding step-up/step-down treatment at home. This is highly applicable to HS, another chronic disease with intermittent flares. Providing HS patients with proper disease education and a written treatment action plan may empower them to manage acute HS flares at home as opposed to seeking care in an acute care setting.

2. Multi-specialty/interdisciplinary HS clinics

   A key component of optimizing current HS management is developing specialized HS treatment centers and multi-specialty HS clinics anchored by the dermatologist, as discussed in Chapter 32.[14] Multi-specialty care can take different forms, including a multidisciplinary clinic with available specialists in one clinic, or referral to a network of specialists interested in and knowledgeable about HS. This comprehensive approach is modeled on the delivery of cancer care. First, those who provide direct care of HS lesions are essential, such as dermatologists, surgeons, nurses, and wound care specialists. Second, access to healthcare providers who care for those with comorbidities, as discussed in Chapter 8, is also key. This includes assessment and treatment by pain specialists, psychologists, psychiatrists, rheumatologists, endocrinologists, cardiologists, primary care physicians, as well as counselors, dietitians, or nutritionists. Patient-led HS support groups established within a specialized HS treatment center can also provide a valuable resource for HS patients and their families, as discussed in Chapter 33.

   Caring for patients in the context of a multi-disciplinary setting can also improve our understanding of the most effective ways to integrate therapeutic approaches for HS management, including conventional medications, physical procedures such as surgery and lasers, and complementary and alternative medicine (CAM). An interdisciplinary approach can also facilitate the timely management of acute flares of HS. Developing multi-disciplinary HS clinical care in areas of higher HS prevalence can also help to reduce health disparities.

3. Clinical, epidemiology, and genetics studies

    Personalized medicine requires knowledge of patient and disease characteristics that guide treatment selection, which can be gained by long-term studies of clinical course, and large-scale epidemiology and genetics studies of HS patients. Earlier chapters have outlined our current knowledge of these areas, but there is still much to be learned. Studies on the role of imaging modalities to facilitate diagnosis, lesion assessment, and treatment planning are also needed. In addition, skin and serum biomarkers may also be useful to guide treatment choice and develop predictors of response, and further investigation in this area of research is warranted.

4. Basic science and translational research

    The current understanding of HS pathogenesis is described in earlier chapters. To expand and accelerate this knowledge, increased basic science and translational research are needed, such as in the fields of genetics, immunology, and the human microbiome. Increased funding for HS research is critical for these efforts.

5. Clinical trials for HS

    Chapter 34 outlined the current pipeline of treatments for HS. To reach our ultimate goal of permanent remission and a cure for HS, greater numbers of clinical trials in all disease stages are needed. Guidance for optimizing clinical trials in HS can be developed in conjunction with physicians, industry partners, regulatory bodies as well as patients. Some key considerations include the design of RCTs and pragmatic clinical studies, choice of comparator arms, dosage regimens, development and implementation of outcomes measures, biomarker studies within clinical trials, and patient recruitment.

Programs & Initiatives to Get Us There

Hidradenitis Suppurativa Foundations

Foundations have a very important role to develop and coordinate many activities to meet the presented goals. There are currently four international foundations for HS, listed as follows:

- United States Hidradenitis Suppurativa Foundation, Inc. (HSF)
- Canadian Hidradenitis Suppurativa Foundation (CHSF)
- European Hidradenitis Suppurativa Foundation (EHSF)
- Asia-Pacific Hidradenitis Suppurativa Foundation (APHiS)

Examples of activities that foundations have conducted and promoted include:

- Foundations play a key role in helping to identify healthcare providers who care for patients with HS and provide this information to the public (such as on the HSF website).
- There is an important role in clinician education for foundations. This can be through the development of treatment guidelines[9,10,15] and providing recommendations for important aspects of HS care including screening of disease co-morbidities and pain management.

- Foundations can host scientific conferences. The EHSF has hosted nine scientific meetings, and the HSF and CHSF have jointly hosted the Symposium on Hidradenitis Suppurativa Advances (SHSA) for the past four years.[16-19] Future education efforts should include healthcare providers from other specialties that are involved in HS care.
- They also play an important role in educating HS patients, friends and families, and the general public. The EHSF, for example, has pioneered an in-person HS School for HS patients and their families that has been well received.[20]
- Foundations can also promote, develop, and support clinical, epidemiology, genetics, basic science, and translational research through grants programs. For example, the HSF offers the Danby HSF Research Grants every year to help investigators generate pilot data to apply for larger funding with research institutes. Foundations can provide infrastructure investments in programs such as registries and biobanks to facilitate future research projects.
- Consensus efforts, such as defining HS lesion morphology, clinical treatment algorithms, treat-to-target paradigms, clinical trials guidance, and practice gaps, can be promoted and conducted by foundations.
- Another important role for foundations is patient advocacy, directed by patients who can guide priorities and lead in this area, supported by healthcare provider allies.
- Foundations can provide much-needed support to patients and families through partnership or sponsorship of support groups. For example, the US-based Hope for HS works closely with the HSF to promote the development of local support groups.
- There is also a potential role for an umbrella international HS Foundation consortium to bring together these national foundations, raise awareness of HS across the world, share processes, and collaborate on activities to reach shared goals.

Patient-Industry-Academia-Physician-Researcher Collaborations

- The International Dermatology Outcome Measures (IDEOM) group established the Hidradenitis SuppuraTiva cORe outcomes set International Collaboration (HISTORIC). This collaborative effort has determined core domains to measure in HS clinical trials: pain, physical signs, HS-specific quality of life, global assessment, progression of course, and symptoms.[21-23] The priority is improved outcome measures for clinical trials, but these instruments will also be extremely useful for clinical care.
- Collaborations between patients, physicians, and researchers also enable education regarding each groups' perspectives and priorities. Global VOICE was an international patient survey conducted by HS physicians' clinics.[24] Another example of a town hall style educational meeting about HS with clinicians, researchers, patients advocates, and patients is archived on the Clinical Directors Network website.
- There are also numerous opportunities for research collaborations. This includes individual principal investigators developing projects with industry partners and industry supporting larger registry and biobanking projects.
- Patient involvement in foundation and research priority setting, education of providers (such as at scientific meetings), and clinical trial design, can also be beneficial for all. Ideally, diverse HS patients are represented in these collaborative projects.

HS Registry and Biobanks

- Registries and biobanks offer powerful opportunities to address many of the gaps and goals discussed.
- The first HS registry established was the European Hidradenitis Suppurativa Registry (HSR).[25] The mission of this registry is to establish a unique database with a large prospective cohort of patients with HS. This registry is designed to collect data on the current status and follow-up of patients with HS.
- The US has recently initiated the Hidradenitis Suppurativa Prospective Observational Registry and Biospecimen Repository (HS PROGRESS).[26] The mission of HS PROGRESS is to facilitate HS research through collaboration between investigators, clinicians, patients, and industry in order to improve the lives of people living with HS. Specific goals include:
  - To develop a longitudinal cohort of HS patients in all stages of disease to understand HS clinical course.
  - To collect biospecimens from HS patients for ongoing and future studies.
  - To establish a cohort of consented patients who can be contacted for future clinical studies.
  - To develop an infrastructure to support pilot projects that can lead to NIH funding.
- Other international groups have started an Italian registry[27] and a Scandinavian registry for HS (HISREG).[28]
- Additional registry efforts are important to expand our knowledge of HS beyond Europe and US populations. Analysis of aggregate data across different registries will also be informative to understand HS in different populations.
- Patients can be recruited to registries from HS and multi-specialty clinics, leading to important real-world data and experience that will direct optimal clinical care and can help generate research questions.

Research Funding

For all these endeavors, research funding is critical. Some sources of funding include the following:
- Foundations. For example, the HSF offers Danby HSF Research Grants every fall. Other programs are in the planning stages for endeavors such as translational research and mentoring grants.
- Federal funding. NIH/NIAMS has offered a Funding Announcement for R21 and R01 grants specifically for HS translational research (excluding clinical trials).
- Industry has partnered with principal investigators at academic centers to perform translational studies to identify therapeutic targets and biomarkers.
- Philanthropic contributions and grassroots campaigns are future sources to be investigated for research funding.

Conclusion

We have presented major obstacles to optimal care of HS patients and suggested initiatives and endeavors to address these gaps. These activities will enable us to achieve the goals of preventing disease progression, optimizing current management, personalizing care, and developing novel therapeutics, with the ultimate goal of attaining permanent remission and cure. Mechanisms to drive and enhance these goals are underway, including active international HS Foundations, numerous collaborations between major stakeholders, formations of HS registries and biobanks, and an improving research funding landscape. From neglect to awareness, we are confident that the future of HS is finally looking promising.

References

1. Kokolakis G, Wolk K, Schneider-Burrus S, et al. Delayed diagnosis of hidradenitis suppurativa and its effect on patients and healthcare system. *Dermatology*. 2020;1–10.
2. Paek SY, Hamzavi I, Danby FW, et al. Disease modification for hidradenitis suppurativa: A new paradigm. *J Am Acad Dermatol*. 2017;76: 772–773.
3. van Vollenhoven R. Treat-to-target in rheumatoid arthritis - are we there yet? *Nat Rev Rheumatol*. 2019;15:180–186.
4. Shukla N, Paul M, Halley M, et al. Identifying barriers to care and research in hidradenitis suppurativa: findings from a patient engagement event. *Br J Dermatol*. 2019.
5. Kimball AB, Okun MM, Williams DA, et al. Two phase 3 trials of adalimumab for hidradenitis suppurativa. *N Engl J Med*. 2016;375: 422–434.
6. Garg A, Wertenteil S, Baltz R, et al. Prevalence estimates for hidradenitis suppurativa among children and adolescents in the United States: A gender- and age-adjusted population analysis. *J Invest Dermatol*. 2018;138:2152–2156.
7. Soliman YS, Hoffman LK, Guzman AK, et al. African American patients with hidradenitis suppurativa have significant health care disparities: A retrospective study. *J Cutan Med Surg*. 2019;23: 334–336.
8. Kwa MC, Silverberg JI. Association between inflammatory skin disease and cardiovascular and cerebrovascular co-morbidities in US adults: Analysis of nationwide inpatient sample data. *Am J Clin Dermatol*. 2017;18:813–823.
9. Alikhan A, Sayed C, Alavi A, et al. North American clinical management guidelines for hidradenitis suppurativa: A publication from the United States and Canadian Hidradenitis Suppurativa Foundations: Part I: Diagnosis, evaluation, and the use of complementary and procedural management. *J Am Acad Dermatol*. 2019;81:76–90.
10. Alikhan A, Sayed C, Alavi A, et al. North American clinical management guidelines for hidradenitis suppurativa: A publication from the United States and Canadian Hidradenitis Suppurativa Foundations: Part II: Topical, intralesional, and systemic medical management. *J Am Acad Dermatol*. 2019;81:91–101.
11. Khalsa A, Liu G, Kirby JS. Increased utilization of emergency department and inpatient care by patients with hidradenitis suppurativa. *J Am Acad Dermatol*. 2015;73:609–614.
12. Agrawal SK, Singh M, Mathew JL, et al. Efficacy of an individualized written home-management plan in the control of moderate persistent asthma: a randomized, controlled trial. *Acta Paediatr*. 2005;94: 1742–1746.
13. Shi VY, Nanda S, Lee K, et al. Improving patient education with an eczema action plan: a randomized controlled trial. *JAMA Dermatol*. 2013;149:481–483.
14. Collier EK, Hsiao JL, Shi VY, et al. Comprehensive approach to managing hidradenitis suppurativa patients. *Int J Dermatol*. 2020.
15. Zouboulis CC, Desai N, Emtestam L, et al. European S1 guideline for the treatment of hidradenitis suppurativa/acne inversa. *J Eur Acad Dermatol Venereol*. 2015;29:619–644.
16. Mehdizadeh A, Alavi A, Alhusayen R, et al. Proceeding report of the Symposium on Hidradenitis Suppurativa Advances (SHSA). *Exp Dermatol*. 2018;27:104–112.
17. Shavit E, Alavi A, Bechara FG, et al. Proceeding report of the Second Symposium on Hidradenitis Suppurativa Advances (SHSA) 2017. *Exp Dermatol*. 2019;28:94–103.
18. Posso-De Los Rios CJ, Sarfo A, Ghias M, et al. Proceeding report of the Third Symposium on Hidradenitis Suppurativa Advances (SHSA) 2018. *Exp Dermatol*. 2019;28:769–775.

19. Narla S, Price KN, Sachdeva M, et al. Proceeding report of the fourth Symposium on Hidradenitis Suppurativa Advances (SHSA) 2019. *J Am Acad Dermatol.* 2020.

20. Zouboulis CC, Del Marmol V, Jemec GBE, et al. Further evidence for the immediate knowledge improvement through EADV Schools on hidradenitis suppurativa/acne inversa. *J Eur Acad Dermatol Venereol.* 2020.

21. Thorlacius L, Garg A, Ingram JR, et al. Towards global consensus on core outcomes for hidradenitis suppurativa research: an update from the HISTORIC consensus meetings I and II. *Br J Dermatol.* 2018; 178:715–721.

22. Thorlacius L, Ingram JR, Garg A, et al. Protocol for the development of a core domain set for hidradenitis suppurativa trial outcomes. *BMJ Open.* 2017;7, e014733.

23. Thorlacius L, Ingram JR, Villumsen B, et al. A core domain set for hidradenitis suppurativa trial outcomes: an international Delphi process. *Br J Dermatol.* 2018;179:642–650.

24. Garg A, Neuren E, Cha D, et al. Evaluating patients' unmet needs in hidradenitis suppurativa: Results from the Global Survey Of Impact and Healthcare Needs (VOICE) Project. *J Am Acad Dermatol.* 2020;82:366–376.

25. Daxhelet M, Suppa M, Benhadou F, et al. Establishment of a European registry for hidradenitis suppurativa/acne inversa by using an open source software. *J Eur Acad Dermatol Venereol.* 2016;30: 1424–1426.

26. Naik HB, Lowes MA. A call to accelerate hidradenitis suppurativa research and improve care-moving beyond burden. *JAMA Dermatol.* 2019.

27. Bettoli V, Pasquinucci S, Caracciolo S, et al. The hidradenitis suppurativa patient journey in Italy: current status, unmet needs and opportunities. *J Eur Acad Dermatol Venereol.* 2016;30:1965–1970.

28. Ingvarsson G, Dufour DN, Killasli H, et al. Development of a clinical Scandinavian registry for hidradenitis suppurativa; HISREG. *Acta Derm Venereol.* 2013;93:350–351.

Note: Page numbers followed by *f* indicate figures, *t* indicate tables, and *b* indicate boxes.

Radiotherapy, 255–256
  in HS, 327
  non-excision procedures, office-based, 220–221
Reactive oxygen species (ROS), 321
Recurrence, 24, 243
Reflectance confocal microscopy (RCM), 48
Registries, 335
Regular (typical) phenotypes, 24
Reimbursement, office-based excision, 244
Release neutrophil extracellular traps (NETs), 321
Research funding, 335
Resorcinol (m-dihydroxybenzene), 132, 150, 221,
  256, 327
  topical, 326–327
Retinoids, 132, 150
  oral, 174
Rifampin, 157–158
Rizankizumab, 325

S
Safety and Efficacy of Humira (Adalimumab) for HS
  Peri-Surgically (SHARPS Study), 328
Sarcoidosis of vulva, 32
Sartorius score, 123–124
  modified, 124, 124t
Scars, 19f, 20, 21–22f, 79, 79f
  atrophic, 22f
  contracture, office-based excision, 243
  folliculitis (atypical) phenotypes, 24
  hypertrophic, 22f
  keloidal, 22f
Science and translational research, 334
Scrofuloderma, 34f
Second intention healing, excision and, 235
Secukinumab (anti-IL-17), 139, 186, 324–325
Sepsis, 83
Serious infection, 83
Severity and Area Score for Hidradenitis (SASH), 126
Severity-guided antibiotic management, 162–165
Sex hormone binding globulin (SHBG), 170, 171f
Sexual dysfunction (SD), 84
Sexual health, 84
  QoL in HS patients, 211–212
Sexually transmitted diseases, 30
Shelley, W., 5–6
Side-to-side repair, excision, 234
Silver, 205
Single nucleotide polymorphisms (SNPs), 107
Single oral antibiotics, 156–157
Sinus tract exteriorization, 218–220
Sinus tracts, 77–78, 77f
Skin color and HS
  access to adequate and empathetic care, 293–294
  adalimumab, 291
  clinical presentation, 291f
  clinical trials, 290–291
  comorbidities, 292–293
    inflammatory bowel disease, 292–293
    metabolic syndrome, 292
    psychiatric comorbidity, 293
    squamous cell carcinoma, 293
  genetics and anatomy, 292
  keloids, 292
  light/laser, 291
  prevalence, 290
Skin fold occlusion, 91
Skin grafting, wound closure and reconstruction,
  228–229, 229f
Skin microbiota
  alterations, 101–102
  perturbations, hidradenitis suppurativa
    lesional skin, 101
    nonlesional skin, 102
Sleep disturbance and daytime somnolence, 212
Smoking cessation, 269

Social isolation, 84
Social media use, support groups, 316
Socioeconomic factors during visits, 66
Sodium, 266–267
Sodium hypochlorite (Bleach), 151
Somatic diseases and infertility, 298–299
Sonographic scoring system of HS (SOS-HS), 46
Spironolactone, 139, 171–172, 298, 326–327
Split thickness skin graft (STSG), 228, 229f
  excision with, 235
Spondyloarthritis, 72
Squamous cell carcinoma, 33, 79–80, 79f, 293
  multinodular ulcerated, 34f
Stigma, 84
Stress management, 270
Subcutis
  cutaneous structure and cellular composition, 39
  histological changes in HS, skin structures, 42
Suboptimal access, HS management, 332
Substance abuse disorders (SUD), 72
  alcohol, 211
  cannabinoids, 211
  opioids, 211
Sudoral glands, necrosis, 5
Suicide, 72, 83–84
  QoL in HS patients, 210
Superabsorbent dressings, HS lesions, 202
Superficial folliculitis, 27
Support groups, 314
  attendance, 316
  community perception and transparency, 317
  hidradenitis suppurativa community perspectives,
    317
  hidradenitis suppurativa provider perspective, 317
  informal peer support, 316
  initial steps, 315f
  meeting format, 315f
  mental health, 317
  online, 316
  participant perspectives, 317
  social media use in, 316
Surgery, 310
  excision, recalcitrant structural disease,
    327–328
  office-based excision, 234–236
    electrocutting, 234
    excision and primary intention healing (per
      primam intentionem), 234–236
    incision and drainage, 234
    lasers, 234
    unroofing, 234
  procedures, 142
Symposium on Hidradenitis Suppurativa Advances
  (SHSA), 334
Symptoms, hidradenitis suppurativa
  family history, 63
  initial, 62
  lesions, 23–24
Syndromic hidradenitis suppurativa, 25, 25t
Systemic amyloidosis, 80–83
Systemic complications
  anemia, 80
  chronic pain, 83
  mortality rate and mortality associations, 83
  nephrotic syndrome, 80–83
  psychological and social complications, 83–84
  sepsis, 83
  serious infection, 83
  systemic amyloidosis, 80–83
Systemic immunomodulators
  colchicine, 174
  dapsone, 175
  methotrexate, 174–175
Systemic retinoids, antibiotics and, 165
Systemic subclinical inflammation, 93

Systemic therapies, 134–138t
  adalimumab, 139
  anakinra, 139
  antibiotics, 132
  biologics and immunomodulators, 132–139
  canakinumab, 139
  etanercept, 139
  infliximab, 139
  retinoids, 132
  secukinumab, 139
  ustekinumab, 139

T
Tape irritation, office-based excision, 243
Tetracyclines, 156–157
TH17 feed-forward inflammation, 94
Third intention healing, excision and, 235
Thomsen, B., 6
Tie1, 92
Tissue examination of HS, 243
Tobacco smoking, 71
Tofacitinib (JAK inhibitor), 187
Toll-like receptors (TLRs), 197–198
Topical therapy, 145, 146–147t
  analgesics, 131
  antibiotics, 145–149
    clindamycin, 145–147
    dapsone, 147–148
    fusidic acid (FA), 147
    gentamicin, 148–149
  antiseptics
    ammonium bituminosulfate (ichthammol), 150
    benzoyl peroxide (BPO), 149
    chlorhexidine, 149
    triclosan, 149–150
    zinc pyrithione, 149
  bathing additives, 150–151
    bleach baths, 151
    magnesium sulfate baths, 151
  cannabidiol oil, 151
  complementary therapies, 151
  keratolytics, 150
    azelaic acid, 150
    resorcinol, 150
    retinoids, 150
  modalities, 133t
    antiseptics, 132
    clindamycin, 132
    keratolytics, 132
    resorcinol, 132
    turmeric, 151
Total Work Productivity Impairment (TWPI)
  questionnaire, 14
Traditional immunosuppressive agents, 139
Tramadol, 132
Treatment modality, HS management, 131
  algorithm, 309
  antiandrogens, 139
  approaches
    antibiotic toolbox, 161–162
    pre-antibiotic evaluation and follow-up of
      patients, 160–161
    severity-guided antibiotic management, 162–165
  based on HS disease level of severity, 66–67
  carbon dioxide (CO_2) ablative laser, 142
  comorbidities, 67
  deroofing, 142
  hormonal modulators, 139
  incision and drainage (I&D), 142
  initiation and baseline labs, 67
  intense pulsed light (IPL), 142
  intralesional corticosteroids, 139–142
  lasers, 140–141t, 142
  light-based therapy, 142
  metformin, 139